Dictionary
of Medical
Acronyms &
Abbreviations

Dictionary of Medical Acronyms & Abbreviations

5th Edition

Compiled and edited by
Stanley Jablonski

ELSEVIER
SAUNDERS

10/30/04

ELSEVIER
SAUNDERS

The Curtis Center
170 S Independence Mall W 300E
Philadelphia, Pennsylvania 19106

Dictionary of Medical Acronyms & Abbreviations   ISBN 1-56053-632-2

Library of Congress Control Number: 2004108494

Previous editions copyrighted 2001, 1997, 1992, 1987 by Elsevier.

International Standard Book Number 1-56053-632-2

Acquisitions Editor: Linda Belfus
Chief Lexicographer: Douglas M. Anderson
Publishing Services Manager: Tina Rebane
Project Manager: Norman Stellander
Designer: Gene Harris

Printed in the United States of America

Last digit is the print number: 9 8 7 6 5 4 3 2 1

Preface to the First Edition

Acronyms and abbreviations are used extensively in medicine, science and technology for good reason—they are more essential in such fields. It would be difficult to imagine how one could write down chemical and mathematical formulas and equations without using abbreviations or symbols. In medicine, they are used as a convenient shorthand in writing medical records, instructions, and prescriptions, and as space-saving devices in printed literature. It is easier and more economical to write down the acronyms HETE and RAAS than their full names 12-L-hydroxy-5,8,10,14-eicosatetraenoic acid and renin-angiotensin-aldosterone system, respectively.

The main reason for abbreviations is said to be economy. Some actually save space in print, such as acronyms for the names of institutions and organizational units, as well as being convenient to use. Many are used for other reasons, as for instance, when trying to be delicate, we may euphemistically refer to bowel movement as BM, an unprinicipled individual as SOB, and body odor as BO. Also, it is sometimes difficult to fathom the reasoning of bureaucratic acronym makers, who have created some tongue-twisting monstrosities, such as AD-COMSUBORDCOMPHIBSPAC (for Administrative Command, Amphibious Forces, Pacific Fleet, Subordinate Command).

Abbreviations and acronyms used in medicine can be grouped into two broad categories. The first consists of official abbreviations and symbols used in chemistry, mathematics, and other sciences, and those designating weights and measures, whose exact form, capitalization, and punctuation have been determined by official governing bodies. In this category, they mean only one thing (e.g., kg is the symbol for kilogram and Hz for hertz), and their form, capitalization, and punctuation have been established by the International System of Units (Système International d'Unités). Abbreviations in the second group, on the other hand, may appear in a variety of forms, the same abbreviation having a different number of letters, sometimes capitalized, at other times not, with or without punctuation. Moreover, they may also have numerous meanings. The abbreviation AP may mean alkaline phosphatase, acid phosphatase, action potential, angina pectoris, and many other things.

Editors of individual scientific publications make an effort to standardize the form of abbreviations and symbols in their journals and books, but they generally vary from one publication to another.

This dictionary lists acronyms and abbreviations occurring with a reasonable frequency in the medical literature that were identified by a systematic scanning of collections of books and periodicals at the National Library of Medicine. Except as they take the form of Greek letters, pure geometric symbols are not included. Although we have attempted to be as inclusive as possible, a book such as this one can never be complete, in spite of the most diligent effort, and it is expected that some abbreviations and acronyms may have escaped detection and others may have been introduced since completion of the manuscript.

Stanley Jablonski

Preface to the Fifth Edition

In the four years since the publication of the fourth edition of the *Dictionary of Medical Acronyms & Abbreviations*, the coining of acronyms has continued at its usual furious pace, and the work of sifting through the enormous volume of candidates for inclusion remains a challenging task. This new fifth edition, although compiled with constant reference to its purpose as a convenient source for the most commonly used acronyms and abbreviations, has nonetheless grown by about 12,000 new entries.

Some long-time users of the book may notice that the familiar Hanley & Belfus imprint has been replaced by Elsevier's Saunders imprint. No matter what the imprint, however, the same care as always has been taken in the selection of entries and the verification of their accuracy. The familiar format of boldface acronyms and abbreviations followed by run-in meanings has been retained, allowing the book to be kept to a convenient size. New terms have been drawn especially from the areas of virology, clinical trials, new technology, and medical informatics. An important enhancement, not visible in this volume but important for the maintenance of the text in the future, is the addition of the contents to the database that houses the well-known *Dorland's Illustrated Medical Dictionary*, so that the same resources that help to make *Dorland's* the world's leading medical dictionary can be used for the *Dictionary of Medical Acronyms & Abbreviations*.

It is an unfortunate fact that the use of abbreviations, although a helpful time-saver, occasionally leads to ambiguity in interpretation. In some cases, especially in handwritten notes, this ambiguity rises to the level of causing serious concern for patient safety, and for this reason the Joint Commission on Accreditation of Healthcare Organizations (JCAHO) has created a list of abbreviations that are considered dangerous and should not be used in a healthcare setting. The abbreviations included in this edition have been compared with JCAHO's "Do not use" list, and those that occur on the list are so identified.

Even as this fifth edition is being prepared for publication, new acronyms and abbreviations are being added to the already existing body, so that no compilation can ever be complete. I invite you to submit your own suggestions for the next edition; this can be done over the Internet at *http://www.dorlands. com*; just click on the link "Suggest a Word." Be sure that in doing so you will have performed a great service to the ranks of grateful users (not to mention the grateful author and publisher) of the *Dictionary of Medical Acronyms & Abbreviations!*

Stanley Jablonski

Acknowledgments

The author would like to thank Christopher Peterson, MD, PhD, of Rio de Janeiro, Brazil, for his continuing interest in the book and for supplying several hundred new entries for this edition. The work of Tsung O. Cheng, MD, of Washington, DC, was extremely useful for verifying acronyms for cardiology trials and is gratefully acknowledged: Cheng TO: Acronyms of clinical trials in cardiology—1998. American Heart Journal 137:726–765, 1999.

Symbols

°	degree		τ	life (time)
′	foot		$\tau\frac{1}{2}$	half-life (time)
″	inch		λ	wavelength
/	per		@	at
%	per cent		$\bar{a}$	before
:	ratio		$\bar{c}$	with
∞	infinity		$\sqrt{c}$	check with
+	positive		$\bar{p}$	after
−	negative		$\bar{s}$	without
±	positive or negative		24°	24 hours
#	number; fracture; pound		Δt	time interval
÷	divided by		2d	second
×	multiplied by; magnification		1°	primary
=	equals		2°	secondary to
≠	does not equal		♀	female
~	approximate		♂	male
↓	decreased		ℨ	dram
↑	increased		℥	ounce
→	to (in direction of)		−ve	negative
∅	normal		+ve	positive
∨	systolic blood pressure		D_x	diagnosis
∧	diastolic blood pressure		R_x	treatment or therapy
∠	angle		†	deceased
∡	angle of entry		◇	lozenge; sex unknown or unspecified
∢	angle of exit		Ⓐ , ⓐx	axilla (temperature)
∟	right lower quadrant		Ⓗ , ⓗ	hypodermically
⌐	right upper quadrant		Ⓜ	intramuscularly
⌐|	left upper quadrant		Ⓥ	intravenously
⌐|	left lower quadrant		Ⓛ	left
>	greater than		Ⓜ	murmur
<	less than		ⓜ	by mouth, murmur
Δ	change		Ⓞ	by mouth, orally
$\sqrt{}$	root; square root		Ⓡ	rectally, registered trademark, right
χ^2	chi square (test)		Ⓧ	end of anesthesia, end of operation
σ	1/1000 of a second standard deviation			
Σ	sum of			
π	3.1415—ratio of circumference of a circle to its diameter			

Genetic Symbols

Symbol	Meaning	Symbol	Meaning
□	male	(□)(○)	adopted
○	female		half siblings
◇	sex unspecified		stillbirth or abortion
□—○	mating or marriage		no offspring
□—○	consanguinity	■ ●	affected offspring
□⫲○	illegitimate offspring	■ ●	proband, propositus, or index case
□⫽○	divorce	◨ ◖	heterozygotes for autosomal recessive
□—○—□	multiple marriage	⊙	carrier of sex-linked recessive
	dizygotic twins	⊘ ∅	death
	monozygotic twins		
④ ③	number of children of sex indicated		

Greek Alphabet and Symbols

α	A	alpha	ω	Ω	omega
β	B	beta	o	O	omicron
χ	X	chi	φ	Φ	phi
δ	Δ	delta (diagnosis; change)	π	Π	pi
ε	E	epsilon	ψ	Ψ	psi
η	H	eta	ρ	P	rho
γ	Γ	gamma	σ	Σ	sigma
ι	I	iota	τ	T	tau
κ	K	kappa	θ	Θ	theta
λ	Λ	lambda	υ	Y	upsilon
μ	M	mu	ξ	Ξ	xi
ν	N	nu	ζ	Z	zeta

A

A abnormal; abortion; absolute temperature; absorbance; acceptor; accommodation; acetone; acetum; achondroplasia; acid; acidophil, acidophilic; acromion; actin; *Actinomyces*; activity [radiation]; adenine; adenoma; adenosine; admittance; adrenalin; Adriamycin; adult; age; akinetic; alanine; albino [guinea pig]; albumin; allergologist, allergy; alpha [cell]; alveolar gas; ambulation; ampere; amphetamine; ampicillin; amplitude; anaphylaxis; androsterone; anesthetic; angstrom, Ångström unit; anode; *Anopheles*; antagonism; anterior; antibody; antrectomy; apical; aqueous; area; argon; artery [Lat. *arteria*]; atomic weight; atrium; atropine; auricle; auscultation; axial; axilla, axillary; before [Lat. *ante*]; blood group A; ear [Lat. *auris*]; mass number; subspinale; total acidity; tumor limited to the bowel [Dukes classification]; tumor limited to the mucosa [Astler-Coller classification]; water [Lat. *aqua*]; year [Lat. *annum*]

A [band] the dark-staining zone of a striated muscle

A1 aortic first sound; prostatic tumor less than 5% [Jewett staging system]

A-1, 2, 3, 4, 5 anterior cerebral artery segments 1, 2, 3, 4, 5

AI, AII, AIII angiotensin I, II, III

A2 prostatic tumor more than 5% [Jewett staging system]

A₂ aortic second sound

Å Ångström unit

Ã cumulated activity; antinuclear antibody

a absorptivity; acceleration; accommodation; acidity; activated; ampere; anode; anterior; area; arterial blood; arterial; artery [Lat. *arteria*]; atto-; autopsy; before [Lat. *ante*]; thermodynamic activity; total acidity; water [Lat. *aqua*]

a- atto- [10^{-18}]

a sample y intercept of straight line

ā before [Lat. *ante*]

α see *alpha*

AA abampere; abdominal aorta; acetabular anteversion; acetic acid; achievement age; active alcoholic; active assistive [range of motion]; active avoidance; acupuncture analgesia; acute appendicitis; adenine arabinoside; adenylic acid; adjuvant arthritis; adrenal androgen; adrenocortical autoantibody; African American; aggregated albumin; [bacterial] aggregative adherence; agranulocytic angina; alcohol abuse; Alcoholics Anonymous; allergic alveolitis; alopecia areata; alveolo-arterial; aminoacetone; amino acid; aminoacyl; amyloid A; anaplastic astrocytoma; anti-arrhythmic agent; anticipatory avoidance; antigen aerosol; aortic amplitude; aortic aneurysm; aortic arch; aplastic anemia; arachidonic acid; arteries; ascending aorta; atlantoaxial; atomic absorption; Australia antigen; autoanalyzer; automobile accident; axonal arborization

2AA 2-aminoanthracene

A&A aid and attendance; awake and aware

A-a alveolar-arterial; alveolar-atrial

aA abampere

aa amino acid; arteries [Lat. *arteriae*]

AAA abdominal aortic aneurysm/aneurysmectomy; acne-associated arthritis; acquired aplastic anemia; acute anxiety attack; alacrimia-achalasia-addisonianism [syndrome]; American Academy of Addictionology; American Academy of Allergy; American Association of Anatomists; androgenic anabolic agent; aneurysm of ascending aorta; angiography of abdominal aorta; Area Agency on Aging; aromatic amino acid; arrest after arrival

AAAD aromatic amino acid decarboxylase

AA/AD alcohol abuse/alcohol dependence

AAAE amino acid activating enzyme

AAAHC Accreditation Association for Ambulatory Health Care

AAAHE American Association for the Advancement of Health Education

AAAI American Academy of Allergy and Immunology; American Association of Artificial Intelligence

AAALAC American Association for Accreditation of Laboratory Animal Care

AAAM Association for the Advancement of Automotive Medicine

AAAS American Association for the Advancement of Science

AAASPS African-American Antiplatelet Stroke Prevention Study

AAAV avian adeno-associated virus

AAB American Association of Bioanalysts; aminoazobenzene

AABB American Association of Blood Banks; axis-aligned bounding boxes

AABCC alertness (consciousness), airway, breathing, circulation, cervical spine

AABS automobile accident, broadside

AABV *Ascogaster argentifrons* bracovirus

AAC antibiotic-associated [pseudomembranous] colitis; antimicrobial agent–induced colitis; augmentative and alternative communication

AACA acylaminocephalosporanic acid

6′AAC-2″APH 6′-acetyltransferase-2″-phosphotransferase

AACC American Association for Clinical Chemistry

AACCN American Association of Critical Care Nurses

AACD aging-associated cognitive decline

AACE acute acquired comitant esotropia

AACEM Association of Academic Chairs in Emergency Medicine

AACG acute angle closure glaucoma

AACHP American Association for Comprehensive Health Planning

AACIA American Association for Clinical Immunology and Allergy

AACN American Association of Colleges of Nursing; American Association of Critical-Care Nurses

AACOM American Association of Colleges of Osteopathic Medicine

AACP American Academy of Cerebral Palsy; American Association of Colleges of Pharmacy

AACPDM American Academy for Cerebral Palsy and Developmental Medicine

AACS American Academy of Cosmetic Surgery

AACSH adrenal androgen corticotropic stimulating hormone

AACT American Academy of Clinical Toxicology

AACVPR American Association of Cardiovascular and Pulmonary Rehabilitation

AAD acute agitated delirium; acute aortic dissection; alcohol abuse or dependence; alloxazine adenine dinucleotide; alpha-1-antitrypsin deficiency; American Academy of Dermatology; antiarrhythmic drug; antibiotic-associated diarrhea; aromatic acid decarboxylase; average absolute deviation

7-AAD 7-amino-actinomycin D

AADC amino acid decarboxylase; L-aromatic amino acid decarboxylase

AADE American Association of Dental Editors; American Association of Dental Examiners

AADGP American Academy of Dental Group Practice

AADH alopecia-anosmia-deafness-hypogonadism [syndrome]

(A-a)D$_{N_2}$ alveolo-arterial nitrogen tension difference

AaDNV *Aedes aegypti* densovirus

AAD$_{O_2}$, (a-A) D$_{O_2}$ arterio-alveolar oxygen tension difference

AADP American Academy of Denture Prosthetics; amyloid A-degrading protease

AADPA American Academy of Dental Practice Administration

AADR American Academy of Dental Radiology

AADS American Academy of Dental Schools

AAE active assistive exercise; acute allergic encephalitis; American Association of Endodontists; annuloaortic ectasia

AAEE American Association of Electromyography and Electrodiagnosis

AAEM American Academy of Emergency Medicine; American Academy of Environmental Medicine; American Association of Electrodiagnostic Medicine

AAEV *Aedes aegypti* entomopoxvirus

AA ex active assistive exercise

AAF acetylaminofluorene; aggregative adherence fimbriae; aortic arch flush; ascorbic acid factor

2-AAF *N*-2-fluorenylacetamide

AAFP American Academy of Family Physicians; American Academy of Family Practice

AAFPRS American Academy of Facial Plastic and Reconstructive Surgery

AAFT amplitude-adjusted Fourier transform

AAG 3-alkaladenine deoxyribonucleic acid glycosylase; allergic angiitis and granulomatosis; alpha-1-acid glycoprotein; alveolar arterial gradient; autoantigen

17AAG 17-allylamino-17-demethoxygeldanamycin

AAGL American Academy of Gynecologic Laparoscopists

AAGP American Academy of General Practice; American Association for Geriatric Psychiatry

AAH Academy of Architecture for Health

AAHA American Academy of Hospital Attorneys; American Association of Homes for the Aging

AAHC American Academy of Healthcare Consultants; American Accreditation HealthCare Commission; Association of Academic Health Centers

AAHD American Association of Hospital Dentists

AAHE Association for the Advancement of Health Education

AAHP American Association of Health Plans

AAHPER American Association for Health, Physical Education, and Recreation

AAHRPP Association for the Accreditation of Human Research Protection Programs

AAHS American Association for Hand Surgery

AAHSL Association of Academic Health Sciences Libraries

AAHSLD Association of Academic Health Sciences Library Directors

AAI acute alveolar injury; Adolescent Alienation Index; American Association of Immunologists; atrial inhibited [pacemaker]

AAIB alpha-1-aminoisobutyrate

AAID American Academy of Implant Dentures

AAIN American Association of Industrial Nurses

AAK allo-activated killer

AAL ambient air level; anterior axillary line

AALAC American Association for Laboratory Animal Care

AALAS American Association of Laboratory Animal Science

AALib amino acid library

AALL American Association for Labor Legislation

AALNC American Association of Legal Nurse Consultants

AAM acute aseptic meningitis; American Academy of Microbiology; amino acid mixture

AAm acrylamide

AAMA American Academy of Medical Administrators; American Association of Medical Assistants

AAMC American Association of Medical Clinics; Association of American Medical Colleges

AAMD American Academy of Medical Directors; American Association of Mental Deficiency

AAME acetylarginine methyl ester

AAMFT American Association for Marriage and Family Therapy

AAMI Association for the Advancement of Medical Instrumentation

AAMIH American Association for Maternal and Infant Health

AAMMC American Association of Medical Milk Commissioners

AAMP American Academy of Maxillofacial Prosthetics; American Academy of Medical Prevention

AAMR American Academy of Mental Retardation

AAMRL American Association of Medical Record Librarians

AAMRS automated ambulatory medical record system

AAMS acute aseptic meningitis syndrome

AAMSI American Association for Medical Systems and Informatics

AAMT American Association for Medical Transcription

AAMU 5-acetylamino-6-amino-methyluracil

AAN AIDS-associated nephropathy; alpha-amino nitrogen; American Academy of Neurology; American Academy of Nursing; American Academy of Nutrition; American Association of Neuropathologists; amino acid nitrogen; analgesic-associated nephropathy; attending's admission notes

AANA American Association of Nurse Anesthetists

AANE American Association of Nurse Executives

AANM American Association of Nurse-Midwives

AANPI American Association of Nurses Practicing Independently

AAO American Academy of Ophthalmology; American Academy of Optometry; American Academy of Osteopathy; American Academy of Otolaryngology; American Association of Ophthalmologists; American Association of Orthodontists; amino acid oxidase; ascending aorta; awake, alert, and oriented

AAo ascending aorta

A-a O_2 alveolar-arterial oxygen gradient; alveolo-arterial oxygen tension

AAOC antacid of choice

AAofA Ambulance Association of America

AAOHN American Association of Occupational Health Nurses

AAOM American Academy of Oral Medicine

AAOMS American Association of Oral and Maxillofacial Surgery

AAOO American Academy of Ophthalmology and Otolaryngology

AAOP American Academy of Oral Pathology

AAOPP American Association of Osteopathic Postgraduate Physicians

AAOS American Academy of Orthopedic Surgeons; American Association of Osteopathic Specialists

AAP acute abdominal pain; acute appendicitis; air at atmospheric pressure; American Academy of Pediatrics; American Academy of Pedodontics; American Academy of Periodontology; American Academy of Psychoanalysts; American Academy of Psychotherapists; American Association of Pathologists; Association for the Advancement of Psychoanalysis; Association for the Advancement of Psychotherapy; Association of Academic Physiatrists; Association of American Physicians

AAPA American Academy of Physician Assistants; American Association of Pathologist Assistants

AAPB American Association of Pathologists and Bacteriologists

AAPC antibiotic-associated pseudomembranous colitis; average annual percent change

AAPCC adjusted annual per capita cost; adjusted average per capita costs; American Association of Poison Control Centers

AaP$_{CO_2}$, (A-a)P$_{CO_2}$ alveolo-arterial carbon dioxide tension difference

AAPF anti-arteriosclerosis polysaccharide factor

AAPH 2,2'-azobis-(2-amidinopropane) hydrochloride

AAPHD American Association of Public Health Dentists

AAPHP American Association of Public Health Physicians

AAPL American Academy of Psychiatry and the Law

AAPM American Association of Physicists in Medicine

AAPMC antibiotic-associated pseudomembranous colitis

AAPM&R American Academy of Physical Medicine and Rehabilitation

AaP$_{O_2}$, (A-a) P$_{O_2}$ alveolo-arterial oxygen tension difference

AAPP American Academy on Physician and Patient

AAPPO American Association of Preferred Provider Organizations

AAPS American Association of Pharmaceutical Scientists; American Association of Plastic Surgeons; Arizona Articulation Proficiency Scale; Association of American Physicians and Surgeons

AAPT Adolescent Alcohol Prevention Trial

AAR active avoidance reaction; acute articular rheumatism; antigen-antiglobulin reaction

aar against all risks

AARC American Association for Respiratory Care

AARE automobile accident, rear end

AARNet Australian Academic and Research Network

AAROM active assertive range of motion; active-assisted range of motion

AARP American Association of Retired Persons

AART American Association for Rehabilitation Therapy; American Association for Respiratory Therapy

AAS Aarskog-Scott [syndrome]; acid aspiration syndrome; alcoholic abstinence syndrome; American Academy of Sanitarians; American Analgesia Society; aneurysm of atrial septum; anthrax antiserum; aortic arch syndrome; atomic absorption spectrophotometry

AASD American Academy of Stress Disorders

aa seq amino acid sequence

AASH adrenal androgen stimulating hormone; American Association for the Study of Headache

AASK African American Study of Kidney Disease and Hypertension Pilot Study

AASP acute atrophic spinal paralysis; American Association of Senior Physicians; ascending aorta synchronized pulsation

AASS American Association for Social Security

AAST American Association for the Surgery of Trauma

AAT Aachen Aphasia Test; academic aptitude test; Accolate Asthma Trial; alanine aminotransferase; alkylating agent therapy; alpha-1-antitrypsin; atrial triggered [pacemaker]; auditory apperception test; automatic atrial tachycardia

A1AT α_1-antitrypsin

α_1AT α_1-antitrypsin

AATB American Association of Tissue Banks

AATS American Association for Thoracic Surgery

AAU acute anterior uveitis

AAUT actual amount of use test

AAV adeno-associated virus

AaV *Acherontia atropas* virus; *Allomyces arbuscula* virus

AAVMC Association of American Veterinary Medical Colleges

AAVP American Association of Veterinary Parasitologists

AAW anterior aortic wall

AB abdominal; able body; abnormal; abortion; Ace bandage; active bilaterally; aid to the blind; airbag; alcian blue; alertness behavior; antibiotic; antibody; antigen binding; apex beat; asbestos body; asthmatic bronchitis; axiobuccal; Bachelor of Arts [Lat. *Artium Baccalaureus*]; blood group AB

A/B acid-base ratio

A&B apnea and bradycardia

A>B air greater than bone [conduction]

Ab abortion; antibiotic; antibody; antivenom

A$_b$ amount in body

aB azure B

ab aberration; abortion; antibody; from [Lat.]

3AB 3-aminobenzamide

ABA abscissic acid; allergic bronchopulmonary aspergillosis; American Board of Anesthesiologists; American Burn Association; antibacterial activity; arrest before arrival; autonomic blocking agent

ABACAS Adjunctive Balloon Angioplasty Following Coronary Atherectomy Study

AB/AM antibiotic/antimycotic

ABAT American Board of Applied Toxicology

ABAV Abadina virus

ABB Albright-Butler-Bloomberg [syndrome]; American Board of Bioanalysis

ABBI advanced breast biopsy instrument

ABBQ AIDS Beliefs and Behavior Questionnaire

abbr abbreviation, abbreviated

ABC abacavir; absolute basophil count; absolute bone conduction; acalculous biliary colic; acid balance control; aconite-belladonna-chloroform; adenosine triphosphate [ATP] binding cassette; airway, breathing, and circulation; alignment, blue, calcium [synovial fluid pearls in gout and pseudogout]; Alpha Beta Canadian [trial]; alternative birth center; alum, blood, and charcoal [purification and deodorizing method]; alum, blood, and clay [sludge deodorizing method]; American Blood Commission; aneurysmal bone cyst; antigen-binding capacity; antigen-binding cell; apnea, bradycardia, cyanosis; aspiration biopsy cytology; assessment of basic competency; atomic, biological, and chemical [warfare]; axiobuccocervical; autism behavior checklist; avidin-biotin peroxidase complex

A&BC air and bone conduction

ABCA1 ATP-binding cassette A1

ABCC Atomic Bomb Casualty Commission

ABCD airway, breathing, circulation, differential diagnosis (or defibrillate) [in cardiopulmonary resuscitation]; amphotericin B colloidal dispersion; appropriate blood pressure control in diabetes; asymmetry, borders are irregular, color variegated, diameter > 6 mm [biopsy in melanoma]

ABCDE airway, breathing, circulation, disability, exposure [in trauma patients]; botulism toxin pentavalent

ABCDES abnormal alignment, bones-periarticular osteoporosis, cartilage-joint space loss, deformities, marginal erosions, soft tissue swelling [x-ray features in rheumatoid arthritis]; adjust medication, bacterial prophylaxis, cervical spine disease, deep vein thrombosis prophylaxis, evaluate extent and activity of disease, stress-dose steroid coverage [preoperative evaluation in rheumatoid diseases]; alignment, bone mineralization, calcifications, distribution of joints, erosions, soft tissue and nails [x-ray features in arthritis]; ankylosis, bone osteoporosis, cartilage destruction, deformity of joints, erosions, swelling of soft tissues [x-ray features of septic arthritis]

ABCIC airway, breathing, circulation, intravenous crystalloid

ABCIL antibody-mediated cell-dependent immunolympholysis

ABC-M chemical-biological aircraft mask

ABCN American Board of Clinical Neuropsychology

ABD abdomen; aged, blind, and disabled; aggressive behavioral disturbance; aortic barodenervated [rat]; automatic border detection; automatic boundary detection; average body dose

Abd, abd abdomen, abdominal; abduct, abduction, abductor

abdom abdomen, abdominal

ABDPH American Board of Dental Public Health

ABE acute bacterial endocarditis; American Board of Endodontics; botulism equine trivalent antitoxin

ABEM American Board of Emergency Medicine

ABEPP American Board of Examiners in Professional Psychology

ABER abducted and externally rotated; auditory brainstem evoked response

aber aberrant

A-β amyloid beta-peptide

ABF aortic blood flow; aortobifemoral

ABG arterial blood gas; axiobucco-gingival

ABGC American Board of Genetic Counseling

ABI ankle/brachial index; atherothrombotic brain infarct

ABIC Adaptive Behavior Inventory for Children; antibody excess immune complex

ABIM American Board of Internal Medicine

ABIMCE American Board of Internal Medicine certifying examination

ABIT assertive behavior inventory tool

ABK aphakic bullous keratopathy

ABL Abelson proto-oncogene; abetalipoproteinemia; acceptable blood loss; acute basophilic leukemia; African Burkitt lymphoma; Albright-Butler-Lightwood [syndrome]; allograft-bound lymphocyte; angioblastic lymphadenopathy; antigen-binding lymphocyte; Army Biological Laboratory; automated biological laboratory; axiobuccolingual

Abl ablation

ABLB alternate binaural loudness balance

ABLC amphotericin B lipid complex

ABLES Adult Blood Lead Epidemiology and Surveillance

ABM abamectin; adjusted body mass; alveolar basement membrane; autologous bone marrow

ABMG American Board of Medical Genetics

ABMI autologous bone marrow infusion

AbMLV Abelson murine leukemia virus

ABMM American Board of Medical Management

ABMS American Board of Medical Specialties

ABMT American Board of Medical Toxicology; autologous bone marrow transplantation

ABMV Above Maiden virus; Abu Mina virus

AbMV Abutilon mosaic virus

AbN antibody nitrogen

Abn, abn abnormal; abnormality(ies)

ABNMP alpha-benzyl-*N*-methyl phenethylamine

ABNO anatomic abnormality [UMLS]

abnor abnormal

ABO abortion; absent bed occupancy; American Board of Orthodontists; blood group system consisting of groups A, AB, B, and O

ABOHN American Board for Occupational Health Nurses

ABOMS American Board of Oral and Maxillofacial Surgery

ABOP American Board of Oral Pathology

Abor, abor abortion

ABOS American Board of Orthopaedic Surgery

ABOVE Acute Bleeding Oesophageal Variceal Episodes [study]

ABP actin-binding protein; acute biliary pancreatitis; ambulatory blood pressure; American Board of Pedodontics; American Board of Periodontology; American Board of Prosthodontists; aminobiphenyl; androgen-binding protein; antigen-binding protein; arterial blood pressure; automatic systolic blood pressure measurement; avidin-biotin peroxidase

aBP arterial blood pressure

ABPA actin-binding protein, autosomal form; allergic bronchopulmonary aspergillosis

ABPC antibody-producing cell

ABPE acute bovine pulmonary edema

ABPM ambulatory blood pressure monitoring

ABPM&R American Board of Physical Medicine and Rehabilitation

ABPS American Board of Plastic Surgery

ABR abortus Bang ring [test]; absolute bed rest; American Board of Radiology; arterial baroreflex; auditory brainstem response

ABr agglutination test for brucellosis

Abr, Abras abrasion

ABRV Abras virus; Arbroath virus

ABS abdominal surgery; acidic ammonium bisulfate; acute brain syndrome; Adaptive Behavior Scale; admitting blood sugar; adult bovine serum; aging brain syndrome; alkylbenzene sulfonate; aloin, belladonna, strychnine; American Board of Surgery; amniotic band sequence; amniotic band syndrome; anti-B serum; Antley-Bixler syndrome; arterial blood sample; at bed side; Australian Bureau of Statistics

Abs absorption

abs absent; absolute

AB-SAAP autologous blood selective aortic arch perfusion

absc abscess; abscissa

abs conf absolute configuration

ABSe ascending bladder septum

abs feb while fever is absent

ABSITE American Board of Surgery In-Training Examination

absorp absorption

AbSR abnormal skin reflex

abst, abstr abstract

ABSV Absettarov virus

ABT abstract behavioral type; autologous blood transfusion; lopinavir

abt about

ABU asymptomatic bacteriuria

ABV actinomycin D-bleomycin-vincristine; *Agaricus bisporus* virus; Aglaonema bacilliform virus; Aransas Bay virus; arthropod-borne virus

AbV *Agaricus bisporus* virus

ABVD Adriamycin, bleomycin, vinblastine, and dacarbazine

ABW average body weight

ABX abciximab; antibiotics

ABY acid bismuth yeast [medium]

AbYV Abutilon yellow virus

AC abdominal circumference; abdominal compression; ablation catheter; abrupt closure; absorption coefficient; abuse case; acetate; acetylcholine; acidified complement; *Acinetobacter calcoaceticus*; acromioclavicular; activated charcoal; acupuncture clinic; acute; acute cholecystitis; adenocarcinoma; adenylate cyclase; adherent cell; adrenal cortex; adrenocorticoid; Adriamycin/cyclophosphamide; air chamber; air conditioning; air conduction; alcoholic cirrhosis; alternating current; alveolar crest; ambulatory care; anesthesia circuit; angiocellular; anodal closure; antecubital; anterior chamber; anterior column; anterior commissure; antibiotic concentrate; anticholinergic; anticoagulant; anticomplement; antiphlogistic corticoid; aortic closure; aortic compliance; aortocoronary; arm circumference; ascending colon; assist control [ventilation]; atriocarotid; autocorrelation; axiocervical; hydrogen cyanide [war gas]

A-C acromioclavicular; adult-versus-child; aortocoronary bypass

A/C albumin/coagulin [ratio]; anterior chamber of eye; assist control [ventilation]

A2C apical two-chamber [view]

A4C apical four-chamber [view]

Ac accelerator [globulin]; acetate; acetyl; actinium; anticoagulant, anticoagulation; aortic closure; arabinosyl cytosine

aC abcoulomb; arabinosyl cytosine

ac acceleration; acetyl; acid; acromioclavicular; acute; alternating current; antecubital; anterior chamber; atrial contraction; axiocervical

5-AC azacitidine

ACA abnormal coronary artery; acrodermatitis chronica atrophicans; acute cerebellar ataxia; adenocarcinoma; adult child of an alcoholic; American Chiropractic Association; American College of Allergists; American College of Anesthesiologists; American College of Angiology; American College of Apothecaries; American Council on Alcoholism; American Counseling Association; aminocephalosporanic acid; ammonia, copper, and acetate; amyotrophic choreo-acanthocytosis; anisotropic conductive adhesive; anterior cerebral artery; anterior communicating aneurysm [or artery]; anticapsular antibody; anticardiolipin antibody; anticentromere antibody; anticollagen antibody; anticomplement activity; anticytoplasmic antibody; arrhythmic cardiac arrest; automatic chemical agent alarm; Automatic Clinical Analyzer

AC/A accommodative convergence/accommodation [ratio]

ACAAI American College of Allergy, Asthma and Immunology

ACAC acetyl-coenzyme A cocarboxylase; activated charcoal artificial cell

ACACN American Council of Applied Clinical Nutrition

ACACT acyl-coenzyme A:cholesterol acyl transferase

ACAD asymptomatic coronary artery disease; atherosclerotic carotid artery disease; Azithromycin in Coronary Artery Disease [study]

Acad academy

ACADEMIC Azithromycin in Coronary Artery Disease Elimination of Myocardial Infection with Chlamydia [study]

A-CAH autoimmune chronic active hepatitis

ACAM American College for Advancement in Medicine

ACAO acyl coenzyme A oxidase

ACAPS Asymptomatic Coronary Artery Plaque Study; Asymptomatic Coronary Artery Progression Study

ACAS adaptive cluster analysis system

ACAT acetyl coenzyme A acetyltransferase; automated computerized axial tomography

ACAV Acara virus; American Committee on Arthropod-Borne Viruses

ACB antibody-coated bacteria; aortocoronary bypass; arterialized capillary blood; asymptomatic carotid bruit

ACBaE air contrast barium enema

ACBC aminocyclobutanecarboxylic acid

AC/BC air conduction/bone conduction [time ratio]

ACBE air contrast barium enema

ACBG aortocoronary bypass graft

ACBS Asymptomatic Cervical Bruit Study

ACC accommodation; acetyl coenzyme A carboxylase; acinic cell carcinoma; actinomycin C; acute care center; adenoid cystic carcinoma; administrative control center; adrenocortical carcinoma; agenesis of corpus callosum; alveolar cell carcinoma; ambulatory care center; American College of Cardiology; anodal closure contraction; anterior cingulate cortex; antitoxin-containing cell; aplasia cutis congenita; articular chondrocalcinosis; automated cell count; automated cell counter

Acc acceleration; adenoid cystic carcinoma

acc acceleration, accelerator; accident; accommodation

ACCA Advisory Committee on Casualty Assessment [Canada]; American College of Cardiovascular Administrators

ACC/AHA American College of Cardiology/American Hospital Association [Task Force]

ACCE American College of Clinical Engineering

ACCEPT Accupril Canadian Clinical Evaluation and Patient Teaching; American College of Cardiology Electrocardiogram Proficiency Test; American College of

Cardiology Evaluation of Preventive Therapies [study]

ACCESS A Comparison of Percutaneous Entry Sites for Coronary Angioplasty; Acute Candesartan Cilexetil Evaluation in Stroke Survivors; Ambulatory Care Clinic Effectiveness Systems Study; Atorvastatin Comparative Cholesterol Efficacy and Safety Study; automated cervical cell screening system

ACCH Association for the Care of Children's Health

AcCh acetylcholine

AcChR acetylcholine receptor

AcCHS acetylcholinesterase

accid accident, accidental

acc insuff accommodation insufficiency

ACCISM Association of City and County Information System Managers

ACCL, Accl anodal closure clonus

ACCME Accreditation Council for Continuing Medical Education

ACCN accession number

AcCoA acetyl coenzyme A

accom accommodation

ACCP American College of Chest Physicians; American College of Clinical Pharmacology; American College of Clinical Pharmacy

AcCPV *Arctia caja* cypovirus

ACCR amylase-creatinine clearance ratio

ACCS American-Canadian Cooperative Study

ACCT Amlodipine Cardiovascular Community Trial

accum accumulation

accur accurately [Lat. *accuratissime*]

ACD absolute cardiac dullness; absolute claudication distance; acid-citrate-dextrose [solution]; actinomycin D; active compression-decompression; adult celiac disease; advanced care directive; allergic contact dermatitis; alopecia-contractures-dwarfism [syndrome]; American College of Dentists; ammonium citrate dextrose; angiokeratoma corporis diffusum; annihilation coincidence detection; anterior chamber depth; anterior chest diameter; anticoagulant citrate dextrose; anticonvulsant drug; area of cardiac dullness; Available Chemicals Directory

AcDB A *C. elegans* Database [gene expression]

AC-DC, ac/dc alternating current or direct current

ACD-CPR active compression-decompression cardiopulmonary resuscitation

ACD-PCR active compression-decompression post-compression remodeling

ACDV Acado virus

ACE acetonitrile; acetylcholine esterase; acute cerebral encephalopathy; acute coronary event; adrenocortical extract; Adverse Childhood Experience [study]; alcohol, chloroform, and ether; analytic continuum electrostatics; angiotensin-converting enzyme; annealed competition of experts [algorithm]; Aspirin and Carotid Endarterectomy [trial]

ace acentric; acetone

ACED anhidrotic congenital ectodermal dysplasia

AceDB A *C. elegans* Database [gene expression]

ACEDS angiotensin-converting enzyme dysfunction syndrome

ACEH acid cholesterol ester hydrolase

ACEI angiotensin-converting enzyme inhibitor

ACEIT applied current electrical impedance tomography

ACEP American College of Emergency Physicians

ACES Alternans Cardiac Electrical Safety [study]; Azithromycin and Coronary Events Study

AcEst acetyl esterase

ACET Advisory Committee for the Elimination of Tuberculosis; Azmacort Cost Effectiveness Trial

ACET, acet acetone; vinegar [Lat. *acetum*]

acetab acetabular, acetabulum

acetyl-CoA acetyl coenzyme A

ACEV *Anomala cuprea* entomopoxvirus

ACF accessory clinical findings; active case finding; acute care facility; advanced communication function or facility; anisotropic conductive film [computer-assisted radiology]; anterior cervical fusion; anterior cranial fossa; area correction factor; asymmetric crying facies; autocorrelation function

ACf autocorrelation function

ACFAO American College of Foot and Ankle Orthopedics and Medicine

ACFAS American College of Foot and Ankle Surgeons

ACG accelerator globulin; adjusted clinical group; alternative care grant; ambulatory care group; American College of Gastroenterology; angiocardiography, angiocardiogram; aortocoronary graft; apexcardiogram

AC-G, AcG, ac-g accelerator globulin

ACGIH American Conference of Governmental Industrial Hygienists

ACGME Accreditation Council for Graduate Medical Education

ACGP American College of General Practitioners

ACGPOMS American College of General Practitioners in Osteopathic Medicine and Surgery

ACGT antibody-coated grid technique

ACH acetylcholine; achalasia; active chronic hepatitis; adrenocortical hormone; air change per hour; amyotrophic cerebellar hypoplasia; arm girth, chest depth, and hip width [nutritional index]

ACh acetylcholine

ACHA American College Health Association; American College of Hospital Administrators

AChA anterior choroidal artery

ACHD atherosclerotic coronary heart disease

ACHE American College of Healthcare Executives; American Council for Headache Education

AChE acetylcholinesterase

ACHIEVE Accupril Congestive Heart Failure Investigation and Economic Variable Evaluation

ACHOO autosomal dominant compelling helio-ophthalmic outburst [syndrome]

ACHPER Australian Council for Health, Physical Education and Recreation [survey]

ACHPR Agency for Health Care Policy and Research

AChR acetylcholine receptor

AChRAb acetylcholine receptor antibody

AChRP acetylcholine receptor protein

ACHS Australian Council on Healthcare Standards

AcHV acciptrid herpesvirus

ACI acceleration index; acoustic comfort index; acute cardiac ischemia; acute coronary infarction; acute coronary insufficiency; adenylate cyclase inhibitor; adrenocortical insufficiency; anticlonus index

ACID Arithmetic, Coding, Information, and Digit Span

ACIF acute care index of functions; anterior cervical interbody fusion; anticomplement immunofluorescence

AciHV Acipenserin herpesvirus

AcINH acid labile isonicotinic acid hydrazide

ACIP acute canine idiopathic polyneuropathy; Advisory Committee on Immunization Practices [CDC]; ambulatory care incentive payment; Asymptomatic Cardiac Ischemia Pilot Study

ACIR Australian Clinical Immunisation Register; Automotive Crash Injury Research

ACIS ambulatory care information system; automated clinical information system

ACIT Asymptomatic Cardiac Ischemia Trial

ACI-TIPI acute cardiac ischemia-time insensitive predictive instrument

AcK francium [actinium K]

ACKD acquired cystic kidney disease

ACL access control list; Achievement Check List; acromegaloid features, cutis verticis gyrata, corneal leukoma [syndrome]; American cutaneous leishmaniasis; anterior chamber lens; anterior cruciate ligament; Association for Computational Linguistics

ACl aspiryl chloride

aCL anticardiolipin [antibody]

ACLA American Clinical Laboratory Association

ACLC Assessment of Children's Language Comprehension

ACLD Association for Children with Learning Disabilities

ACLE acute cutaneous lupus erythematosus

ACLF adult congregate living facility

ACLI American Council on Life Insurance

ACLM American College of Legal Medicine

ACLPS Academy of Clinical Laboratory Physicians and Scientists

ACLR anterior capsulolabral reconstruction

ACLS acrocallosal syndrome; advanced cardiac life support; Assessment of Children's Language Comprehension

AcLV avian acute leukemia virus

ACM access control matrix; acetaminophen; acute cerebrospinal meningitis; adaptive fuzzy c-means algorithm; Adriamycin, cyclophosphamide, methotrexate; albumin-calcium-magnesium; alcoholic cardiomyopathy; alveolar capillary membrane; anticardiac myosin; Arnold-Chiari malformation; asbestos-containing material; Association of Computing Machinery; automated cardiac flow measurement

ACMC Association of Canadian Medical Colleges

ACMD associate chief medical director

ACME Advisory Council on Medical Education; Angioplasty Compared to Medicine [study]; assessing changes in medical education; Automated Classification of Medical Entities

ACMF arachnoid cyst of the middle fossa

ACMG American College of Medical Genetics

ACMHV avian carcinoma Mill Hill virus

ACMI age-consistent memory impairment; American College of Medical Informatics

ACML atypical chronic myeloid leukemia

AcMNPV *Autographa californica* multicapsid nucleopolyhedrovirus

ACMP alveolar-capillary membrane permeability

ACMR Advisory Committee on Medical Research

ACMS American Chinese Medical Society

ACMT artificial circus movement tachycardia

ACMV assist-controlled mechanical ventilation

ACN acute conditioned neurosis; Ambulatory Care Network; American College of Neuropsychiatrists; American College of Nutrition

ACNM American College of Nuclear Medicine; American College of Nurse-Midwives

ACNP acute care nurse practitioner; American College of Nuclear Physicians

ACO acute coronary occlusion; alert, cooperative, and oriented; anodal closure odor

ACOA adult children of alcoholics

ACoA anterior communicating artery

ACODENIC Advisory Committee on Dental Electronic Nomenclature, Indexing and Classification

ACOEM American College of Occupational and Environmental Medicine

ACOEP American College of Osteopathic Emergency Physicians

ACOEV *Araphia conspersa* entomopoxvirus

ACOG American College of Obstetricians and Gynecologists

ACOHA American College of Osteopathic Hospital Administrators

ACO-HNS American Council of Otolaryngology-Head and Neck Surgery

ACOI American College of Osteopathic Internists

ACOM American College of Occupational Medicine; anterior communicating [artery]

AComA anterior communicating artery

ACOMS American College of Oral and Maxillofacial Surgeons

ACOOG American College of Osteopathic Obstetricians and Gynecologists

ACOP American College of Osteopathic Pediatricians; approved code of practice

ACORDE A Consortium on Restorative Dentistry Education

ACOS American College of Osteopathic Surgeons; associate chief of staff

ACOS/AC associate chief of staff for ambulatory care

Acous acoustics, acoustic

ACOX acetyl coenzyme A [CoA] oxidase

ACP accessory conduction pathway; acid phosphatase; acyl carrier protein; American College of Pathologists; American College of Pharmacists; American College of Physicians; American College of Prosthodontists; American College of Psychiatrists; Animal Care Panel; anodal closure picture; aspirin-caffeine-phenacetin; Association for Child Psychiatrists; Association of Clinical Pathologists; Association of Correctional Psychologists; Asymptomatic Cardiac Ischemia Pilot Study; atom class pair

ACPA American Cleft Palate Association

AcPase acid phosphatase

ACPC aminocyclopentane carboxylic [acid]

AC-PC anterior commissure-posterior commissure

ACPE American College of Physician Executives

AC-PH, ac phos acid phosphatase

ACPM American College of Preventive Medicine

ACPP adrenocortical polypeptide; prostate-specific acid phosphatase

ACPS acrocephalopolysyndactyly

ACQUIP Ambulatory Care Quality Improvement Project

ACR abnormally contracting region; absolute catabolic rate; acriflavine; acute-to-chronic ratio; adenomatosis of colon and rectum; adjusted community rate; ambulance call report; American College of Radiology; American College of Rheumatology; anticonstipation regimen; axillary count rate

Acr acrylic

ACRE Appropriateness of Coronary Revascularization [study]

ACRF acute-on-chronic respiratory failure; ambulatory care research facility

ACRM American Congress of Rehabilitation Medicine

ACR/NEMA American College of Radiology/National Electrical Manufacturers' Association [standard for transferring radiologic images]

ACS access control system; acrocallosal syndrome; acrocephalosyndactyly; acute chest syndrome; acute confusional state; acute coronary syndrome; Alcon Closure System; ambulatory care-sensitive [condition]; American Cancer Society; American Chemical Society; American College of Surgeons; anodal closure sound; antireticular cytotoxic serum; aperture current setting; Association of Clinical Scientists; automatic corneal shaper

ACs air changes

ACSA adenylate cyclase-stimulating activity

ACSCEPT Assessment for Carotid Stenosis: Correlation with Endarterectomy Specimen Trial

ACS CPS American Cancer Society Cancer Prevention Studies

ACSE association control service element

ACSF artificial cerebrospinal fluid

aCSF artificial cerebrospinal fluid

AC/SIUG ambulatory care special-interest user group

ACSM American College of Sports Medicine

ACSML arbitration and control state machine logic

ACSP adenylate cyclase-stimulating protein

ACSSuT ampicillin, chloramphenicol, streptomycin, sulfonamides, and tetracyclines

ACST Asymptomatic Carotid Surgery Trial

ACSV aortocoronary saphenous vein

ACSVBG aortocoronary saphenous vein bypass graft

ACT abdominal computed tomography; ablation catheter tip; achievement through counseling and treatment; actin; actinomycin; action class torsion; activated clotting time; adaptive current tomography; advanced coronary treatment; Angioplasty Compliance Trial; anterocolic transposition; antichymotrypsin; anticoagulant therapy; anxiety control training; artemisinin combination therapy [malaria]; Association of Cytogenetic Technologists; asthma care training; atropine coma therapy; Attacking Claudication with Ticlopidine [study]; Australian Capital Territory [heroin trial]

AcT acceleration time

Act activity

act actinomycin; activity, active

ACTA American Cardiology Technologists Association; automatic computerized transverse axial [scanning]

Act-C actinomycin C

ACTC alpha-actin, cardiac muscle

Act-D actinomycin D

ACT/DB Adaptable Clinical Trials Database

ACTe anodal closure tetanus

ACTG AIDS Clinical Trial Group [study]

ACTH adrenocorticotropic hormone

ACTH-LI adrenocorticotropin-like immunoreactivity

ACTHR adrenocorticotropic hormone receptor

ACTHR/MC-2 adrenocorticotropin receptor/melanocortin receptor 2

ACTH-RF adrenocorticotropic hormone releasing factor

ACTION A Coronary Disease Trial Investigating Outcome with Nifedipine GITS; Assisting Carriers Using Telematics Interventions to Meet Older Persons Needs [Ireland]

ACTIS [NLM database] Acquired Immunodeficiency Syndrome [AIDS] Clinical Trials Information Service

activ active, activity

ACTN adrenocorticotropin

ACTOBAT Australasian Clinical Trial of Betamethasone and Thyroid-Releasing Hormone

ACTP adrenocorticotropic polypeptide

ACT/PD actual nursing hours per patient/day

ACTR American Club of Therapeutic Radiologists

ACTS acute cervical traumatic sprain or syndrome; advanced communication technology satellite; advanced computational testing and simulation [toolkit]; American-Canadian Thrombosis Study; American College Testing Services; Auditory Comprehension Test for Sentences

ACTUR Automated Central Tumor Registry

ACTV Acatinga virus; activity [UMLS]

ACU acquired cold urticaria; acute care unit; agar colony-forming unit; ambulatory care unit

ACURP American College of Utilization Review Physicians

ACUTE Analysis of Coronary Ultrasound Thrombolysis Endpoints; Assessment of Cardioversion Utilizing Transesophageal Echocardiography [pilot study]

ACV acute cardiovascular [disease]; acyclovir; assisted controlled ventilation; atrial/carotid/ventricular; autonomic conduction velocity

ACVB aortocoronary venous bypass

ACVD acute cardiovascular disease, atherosclerotic cardiovascular disease

ACx anomalous circumflex [coronary artery]

AD abductor digiti minimi [muscle]; above diaphragm; absorbed dose; acceptable daily intake; accident dispensary; accidental death; acetabular depth; acetate dialysis; active disease; active domain; acute dermatomyositis; addict, addiction; adenoid degeneration [agent]; adjuvant disease; admitting diagnosis; adrenodoxin; adrenostenedione; adult disease; advanced directive; aerosol deposition; affective disorder; after discharge; alcohol dehydrogenase; Aleutian disease; alveolar diffusion; alveolar duct; Alzheimer dementia; Alzheimer disease; analgesic dose; analog device; anodal duration; anterior division; antigenic determinant; appropriate disability; arthritic dose; associate degree; atopic dermatitis; attentional disturbance; Aujeszky disease; autistic disorder; autonomic dysreflexia; autosomal dominant; average deviation; average difference; axiodistal; axis deviation; right ear [Lat. *auris dextra*; JCAHO unapproved abbreviation]

A/D analog-to-digital

A&D admission and discharge; ascending and descending

Ad adenovirus; adrenal; anisotropic disk

ad add [Lat. *adde*]; let there be added [up to a specified amount, Lat. *addetur*]; axiodistal; right ear [Lat. *auris dextra*]

AD1 Alzheimer disease type I

ADA adenosine deaminase; American Dental Association; American Dermatological Association; American Diabetes Association; American Dietetic Association; Americans with Disabilities Act; anterior descending artery; antideoxyribonucleic acid antibody; approved dietary allowance

ADAA American Dental Assistants Association

ADACS automatic data acquisition and control system

ADAM adduct detection by acylation with ^{35}S-methionine; amniotic deformity, adhesion, mutilation [syndrome]; A disintegrin and A metalloprotease; Amsterdam Duration of Antiretroviral Medication [study]

ADAMHA Alcohol, Drug Abuse, and Mental Health Administration

ADAP American Dental Assistants' Program; Assistant Director of Army Psychiatry

ADAPC alcohol and drug abuse prevention and control

ADAPT American Disabled for Attendant Programs Today [organization]; Association for Drug and Alcohol Prevention and Treatment; Automated Data Analysis and Pattern Recognition Toolkit

ADAPTS acute directional atherectomy prior to stenting

ADAS Alzheimer's Disease Assessment Scale

ADAS-COG cognitive portion of the Alzheimer's Disease Assessment Scale

AdASDiM Adaptive Advisory System for Diabetic Management

ADase adenosine deaminase

ADAU adolescent drug abuse unit

ADB accidental death benefit; archival database

ADC adenylate cyclase; adult day care [facility]; affective disorders clinic; Aid to [Families with] Dependent Children; AIDS-dementia complex; albumin, dextrose, and catalase [medium]; ambulance design criteria; analog-to-digital converter; anodal duration contraction; apparent diffusion coefficient; audio-to-digital conversion; average daily census; axiodistocervical

AdC adenylate cyclase; adrenal cortex

ADCA autosomal dominant cerebellar ataxia

ADCC acute disorder of cerebral circulation; antibody-dependent cell-mediated cytotoxicity

ADCH autosomal dominant cyclic hematopoiesis

AD-CHF acutely decompensated congestive heart failure

ADCMC antibody-dependent complement-mediated cytotoxicity

AdCMVHSV-TK adenovirus carrying the gene for herpes simplex thymidine kinase

ADCP adenosine deaminase complexing protein

AD-CPEO autosomal dominant chronic progressive external ophthalmoplegia

ADCS Argonz del Castillo syndrome

ADCY adenyl cyclase

ADD acceptable daily dose; adduction; adenosine deaminase; Anti-Epileptic Drug Development [program]; attention deficit disorder; auditory discrimination in depth; average daily dose

add addition; adductor, adduction; let there be added [Lat. *addatur*]

ADDH attention deficit disorder with hyperactivity

ADD/HA attention deficit disorder/hyperactivity

addict addiction, addictive

AdDNV *Aceta domestica* densovirus

add poll adductor pollicis

ADDS American Digestive Disease Society

ADDU alcohol and drug dependence unit

ADE acute disseminated encephalitis; adaptive delay estimation; advanced large-scale integrated computational environment [ALICE] differencing engine; adverse drug event; antibody-dependent enhancement; apparent digestible energy

Ade adenine

ADEAR Alzheimer Disease Education and Referral [center]

AdeCbl adenosyl cobalamine

ADEE age-dependent epileptic encephalopathy

ADEG Antiarrhythmic Drug Evaluation Group [trial]

ADEM academic department of emergency medicine; acute disseminated encephalomyelitis

AdenCa adenocarcinoma

ADEP Atherosclerotic Disease Evolution by Picotamide [study]

ADEPT Applying Diagnosis, Etiology, Prognosis, and Therapy [program]

adeq adequate

ADF adaptive filter; administrative determination of fault; average duration of failures

ADFVd Apple dimple fruit viroid

AD/FHD acetabular depth/femoral head diameter

ADFN albinism-deafness [syndrome]

ADFR activate, depress, free, repeat [coherence therapy]

ADFS alternative delivery and financing system

AD-FSP autosomal dominant familial spastic paraplegia

ADG ambulatory diagnostic group; atrial diastolic gallop; axiodistogingival

ADH Academy of Dentistry for the Handicapped; adhesion; alcohol dehydrogenase; antidiuretic hormone; arginine dihydrolase; atypical ductal hyperplasia

adh adhesion, adhesive; antidiuretic hormone

ADHA American Dental Hygienists Association

ADH/CA atypical ductal hyperplasia with adjacent ductal cancer

ADHD attention deficit-hyperactivity disorder

ADHDP action-dependent dual heuristic programming

ADI Academy of Dentistry International; acceptable daily intake; AIDS-defining illness; allowable daily intake; alternating direction implicit; alternating directions implicit [method]; artificial diverticulum of the ileum; atlas-dens interval; autism diagnostic interview; average daily intake; axiodistoincisal

adj adjacent; adjoining; adjuvant

ADK adenosine kinase

ADKC atopic dermatitis with keratoconjunctivitis

ADL active digital library; activities of daily living; advanced distributed learning; Amsterdam Depression List; annual dose limit

ADLAR advanced design linear accelerator radiosurgery

ADLC antibody-dependent lymphocyte-mediated cytotoxicity

ad lib as desired [Lat. *ad libitum*]

ADLS Activities of Daily Living Survey

ADM abductor digiti minimi; add-drop multiplexer; administrative medicine; admission; Adriamycin; Alcohol, Drug Abuse and Mental Health [grant of US Department of Health and Human Services]

AdM adrenal medulla

adm administration; admission; apply [Lat. *admove*]

Adm Dr admitting doctor

ADME [drug] absorption, distribution, metabolism, and excretion

Admin administration

ADMIRE AMP 579 Delivery for Myocardial Infarction Reduction

ADMIT Arterial Disease Multiple Intervention Trial

AdML adenovirus major late promoter

Adm Ph admitting physician

ADMR average daily metabolic rate

ADMS analysis of disorders of masticatory system; atmospheric dispersion modeling system

ADMX adrenal medullectomy

ADN antideoxyribonuclease; aortic depressor nerve; associate degree in nursing

ad naus to the point of producing nausea [Lat. *ad nauseam*]

ADN-B antideoxyribonuclease B

ADO active data object; adenosine; adolescent medicine; allele drop-out; axiodisto-occlusal

Ado adenosine

ADOA autosomal dominant ocular albinism

AdoCbl 5'-adenosylcobalamin

ADOD arthrodentosteodysplasia

AdoDABA adenosyldiaminobutyric acid

AdoHcy *S*-adenosylhomocysteine

adol adolescence, adolescent

AdoMet *S*-adenosylmethionine

ADOPT Accupril Decision on Pharmacotherapy [trial]

ADOS autism diagnostic observation scale; autosomal dominant Opitz syndrome

ADOTS affective disorder outpatient telephone screening

Adox oxidized adenosine

ADP adenopathy; adenosine diphosphate; adenovirus death protein; administrative psychiatry; approved drug product; approximate dynamic programming; area diastolic pressure; automatic data processing

AdP adductor pollicis

ADPase adenosine diphosphatase

ADPK autosomal dominant polycystic kidney [disease]

ADPKD autosomal dominant polycystic kidney disease

ADPL average daily patient load

ADPR adenosine diphosphate ribose

ADPRT adenosine diphosphate ribosyltransferase

ADQ abductor digiti quinti; adolescent drinking questionnaire

ADR activation, depression, repetition [in bone remodeling]; adrenalin; adrenals;

adrenergic receptor; adrenodoxin reductase; Adriamycin; adverse drug reaction; airway dilation reflex; alternative dispute resolution; arrested development of righting response; ataxia-deafness-retardation [syndrome]

Adr adrenalin; Adriamycin

adr adrenal, adrenalectomy

ADRA1A alpha-1A-adrenergic receptor

ADRA1B beta-1B-adrenergic receptor

ADRAC Adverse Drug Reactions Advisory Committee [Australia]

ADRA1C alpha-1C-adrenergic receptor

ADRA2C alpha-2C-adrenergic receptor

ADRAR alpha-2-adrenergic receptor

ADRBK beta-1-adrenergic receptor kinase

ADRBR adrenergic beta-receptor

ADRC Alzheimer Disease Research Center

ADRDA Alzheimer Disease and Related Disorders Association

ADRP adipose differentiation-related protein; autosomal dominant retinitis pigmentosa

ADRT approximate discrete radon transform

ADS acute death syndrome; acute diarrheal syndrome; adenocarcinoma dataset; Alcohol Dependence Scale; alternative delivery system; anatomical dead space; anonymous donor's sperm; antibody deficiency syndrome; antidiuretic substance; Army Dental Service

ADSD adductor spasmodic dysphonia

ADSL adenylosuccinate lyase; asymmetrical digital single line; asymmetrical digital subscription line

ADSP analog devices digital signal processor

ADSS adenylosuccinate synthetase

ADSTGD Stargardt-like muscular dystrophy

ADSV Arborea virus

ADT Accepted Dental Therapeutics; adenosine triphosphate; admission, discharge, and transfer; agar-gel diffusion test; alternate-day therapy; any, what you desire, thing (a placebo); Alzheimer-type dementia; Auditory Discrimination Test

ADTA American Dental Trade Association

ADTe anodal duration tetanus

ADU alkaline deoxyribonucleic acid unwinding

AD&U acid dissociation and ultrafiltration

ADV adenovirus; adventitia; Aleutian disease virus; Aujeszky disease virus

AdV adenovirus

Adv adenovirus

adv advanced; against [Lat. *adversum*]

ADVENT antithrombin for deep venous thrombosis

ADVIRC autosomal dominant vitreo-retinochoroidopathy

ADVS activities of daily vision survey

ADW assault with deadly weapon

A5D5W alcohol 5%, dextrose 5%, in water

ADX adrenalectomized; adrenodoxin

AE above-elbow [amputation]; acrodermatitis enteropathica; activation energy; adult erythrocyte; adverse event; aftereffect; agarose electrophoresis; air embolism; air entry; alcoholic embryopathy; aminoethyl; anion exchange; anoxic encephalopathy; antiepileptic; antitoxic unit [Ger. *Antitoxineinheit*]; apoenzyme; aryepiglottic; atherosclerotic encephalopathy; atrial ectopic [heart beat]; avian encephalomyelitis

A&E accident and emergency [department]

A + E accident and emergency [department]; analysis and evaluation

A/E above elbow [amputation]

AEA acquired epileptic aplasia; alcohol, ether, and acetone [solution]

AEB acute erythroblastopenia; avian erythroblastosis

AEC aminoethylcarbazole; ankyloblepharon, ectodermal defects, and cleft lip [syndrome]; at earliest convenience; Atomic Energy Commission; automatic exposure control

AECB acute exacerbation of chronic bronchitis

AECD allergic eczematous contact dermatitis

AECE-6-AZUMP 5-[2-(aminoethyl) carbamyl]-6-azauridine-5′monophosphate

AECGM ambulatory electrocardiography monitoring

AECS acute exacerbation of chronic sinusitis

AED academic emergency department; antiepileptic drug; antihidrotic ectodermal dysplasia; anxious ego dissolution; automated external defibrillator

AEDP automated external defibrillator pacemaker

AEE Atomic Energy Establishment

AEF allogenic effect factor; amyloid enhancing factor; aorto-enteric fistula

AEFB aerobic endospore-forming bacterium

A$_{EFF}$ effective area

AEFI adverse events following immunization

AEFV acceleration of early flow velocity

AEG acute erosive gastritis; air encephalography, air encephalogram; atrial electrogram

AEGIS Aid for the Elderly in Government Institutions

AEI arbitrary evolution index; atrial emptying index; atrial escape interval

AEL acute erythroleukemia

AELV avian entero-like virus

AEM Academic Emergency Medicine [journal]; ambulatory electrocardiographic monitoring; analytical electron microscopy; ataxia episodica with myokymia; avian encephalomyelitis

AEMG abdominal electromyography

AEMIS Aerospace and Environmental Medicine Information System

AEMK ataxia episodica with myokymia

A-EMT advanced emergency medical technician

AEN anal epithelial neoplasia; aseptic epiphyseal necrosis

AEP acute edematous pancreatitis; artificial endocrine pancreas; auditory evoked potential; average evoked potential

AEq age equivalent

AER abduction/external rotation; acoustic evoked response; acute exertional rhabdomyolysis; agranular endoplasmic reticulum; albumin excretion rate; aldosterone excretion rate; apical ectodermal ridge; auditory evoked response; average electroencephalic response; average evoked response

AERE Atomic Energy Research Establishment

Aero *Aerobacter*

AERP aircrew air and respiratory protection; antegrade effective refractory period; atrial effective refractory period; auditory event related potential

AERPAP antegrade effective refractory period accessory pathway

AERS acute equine respiratory syndrome

AES acetone-extracted serum; ambulatory encounter system; American Electroencephalographic Society; American Encephalographic Society; American Endocrine Society; American Endodontic Society; American Epidemiological Society; American Equilibration Society; anterior esophageal sensor; anti-embolic stockings; antral ethmoidal sphenoidectomy; aortic ejection sound; Auger's electron spectroscopy; auto-erythrocyte sensitization

AEs adverse events

AesoNPV *Aedes sollicitans* nucleopolyhedrovirus

AEST aeromedical evacuation support team

AET absorption-equivalent thickness; *S*-(2-aminoethyl) isothiuronium

AETT acetylethyltetramethyltetralin

AEV arthritis encephalitis virus; avian encephalomyelitis-like virus; avian erythroblastosis virus

AeV *Antheraea eucalypti* virus

AEZ acrodermatitis enteropathica, zinc deficient

AF abnormal frequency; acid-fast; actin filament; active force; adult female; afebrile; affected female; aflatoxin; albuminfree; albumose-free; alcoholic female; aldehyde fuchsin; amaurosis fugax; aminofluorine; aminophylline; amniotic fluid; angiogenesis factor; anteflexion; anterior fontanelle; antibody-forming; anti-fog; aortic flow; Arthritis Foundation; artificial feeding; ascitic fluid; atrial fibrillation; atrial flutter; atrial fusion; attenuation factor; attributable fraction; audio frequency

aF abfarad

af audio frequency

AFA acromegaloid facial appearance [syndrome]; advanced first aid; alcohol-formaldehyde-acetic acid [fixative]

AFAFP amniotic fluid alpha-fetoprotein

AFAR American Foundation for Aging Research

AFASAK Atrial Fibrillation, Aspirin, Anticoagulation [trial]

AFB acid-fast bacillus; aflatoxin B; aflatoxin biomarker; air fluidized bed; aortofemoral bypass

AFBAC affected family-based control test

AFBG aortofemoral bypass graft

AFC adult foster care; alternative forced choice; amplitude frequency characteristics; antibody-forming cell

AFCAPS Air Force Coronary Atherosclerosis Prevention Study

AFCI acute focal cerebral ischemia

AFCR American Federation for Clinical Research

AfCVd Apple fruit crinkle viroid

AFD accelerated freeze drying; acrofacial dysostosis

AFDC Aid to Families with Dependent Children

AFDH American Fund for Dental Health

AFDM adaptive focus deformable model

AFDSM adaptive focus deformable statistical model

AFDW ash-free dry weight

AFE amniotic fluid embolism

afeb afebrile

AFEDI Association Francophone Europeenne des Infirmiers [Canada]

AFF atrial fibrillation and flutter; atrial filling fraction

aff afferent

AFFIRM Atrial Fibrillation Follow-Up Investigation of Rhythm Management

AFFN acrofrontofacionasal [dysostosis]

AFG aflatoxin G; amniotic fluid glucose; arbitrary function generator

aFGF acidic fibroblast growth factor

AFH angiofollicular hyperplasia; anterior facial height

AFI amaurotic familial idiocy; Atrial Fibrillation Investigators [1993 pooled study]

AFib atrial fibrillation

AFIB Atrial Fibrillation Investigation with Bidisomide [trial]

AFIB/FL atrial fibrillation/flutter

AFIP Armed Forces Institute of Pathology

AFIPS American Federation of Information Processing Societies

AFIRME antagonist of the fibrinogen receptor after myocardial events

AFIS amniotic fluid infection syndrome

AFL antifibrinolysin; artificial limb; atrial flutter

AFLNH angiofollicular lymph node hyperplasia

AFLP acute fatty liver of pregnancy; amplified fragment length polymorphism

AFM aflatoxin M; after fatty meal; American Federation of Musicians; atomic force microscopy

AFMA automated fabrication of modality aids

AFMU 5-acetylamino-6-formylamino-3-methyluracil

AFN afunctional neutrophil; antegrade femoral nail

AFNC Air Force Nurse Corps

AFND acute febrile neutrophilic dermatosis

AFO ankle/foot orthotic [brace or cast]; ankle-foot orthosis

AFORMED alternating failure of response, mechanical, [to] electrical depolarization

AFP acute flaccid paralysis; alpha-fetoprotein; anterior faucial pillar; atypical facial pain

AFPP acute fibropurulent pneumonia

AFQ aflatoxin Q

AFR aqueous flare response; ascorbic free radical

AFRAX autism-fragile X [syndrome]

AFRD acute febrile respiratory disease

AFRI acute febrile respiratory illness

AFROC Association for Freestanding Radiation Oncology Centers

AFS acquired or adult Fanconi syndrome; alternative financing system; American Fertility Society; antifibroblast serum

AFSAM Air Force School of Aviation Medicine

AFSCME American Federation of State, County and Municipal Employees

AFSM adaptive Fourier series modeling

AFSP acute fibrinoserous pneumonia

AFT aflatoxin; agglutination-flocculation test

AFTA American Family Therapy Association

AFTER Anistreplase Following Thrombolysis Effect on Reocclusion [study]; Aspirin/Anticoagulants Following Thrombolysis with Eminase in Recurrent Infarction [study]; Aspirin/Anticoagulants Following Thrombolysis with Eminase Results [study]

AFTN autonomously functioning thyroid nodule

AFV amniotic fluid volume; aortic flow velocity; *Aspergillus foetidus* virus

AFV-F *Aspergillus foetidus* virus F

AFV-S *Aspergillus foetidus* virus S

AFX atypical fibroxanthoma

AG abdominal girth; acidophilic granulocyte; agarose; aminoglutethimide; analytical grade; angular gyrus; anion gap; antigen; antigenomic; antiglobulin; antigravity; atrial gallop; attached gingiva; autograft; axiogingival; azurophilic granule

AG, A/G albumin-globulin [ratio]

Ag antigen; silver [Lat. *argentum*]

Ag* labeled antigen

ag androgenetic; antigen

AGA accelerated growth area; allergic granulomatosis and angiitis; American Gastroenterological Association; American Genetic Association; American Geriatrics Association; American Goiter Association; antigliadin antibody; antiglomerular antibody; anti-IgG autoantibody; appropriate for gestational age [birthweight]; aspartylglucosamidase

Ag-Ab antigen-antibody complex

AGAC aminoglycoside-aminocyclitol

AGAG acidic glycosaminoglycans

AGAR Australian Group on Antimicrobial Resistance [study]

AGBAD Alexander Graham Bell Association for the Deaf

AGC absolute granulocyte count; anatomically graduated component; atypical glandular cell; automatic gain control

AGC-FN atypical glandular cell-favor neoplasia

AGC-FR atypical glandular cell-favor reactive

AgCPV *Abraxas grossulariata* cypovirus; *Autographa gamma* cypovirus

AGCT antiglobulin consumption test; Army General Classification Test

AGC-U atypical glandular cell-unqualified

AGD agar gel diffusion; agarose diffusion; alpha-ketoglutarate dehydrogenase

AGDD agar gel double diffusion

AGE acrylamide gel; acute gastroenteritis; advanced glycosylation end-product; agarose gel electrophoresis; angle of greatest extension; arterial gas embolism

AGED automated general experimental device

AGEG age group

AGE-IEF agarose gel-isoelectric focusing [electrophoresis]

AGEPC acetyl glyceryl ether phosphorylcholine

AGES age grade extension size [thyroid tumor]

AGF adrenal growth factor; angle of greatest flexion

AGG agammaglobulinemia

agg agglutination; aggravation; aggregation

aggl, agglut agglutination

aggrav aggravated, aggravation

aggreg aggregated, aggregation

AGGS anti-gas gangrene serum

AGI adjusted gross income

AGID agar gel immunodiffusion

AGIS Advanced Glaucoma Intervention Study

agit agitated, agitation

AGIV *Anticarisia gemmatalis* iridescent virus

AGL acute granulocytic leukemia; agglutination; aminoglutethimide; anterior glenoid labrum

AGM absorbent gelling material

AGMK African green monkey kidney [cell]

AGMkK African green monkey kidney [cell]

AgMNPV *Anticarisia gemmatalis* multiple nucleopolyhedrovirus

AGMPyV African green monkey polyoma virus

AGN acute glomerulonephritis; agnosia

VIIIAGN factor VIII antigen

agn agnosia

AGNB aerobic gram-negative bacillus

AgNOR silver-staining nucleolar organizer region

AGOS American Gynecological and Obstetrical Society

AGP acid glycoprotein; agar gel precipitation; ambulatory glucose profile; azurophil granule protein

AGPA American Group Practice Association; American Group Psychotherapy Association

AGPI agar gel precipitin inhibition

AGPT agar-gel precipitation test

AGR aniridia-ambiguous genitalia-mental retardation [syndrome]; anticipatory goal response

agr accessory gene regulator

agri agriculture

AGRP agouti-related protein

AGS adrenogenital syndrome; Alagille syndrome; American Geriatrics Society; audiogenic seizures

AGSP Australian Gonococcal Surveillance Programme

AGT abnormal glucose tolerance; activity group therapy; acute generalized tuberculosis; alkylguanine deoxyribonucleic acid alkyltransferase; angiotensin; aniline/glyoxylate aminotransferase; antiglobulin test; Association of Genetic Technologists

agt agent

AGTH adrenoglomerulotropic hormone

AGTr adrenoglomerulotropin

AGTT abnormal glucose tolerance test

AGU aspartylglucosaminuria

AGUS atypia of gland cells of undetermined significance

AGUV aguacate virus

AGV aniline gentian violet

AGVd Australian grapevine viroid

AH abdominal hysterectomy; absorptive hypercalciuria; accidental hypothermia; acetohexamide; acid hydrolysis; acute hepatitis; adrenal hypoplasia; affected hemisphere; after-hyperpolarization; agnathia-holoprosencephaly; alcoholic hepatitis; amenorrhea and hirsutism; aminohippurate; anterior heel; anterior hypothalamus; antihyaluronidase; arcuate hypothalamus; Army Hospital; arterial hypertension; artificial heart; aryl hydrocarbon; ascites hepatoma; assisted hatching; astigmatic hypermetropia; ataxic hemiparesis; atypical hyperplasia; autoimmune hepatitis; autonomic hyperreflexia; axillary hair

A/H amenorrhea-hyperprolactinemia

A + H accident & health [policy]

A·h ampere-hour

Ah ampere hour

aH abhenry

ah hyperopic astigmatism

AHA acetohydroxamic acid; acquired hemolytic anemia; acute hemolytic anemia; American Heart Association; American Hospital Association; anterior hypothalamic area; anti-heart antibody; antihistone antibody; area health authority; arthritis-hives-angioedema [syndrome]; aspartyl-hydroxamic acid; autoimmune hemolytic anemia

AHA/ACC American Heart Association/American College of Cardiology [Task Force]

AHB alpha-hydroxybutyric acid

AHC academic health care; academic health center; acute hemorrhagic conjunctivitis; acute hemorrhagic cystitis; adrenal hypoplasia congenita; antihemophilic factor C

AHCA Agency for Health Care Administration; American Health Care Association

AHCD acquired hepatocellular degeneration

AHC/HHG adrenal hypoplasia congenita-hypogonadotropic hypogonadism [syndrome]

aHCl aqueous solution of hydrogen chloride

AHCN American Housecall Network [consumer health information]

AHCP allied health care professional

AHCPR Agency for Health Care Policy and Research (see AHRQ)

AhCPV *Agrochola helvolva* cypovirus

AHCy adenosyl homocysteine

AHD acquired hepatocerebral degeneration; acute heart disease; antihyaluronidase; antihypertensive drug; arterio-hepatic dysplasia; arteriosclerotic heart disease; atherosclerotic heart disease; autoimmune hemolytic disease

AHDMS automated hospital data management system

AHDP azacycloheptane diphosphonate

AHDS Allan-Herndon-Dudley syndrome

AHE acute hazardous events [database]; acute hemorrhagic encephalomyelitis

AHEA area health education activity

AHEAD Asset and Health Dynamics

AHEC area health education center

AHES artificial heart energy system

AHF acute heart failure; American Health Foundation; American Hepatic

Foundation; American Hospital Formulary; antihemolytic factor; antihemophilic factor; Argentinian hemorrhagic fever; Associated Health Foundation

AHFS American Hospital Formulary Service

AHF SCENE Advanced Heart Failure Shared Clinical Experience Network

AHG aggregated human globulin; antihemophilic globulin; antihuman globulin; arterial hypertension group

AHGG aggregated human gammaglobulin; antihuman gammaglobulin

AHGS acute herpetic gingival stomatitis

AHH alpha-hydrazine analog of histidine; anosmia and hypogonadotropic hypogonadism [syndrome]; arylhydrocarbon hydroxylase; Association for Holistic Health

AHI acromiohumeral interval; active hostility index; Animal Health Institute; apnea-plus-hypopnea index; applied health informatics

AHIMA American Health Information Management Association

AHIP assisted health insurance plan

AHIS automated hospital information system

AHJ artificial hip joint

AHL apparent half-life

AHLE acute hemorrhagic leukoencephalitis

AHLG antihuman lymphocyte globulin

AHLS antihuman lymphocyte serum

AHM allied health manpower; ambulatory Holter monitor

AHMA American Holistic Medicine Association; antiheart muscle autoantibody

AHMC Association of Hospital Management Committees

AHMD alcoholic heart muscle disease

AHN Army Head Nurse; assistant head nurse

AHNS American Head and Neck Society

AHO acute hematogenous osteomyelitis; Albright hereditary osteodystrophy

AHP accountable health plan or partnership; acute hemorrhagic pancreatitis; afterhyperpolarization; air at high pressure; aminohydroxyphenylalanine; analytic hierarchy process; approved health plan; Assistant House Physician; hyperpolarizing afterpotential

AHPA American Health Planning Association

AHPO anterior hypothalamic preoptic [area]

AHPSR Alliance for Health Policy and Systems Research

AHR antihyaluronidase reaction; aryl hydrocarbon receptor; Association for Health Records; atrial heart rate

AhR aryl hydrocarbon receptor

AHRA American Hospital Radiology Administration

AHRF acute hypoxemic respiratory failure; American Hearing Research Foundation

AHRQ Agency for Healthcare Research and Quality [formerly Agency for Health Care Policy and Research]

AHRTAG Appropriate Health Resources and Technologies Action Group

AHS Academy of Health Sciences; Adventist Health Study; African horse sickness; alveolar hypoventilation syndrome; American Hearing Society; American Hospital Society; area health service; assistant house surgeon

AHSA American Health Security Act

AHSDF area health service development fund

AHSG alpha-2HS-glycoprotein

AHSN Assembly of Hospital Schools of Nursing

AHSP AIDS Health Services Program [of the Robert Wood Johnson Foundation]

AHSR Association for Health Services Research

AHSV African horse sickness virus

AHT aggregation half-time; antihyaluronidase titer; augmented histamine test; autogenous hamster tumor

AHTG antihuman thymocyte globulin

AHTP antihuman thymocyte plasma

AHTS antihuman thymus serum

AHU acute hemolytic uremic [syndrome]; air handling unit; arginine, hypoxanthine, and uracil

AHuG aggregated human IgG

AHV Abu Hammad virus; avian herpes virus

AhV *Atkinsonella hypoxylon* virus

AI accidental injury; accidentally incurred; active ingredient; adiposity index; aggregation index; allergy and immunology; amylogenesis imperfecta; anaphylatoxin inactivator; angiogenesis inhibitor; angiotensin I; anxiety index; aortic incompetence; aortic insufficiency; apical impulse; articulation index; artificial insemination; artificial intelligence; atherogenic index; atrial insufficiency; autoimmune, autoimmunity; avidity index; axio-incisal; first meiotic anaphase

A&I allergy and immunology

ai active ingredient

AIA allylisopropylacetamide; amylase inhibitor activity; anti-immunoglobulin antibody; anti-insulin antibody; aortoiliac aneurysm; aspirin-induced asthma; automated image analysis

AIB aminoisobutyrate; avian infectious bronchitis

AIBA aminoisobutyric acid

AIBS American Institute of Biological Sciences

AIC Akaike information criterion [a goodness-of-fit measure]; aminoimidazole carboxamide; Association des Infirmières Canadiennes

A-IC average integrated concentration

AICA anterior inferior cerebellar artery; anterior inferior communicating artery

AI-CAH autoimmune-type chronic active hepatitis

AICAR aminoimidazole carboxamide ribonucleotide

AICD activation-induced cell death; automatic implantable cardioverter-defibrillator

AICE angiotensin I converting enzyme

AICF adaptive impulse correlated filtering; autoimmune complement fixation

AICG appraisal instrument for clinical guidelines

AI/COAG artificial intelligence hemostasis consultant system

AICPV *Aporophyla lutulenta* cypovirus

AICS acute ischemic coronary syndrome; artery of inferior cavernous sinus

AID acquired immunodeficiency disease; acute infectious disease; acute ionization detector; Agency for International Development; argon ionization detector; artificial insemination by donor; autoimmune deficiency; autoimmune disease; automatic implantable defibrillator; average interocular difference

AIDA automatic interpretation for diagnostic assistance; automatic interpretation of data analysis

AIDCI angle independent Doppler color imaging

AIDH atypical intraductal hyperplasia

AIDNV *Aedes albopictus* densovirus

AIDP acute idiopathic demyelinating polyneuropathy

AIDS acquired immune deficiency or immunodeficiency syndrome

AIDSDRUGS Clinical Trials of AIDS drugs [National Library of Medicine (NLM) database]

AIDS-KS acquired immuno deficiency syndrome with Kaposi's sarcoma

AIDSLINE on-line information on acquired immunodeficiency syndrome [MEDLARS data base]

AIDSPIT Artificial Insulin Delivery System Pancreas and Islet Transplantation [study]

AIDSTRIALS clinical trials of acquired immunodeficiency syndrome drugs [MEDLARS data base]

AIE acute inclusion-body encephalitis; acute infectious encephalitis; acute infective endocarditis

AIEP amount of insulin extractable from pancreas

AIF anemia-inducing factor; anti-inflammatory; anti-invasion factor

AIFD acute intrapartum fetal distress

AIG anti-immunoglobulin

AIgE anti-immunoglobulin E antibody

AIH amelogenesis imperfecta, hypomaturation type; American Institute of Homeopathy; artificial insemination, homologous; artificial insemination by husband; autoimmune hemolysis

AIHA American Industrial Hygiene Association; American International Health Alliance; autoimmune hemolytic anemia

AIHC American Industrial Health Conference

AIHD acquired immune hemolytic disease

AIHV alcelaphine herpesvirus

AII acute intestinal infection; angiotensin II; second meiotic anaphase

AIIS anterior inferior iliac spine

AIIT amiodarone-iodine-induced thyrotoxicosis

AIL acute infectious lymphocytosis; angiocentric immunoproliferative lesion; angioimmunoblastic lymphadenopathy

AILA angioimmunoblastic lymphadenopathy

AILD alveolar interstitial lung disease; angioimmunoblastic lymphadenopathy with dysproteinemia

AIM Abridged Index Medicus; acquisition interface module; acuity index method; advanced informatics and medicine; all in medicine; applications integration mechanism [software]; area of interest magnification; artificial intelligence in medicine; associate in internal medicine; atypical immature squamous metaplasia

AIMBE American Institute for Medical and Biological Engineering

AIMD abnormal involuntary movement disorder; active implantable medical device

AIMS abnormal involuntary movement scale; Acylated Plasminogen-Streptokinase Activator Complex [APSAC] Intervention Mortality Study; aid for the impaired medical student; Arthritis Impact Measurement Scale; Automated Immunization Management System; automated indexing management system

AIMV alfalfa mosaic virus

AIN acute interstitial nephritis; American Institute of Nutrition; anal intraepithelial neoplasia; anterior interosseous nerve

AINA automated immunonephelometric assay

AINOV Aino virus

AINS anterior interosseous nerve syndrome; anti-inflammatory nonsteroidal

AIOD aortoiliac occlusive disease

AION anterior ischemic optic neuropathy

AIOS Acute Illness Observation Scale

AIP acute idiopathic pericarditis; acute infectious polyneuritis; acute intermittent porphyria; acute interstitial pneumonia; aldosterone-induced protein; American Institute of Physics; automated immunoprecipitation; average intravascular pressure; integral anatuberculin, Petragnani

AIPE acute interstitial pulmonary emphysema; alcoholism intervention performance evaluation

AIPFP acute idiopathic peripheral facial nerve palsy

AIPRI ACE Inhibition in Progressive Renal Insufficiency [study]

AIPS American Institute of Pathologic Science

AIR acute insulin response; airway responsiveness; amino-imidazole ribonucleotide; aortoiliac reconstruction; automated image registration; average impairment rating

AIRA anti-insulin receptor antibody

AIRE Acute Infarction Ramipril Efficacy [study]; Acute Infarction Ramipril Efficacy [trial]; Acute Infarction Reperfusion Efficacy [study]

AIREX Acute Infarction Ramipril Efficacy Extension [study]

AIRF alterations in respiratory function

AI/RHEUM artificial intelligence rheumatology consultant system

AIRIO Agency for Intramural Research Integrity Office [NIH]

AIR-L Association of Internet Researchers List [listserv]

AIRS Amphetamine Interview Rating Scale

AIS Abbreviated Injury Scale; absolute increase in survival; acute ischemic stroke; acute ischemic syndrome; adenocarcinoma in situ; administrative information system; adolescent idiopathic scoliosis; aggregate injury score; amniotic infection syndrome; analyzer of interrated sequences [model of a beating ventricle]; androgen insensitivity syndrome; anterior interosseous nerve syndrome; anti-insulin serum; automatic information system; automotive injury score

AISA acquired idiopathic sideroblastic anemia

AISI African Information Society Initiative

AIS/MR Alternative Intermediate Services for the Mentally Retarded

AIT acute intensive treatment; aeromedical isolation team

AITD autoimmune thyroid disease

AITIA aspirin in transient ischemic attacks

AITIAIS Aspirin in Transient Ischemic Attacks Italian Study

AITP autoimmune idiopathic thrombocytopenic purpura

AITT arginine insulin tolerance test; augmented insulin tolerance test

AIU absolute iodine uptake; antigen-inducing unit

AIUM American Institute of Ultrasound in Medicine

AIV AI chi virus

AIVC Australian Influenza Vaccine Committee

AIVR accelerated idioventricular rhythm

AIVV anterior internal vertebral vein

AJ adherens junction

AJ, A/J ankle jerk

AJCC American Joint Committee on Cancer

AJCCS American Joint Committee on Cancer Staging

AJDL arteriojugular venous lactate content difference

AJDO₂ arteriojugular venous oxygen content difference

AJR abdominojugular reflux maneuver

AJS acute joint syndrome

AJT automatic junctional tachycardia

AK above knee; acetate kinase; actinic keratosis; adenosine kinase; adenylate kinase; artificial kidney

A/K, ak above knee [amputation]

A→K ankle to knee

AKA above-knee amputation; alcoholic ketoacidosis; also known as; antikeratin antibody

aka also known as

AK amp above-knee amputation

AKAV Akabane virus

AKBR arterial ketone body ratio

AKE acrokeratoelastoidosis

A/kg amperes per kilogram

AKP alkaline phosphatase

AKRMLV AKR murine leukemia virus

AKS alcoholic Korsakoff syndrome; auditory and kinesthetic sensation

AKU alkaptonuria

AL absolute latency; acinar lumen; acute leukemia; adaptation level; albumin; alcoholism [and other drug dependence services]; alignment; amyloid L; amyloidosis; analyzer and loader; anatomic location, anatomical localizer; anterior leaflet; anterolateral; antihuman lymphocytic [globulin]; argininosuccinate lyase; avian leukosis; axial length; axillary loop; axiolingual; left ear [Lat. *auris laeva*]

A_L angiographic area of lateral projection

Al allantoic; allergic; allergy; aluminum

al left ear [Lat. *auris laeva*]

ALA amebic liver abscess; American Laryngological Association; American Lung Association; aminolevulinate; aminolevulinic acid; axiolabial

ALa axiolabial

Ala alanine

ala alanine

AL-Ab antilymphocyte antibody

ALAD abnormal left axis deviation

ALAD, ALA-D aminolevulinic acid dehydrase

ALADH delta-aminolevulinate dehydratase

ALADP aminolevulinic acid dehydrogenase deficiency porphyria

ALAG, ALaG axiolabiogingival

A-LAK adherent lymphokine-activated killer [cell]

ALAL, ALaL axiolabiolingual

A_LAO angiographic area of left anterior oblique projection

AlaP, ala-P alafosfalin

ALARA as low as reasonably achievable [radiation exposure]

ALARM adjustable leg and ankle repositioning mechanism

ALARP as low as reasonably possible

ALAS delta-aminolevulinate synthase

ALASH delta-aminolevulinate synthase, housekeeping type

ALAT alanine aminotransferase

ALB albumin; avian lymphoblastosis

alb albumin; white [Lat. *albus*]

ALBC albumin clearance

ALB/GLOB albumin/globulin [ratio]

ALC absolute lymphocyte count; acute lethal catatonia; aided living center; alternate level of care; Alternative Lifestyle Checklist; approximate lethal concentration; avian leukosis complex; axiolinguo-cervical

alc alcohol, alcoholic, alcoholism

ALCA anomalous left coronary artery

ALCAPA anomalous origin of left coronary artery from pulmonary artery

ALCAR acetyl-L-carnitine

ALCEQ Adolescent Life Change Event Questionnaire

ALCL anaplastic large cell lymphoma

ALCO Anonymous Fighters Against Obesity

alcoh alcohol, alcoholic, alcoholism

AlCPV *Agrochola lychnidis* cypovirus; *Aporophyla lutulenta* cypovirus

AlcR, alcR alcohol rub

AlCr aluminum crown

ALD adrenoleukodystrophy; alcoholic liver disease; aldehyde dehydrogenase; aldolase; aldosterone; anterior latissimus dorsi; Appraisal of Language Disturbance; approximate lethal dose; assistive listening device

Ald aldolase; aldosterone

ALDA aldolase A

ALDB aldolase B

ALDC aldolase C

ALDF American Lyme Disease Foundation

ALDH aldehyde dehydrogenase

Aldo aldosterone

ALDOA aldolase A

ALDOC aldolase C

ALDOST aldosterone

ALDP adrenoleukodystrophy protein

ALDR aldose reductase

ALDS albinism-deafness syndrome

ALDUSA aspirin low dosage in unstable angina

ALE active life expectancy; adaptive line enhancer; allowable limits of error; amputated lower extremity

ALEC artificial lung-expanding compound

ALEP atypical lymphoepithelioid cell proliferation

ALERT Amiodarone vs Lidocaine Inpatient Emergency Resuscitation Trial; Assessment of Lescol in Renal Transplantation [to reduce coronary event]

ALEV Alenquer virus

ALF acute liver failure; advance laser flowmeter; American Liver Foundation; assisted living facilities; automated laser fluorescence

ALFT abnormal liver function test

ALFV Alfuy virus

ALG antilymphocytic globulin; axiolinguogingival

alg allergy

ALGOL algorithmic oriented language

ALH angiolymphoid hyperplasia; anterior lobe hormone; anterior lobe of hypophysis

ALHE angiolymphoid hyperplasia with eosinophilia

ALHV alcelaphine herpesvirus

ALI acute lung injury; annual limit of intake; average lobe index

ALICE advanced large-scale integrated computational environment

ALIF anterior lumbar interbody fusion

ALIP abnormal localized immature myeloid precursor

ALIVE Adenosine Lidocaine Infarct Zone Viability Enhancement [trial]; Amiodarone vs Lidocaine in Prehospital Refractory Ventricular Fibrillation [study]; Azimilide Postinfarction Survival Evaluation [trial]

ALJV Alajuela virus

ALK automated lamellar keratoplasty

ALK, alk alkaline; alkylating

ALK-P alkaline phosphatase

ALL acute lymphoblastic leukemia; acute lymphocytic leukemia; Antihypertensive and Lipid-Lowering [study]

all allergy, allergic

ALLA acute lymphocytic leukemia antigen

ALLHAT Antihypertensive and Lipid-Lowering Treatment to Prevent Heart Attack Trial

ALLO atypical *Legionella*-like organism

ALM aerial lentiginous melanoma; alveolar living material

ALME acetyl-lysine methyl ester

ALMI anterior lateral myocardial infarct

ALMV Almeirim virus; Almpiwar virus; anterior leaflet of the mitral valve

AlMV alfalfa mosaic virus

ALN allylnitrile; anterior lymph node; axillary lymph node

ALO average lymphocyte output; axiolinguo-occlusal

ALOS average length of stay

ALOSH Appalachian Laboratory for Occupational Safety and Health

ALOX aluminum oxide

ALP acute leukemia protocol; acute lupus pericarditis; alkaline phosphatase; alveolar proteinosis; anterior lobe of pituitary; antileukoproteinase; antilymphocytic plasma; argon laser photocoagulation; automated linkage preprocessor

AlPase alkaline phosphatase

ALPG alkaline phosphatase, germ-cell

α Greek letter *alpha*; angular acceleration; first [carbon atom next to the carbon atom bearing the active group in organic compounds]; optical rotation; probability of type I error; solubility coefficient

alpha₂-AP alpha₂-antiplasmin

α₁-AT alpha₁-antitrypsin

α error type I error [statistics]

alpha-GLUC alpha-glucosidase

alpha₂M alpha₂-macroglobulin

α₂ PIPC α₂-plasmin inhibitor–plasmin complex

ALPL alkaline phosphatase, liver

ALPP alkaline phosphatase, placental

ALPPL alkaline phosphatase-like, placental

ALPS angiolymphoproliferative syndrome; Aphasia Language Performance Scale; attitudinal listening profile system

ALPSA anterior labroligamentous periosteal sleeve avulsion

ALPV aphid lethal paralysis virus

ALR aldehyde reductase

ALRI anterolateral rotatory instability

ALROS American Laryngological, Rhinological, and Otological Society

ALS acute lateral sclerosis; advanced life support; afferent loop syndrome; alkali-labile site; amyotrophic lateral sclerosis; angiotensin-like substance; anterolateral sclerosis; anticipated life span; antilymphocyte serum

ALSD Alzheimer-like senile dementia

ALSPAC Avon Longitudinal Study of Pregnancy and Childhood

ALS-PD amyotrophic lateral sclerosis-parkinsonism-dementia [complex]

AlStV Alstroemeria streak virus

AL-SV avian leukosis sarcoma virus

ALT alanine aminotransferase; argon laser trabeculoplasty; autolymphocyte therapy; avian laryngotracheitis

AlT aluminum tartrate

Alt, alt alternate; altitude; aluminum tartrate

ALTB acute laryngotracheobronchitis

ALTE apparent life-threatening event

ALTEE acetyl-ʟ-tyrosine ethyl ester

ALTS acute lumbar traumatic sprain or syndrome

ALTV Altamira virus

ALU arithmetic and logic unit

ALV Abelson leukemia virus; adeno-like virus; alveolar, alveolus; American latent virus; Arracacha latent virus; ascending lumbar vein; avian leukosis virus

Alv alveolus, alveolar

ALV-A avian leukosis virus A

ALVAD abdominal left ventricular assist device

ALVF acute left ventricular failure

ALV-HPRS103 avian leukosis virus-HPRS103

ALV M alveolar mucosa

ALVT aortic and left ventricular tunnel

alv vent alveolar ventilation

ALVX alveolectomy

ALW arch-loop whorl

ALWMI anterolateral wall myocardial infarct

AM Academic Medicine [journal]; actomyosin; acute myelofibrosis; adult male; adult monocyte; aerospace medicine; affected male; akinetic mutism; alcoholic male; alveolar macrophage; alveolar mucosa; amacrine cell; ambulatory; amethopterin; ametropia; ammeter; amperemeter; ampicillin; amplitude modulation; amyl; anovular menstruation; anterior mitral leaflet; antimycotic; arithmetic mean; arousal mechanism; articular manipulation; aviation medicine; axiomesial; meter angle; myopic astigmatism

Am americium; amnion; amyl

A/m amperes per meter

A-m² ampere-square meter

am ametropia; amyl; amplitude; meter angle; myopic astigmatism

AMA against medical advice; alkaline membrane assay; American Management Association; American Medical Association; analog multiplexer array; antimitochondrial antibody; antimyosin antibody; antithyroid microsomal antibody; apocrine membrane antigen; arm muscle area; Australian Medical Association

AMA-DE American Medical Association Drug Evaluation

AMAL Aero-Medical Acceleration Laboratory

AMANET, AMA/Net American Medical Association Network

AMAP American Medical Accreditation Program; as much as possible

A-MAT amorphous material

AMAV Amapari virus

AMB amphotericin B; anomalous muscle bundle; anteromedial bundle; avian myeloblastosis

Amb ambulance; ambulatory, ambulation

amb ambient; ambiguous; ambulance; ambulatory

AMBER advanced multiple-beam equalization radiography; assisted model building with energy refinement

ambig ambiguous

AMBL acute megakaryoblastic leukemia

AMbL acute myeloblastic leukemia

AMBRE atraumatic multidirectional bilateral rehabilitation [shoulder]

AMBRI atraumatic, multidirectional, bilateral radial instability

AMBU air mask bag unit

ambul ambulatory

AMBV Anhembi virus

AMC academic medical center; acetylmethyl carbinol; Animal Medical Center; antibody-mediated cytotoxicity; antimalaria campaign; arm muscle circumference; Army Medical Corps; arthrogryposis multiplex congenita; ataxia-microcephaly-retardation [syndrome]; automated mixture control; axiomesiocervical

AMCAS American Medical College Application Service

AMCD Aeromedical Certification Division

AMCHA aminomethylcyclohexane-carboxylic acid

AMCN anteromedial caudate nucleus

AmCPV *Antheraea mylitta* cypovirus

AMCRA American Managed Care and Review Association

AMCV avian myelocytomatosis virus

AMD acid maltase deficiency; acromandibular dysplasia; actinomycin D; *S*-adenosylmethionine decarboxylase; adrenomyelodystrophy; advance medical directives; age-related macular degeneration; Aleutian mink disease; alpha-methyldopa; Association for Macular Diseases; axiomesiodistal

AMDA American Medical Directors Association

AMDF average magnitude difference function

AMDGF alveolar macrophage-derived growth factor

AMDS Association of Military Dental Surgeons

AMDV Aleutian mink disease virus

AME amphotericin methyl ester; apparent mineralocorticoid excess; aseptic meningoencephalitis

AMEA American Medical Electroencephalographic Association

AMEAE acute monophasic experimental autoimmune encephalomyelitis

AMED Allied and Alternative Medicine Database [UK]; Army Medical Department

AMEDD Army Medical Department

AMEDS Army Medical Service

AMEGL, AMegL acute megakaryoblastic leukemia

AMEND Aiding Mothers and Fathers Experiencing Neonatal Death

AMES age metastasis extension size

AMet adenosyl-L-methionine

AMETHIST Ambroxol Efficacy and Tolerability on Hypersecretion, Italian Study

AMEV *Amsacta moorei* entomopoxvirus

AMF antimuscle factor

Amf amniotic fluid

AMFAR American Foundation for AIDS Research

AM/FM automated mapping and facility management

AMFPI active matrix flat panel imager

AMG alpha-2-macroglobulin; amyloglucosidase; antimacrophage globulin; arterial migraine grinder; axiomesiogingival

A₂MG alpha-2-macroglobulin

AMH Accreditation Manual for Hospitals; anti-müllerian hormone; automated medical history

Amh mixed astigmatism with myopia predominating over hyeropia

AMHA Association of Mental Health Administrators

AMHIS Alberta Mental Health Information System

AMHT automated multiphasic health testing

AMI acquired monosaccharide intolerance; acute myocardial infarction; amitriptyline; anterior myocardial infarct; anterior myocardial infarction; Argatroban in Myocardial Infarction [study]; Association of Medical Illustrators; Athletic Motivation Inventory; axiomesioincisal

AMIA American Medical Informatics Association

AMIABLE Acute Myocardial Infarction Angioplasty Bolus Lysis Evaluation

AMICUS Austrian Multicenter Isradipine cum Spirapril Study

AMIS Ambulatory Medical Information System; Aspirin in Myocardial Infarction Study; Automated Management Information System

AMISTAD Acute Myocardial Infarction Study of Adenosine

AMKL acute megakaryoblastic leukemia

AML acute monocytic leukemia; acute mucosal lesion; acute myeloblastic leukemia; acute myelocytic leukemia; acute myelogenous leukemia; anatomic medullary locking; angiomyolipoma; anterior mitral leaflet; automated multitest laboratory

AMLB alternate monaural loudness balance

AMLC adherent macrophage-like cell; autologous mixed lymphocyte culture

AMLCD active matrix liquid crystal display

AMLR autologous mixed lymphocyte reaction

AMLS antimouse lymphocyte serum

AMLSGA acute myeloblastic leukemia surface glycoprotein antigen

AMM agnogenic myeloid metaplasia; ammonia; antibody to murine cardiac myosin; Association of Medical Microbiologists [UK]; World Medical Association [Fr. *Association Médicale Mondiale*]

amm ammonia

AMML acute myelomonocytic leukemia

AMMoL acute myelomonocytic or myelomonoblastic leukemia

ammon ammonia

AMN adrenomyeloneuropathy; alloxazine mononucleotide; aminonucleoside; anterior median nucleus

AMNS aminonucleoside

AMO assistant medical officer; axiomesio-occlusal

AmO alarm object

amo, amor amorphous

A-mode amplitude mode; amplitude modulation

AMOG adhesion molecule on glia

AMOL, AMoL acute monocytic or monoblastic leukemia

AMP accelerated mental processes; acid mucopolysaccharide; adenosine monophosphate; Aerospace Medical Panel; 2,3-aminophenazine; 2-amino-2,1-propanol; amphetamine; ampicillin; ampule; amputation; average mean pressure

amp ampere; amplification; amplitude; ampule; amputation, amputee

AMPA alpha-amino-3-hydroxy-5-methyl-4-isoxazolepropionate; American Medical Publishers Association; aminoisopropyl propionic acid

AMPAC American Medical Political Action Committee

AMPAR alpha-amino-3-hydroxy-5-methyl-4-isoxazole propionate receptor

AMP-c cyclic adenosine monophosphate

AMPH, amphet amphetamine

amp-hr ampere-hour

AMPI APSAC in Acute Myocardial Infarction Placebo Controlled Investigation

ampl large [Lat. *amplus*]

AMPLE allergies, medications, past medical history, last meal, events preceding present condition

A-M pr Austin-Moore prosthesis

Amp-RT amplified reverse transcriptase

AMPS abnormal mucopolysacchariduria; acid mucopolysaccharide

AMPT active mouse protection test; alpha-methylparatyrosine

ampul ampule

AMR acoustic muscle reflex; activity metabolic rate; acute mitral regurgitation; alopecia-mental retardation [syndrome]; alternate motion rate; alternating motion reflex; ambulatory medical record

AMRA American Medical Record Association

AMRF American Medical Resources Foundation

AMRI anteromedial rotatory instability

AMRL Aerospace Medical Research Laboratory

AMRNL Army Medical Research and Nutrition Laboratory

AMRO Amsterdam-Rotterdam Trial Comparing Excimer Laser and Percutaneous Transluminal Coronary Angioplasty

AMRS ambulatory medical records system; automated medical record system

AMS ablepharon-microstomia syndrome; accelerator mass spectrometry; act management system; acute mountain sickness; adenosylmethionine synthetase; advanced large-scale integrated computational environment [ALICE] memory snooper; advanced medical systems [fetal monitor]; aggravated in military service; altered mental status; American Microscopical Society; amount of substance; amylase; antimacrophage serum; Army Medical Service; aseptic meningitis syndrome; Association of Military Surgeons; auditory memory span; automated multiphasic screening

ams amount of a substance

AMSA acridinylamine methanesulfon-*m*-anisidide; American Medical Society on Alcoholism; American Medical Students Association; amsacrine

AMSAODD American Medical Society on Alcoholism and Other Drug Dependencies

AMSC Army Medical Specialist Corps

AMSP Association of Medical School Pharmacology

AMSRDC Army Medical Service Research and Development Command

AMSU ambulatory minor surgery unit

AMT acute miliary tuberculosis; Adenosine Scan Multicenter Trial; alpha-methyltyrosine; American Medical Technologists; amethopterin; amitriptyline; amniotic membrane transplantation; amphetamine; anxiety management training; atherogenic metabolic triad

amt amount

AMTV Arumowot virus

amt/vol amount/volume

AMU Army Medical Unit

amu atomic mass unit

AmuLV Abelson murine leukemia virus; amphotrophic murine leukemia virus

AMV alfalfa mosaic virus; apex to mitral valve; assisted mechanical ventilation; asteroid mosaic virus; avian myeloblastosis virus

AMVF additive multiattribute value function

AMVI acute mesenteric vascular insufficiency

aMVL anterior mitral valve leaflet

AMWA American Medical Women's Association; American Medical Writers' Association

AMX advanced multiprocessor extension; amoxicillin

AMY, amy amylase

AMyA antimyocardial antibody

AN acanthosis nigricans; acetylnitrile; acne neonatorum; adult, normal; ala nasi; amyl nitrate; aneurysm; anisometropia; anode; anorexia nervosa; antenatal; anterior; antineuraminidase; aseptic necrosis; atmosphere normal; atrionodal; autonomic neuropathy; avascular necrosis

A/N antenatal; as needed

An actinon; anisometropia; anode, anodal; antigen; *Aspergillus niger*; atmosphere normal

A$_n$ atmosphere normal

A1-NA A1 area of the nucleus ambiguus

ANA acetylneuraminic acid; American Narcolepsy Association; American Neurological Association; American Nurses Association; anesthesia [anaesthesia]; antibody to nuclear antigens; antinuclear antibody; aspartyl naphthylamide

Ana anaplastic

ANAD anorexia nervosa with associated disorders

ANAE alpha-naphthyl acetate esterase

ANAG acute narrow angle glaucoma

AnalNH anaphylotoxin inhibitor

ANAL, anal analgesia, analgesic; analysis, analytic

ANAM automated neuropsychological assessment metrics

ANAP agglutination negative, absorption positive [reaction]

ANAS anastomosis; auditory nerve activating substance

ANASCD American Nurses Association Steering Committee on Databases

anast anastomosis

ANAT anatomic structure [UMLS]

Anat, anat anatomy, anatomist

ANAV *Anopheles* A virus

ANB avascular necrosis of bone

ANBN alpha-nitroso-beta-naphthol

ANBP Australian National Blood Pressure [trial]

ANBV *Anopheles* B virus

ANC absolute neutrophil count; acid neutralization capacity; active noise control [MRI]; adaptive or noise canceler; adult neuronal ceroid [lipofuscinosis]; ancestor [UMLS]; antigen-neutralizing capacity; Army Nurse Corps

ANC₁ ancestor, first level in hierarchy [UMLS]

ANCA antineutrophilic cytoplasmic antibody

ANCC, AnCC anodal closure contraction

ANCHR Access to National Claims History Repository [Medicare database]

ANCL adult neuronal ceroid lipofuscinosis

ANCOVA analysis of covariance

ANCR Association of the Nordic Cancer Registries

AND algoneurodystrophy; anterior nasal discharge

ANDA Abbreviated New Drug Application

ANDRO, andro androsterone

ANDTE, AnDTe anodal duration tetanus

ANDV Andasibe virus; Andes virus

anes, anesth anesthesia, anesthetic

ANESR apparent norepinephrine secretion rate

AnEx, an ex anodal excitation

ANF alpha-naphthoflavone; American Nurses' Foundation; antineuritic factor; antinuclear factor; atrial natriuretic factor

AnfaMNPV *Anagrapha* falciform multiple nucleopolyhedrovirus

ANFIS adaptive neuro-fuzzy inference system

ANFO ammonium nitrate-fuel oil [bomb]

ANG angiogenin; angiogram, angiography; angiotensin

Ang II, ANGII angiotensin II

ang angiogram, angiography; angle, angular

ANGEL a new global environment for learning [computer-assisted]

ANGFA antinerve growth factor antibody

Ang GR angiotensin generation rate

AngHV anguillid herpesvirus

Angio angiogram, angiographic; angiography

ang pect angina pectoris

ANH academic nursing home

anh anhydrous

ANHV Anhanga virus

AnHV anatid herpesvirus

ANI acute nerve irritation

ANIA automated nephelometric immunoassay

ANIM animal [UMLS]

ANIMAL automatic nonlinear image matching and anatomical labeling

ANIR Advanced Networking Infrastructure and Research [National Science Foundation]

ANIS Anorexia Nervosa Inventory for Self-rating

aniso anisocytosis

ANIT alpha-naphthyl-isothiocyanate

ANK, Ank ankyrin

ank ankle

ANL acute nonlymphoblastic leukemia

ANLI antibody-negative with latent infection

ANLL acute nonlymphocytic leukemia

ANN artificial neural network

Ann annual

ANNA antineutrophil nuclear antibody

ann fib annulus fibrosus

ANNP artificial neural network processor

ANOC, AnOC anodal opening contraction

ANOCL anodal opening clonus

ANOCOVA analysis of covariance [statistics]

ANOP anophthalmia

ANOV, ANOVA analysis of variance [statistics]

ANP acute necrotizing pancreatitis; adult nurse practitioner; advanced nurse practitioner; ancillary nursing personnel; A-norprogesterone; atrial natriuretic peptide

ANP-A atrial natriuretic peptide A

ANP-B atrial natriuretic peptide B

ANP-C atrial natriuretic peptide C

A-NPP absorbed normal pooled plasma

ANRC American National Red Cross

ANRL antihypertensive neutral renomedullary lipid

ANS acanthion; American National Standards; American Nimodipine Study; American Nutrition Society; 8-anilino-1-naphthalene-sulfonic acid; anterior nasal spine; antineutrophilic serum; antirat neutrophil serum; Army Nursing Service; arterionephrosclerosis; Associate in Nursing Science; autonomic nervous system

ANSCII American National Standard Code for Information Interchange

ANSI American National Standards Institute

ANSI-HISPP American National Standards Institute Healthcare Informatics Standards Planning Panel

AN-SIR advice nurse structured implicit review [telemedicine]

ANSWER Agency for Toxic Substances and Disease Registry/National Library of Medicine's Workstation for Emergency Response

ANT acoustic noise test; adenine nucleotide translocator; aminonitrothiazole; anterior

ant anterior; antimycin

AntA antimycin A

antag antagonist

ANTENOX [Switch to oral] Anticoagulant from Enoxaparin [in treatment of acute deep venous thrombosis]

Anth-Gly anthraquinone-glycine [conjugate]

Anth-IDA anthraquinone-iminodiacetate [conjugate]

anti-HB$_c$ antibody to hepatitis B core antigen

anti-HB$_e$ antibody to hepatitis B early antigen

anti-HB$_s$ antibody to hepatitis B surface antigen

anti-PNM Ab anti-peripheral nerve myelin antibody

AntLV *Anthriscus* latent virus

ANTR apparent net transfer rate

ANTU alpha-naphthylthiourea

ANTV Antequera virus

ANT3Y adenine nucleotide translocator 3 Y

ANU artificial neural unit

ANuA antinuclear antibody

ANUG acute necrotizing ulcerative gingivitis

ANUV Ananindeua virus

ANV avian nephritis virus

AnV-S *Aspergillus niger* virus S

ANX annexin

anx anxiety

ANZ Australia and New Zealand [heart failure collaborative study]

AO abdominal aorta; abdominally obese; achievement orientation; acid output; acridine orange; age of onset; ankle orthosis; anodal opening; anterior oblique; antisense oligonucleotide; aorta; aortic opening; arthro-ophthalmopathy; assessment-object; atelosteogenesis; atomic orbital; atrioventricular [valve] opening; average optical [density]; axio-occlusal

Ao aorta; *Aspergillus ochraceus*

A$_o$ orifice area

A/O atlanto-occipital

A&O, A/O alert and oriented

AOA Administration on Aging; Alpha Omega Alpha Honor Society; American Optometric Association; American Orthopedic Association; American Orthopsychiatric Association; American Osteopathic Association; ascending aorta

AoA age of acquisition

AOAA amino-oxyacetic acid

AOAC Association of Official Agricultural Chemists

AOAP as often as possible

AoArE aortic arch epinephrine

AOAS American Osteopathic Academy of Sclerotherapy

AOB accessory olfactory bulb; alcohol on breath

AOBEM American Osteopathic Board of Emergency Medicine

AOBS acute organic brain syndrome

AOC abridged ocular chart; allyloxycarbonyl; amyloxycarbonyl; anodal opening contraction; area of concern

AOCA American Osteopathic College of Anesthesiologists

AOCD American Osteopathic College of Dermatology

AOCl anodal opening clonus

AOCN advanced oncology certified nurse

AOCPA American Osteopathic College of Pathologists

AOCPR American Osteopathic College of Proctology

AOCR American Osteopathic College of Radiology; American Osteopathic College of Rheumatology

AOD Academy of Operative Dentistry; Academy of Oral Dynamics; adult-onset diabetes; anesthesiologist-on-duty; arterial oxygen desaturation; arteriosclerotic occlusive disease; auriculo-osteodysplasia

AODM adult-onset diabetes mellitus

AODME Academy of Osteopathic Directors of Medical Education

AODP alcohol and other drug problems

AOE admission order entry

AoE aortic epinephrine

AOHA American Osteopathic Hospital Association

AoHV aotine herpesvirus

AOI apnea of infancy

AoIR Association of Internet Researchers

AOIVM angiographically occult intracranial vascular malformation

AOL acro-osteolysis

AOM acute otitis media; alternatives of management; arthroophthalmopathy; azoxymethane

AOMA American Occupational Medical Association

AOMP, AoMP aortic mean pressure

AON anterior olfactory nucleus

AONE American Organization of Nurse Executives

AOO anodal opening odor; atrial asynchronous (competitive, fixed-rate) [pacemaker]

AOP anodal opening picture; aortic pressure

AoP aortic pressure

AOPA American Orthotics and Prosthetics Association

AOPC adult outpatient psychotherapy clinic

AOPW, AoPW aortic posterior wall

AOR adjusted odds ratio; Alvarado Orthopedic Research [instruments]; auditory oculogyric reflex

AORN Association of Operating Room Nurses

AOS American Ophthalmological Society; American Otological Society; anodal opening sound; anterior [o]esophageal sensor

A$_{2\text{-os}}$ aortic second sound, opening snap

AOSF adaptive order statistic filter

AOSSM American Orthopedic Society for Sports Medicine

AOT accessory optic tract; acute occlusive thrombus or thrombosis; Anderson Olsson table; anodal opening tetanus; Association of Occupational Therapists

AOTA American Occupational Therapy Association

AOTe anodal opening tetanus

AOTF American Occupational Therapy Foundation

AOU apparent oxygen utilization

AOV aortic valve

AoV aortic valve; *Aspergillus ochraceus* virus

AP abdominal pain; abdominal [voiding] pressure; abdominoperitoneal; accelerated phase; accessory pathway; accounts payable; acid phosphatase; acinar parenchyma; action plan; action potential; activator protein; active pepsin; active pressure; acute pancreatitis; acute phase; acute pneumonia; acute proliferative; adductor pollicis [muscle]; adenomatous polyposis; adolescent psychiatry; after parturition; agno protein; alkaline phosphatase; alum precipitated; aminopeptidase; aminopyrine; amyloid P-component; amyloid peptide; anatomic profile; angina pectoris; antepartal [Lat. *ante partum*]; anterior pituitary; anteroposterior; antidromic potential; antiplasmin; antipyrine; antiviral protein; antral peristalsis; aortic pressure; aortopulmonary; apical pulse; apothecary; appendectomy; appendicitis; appendix; apurinic acid; apurinic/apyrimidinic [site in DNA]; area postrema; arithmetic progression; arterial pressure; artificial pneumothorax; aspiration pneumonia; assessment and plans; association period; atherosclerotic plaque; atrial pacing; atrioventricular pathway; attending physician; axiopulpal; before parturition [Lat. *ante partum*]

A-P anteroposterior

A&P anterior and posterior; assessment and plans; auscultation and percussion

A/P abdominal/perineal; antepartum; ascites/plasma [ratio]

A$_2$ P$_2$ aortic second sound, pulmonary second sound

4-AP 4-aminopyridine

Ap apex

A$_p$ amount in plasma

aP acellular pertussis [vaccine]

ap anteroposterior; attachment point

APA action potential amplitude; aldosterone-producing adenoma; Ambulatory Pediatric Association; American Pancreatic Association; American Pharmaceutic Association; American Physiotherapy Association; American Podiatric

Association; American Psychiatric Association; American Psychoanalytic Association; American Psychological Association; American Psychopathological Association; American Psychotherapy Association; aminopenicillanic acid; anterior margin of pulmonary artery; antipernicious anemia [factor]; antiphospholipid antibody; antiproliferative antibody; arcuate premotor area; azidophenacyl

ApA adenylyl (3'-5') adenosine; azidophenacyl

APAAP alkaline phosphatase-antialkaline phosphatase [labeling]

APAB antiphospholipid antibody; azidophenacyl bromide

APACHE Acute Physiology, Age, and Chronic Health Evaluation

APACS analog picture archiving and communication system

APAF antipernicious anemia factor

APAMI Asian Pacific Association of Medical Informatics

APAN Asian-Pacific Advanced Network

APAP acetaminophen; adaptive positive airway pressure

APASS Antiphospholipid Antibodies in Stroke Studies

APB abductor pollicis brevis; atrial premature beat

APBD adult polyglucosan body disease

APC acetylsalicylic acid, phenacetin, and caffeine; activated protein C; adenoidal-pharyngeal-conjunctival [agent]; adenomatous polyposis coli; allophyocyanin; all-purpose capsule; angiotensin presenting cell; antigen-presenting cell; antiphlogistic corticoid; aortopulmonary collateral artery; aperture current; apneustic center; argon plasma coagulation; Association for Practitioners in Infection Control; aspirin-phenacetin-caffeine; atrial premature contraction; autologous platelet concentrate

aPC activated protein C

ApCAM aplasia cell adhesion molecule

APCC aspirin-phenacetin-caffeine-codeine

APCD acquired prothrombin complex deficiency [syndrome]; adult polycystic kidney disease

APCF acute pharyngoconjunctival fever

APCG apex cardiogram

Ap4CH apical four-chamber plane

APCKD adult-type polycystic kidney disease

ApCPV *Anaitis plagiata* cypovirus; *Antheraea pernyi* cypovirus

APC-R, APCR activated protein C resistance

APD acquired perforating dermatosis; action potential duration [of heart]; acute polycystic disease; adult polycystic disease; advanced physical diagnosis; airway pressure disconnect; anteroposterior diameter; antipsychotic drug; articulation-phonological disorders; atrial premature depolarization; autoimmune progesterone dermatitis; automated peritoneal dialysis; avalanche photodiodes

APD$_{80}$ action potential duration at 80% repolarization

A-PD anteroposterior diameter

APD$_b$ [heart] action potential duration-baseline beat

APDF amplitude probability density function

APDI Adult Personal Data Inventory

APDIM Association of Program Directors in Internal Medicine

ApDNV *Aedes pseudoscutellaris* densovirus

APD$_p$ [heart] action potential duration-premature stimulus

AP-DRG all patients-diagnosis-related group

APE acetone powder extract; acute polioencephalitis; acute psychotic episode; acute pulmonary edema; airway pressure excursion; aminophylline, phenobarbital, and ephedrine; anterior pituitary extract; asthma of physical effort; avian pneumoencephalitis

APECED autoimmune polyendocrinopathy-candidosis-ectodermal dystrophy

ApEn approximate entropy

APES aminopropyltriethoxysilane

APEUV Apeu virus

APEX automatic programmable electronic matrix

APF acidulated phosphofluoride; adaptive pattern filtering; American Psychological Foundation; anabolism-promoting factor; animal protein factor; antiperinuclear factor; assigned protection factor

APG acid-precipitated globulin; air plethysmography; ambulatory patient group; animal pituitary gonadotropin; antegrade pyelography

APGAR American Pediatric Gross Assessment Record

APGL alkaline phosphatase activity of granular leukocytes

APGO Association of Professors of Gynecology and Obstetrics

APH alcohol-positive history; alternative pathway hemolysis; aminoglycoside phosphotransferase; antepartum hemorrhage; anterior pituitary hormone; Association of Private Hospitals

Aph aphasia

APHA American Protestant Hospital Association; American Public Health Association

APhA American Pharmaceutical Association

APHEA Air Pollution in Health, European Approach

APHIS Animal and Plant Health Inspection Service

APHL Association of Public Health Laboratories

APHP anti-*Pseudomonas* human plasma

API alkaline protease inhibitor; Analytical Profile Index; annual parasitological index; application program interface; applications programming interface; arterial pressure index; atmospheric pressure ionization; Autonomy Preference Index

APIC Acenocoumarin vs Pentoxifylline in Intermittent Claudication [trial]; Association for Practitioners in Infection Control

APIE assessment, plan, implementation, and evaluation

APIM Association Professionnelle Internationale des Médecins

APIP additional personal injury protection

APIS Antihypertensive Patch, Italian Study

APIVR artificial pacemaker-induced ventricular rhythm

aPKC atypical protein kinase C

APKD adult-onset polycystic kidney disease

APL abductor pollicis longus; accelerated painless labor; acute promyelocytic leukemia; animal placenta lactogen; anterior pituitary-like; anterior pulmonary leaflet

aPL antiphospholipid

A-P&L anteroposterior and lateral

APLA, aPLA antiphospholipid antibody

APLAUD Antiplatelet Useful Dose [trial]

APLAUSE Antiplatelet Treatment After Intravascular Ultrasound Guided Optimal Stent Expansion [trial]

APLP amyloid precursor-like protein

APLPV American plum line pattern virus

APLS advanced pediatric life support

APLV Andean potato latent virus

APM Academy of Parapsychology and Medicine; Academy of Physical Medicine; Academy of Psychosomatic Medicine; acid precipitable material; admission pattern monitoring; affected pedigree member; alternating pressure mattress; anterior papillary muscle; anteroposterior movement; apical plasma membrane; aspartame; Association of Professors of Medicine

APML acute promyelocytic leukemia

APMOMS Advisory Panel on the Mission and Organization of Medical Schools

APMoV Andean potato mottle virus

APMR Association for Physical and Mental Retardation

APMV avian paramyxovirus

ApMV apple mosaic virus

APN acute pyelonephritis; advanced practice nurse; average peak noise

APNCU adequacy of prenatal care utilization

APNH antiporter sodium-hydrogen ion

APO abductor pollicis obliquus; acquired pendular oscillation; Adriamycin, prednisone, vincristine; adverse patient occurrence; aphoxide; apolipoprotein; apomorphine; apoprotein

Apo, apo apolipoprotein

APOA, apoA apolipoprotein A

APOB, apoB apolipoprotein B

APOC African Program for Onchocerciasis Control; apolipoprotein C

apoC apolipoprotein C

APOE, apoE apolipoprotein E

APOIV Apoi virus

APOJ, apoJ apolipoprotein J

APORF acute postoperative renal failure

apoth apothecary

APP acute phase protein; alum-precipitated pyridine; aminopyrazolopyrimidine; amyloid peptide precursor; amyloid precursor protein; antiplatelet plasma; aqueous procaine penicillin; automated physiologic profile; average pixel projection; avian pancreatic polypeptide

App, app appendix

APPA American Psychopathological Association; 4-aminophenylacetic acid

appar apparatus

APPC application or advanced program-to-program communication

APPCPT atom and physicochemical property class pair and torsion

APPCR, AP-PCR arbitrarily primed polymerase chain reaction

APPG aqueous procaine penicillin G

APPI Active Persantine in Postischemic Injury [study]

appl appliance; application, applied

APPROACH Alberta Provincial Project for Outcomes Assessment in Coronary Heart Disease

approp appropriate

approx approximate

APPS amyloid precursor protein secretase

APPT Adolescent Pediatric Pain Tool

Appt, appt appointment

appx appendix

appy appendectomy

APR abdominoperineal resection; absolute proximal reabsorption; acute phase reaction or reactant; air-purifying respirator; amebic prevalence rate; anatomic porous replacement; anterior pituitary reaction; average payment rate

APRAIS Acute Phase Reactions and Ischemic Coronary Syndromes

APRAISE Antisense to Prevent Restenosis After Intervention, Stent Evaluation

aprax apraxia

APRICOT Antithrombotics in the Prevention of Reocclusion in Coronary Thrombolysis [trial]; Aspirin vs Coumadin Trial; Aspirin vs Coumadin in the Prevention of Reocclusion and Recurrent Ischemia after Successful Thrombolysis Trial

APRL American Prosthetic Research Laboratory

AProL acute promyelocytic leukemia

APRP acidic proline-rich protein; acute phase reactant protein

APRT adenine phosphoribosyl transferase

APRV airway pressure release ventilation

APS acute physiology score; adenosine phosphosulfate; advanced photon source; American Pain Society; American Pediatric Society; American Physiological Society; American Proctologic Society; American Prosthodontic Society; American Psychological Society; American Psychosomatic Society; aminopropylsilane; ammonium persulfate; analog processing stage; annual person summary [Medicare data file]; antiphospholipid antibody syndrome; attending physician's statement; Australian Psychological Society; autoimmune polyglandular syndrome; automated patent system; prostate-specific antigen

APSAC acylated plasminogen-streptokinase activator complex; anisoylated plasminogen streptokinase activator complex

APSD aorticopulmonary septal defect

APSGN acute poststreptococcal glomerulonephritis

APSIS Angina Prognosis Study in Stockholm; Angina Prognosis Study with Isoptin and Seloken [trial]

APSP assisted peak systolic pressure

APSQ Abbreviated Parent Symptom Questionnaire

APSS Association for the Psychophysiological Study of Sleep

APSU Australian Paediatric Surveillance Unit

APT Ablate and Pace Trial; alum-precipitated toxoid; aminophenylthioether; antiplatelet trials; applied potential tomography; automatic peak tracing

APTA American Physical Therapy Association

APTD Aid to Permanently and Totally Disabled

APTES γ-aminopropyltriethoxysilane

APTF American Physical Therapy Foundation

APTH ambulatory blood pressure monitoring and treatment of hypertension

APTI airway pressure time index

APTT, aPTT activated partial thromboplastin time

APUD amine precursor uptake and decarboxylation

APV abnormal posterior vector; *Acyrthosiphon pisum* virus; amprenavir

aPV acellular pertussis vaccine

APVC anomalous pulmonary venous connection

APW alkaline peptone water

APWS attending physician work station

AQ achievement quotient; acoustic quantification; anthraquinone; any quantity; aphasia quotient

aq aqueous; water [Lat. *aqua*]

AQAB acquired abnormality [UMLS]

AQCESS Automated Quality of Care Evaluation Support System

AQIS Australian Quarantine and Inspection Service

AQL acceptable quality level

AQLQ Asthma Quality of Life Questionnaire

AQMS acute quadriplegic myopathy syndrome

AQP aquaporin

AQS additional qualifying symptoms

aqu aqueous

AR absolute risk; acceptable risk; accounts receivable; achievement ratio; actinic reticuloid [syndrome]; active resistance; acute rejection; acute relapse; adherence ratio; admission rate; admitting room; adrenergic receptor; adrenodoxin reductase; airway resistance; alarm reaction; alcohol related; alkali reserve; allergic rhinitis; allowance region [radiotherapy]; alloy restoration; ambulance report; amphiregulin; amplitude ratio; analytical reagent; androgen receptor; anterior root; aortic regurgitation; apical-radial; Argyll Robertson [pupil]; aromatase; arsphenamine; articulare; artificial respiration; ascorbate reductase; assisted respiration; at risk; atrial rate; atrial reversal; atrophic rhinitis; augmented reality [computer graphics]; autoradiography; autoregressive; autosomal recessive

A₁R adenosine A_1 receptor

Ar argon; articulare

A_r relative atomic mass

ar aromatic

A/R apical/radial

A&R advised and released

ARA Academy of Rehabilitative Audiometry; acetylene reduction activity; adenine regulating agent; American Rheumatism Association; anorectal agenesis; antireticulin antibody; aortic root angiogram; arabinose; Associate of the Royal Academy; Axenfeld-Rieger anomaly

ara arabinose

ara-A adenine arabinoside

Ara-C arabinosylcytidine

ara-C cytosine arabinose; cytosine arabinoside

ARAL adjustment reaction to adult life

ARAM antigen recognition activation motif

ARAMIS American Rheumatism Association Medical Information System

A_RAO angiographic area of right anterior oblique projection

ARAS ascending reticular activating system

ara-U arabinosyluracil

ARAV Araguari virus

ARB adrenergic receptor binder; angiotensin receptor blocker

arb arbitrary unit

ARBD alcohol-related birth defects

ARBV Arbia virus

ARC absolute reticulocyte count; accelerating rate calorimetry; Accreditation Review Council; acquired immunodeficiency syndrome-related complex; active renin concentration; AIDS-related complex; American Red Cross; anomalous retinal correspondence; antigen reactive cell; arcuate; Arthritis Rehabilitation Center; arthrogryposis-renal dysfunction-cholestasis [syndrome]; Association for Retarded Children; atypical reparative changes; automatic exposure control

ARCA acquired red cell aplasia

ARCD age-related cognitive decline

ARCH Amiodarone Reduces Coronary Artery Bypass Grafting Hospitalization [trial]; automated record for child health

ARCI Addiction Research Center Inventory

ARCOS Auckland Region Coronary or Stroke [study]

ARCS Associate of the Royal College of Science; Atherosclerosis Risk in Communities Study

ARC-ST Accreditation Review Council for Educational Programs in Surgical Technology

ARD absolute reaction of degeneration; acute radiation disease; acute respiratory disease; adult respiratory distress; allergic respiratory disease; ancillary report display; anorectal dressing; aortic root diameter; arthritis and rheumatic diseases; atopic respiratory disease

AR-DLMD autosomal recessive Duchenne-like muscular dystrophy

ARDMS American Registry of Diagnostic Medical Sonographers

ARDS acute respiratory distress syndrome; adult respiratory distress syndrome

ARE active-resistive exercises; AIDS-related encephalitis; antioxidant response element

AREDS Age-Related Eye Disease Study

AREDYLD acrorenal field defect, ectodermal dysplasia, lipoatrophic diabetes [syndrome]

AREPA acetazolamide-responsive familial paroxysmal ataxia

ARES antireticulo-endothelial serum

AREV Advanced Revelations [platform for database distribution]

ARF acute renal failure; acute respiratory failure; acute rheumatic fever; Addiction Research Foundation; ambulance report form; area resource file

ARFC active rosette-forming T-cell; autologous rosette-forming cell

ARFD acrorenal field defect

AR-FSP autosomal recessive familial spastic paraplegia

ARG, Arg arginine

arg arginine; silver [Lat. *argentum*]

ARGAMI Argatroban Compared with Heparin in Myocardial Infarction Treated with Recombinant Tissue Plasminogen Activator

ARGS antitrypsin-related gene sequence

ArGV *Artogeia rapae* granulovirus

ARI absolute risk increase; activation-recovery interval; acute renal insufficiency; acute respiratory illness; airway reactivity index; aldolase reductase inhibitor; annual rate of infection; anxiety reaction, intense

ARIA acetylcholine receptor-inducing activity; allergic rhinitis and its impact on asthma; automated radioimmunoassay

ARIC Atherosclerosis Risk in Communities [study]

ARIF Aggressive Research Intelligence Facility [UK]

ARIMA autoregressive integrated moving average

ARIS Andrology Research Information System; Anturan Reinfarction Italian Study; auto-regulated inspiratory support

Ar Kr argon-krypton [laser]

ARKV Arkonam virus

ARL Association of Research Libraries; average remaining lifetime

ARLD alcohol-related liver disease

AR-LGMD autosomal recessive limb muscular dystrophy

ArLV artichoke latent virus

ArLVM artichoke latent virus M

ArLVS artichoke latent virus S

ARM adrenergic receptor material; advanced respiratory mechanics; aerosol rebreathing method; ambulatory renal monitor; anorectal manometry; anxiety reaction, mild; arginine-rich motif; Armenian [hamster]; artificial rupture of membranes; associations rule mining [algorithm]; atomic resolution microscopy

ARMA autoregressive moving average

ARMD age-related muscle degeneration

ARMS access by radial artery multilink stent; adverse reaction monitoring system; amplification refractory mutation system

ARMV Arumateua virus

ARN acute renal necrosis; acute retinal necrosis; arcuate nucleus; Association of Rehabilitation Nurses

ARNMD Association for Research in Nervous and Mental Diseases

ARNP Advanced Registered Nurse Practitioner

ARNSHL autosomal recessive non-syndromic hearing loss

ARNT aryl hydrocarbon nuclear translocator; aryl hydrocarbon receptor nuclear translocator

ARNV Aruana virus

ARO adjusted relative odds; Associate for Research in Ophthalmology

AROA autosomal recessive ocular albinism

AROAV Aroa virus

AROM active range of motion; artificial rupture of membranes

arom aromatic

ARP absolute refractory period; address resolution protocol; American Registry of Pathologists; anticipated recovery path; apolipoprotein regulatory protein; assay reference plasma; assimilation regulatory protein; atrial refractory period; at risk period; automaticity recovery phase

ARPA Advanced Research Projects Agency

ARPANET Advanced Research Projects Agency Network

ARPC Akaike relative power contribution

ARPD autosomal recessive polycystic disease

ARPES angular resolved photoelectron spectroscopy

ARPKD autosomal recessive polycystic kidney disease

ARPT American Registry of Physical Therapists

ARR absolute risk reduction; aortic root replacement

arr arrest, arrested

ARRC Associate of the Royal Red Cross

ARREST Amiodarone in Out-of-Hospital Resuscitation of Refractory Sustained Ventricular Tachyarrhythmia; Amsterdam Resuscitation Study

ARRP autosomal recessive retinitis pigmentosa

ARRS American Roentgen Ray Society

ARRT American Registry of Radiologic Technologists

ARS acquiescence response scale; acute radiation syndrome or sickness; adult Reye's syndrome; alcohol-related seizures; alizarin red S; American Radium Society; American Rhinologic Society; antirabies serum; arsphenamine; arylsulfatase; Atherogenic Risk Study; autonomously replicating sequence

Ars arsphenamine

ARSA American Reye's Syndrome Association; arylsulfatase A

ARSAC Administration of Radioactive Substances Advisory Committee

ARSACS autosomal recessive spastic ataxia of Charlevoix-Saguenay

ARSB arylsulfatase B

ARSC arylsulfatase C; Associate of the Royal Society of Chemistry

ARSM acute respiratory system malfunction

ARSPH Associate of the Royal Society for the Promotion of Health

ART absolute retention time; Accredited Record Technician; Achilles reflex time; acoustic reflex test; acoustic reflex threshold; adaptive resonance theory; algebraic reconstruction technique; algebraic

reconstructive technique; AngioJet Rapid Thrombectomy Catheter Study; antiretroviral therapy; artery; assisted reproductive technique; automated radiation therapy; automated reagin test; automaticity recovery time

art artery, arterial; articulation; artificial

ARTF artificial

arth arthritis

artic articulation, articulated

artif artificial

ARTIS Human Immunodeficiency Virus/ Acquired Immunodeficiency Syndrome [HIV/AIDS] Treatment Information Service [NLM database]

ARTISTIC Angiorad Radiation Technology for In-Stent Restenosis Trial in Coronaries

ARTMAP adaptive resonance theory mapping

Art O$_2$ arterial oxygen flow

ARTS Arterial Revascularization Therapies Study

ARU arthritis rehabilitation unit

ARUAV Aruac virus

ARV acquired immunodeficiency syndrome-related virus; Adelaide River virus; anterior right ventricle; antiretroviral; avian orthoreovirus; avian reovirus

ARV-A aquareovirus A

ARV-B aquareovirus B

ARV-C aquareovirus C

ARVD arrhythmogenic right ventricular dysplasia

ARV-D aquareovirus D

ARV-E aquareovirus E

ARV-F aquareovirus F

ARVP arginine-vasopressin

ARX autoregressive with exogenous input [model]

ARZAP archive zap process [database element]

AS above scale; absence of seizures; access service [to health information]; acetylstrophanthidin; acidified serum; acoustic schwannoma; acoustic stimulation; active sarcoidosis; active sleep; Adams-Stokes [disease]; adolescent suicide; aerosol sensitivity; aerosol sensitization; allele-specific; Alport syndrome; alveolar sac; amphetamine sulfate; amyloid substance; anabolic steroid; anal sphincter; androsterone sulfate; Angelman syndrome; angiosarcoma;

ankylosing spondylitis; anorexia site [database, Italy]; anovulatory syndrome; anterior synechia; anteroseptal; anterosuperior; antiserum; antisocial; antistreptolysin; antral spasm; anxiety state; aortic sound; aortic stenosis; approaching significance [statistical]; aqueous solution; aqueous suspension; archives server; area of stenosis; arteriosclerosis; artificial sweetener; aseptic meningitis; asparagine synthetase; Asperger syndrome; assisted suicide; astigmatism; asymmetric; atherosclerosis; atrial septum; atrial stenosis; atropine sulfate; audiogenic seizure; Auto-Suture; left ear [Lat. *auris sinistra*; JCAHO unapproved abbreviation]

As arsenic; astigmatism; asymptomatic

A(s) asplenia syndrome

As ampere second

A/s ampere per second

A$_s$ shifted ligand concentration [amount/volume]

aS absiemens

as left ear [Lat. *auris sinistra*]

ASA acetylsalicylic acid; active systemic anaphylaxis; acute severe asthma; Adams-Stokes attack; ambulatory services architecture; American Society of Anesthesiologists; American Standards Association; American Surgical Association; aminosalicylic acid; anterior spinal artery; antibody to surface antigen; argininosuccinic acid; arylsulfatase-A; aspirin-sensitive asthma; asthma-nasal polyps-aspirin intolerance [triad]

ASAAC Acetylsalicylic Acid Aorto-Coronary Bypass Surgery; Acetylsalicylic Acid vs Anticoagulants [study]

ASAAD American Society for the Advancement of Anesthesia in Dentistry

ASAC acidified serum-acidified complement

ASAH antibiotic sterilized aortic valve homograft

ASAHP American Society of Allied Health Professions

ASAIO American Society for Artificial Internal Organs

ASAL arginosuccinic acid lyase

ASAP Academic Strategic Alliance Program; Acetylsalicylic Acid Persantine [study]; American Society for Adolescent Psychology; apparatus for sensing accu-

racy of position; arbitrary signatures from amplification profiles; Areawide Stroke Awareness Program; as soon as possible; Azimilide Supraventricular Arrhythmia Program [trial]

ASAPS American Society of Aesthetic Plastic Surgery

ASAS Anderson Symptom Assessment Scale; argininosuccinate synthetase

ASAT aspartate aminotransferase

ASB American Society of Bacteriologists; anencephaly-spina bifida [syndrome]; anesthesia standby; Anxiety Scale for the Blind; asymptomatic bacteriuria

ASBMT American Society for Blood and Marrow Transplantation

ASBS American Society for Bariatric Surgery

ASBV, ASBVd avocado sunblotch viroid

ASC acetylsulfanilyl chloride; acute suppurative cholangitis; altered state of consciousness; ambulatory surgical center; American Society of Cytology; anterior subcapsular cataract; antibody-secreting cell; antigen-sensitive cell; ascorbate, ascorbic acid; asthma symptom checklist; auditory sequence comparison; automatic sensitivity control

asc anterior subcapsular; ascending

ASCAD atherosclerotic coronary artery disease

ASCAo ascending aorta

ASCB Asymptomatic Cervical Bruit [study]

ASCH American Society of Clinical Hypnosis

ASCI Accelerated Strategic Computing Initiative; acute spinal cord injury; American Society for Clinical Investigation; automated stress relaxation and creep indentation

ASCIA American Spinal Cord Injury Association

ASCII American Standard Code for Information Interchange

ASCLT American Society of Clinical Laboratory Technicians

ASCMS American Society of Contemporary Medicine and Surgery

ASCN American Society for Clinical Nutrition

ASCO American Society of Clinical Oncology; American Society of Contemporary Ophthalmology

ASCOT Anglo-Scandinavian Cardiac Outcomes Trial; a severity characterization of trauma

ASCOTA American Student Committee of the Occupational Therapy Association

ASCP American Society of Clinical Pathologists; American Society of Consulting Pharmacists

AsCPV *Actias selene* cypovirus; *Agrotis segetum* cypovirus

ASCR American Society of Chiropodical Roentgenology

ASCS admissions scheduling system

ASCT autologous stem cell transplantation

ASCUS atypia of squamous cells of undetermined significance

ASCUS-H atypical squamous cell of undetermined significance, high-grade squamous intraepithelial lesion

ASCUS-L atypical squamous cell of undetermined significance, low-grade squamous intraepithelial lesion

ASCVD arteriosclerotic cardiovascular disease; atherosclerotic cardiovascular disease

ASD adaptive seating device; aldosterone secretion defect; Alzheimer senile dementia; antisiphon device; argininosuccinic acid synthetase deficiency; arthritis syphilitica deformans; arthroscopic subacromial decompression; atrial septal defect

ASDB Active Substance Database; Annotation and Similarity [protein] Database

A-SDC anomaly-symptomatic deformity complex

ASDC American Society of Dentistry for Children; Association of Sleep Disorders Centers

ASDE Accelerated Strategic Computing Initiative [ASCI] Simulation Development Environment

ASDH acute subdural hemorrhage or hematoma

ASDOS Atrial Septal Defect Occlusion System [study]

ASDP anal sphincter dysplasia

ASDS American Society for Dermatological Surgery

ASE acute stress erosion; American Society of Electrocardiography; application service element; axilla, shoulder, and elbow

ASEX Arizona Sexual Experiences Scale

ASF African swine fever; aniline-sulfur-formaldehyde [resin]

ASFR age-specific fertility rate

ASFV African swine fever virus

ASG advanced cell group; American Society for Genetics; Army Surgeon General; aspermiogenesis

ASGBI Association of Surgeons of Great Britain and Ireland

ASGE American Society for Gastrointestinal Endoscopy

ASGP asialoglycoprotein

AS/GP antiserum, guinea pig

ASGR asialoglycoprotein receptor

ASGV apple stem grooving virus

ASH Action on Smoking and Health; aldosterone-stimulating hormone; American Society of Hematology; ankylosing spinal hyperostosis; antistreptococcal hyaluronidase; asymmetric septal hypertrophy

AsH astigmatism, hypermetropic

A&Sh arm and shoulder

ASHA American School Health Association; American Social Health Association; American Speech and Hearing Association

ASHAC acquired immunodeficiency syndrome self-help and care

ASHBEAMS American Society of Hospital-Based Emergency Aeromedical Services

ASHBM Associate Scottish Hospital Bureau of Management

ASHCRM American Society of Health Care Risk Managers

ASHCSP American Society for Hospital Central Service Personnel [of AHA]

ASHCVD atherosclerotic hypertensive cardiovascular disease

ASHD arteriosclerotic heart disease; atrioseptal heart disease

ASHE American Society for Hospital Engineering

ASHET American Society for Health Manpower Education and Training

ASHFSA American Society for Hospital Food Service Administrators

ASHG American Society for Human Genetics

ASHI Association for the Study of Human Infertility

ASHL Association of Scottish Health Science Librarians

ASHM Australasian Society for Human Immunodeficiency Virus Medicine

ASHN acute sclerosing hyaline necrosis

AS/Ho antiserum, horse

ASHP American Society for Hospital Planning; American Society of Hospital Pharmacists

ASHPA American Society for Hospital Personnel Administration

ASHT American Society of Hand Therapists

ASHV Arctic squirrel hepatitis virus

ASI Addiction Severity Index; anxiety state inventory; anxiety status inventory; arthroscopic screw installation

a-Si amorphous silicon

ASIA American Spinal Injury Association

ASIC acid sensing ion channel; application-specific integrated circuit

aSi/CsI cesium iodide and amorphous silicon [x-ray detector]

ASIF Association for Study of Internal Fixation

ASII American Science Information Institute

ASIM American Society of Internal Medicine

ASIP atypical protein kinase C isotype-specific interacting protein

ASIR age-standardized incidence rate

ASIS American Society for Information Science; American Study of Infarct Survival; Angina and Silent Ischemia Study; average severity of index score; anterior superior iliac spine

ASIST Atenolol Silent Ischemia Trial

ASK anomalous state of knowledge; antistreptokinase; Australian Streptokinase [trial in stroke]

ASL angiosarcoma of liver; antistreptolysin; argininosuccinate lyase

ASLIB Association of Special Libraries and Information Bureau

ASLM American Society of Law and Medicine

ASLN Alport syndrome-like hereditary nephritis

ASLO antistreptolysin O

ASLT antistreptolysin test

ASLV avian sarcoma and leukosis virus

ASM acid sphingomyelinase; active shape model [radiological image]; age-specific mortality; airway smooth muscle; American Society for Microbiology; angular second moment; anterior scalenus muscle

AsM astigmatism, myopic

asm age-specific mortality

ASMA Aerospace Medical Association; antismooth muscle antibody

ASMC arterial smooth muscle cell

ASMD anterior segment mesenchymal dysgenesis; atonic sclerotic muscle dystrophy

ASME Association for the Study of Medical Education

ASMI anteroseptal myocardial infarct

As/Mk antiserum, monkey

ASMPA Armed Services Medical Procurement Agency

ASMR age-standardized mortality ratio

ASMS archival [imaging] storage management system

ASMT acetylserotonin methyltransferase; American Society for Medical Technology

ASMTY acetylserotonin methyltransferase Y

ASN abstract syntax notation; alkali-soluble nitrogen; American Society of Nephrology; American Society of Neurochemistry; arteriosclerotic nephritis; asparagine; Associate in Nursing

Asn, asn asparagine

ASO administrative services only; AIDS service organization; allele-specific oligonucleoside; antistreptolysin O; arteriosclerosis obliterans

ASOD anterior segmental ocular dysgenesis

AS ON antisense oligonucleotide

ASOS American Society of Oral Surgeons

ASOT antistreptolysin-O test

ASP abnormal spinal posture; active server page or pages; active server processor; acute suppurative parotitis; acute symmetric polyarthritis; affected sibling pair; African swine pox; aged substrate plasma; alkali-stable pepsin; American Society of Parasitology; amnesic shellfish poisoning; ankylosing spondylitis; anorectal malformation, sacral bony abnormality, presacral mass [association]; antibody-specific prediction; antisocial

personality; aortic systolic pressure; application service provider; area systolic pressure; asparaginase; aspartic acid

Asp aspartic acid; asparaginase

asp aspartame; aspartate, aspartic acid; aspiration; automatic signal processing

ASPA American Society of Physician Analysts; American Society of Podiatric Assistants; aspartoacylase

ASPAC Asia-Pacific [regional study]

ASPAT antistreptococcal polysaccharide test

ASPCR, AS-PCR allele-specific polymerase chain reaction

ASPD antisocial personality disorder

ASPDM American Society of Psychosomatic Dentistry and Medicine

ASPECT Anticoagulants in Secondary Prevention of Events in Coronary Thrombosis; Approach to Systematic Planning and Evaluation of Clinical Trials

ASPEN American Society for Parenteral and Enteral Nutrition

ASPG antispleen globulin

AS/PI anterior superior/posterior inferior

ASPIRE Action on Secondary Prevention by Intervention to Reduce Events

ASPM American Society of Paramedics

ASPO American Society for Psychoprophylaxis in Obstetrics; American Society of Pediatric Otolaryngology

ASPP Association for Sane Psychiatric Practices

ASPREN Australian Sentinel Practice Research Network

ASPRS American Society of Plastic and Reconstructive Surgeons

ASPS advanced sleep phase syndrome; Australian Swedish Pindolol Study

ASPSOM adaptive structure probabilistic self-organizing map

ASPV apple stem pitting virus

ASPVD atherosclerotic peripheral vascular disease; atherosclerotic pulmonary vascular disease

ASQ Abbreviated Symptom Questionnaire; Anxiety Scale Questionnaire

ASR adrenal/spleen ratio; age-standardized rate; aldosterone secretion rate; antistreptolysin reaction; automated speech recognition

AS/Rab antiserum, rabbit

ASRT American Society of Radiologic Technologists; American Society of Registered Technologists

ASS Aarskog-Scott syndrome; acute serum sickness; acute spinal stenosis; acute stroke study; anterior superior spine; argininosuccinate synthetase; Auckland Stroke Study

ASSA, ASSAS aminopterin-like syndrome sine aminopterin

ASSC acute splenic sequestration crisis

AS-SCORE age, stage of disease, physiological system involved, complications, response to therapy

ASSENT Assessment of the Safety and Efficacy of a New Thrombolytic Agent

ASSERT [improving] Alcohol and Substance Abuse Services and Educating Providers to Refer Patients to Treatment

ASSET Anglo-Scandinavian Study of Early Thrombolysis; Atorvastatin Simvastatin Safety and Efficacy Trial

ASSH American Society for Surgery of the Hand

ASSI Accurate Surgical and Scientific Instruments

ASSIA Applied Social Science Index and Abstracts [UK]

assim assimilate, assimilation

ASSIST American Stop Smoking Intervention Study

ASSO American Society for the Study of Orthodontics

Assoc association, associate

ASSP argininosuccinate synthetase pseudogene

ASSR adult situation stress reaction; auditory steady-state response

ASSURE A Stent vs Stent Ultrasound Remodeling Evaluation

ASSVd Apple scar skin viroid

ASSX argininosuccinate synthetase pseudogene

AST above selected threshold; allele-specific transcript; allergy serum transfer; angiotensin sensitivity test; anterior spinothalamic tract; antimicrobial susceptibility test; antistreptolysin test; aspartate aminotransferase (SGOT); Association of Surgical Technologists; astigmatism; atrial overdrive stimulation rate; audiometry sweep test; Australian Streptokinase Trial

Ast astigmatism

ASTA anti-alpha-staphylolysin

ASTAM American Society for Testing and Materials

ASTECS Antenatal Steroid Therapy in Elective Cesarean Section [study]

ASTH, Asth asthenopia

ASTHO Association of State and Territorial Health Officers; Association of State and Territorial Health Officials

ASTI antispasticity index

ASTM American Society for Testing and Materials

ASTMH American Society of Tropical Medicine and Hygiene

ASTO antistreptolysin O

as tol as tolerated

ASTPHND Association of State and Territorial Public Health and Nutrition Directors

ASTRO American Society for Therapeutic Radiology and Oncology

AstV *Astrovirus*

ASTZ antistreptozyme

ASUB active substance [UMLS]

ASV anodic stripping voltammetry; anti-siphon valve; anti–snake venom; autologous saphenous vein; avian sarcoma virus

ASV-CT10 avian sarcoma virus CT10

ASVO American Society of Veterinary Ophthalmology

ASVPP American Society of Veterinary Physiologists and Pharmacologists

ASW artificial sweetener

ASWC averaged spike and wave complex [EEG]

Asx amino acid that gives aspartic acid after hydrolysis; asymptomatic

asym asymmetry, asymmetric

AT abdominal thrusts; Achilles tendon; Achard-Thiers [syndrome]; achievement test; activity training; acute thrombosis; adaptive thermogenesis; adenine-thymine; adenine-thyronine; adipose tissue; adjunctive therapy; adnexal torsion; air temperature; allergy treatment; amino acid transporter; aminotransferase; aminotriazole; amitriptyline; anaerobic threshold; anaphylotoxin; angiotensin; anterior tibia; antithrombin; antitrypsin; antral transplantation; applanation tonometry; ataxia-telangiectasia; atmosphere; atraumatic; atresia, tricuspid; atrial tachycardia; atrial tumor; atropine; attenuate, attenuation; autoimmune thrombocytopenia; axonal terminal; old tuberculin [Gr. *alt Tuberkulin*]

A-T ataxia-telangiectasia

AT$_1$ angiotensin II type 1

AT$_{10}$ dihydrotachysterol

AT I angiotensin I

AT II angiotensin II

AT III angiotensin III; antithrombin III

At acidity, total; angiotensin; antithrombin; astatine; atrium, atrial

A$_t$ amount in tissue

at air tight; atom, atomic; technical atmosphere

ATA alimentary toxic aleukia; American Telemedicine Association; American Thyroid Association; aminotriazole; antithymic activity; antithyroglobulin antibody; anti-Toxoplasma antibody; atmosphere absolute; aurintricarboxylic acid

ATACS Antithrombotic Therapy in Acute Coronary Syndromes [trial]

ATAI acute traumatic aortic injury

ATB Articulated Total Body [model]; at the time of the bomb [A-bomb in Japan]; atrial tachycardia with block

Atb antibiotic

ATBC Alpha-Tocopherol/Beta Carotene [cancer prevention study]

ATC activated thymus cell; alpha tocopherol; anaplastic thyroid carcinoma; Anatomical Therapeutic Chemical [classification]; around the clock; certified athletic trainer

ATCase aspartate transcarbamoylase

ATCC American Type Culture Collection

ATCL adult T-cell leukemia or lymphoma

ATCS anterior tibial compartment syndrome

ATD Alzheimer-type dementia; androstatrienedione; anthropomorphic test dummy; antithyroid drug; aqueous tear deficiency; asphyxiating thoracic dystrophy

ATDC Association of Thalidomide Damaged Children

ATDNet Advanced Technology Demonstration Network

ATDP Attitude Toward Disabled Persons [scale]

ATE acute toxic encephalopathy; acute toxicity end point; adipose tissue extract; autologous tumor extract

ATEE *N*-acetyl-1-tyrosyl-ethyl ester

ATEM analytic transmission electron microscopy

Aten atenolol

ATEST Atenolol and Streptokinase Trial

ATEV *Aphodius tasmaniae* entomopoxvirus

ATF activating transcription factor; anterior talofibular [ligament]; ascites tumor fluid

At fib atrial fibrillation

ATG adenine-thymidine-guanine; advanced technology group; antihuman thymocyte globulin; antithrombocyte globulin; antithymocyte globulin; antithyroglobulin

ATGAM antithymocyte gamma-globulin

AT/GC adenine-thymine/guanine-cytosine [ratio]

ATH acetyl-tyrosine hydrazide; alkylated thiohydantoin

ATh Associate in Therapy

Athsc atherosclerosis

AtHV ateline herpesvirus

ATI abdominal trauma index; attitude-treatment interaction

ATIAIS Anturane Transient Ischemic Attack Italian Study

ATIME Accupril Titration Interval Management Evaluation [trial]

ATL Achilles tendon lengthening; active template library; acute T-cell leukemia; adult T-cell leukemia; anterior tricuspid leaflet; antitension line; atypical lymphocyte

ATLA adult T-cell leukemia virus-associated antigen; alternatives to laboratory animals

ATLANTIC Angina Treatment, Lasers, and Normal Therapy in Comparison [trial]

ATLANTIS Alteplase Thrombolysis for Acute Noninterventional Therapy in Ischemic Stroke

ATLAS Adolescents Training and Learning to Avoid Steroids; Aspirin and Ticlid vs Anticoagulants for Stents [study]; Assessment of Treatment with Lisinopril and Survival [trial]

ATLAST Antiplatelet Therapy vs Lovenox Plus Antiplatelet Therapy for Patients with Increased Risk of Stent Thrombosis; Aspirin/Ticlopidine vs Low-Molecular-Weight Heparin/Aspirin/Ticlopidine Stent Trial

ATLL adult T-cell leukemia/lymphoma

ATLP anterior titanium thoracolumbar locking plate

ATLS acute tumor lysis syndrome; Advanced Tool for Learning Anatomical Structures; advanced trauma life support

ATLV adult T-cell leukemia virus

ATM abnormal tubular myelin; acute transverse myelopathy; adaptive template moderated; advanced trauma management; Arizona Asynchronous Transfer Mode [network]; asynchronous transfer mode; asynchronous transfer protocol; ataxia-telangiectasia-mutated [protein]; atmosphere; average time of maintenance

atm standard atmosphere

ATMA Amiodarone Trials Meta Analysis; antithyroid plasma membrane antibody

ATMI application transaction manager interface

atmos atmospheric

ATMTN asynchronous transfer mode teleradiology network

ATN acute tubular necrosis; Adolescent Trials Network; augmented transition network

ATNC atraumatic normocephalic

at no atomic number

ATNR asymmetric tonic neck reflex

A-to-D analog-to-digital

A$_{TOT}$ total anions

ATP addiction treatment program; adenosine triphosphate; ambient temperature and pressure; annual transmission potential; antitachycardia pacing; Arizona Telemedicine Program; autoimmune thrombocytopenic purpura

A-TP adsorbed test plasma

AT-P antitrypsin-Pittsburgh

AtP attending physician

ATPA 2-amino-3-(hydroxy-5-*tert*-butyl-isoxazol-4-yl) propanoic acid

AT-PAS aldehyde-thionine–periodic acid Schiff [test]

ATPase adenosine triphosphatase

ATPD dried at ambient temperature and pressure

ATP-2Na adenosine triphosphate disodium

ATPS ambient temperature and pressure, saturated

ATR Achilles tendon reflex; Achilles tendon rupture; acid-tolerance response; alpha-thalassemia-mental retardation [syndrome]; ataxia-telangiectasia and rad3-related [protein]; attenuated total reflectance; automatic term recognition; axial trunk rotation

atr atrophy

ATR1 alpha-thalassemia mental retardation [syndrome] type 1

ATR2 alpha-thalassemia mental retardation [syndrome] type 2

ATRA all-*trans*retinoic acid

ATRAMI Autonomic Tone and Reflexes After Myocardial Infarction [trial]

ATRAS Adrenal Test Retrieval and Analysis System

Atr fib atrial fibrillation

ATRX, ATR-X X-linked alpha-thalassemia mental retardation [syndrome]

ATS Achard-Thiers syndrome; acid test solution; alpha-D-tocopherol acid succinate; American Thoracic Society; American Trauma Society; American Trudeau Society; antirat thymocyte serum; antitetanus serum; antithymocyte serum; anxiety tension state; arteriosclerosis; autologous transfusion system

ATSDR Agency for Toxic Substances and Disease Registry

ATT arginine tolerance test; aspirin tolerance time

att attending

atten attenuated

ATTMH Australian Therapeutic Trial of Mild Hypertension

ATTRACT application of telemedicine taking rapid advantage of cable television

ATV Abelson virus transformed; *Ambystoma tigrinum stebbinsi* virus; antisense target validation; atazanavir; avian tumor virus

at vol atomic volume

at wt atomic weight

ATX associated expressions [UMLS]

ATx adult thymectomy

atyp atypical

ATZ acetazolamide; atypical transformation zone

AU allergenic unit; Alzheimer unit; Ångström unit; antitoxin unit; arbitrary unit; Australia antigen; azauridine; both ears [Lat. *aures unitas*; JCAHO unapproved abbreviation]; each ear [Lat. *auris uterque*; JCAHO unapproved abbreviation]

Au Australia [antigen]; authorization

AUA American Urological Association; asymptomatic urinary abnormalities

Au Ag Australia antigen

AUB abnormal uterine bleeding

AUC area under the curve

AUC$_{extra}$ extrapolated area under the curve

AuCPV *Aglais urticae* cypovirus

AUC$_{SS}$ steady-state area under the curve

AUD arthritis of unknown diagnosis

aud auditory

AUDEX automated urologic diagnostic expert [ultrasonographic imaging]

AUDIT alcohol use disorders identification test

AUDIT-C alcohol use disorders identification test-alcohol consumption questions

aud-vis audiovisual

AUG acute ulcerative gingivitis; adenosine-uracil-guanine

AUGH acute upper gastrointestinal hemorrhage

AuHAA Australia hepatitis-associated antigen

AUI Alcohol Use Inventory

AUL acute undifferentiated leukemia

AUMC area under the first moment curve

AUMC$_{extra}$ extrapolated area under the first moment curve

AUO amyloid of unknown origin

AuP Australian antigen protein

AUPHA Association of University Programs in Health Administration

AUR Association of University Radiologists

aur, auric auricle, auricular

AURAV Aura virus

AURT Association of University Radiologic Technicians

AUS acute urethral syndrome; artificial urinary sphincter

AuS Australia serum hepatitis

aus, ausc auscultation

AuSH Australia serum hepatitis

AUST Australian Urokinase Stroke Trial

AUT authentication

AutoCAD auto-computer assisted diagnosis [software]

Auto-PEEP self-controlled positive end-expiratory pressure

AUV anterior urethral valve

aux auxiliary

AV adeno-associated virus; adenovirus; Adriamycin and vincristine; air velocity; allergic vasculitis; anteroventral; anteversion; anticipatory vomiting; antivirin; aortic valve; arenavirus; arteriovenous; artificial ventilation; ascovirus; asparagus virus; assisted ventilation; atrioventricular; audiovisual; augmented vector; average; aviation medicine; avoirdupois

A-V arteriovenous; atrioventricular

A/V ampere/volt; arteriovenous

Av average; avoirdupois

aV abvolt

av air velocity; average; avulsion

AVA activity vector analysis; anthrax vaccine adsorbed; antiviral antibody; aortic valve annulus; aortic valve area; aortic valve atresia; Arracacha virus A; arteriovenous anastomosis

AvaCPV *Agraulis vanillae* cypovirus

AV/AF anteverted, anteflexed

AVAV Avalon virus

AVB Arracacha virus B; atrioventricular block

AVC aberrant ventricular conduction; Academy of Veterinary Cardiology; aortic valve closure; arteriovenous communication; Association of Vitamin Chemists; associative visual cortex; atrioventricular canal; automatic volume control

AVCN anteroventral cochlear nucleus

AVCO$_2$R arteriovenous carbon dioxide removal

AVCS atrioventricular conduction system

AVCx atrioventricular circumflex branch

AVD aortic valvular disease; apparent volume of distribution; Army Veterinary Department; atrioventricular dissociation

AvDNV *Agraulis vanillae* densovirus

AVDO$_2$ arteriovenous oxygen saturation difference

AVDO$_2$B arteriovenous oxygen saturation difference, basal

AVDP average diastolic pressure

avdp avoirdupois

AVE aortic valve echocardiogram

ave, aver average

AVED ataxia with vitamin E deficiency

AVERT Atorvastatin vs Revascularization Treatment [trial]

AVEU AIDS Vaccine Evaluation Unit

AVF antiviral factor; arteriovenous fistula

aVF automated volt foot

aV$_F$ unipolar limb lead on the left leg in electrocardiography

AVG ambulatory visit group; aortic valve gradient

avg average

AVH acute viral hepatitis

AVHD acquired valvular heart disease

AVHS acquired valvular heart syndrome

AVI air velocity index; Association of Veterinary Inspectors; atrioventricular interval; audio-video interleave

AviCPV *Arctia villica* cypovirus

AVID Amiodarone vs Implantable Defibrillators [trial]; Angiography vs Intravascular Ultrasound Directed Coronary Stent Placement [trial]; Antiarrhythmics vs Implantable Defibrillators [study]

AVIR aortic valve replacement

AVJ atrioventricular junction

AVJR atrioventricular junction rhythm

AVJRe atrioventricular junctional reentrant

AVL automatic vehicle locator

aVL automated volt left

aV$_K$ unipolar limb lead on the left arm in electrocardiography

AVLINE Audiovisuals Online [NLM database]

AVLJ absolute value of logarithm of Jacobian

AVM arteriovenous malformation; atrioventricular malformation; avermectin; aviation medicine

AVMA American Veterinary Medical Association

AVN acute vasomotor nephropathy; atrioventricular nodal [conduction]; atrioventricular node; avascular necrosis

AVNA atrioventricular node artery

AVND atrioventricular node dysfunction

AVNFH avascular necrosis of the femoral head

AVNFRP atrioventricular node functional refractory period

AVNR atrioventricular nodal reentry

AVNRT atrioventricular node reentry tachycardia

AVO aortic valve opening; aortic valve orifice; atrioventricular opening

AVO₂ arteriovenous oxygen ratio

AVOA amorphous vascular occluding agent

AVP abnormal vasopressin; actinomycin-vincristine-Platinol; ambulatory venous pressure; antiviral protein; aortoventriculoplasty; aqueous vasopressin; arginine-vasopressin; arteriovenous passage time

AVP-NPII arginine vasopressin-neurophysin II

AVPU alert, verbal, painful, unresponsive [neurologic test]

AVR accelerated ventricular rhythm; antiviral regulator; aortic valve replacement

aVR automated volt right

aV$_R$ unipolar limb lead on the right arm in electrocardiography

AVREO avian reovirus

AVRI acute viral respiratory infection

AVRP atrioventricular refractory period

AVRR antiviral repressor regulator

AVRT atrioventricular reciprocating tachycardia; atrioventricular reentrant tachycardia; atrioventricular reentry

AVS Advanced Visual Systems; aortic valve stenosis; application visualization system; arteriovenous shunt; auditory vocal sequencing

AVSD atrioventricular septal defect

AVSV aortic valve stroke volume

AVT Allen vision test; arginine vasotocin; Aviation Medicine Technician

AVV atrioventricular valve

AvV *Agraulis vanillae* virus

Av3V anteroventral third ventricle

AVVM angiographically visualized vascular malformation

AVY Arracacha virus Y

AVZ avascular zone

AW able to work; above waist; abrupt withdrawal; airways; alcohol withdrawal; alveolar wall; anterior wall; atomic warfare; atomic weight

A&W alive and well

aw airway; water activity

AWAR anterior wall of aortic root

AWBM alveolar wall basement membrane

AWBV Ahlum waterborne virus

AWD alive with disease

AWESOME Angina with Extremely Serious Operative Mortality Evaluation

AWFM adaptive Walsh function modeling

AWG American Wire Gauge

AWGN additive white gaussian noise [telemedicine]

AWHILES All-Wales Health Information and Library Extension Service

AWI anterior wall infarction

AWIGS advanced workplace for image-guided surgery

AWL active waiting list

AWM abnormal wall motion

AWMI anterior wall myocardial infarction

AWMN Acid Waters Monitoring Network [UK]

AWMV amplitude-weighted mean velocity

AWO airway obstruction

AWOL absent without official leave

AWP airway pressure; any willing provider; average of the wholesale prices; average wholesale price

AWR absolute weighted residual; airway restriction

AWRS anti-whole rabbit serum

AWRU active wrist rotation unit

AWS Alagille-Watson syndrome; alcohol withdrawal syndrome

AWTA aniridia-Wilms tumor association

awu atomic weight unit

ax axillary; axis, axial

AxCPV anti-xanthomista cypovirus

AXD axillary dissection

AXF advanced x-ray facility

AXG adult xanthogranuloma

AXL anexelekto [oncogene]; axillary lymphoscintigraphy

AXR abdominal x-ray [examination]

AXT alternating exotropia

AYA acute yellow atrophy

AYF antiyeast factor

AYP autolyzed yeast protein

AYV Anthriscus yellows virus

AZ Aschheim-Zondek [test]; 5-azacytidine; azathioprine

Az nitrogen [Fr. *azote*]

AZA azathioprine; azelaic acid

AzC azacytosine

AZEV *Acrobasis zelleri* entomopoxvirus

AZF azoospermia factor
AzG, azg azaguanine
AZGP zinc-alpha-2-glycoprotein
AZO [indicates presence of the group —N:N—]
AZOA azaorotic acid
AZQ diaziquone
AZR alizarin
AZT Aschheim-Zondek test; azidothymidine; 3′-azido-3′-deoxythymidine; zidovudine (azidothymidine)

AZTEC amplitude zone time epoch coding [in ECG]
AZTMP azidothymidine monophosphate
AZT-R azidothymidine-resistant
AZT-S azidothymidine-susceptible or sensitive
AZTTP azidothymidine trithiophosphate
AZT-TP 3′-azido-3′-deoxythymidine triphosphate
AZU azauracil; azurocidin
AzUr 6-azauridine

B

B bacillus; bands; barometric; base; basophil, basophilic; bath [Lat. *balneum*]; Baumé scale; behavior; bel; Benoist scale; benzoate; beta; biscuspid; black; blood, bloody; blue; body; boils at; Bolton point; bone marrow-derived [cell or lymphocyte]; born; boron; bound; bovine; break; bregma; bronchial, bronchus; brother; *Brucella*; bruit; buccal; Bucky [film in cassette in Potter-Bucky diaphragm]; Bucky factor; bursa cells; burst [pacemaker]; bypass; byte; colorectal tumor extending into adipose tissue [Dukes classification]; magnetic induction; minimal detectable blurring; supramentale [point]

B₀ constant magnetic field in nuclear magnetic resonance

B1 palpable one lobe prostatic tumor less than 1.5 cm [Jewett staging system]; tumor extending into muscularis propria [Astler-Coller classification]

B₁ induced field in nuclear magnetic resonance; radiofrequency magnetic field in nuclear magnetic resonance; thiamine

B2 palpable two-lobe prostatic tumor larger than 1.5 cm [Jewett staging system]; tumor extending into perirectal adipose tissue [Astler-Coller classification]

B₂ riboflavin

B₆ pyridoxine

B₇ biotin

B₈ adenosine phosphate

B₁₂ cyanocobalamin

b barn; base; boils at; born; brain; branched; [chromosome] break; supramentale [point]; twice [Lat. *bis*]

b sample regression coefficient [statistics]

b⁺ positron emission

b⁻ beta emission

β see *beta*

BA Bachelor of Arts; backache; bacterial agglutination; bactericidal activity; barbituric acid; basion; benz[*a*]anthracene; benzyladenine; best amplitude; beta adrenergic; betamethasone acetate; bilateral asymmetrical; bile acid; biliary atresia; biological activity; blocking antibody; blood agar; blood alcohol; bone age; boric acid; bovine albumin; brachial artery; breathing apparatus; bronchial asthma; buccoaxial; buffered acetone

Ba barium; barium enema; basion

ba basion

BAA benzoylarginine amide; branched amino acid

BAAP bone-anchored auricular prosthesis

BAATAF Boston Area Anticoagulation Trial for Atrial Fibrillation

BAAV bovine adeno-associated virus

BAB blood agar base

Bab Babinski's reflex; baboon

BabK baboon kidney

BABs born after the ban cases [see BSE]

BABV Babahoya virus

BAC baclofen; bacterial adherent colony; bacterial antigen complex; bacterial artificial chromosome; blood alcohol concentration; British Association of Chemists; bronchoalveolar carcinoma; bronchoalveolar cells; buccoaxiocervical

Bac, bac *Bacillus*

BACT bacterium [UMLS]; best available control technology

Bact, bact *Bacterium*; bacterium, bacteria

BACUS Balloon Angioplasty Compliance Ultrasound Study

BAD biological aerosol detection; biologically active dose; British Association of Dermatologists

BADE [Thoracic] Bioimpedance as an Adjunct to Dobutamine Echocardiography [study]

BADS black locks-albinism-deafness syndrome

BAdV bovine adenovirus

BAdV-A, B, C bovine adenovirus A, B and C

BAE bovine aortic endothelium; bronchial artery embolization

BaE barium enema

BAEC bovine aortic endothelial cell

BAEDP balloon aortic end-diastolic pressure

BAEE benzoylarginine ethyl ester

BaEn barium enema

BAEP brainstem auditory evoked potential

BAER brainstem auditory evoked response

BaEV baboon endogenous virus

BaFBr:Eu europium-activated barium fluorohalide

BAG buccoaxiogingival

BAGG buffered azide glucose glycerol

BAGV Bagaza virus

BAHA® bone-anchored hearing aid

BAHAMA Baragwanath Hypertension Ambulatory Blood Pressure Monitoring Multiarm

BA/HPCC biomedical application of high performance computing and communication

BAHS Boston Area Health Study; butoctamide hydrogen succinate

BAHV Bahig virus

BAI beta-aminoisobutyrate

BAIB beta-aminoisobutyric [acid]

BAIF bile acid independent flow

BAIT bacterial automated identification technique

BAKUV Baku virus

BAKV Bakel virus; Bakau virus

BAL bio-artificial liver; blood alcohol level; British anti-lewisite; bronchoalveolar lavage

bal balance; balsam

BALB binaural alternate loudness balance

BALF broncho-alveolar lavage fluid

bals balsam

BALT bronchus-associated lymphoid tissue

BAM Bacteriological Analytical Manual; basilar artery migraine; bilateral augmentation mammoplasty; brachial artery mean [pressure]

BaM barium meal

Bam benzamide

BAME benzoylarginine methyl ester

BaMMV barley mild mosaic virus

BaMV bamboo mosaic virus

BAN British Approved Name; British Association of Neurologists

BANS back, arms, neck, and scalp

BANTER Bayesian Network Tutoring and Explanation

BANV Banzi virus

BAO basal acid output; brachial artery output

BAO-MAO basal acid output to maximal acid output [ratio]

BAP bacterial alkaline phosphatase; Behavior Activity Profile; beta-amyloid peptide; blood-agar plate; bovine albumin in phosphate buffer; brachial artery pressure; brightness area product

BAPhysMed British Association of Physical Medicine

BAPI barley alkaline protease inhibitor

BAPN beta-aminoproprionitrile

BAPO British Association of Paediatric Otorhinolaryngologists

BAPP beta amyloid precursor protein

BAPS biomechanical ankle platform system; bovine albumin phosphate saline; British Association of Paediatric Surgeons; British Association of Plastic Surgeons

BAPT British Association of Physical Training

BAPTA 1,2-bis (aminophenoxy) ethane-N,N,N',N'-tetraacetic acid

BAPV bovine alimentary papillomavirus

BAQ brain-age quotient

BAR bariatrics; barometer, barometric; beta-adrenergic receptor

βAR beta adrenergic receptor

bar barometric

BARASTER Balloon Angioplasty vs Rotational Atherectomy for Stent Restenosis

Barb, barb barbiturate, barbituric

BARI Bypass Angioplasty Revascularization Investigation [trial]

BARK beta-adrenergic receptor kinase

BARN bilateral acute retinal necrosis; Body Awareness Resource Network

BAROCCO Balloon Angioplasty vs Rotacs for Total Chronic Coronary Occlusion [trial]

BARS behaviorally anchored rating scale

BART blood-activated recalcification time

BARV Barur virus

BarV barley virus

BarV-B1 barley virus B1

BAS balloon atrial septostomy; battalion aid station; benzyl anti-serotonin; beta-adrenergic stimulation; boric acid solution; Bronx Longitudinal Aging Study

BaS barium swallow

bas basilar; basophil, basophilic

BASA Boston Assessment of Severe Aphasia

BASC Blood Pressure in Acute Stroke Collaboration

BASE B27-arthritis-sacroiliitis-extra-articular features [syndrome]

BASH body acceleration synchronous with heart rate

BASIC Beginner's All-Purpose Symbolic Introduction Code

BASIS Basel Antiarrhythmic Study of Infarct Survival

baso basophil

BASOC boundary at the scale of the core [imaging]

BAstV bovine astrovirus

BaSV Bajra streak virus

BAT basic aid training; best available technology; blunt abdominal trauma; bright acuity test; brown adipose tissue

BATV Batai virus

BAUP Bovie-assisted uvulopalatoplasty

BAUS British Association of Urological Surgeons

BAUV Bauline virus

BAV banana virus; bicuspid aortic valve; Bivens arm virus

BaV Barramundi virus

BAV-CH banana virus-China

BAVCP bilateral abductor vocal cord paralysis

BAVFO bradycardia after arteriovenous fistula occlusion

BAW bronchoalveolar washing

BaYMV barley yellow mosaic virus

BAYV bayou virus

BB bad breath; bed bath; beta blockade, beta blocker; biceps brachii; BioBreeding [rat]; blanket bath; blood bank; blood buffer; blow bottle; blue bloaters [emphysema]; bombesin; borderline; Bortfeld/Boyer [radiotherapy]; both bones; breakthrough bleeding; breast biopsy; bronchial blocker [tube]; brush border; buffer base; bundle branch; isoenzyme of creatine kinase containing two B subunits

B&B branch and bound [algorithm]

bb Bolton point; both bones

BBA born before arrival

BBB blood-brain barrier; blood buffer base; bundle-branch block

BBBB bilateral bundle-branch block

BBBD blood brain barrier disruption

BBC bromobenzycyanide; buccal bifurcation cyst

BbCPV *Biston betularia* cypovirus

BBD benign breast disease

BB3DI broad beam 3-dimensional irradiation

BBE *Bacteroides* bile esculin [agar]

BBEP biotechnology, biologics, and environmental protection; brush border endopeptidase

BBF bronchial blood flow

BBI Biomedical Business International; Bowman-Birk soybean inhibitor

BBM banked breast milk; brush border membrane

BBMV broad bean mottle virus; brush border membrane vesicle

BBN broad band noise

BBNV broad bean necrosis virus

BBOT 2,5-bis(5-t-butylbenzoxalol-2-yl)-thiophene

BBOV Bimbo virus

BBPP Beta-Blocker Pooling Project

BBR bibasilar rate; bundle branch reentry

BBRS Burks' Behavior Rating Scale

BBR-VT bundle branch reentry-ventricular tachycardia

BBs both bones

BBS Barolet-Biedl syndrome; bashful bladder syndrome; benign breast syndrome; bilateral breath sounds; bombesin; borate-buffered saline; brown bowel syndrome; bulletin board software

BBScV blueberry scorch virus

BBSV broad bean stain virus

BBT basal body temperature

BBTD baby bottle tooth decay

BBTMV broad bean true mosaic virus

BBTV banana bunchy top virus

BBV Berkeley bee virus; black beetle virus; Bukalasa bat virus

BB/W BioBreeding/Worcester [rat]

BBWV broad bean wilt virus

BC Bachelor of Surgery [Lat. *Baccalaureus Chirurgiae*]; back care; bactericidal concentration; basal cell; basket cell; battle casualty; bicarbonate; biliary colic; bipolar cell; birth control; blastic crisis; blood count; blood culture; Blue Cross [plan]; board certified; bone conduction; brachiocephalic; brain contour; breast cancer; bronchial carcinoma; buccal cartilage; buccocervical; buffy coat

B&C biopsy and curettage

Bc *Bacillus cereus*

b/c benefit/cost [ratio]

BCA balloon catheter angioplasty; bell clapper anomaly; bicinchoninic acid; blood color analyzer; Blue Cross Association; branchial cleft anomaly; Breast

Cancer Action; breast cancer antigen; bromochloroacetic acid

BCAA branched chain amino acid

bCaCC bovine calcium-sensitive chloride channel

BCAEC bovine coronary artery endothelial cell

BCaMV bean calico mosaic virus

BCAPS Beta-Blocker Cholesterol-Lowering Asymptomatic Plaque Study

BCAT brachiocephalic arterial trunk

BCB blood-cerebrospinal fluid barrier; brilliant cresyl blue

BCBR bilateral carotid body resection

BC/BS Blue Cross/Blue Shield [plan]

BCBSA Blue Cross and Blue Shield Association

BCC basal-cell carcinoma; bedside communication controller; biliary cholesterol concentration; birth control clinic; business card computer

bcc body-centered-cubic

BC-CFC blast cell colony-forming cell

BCCG British Cooperative Clinical Group

BCCP biotin carboxyl carrier protein

BCCV Black Creek Canal virus

BCD binary-coded decimal; bleomycin, cyclophosphamide, dactinomycin

BCDDP Breast Cancer Detection Demonstration Project

BCDF B-cell differentiation factor

BCDL Brachmann-Cornelia de Lange [syndrome]

BCDRS Brief Carroll Depression Rating Scale

BCDS Bulimia Cognitive Distortions Scale

BCDSP Boston Collaborative Drug Surveillance Program

BCE basal cell epithelioma; benign childhood epilepsy; bubble chamber equipment

BCECT benign childhood epilepsy with centrotemporal [spikes]

BCEI breast cancer estrogen-inducible

BCEOP benign partial epilepsy with occipital paroxysms

BCF basic conditioning factor; basophil chemotactic factor; bioconcentration factor; breast cyst fluid

BCFP breast cyst fluid protein

BCG bacille Calmette-Guérin [vaccine]; ballistocardiography, ballistocardiogram; bicolor guaiac test; bromcresol green

BCGF B-cell growth factor

BCGM bi-conjugate gradient method

BCH basal cell hyperplasia

BCh Bachelor of Surgery [Lat. *Baccalaureus Chirurgiae*]

BChD Bachelor of Dental Surgery

BCHE butyrylcholinesterase

BChir Bachelor of Surgery [Lat. *Baccalaureus Chirurgiae*]

Bchl, bChl bacterial chlorophyll

BCHS Bureau of Community Health Services

BCI behavioral cues index; brain-computer interface

BCIA Biomedical Clinical Instrumentation Association

BCIP 5-bromo-4-chloro-3-inodolyl phosphate

BCIRG Breast Cancer International Research Group

BCIS British Cardiovascular Intervention Society

BCKA branched-chain keto acid

BCKD branched-chain alpha-keto acid dehydrogenase

BCL basic cycle length; B-cell leukemia/lymphoma

BCLD B-cell lymphoproliferative disease

BCLL B-cell chronic lymphocytic leukemia

BCLM below critical length material

BCLP bilateral cleft of lip and palate

BCLS basic cardiac life support

BCM B-cell maturation; beclomethasone; birth control medication; blood-clotting mechanism; body cell mass; body control and movement

BCME bis-chloromethyl ether

BCMF B-cell maturation factor

BCMNV bean common mosaic necrosis virus

BCMS Bioethic Citation Maintenance System

BCN basal cell nevus; bilateral cortical necrosis; breast care nursing

BCNS basal cell nevus syndrome

BCNU 1,3-bis-(2-chloroethyl)-1-nitrosourea

BCO biliary cholesterol output

BCOC bowel care of choice

BCoV bovine coronavirus

BCP basic calcium phosphate; birth control pill; blue cone pigment; Blue Cross Plan; bromcresol purple

BCPD bromcresol purple deoxylate

BCPR bystander cardiopulmonary resuscitation

BCPT Breast Cancer Prevention Trial

BCPV bovine cutaneous papillomavirus

BCQ breast cancer questionnaire

BCR B-cell reactivity; birth control regimen; breakpoint cluster region; bromocriptine; bulbocavernosus reflex

bcr breakpoint cluster region

BCRS brief cognitive rating scale

BCRx birth control drug

BCS battered child syndrome; blood cell separator; bovine calf serum; breast cancer screening; British Cardiac Society; Budd-Chiari syndrome

BCSFB blood-cerebrospinal fluid barrier

BCSI breast cancer screening indicator

BCSP Bavarian Cholesterol Screening Project

BCT brachiocephalic trunk; branched-chain amino acid transferase; breast conservation therapy

BCTF Breast Cancer Task Force

BCtg bovine chymotrypsinogen

BCtr bovine chymotrypsin

BCTV beet curly top virus

BCV Batu Cave virus; beet cryptic virus; between class variance; blue crab virus; Bunyip Creek virus

BCVA best corrected visual acuity

BCVd blister canker viroid

BCW biological and chemical warfare

BCYE buffered charcoal-yeast extract [agar]

BD barbital-dependent; barbiturate dependence; base deficit; base of prism down; basophilic degeneration; Batten disease; behavioral disorder; Behçet disease; belladonna; below diaphragm; Bessel distribution; bicarbonate dialysis; bile duct; binding domain; binocular deprivation; birth date; black death; bladder drainage; block design [test]; blood donor; blue diaper [syndrome]; borderline dull; bound; brain damage; brain dead, brain death; Briquet disorder; bronchodilation, bronchodilator; buccodistal; Byler disease

B-D Becton-Dickinson

Bd board; buoyant density

bd band; bundle

BDA balloon dilation angioplasty; British Dental Association

BDAC Bureau of Drug Abuse Control

BDAE Boston Diagnostic Aphasia Examination

BDAV Bandia virus

BDC Bazex-Dupré-Christol [syndrome]; burn-dressing change

BDE balanced differential expression [microarray analysis]; bile duct examination

BDentSci Bachelor of Dental Science

BDG buccal developmental groove; buffered desoxycholate glucose

BDGF brain-derived growth factor

BDHI Buss-Durkee Hostility Inventory

BDI Beck Depression Inventory

BDIP biomedical digital image processing

BDIS Becton-Dickinson immunocytometry system; Birth Defects Information Service

BDL behaviors of daily living; below detectable limits; bile duct ligation

BDLS Brachmann-de Lange syndrome

BDM Becker's muscular dystrophy; border detection method; 2,3-butanedione 2-monoxime

BDMS Bureau of Data Management Strategy [Health Care Financing Administration (HCFA)]

BDMV bean dwarf mosaic virus

bDNA branched deoxyribonucleic acid [DNA]

BDNF brain-derived neurotrophic factor

BDO battle dress overgarment

BDOH broad determinants of health

BDP beclomethasone dipropionate; benzodiazepine; bilateral diaphragmatic paralysis; Biological Department, Porton [UK]; bronchopulmonary dysplasia

BDQ bowel disease questionnaire

BDR background diabetic retinopathy

BDRP Biological Defense Research Program

BDRS Blessed Dementia Rating Scale

BDS Bachelor of Dental Surgery; biological detection system; Blessed Dementia Scale

BdS blood pressure-depressing substance

BDSc Bachelor of Dental Science

BDT binary distance transformation [imaging]

BDUR bromodeoxyuridine

BDV border disease virus; Borna disease virus; bushy dwarf virus

BDW biphasic defibrillation waveform; buffered distilled water

BE bacillary emulsion; bacterial endocarditis; barium enema; Barrett's esophagus; base excess; below-elbow; bile-esculin [test]; bioequivalence; biological effect; biologically effective; biologically equivalent; bovine enteritis; brain edema; bread equivalent; breast examination; bronchiectasis; bronchoesophagology

B/E below-elbow

B&E brisk and equal

Be beryllium

Bé Baumé scale

BEA below-elbow amputation; bioelectrical activity; bromoethylamine

BEAM brain electrical activity monitoring

BEAP bronchiectasis, eosinophilia, asthma, pneumonia

BEAR biological effects of atomic radiation

BEB Biomedical Engineering Branch [of US Army]

BEBV Bebaru virus

BEC bacterial endocarditis; behavioral emergency committee; biliary epithelial cells; blood ethyl alcohol content; bromoergocryptine; buccal epithelial cells

BECAIT Bezafibrate Coronary Atherosclerosis Intervention Trial

BECF blood extracellular fluid

BED binge eating disorder; biologically effective dose; biologically equivalent dose [radiation]

BEE basal energy expenditure

BEFV bovine ephemeral fever virus

beg begin, beginning

BEH benign exertional headache

beh behavior, behavioral

BEHA behavior [UMLS]

BEI back-scattered electron imaging; biological exposure indexes; butanol-extractable iodine

BEIR biological effects of ionizing radiation

BEK bovine embryonic kidney [cells]

BEL blood ethanol level; bovine embryonic lung

BELIR beta-endorphin-like immunoreactivity

BELTV Belterra virus

BELV Belmont virus; Bermuda grass etched line virus

BEM boundary element method

BEMS Bioelectromagnetics Society

BeMV belladonna mottle virus

BEN Balkan endemic neuropathy

bENaC bovine epithelial sodium channel

BENAR blood eosinophilic non-allergic rhinitis

BENEDICT Bergamo Nephrologic Diabetes Complications Trial

BENESTENT Belgian-Netherlands Stent [study]

BENV Benevides virus; Benfica virus

Benz, benz benzene; benzidine; benzoate

BEP basic element of performance; brain evoked potential

B-EP β-endorphin

BEPS Belgian Eminase Prehospital Study

BEPT biliary endoscopic papillotomy

BER base encoding rule; base excision repair; basic electrical rhythm

BERA brainstem evoked response audiometry

BERG balloon-assisted endoscopic retroperitoneal gasless [approach]

BERNWARD building essential concept representations in well-arranged restricted domains

BERT Beneficiary Enrollment Retrieval System [Medicare]; Beta Energy Restenosis Trial

BERV Bertioga virus

BES balanced electrolyte solution; Baltimore Eye Study

BESA brain electric source analysis

BESC bronchitis emphysema symptom checklist

BESM bovine embryonic skeletal muscle

BESMART Bestent in Small Arteries Study

BESP bovine embryonic spleen [cells]

BESS Berlin Pacemaker Study on Syncope; Part B Extract and Summary System [Medicare]

BESSAMI Berlin Stent Study in Acute Myocardial Infarction

BEST Beta-blocker Evaluation of Survival Trial; Beta-blocker Stroke Trial; Beta-Cath System Trial; Bolus Dose Escalation Study of Tissue-Type Plasminogen Activator; Bucindolol Evaluation of Survival Trial; Medtronic Bestent Coronary Stent vs Palmaz-Schatz Coronary Stent

BET benign epithelial tumor; Brunauer-Emmet-Teller [method]
BETA Biomedical Electronics Technicians Association
β [Greek letter *beta*] an anomer of a carbohydrate; buffer capacity; carbon separated from a carboxyl by one other carbon in aliphatic compounds; a constituent of a plasma protein fraction; probability of Type II error; a substituent group of a steroid that projects above the plane of the ring
1−*β* power of statistical test
β **error** Type II error
*β*₂**m** beta₂-microglobulin
BEV baboon endogenous virus; beam's eye view; Berne virus; bleeding esophageal varix; bovine enterovirus
BeV, Bev billion electron volts
bev beverage
BeYDV bean yellow dwarf virus
BF Barmah Forest [virus]; bentonite flocculation; bile flow; biofeedback; black female; blastogenic factor; blister fluid; blood flow; body fat; bouillon filtrate [tuberculin Fr. *bouillon filtré*]; brain factor; breakfast fed; breast feeding; buffered; burning feet [syndrome]; butter fat
B/F black female; bound/free [antigen ratio]
B3F band 3 cytoplasmic fragment
bf black female; bouillon filtrate [tuberculin]
BFA bifemoral angiography; brefeldin A
BFB biological feedback; bronchial foreign body
BFC benign febrile convulsion
BFDI bronchodilation following deep inspiration
BFDV beak and feather disease virus
BFE blood flow energy; bulk fluid endocytosis
BFEC benign focal epilepsy of childhood
bFGF basic fibroblast growth factor
BFGS Broyden-Fletcher-Goldfarb-Shanno [algorithm]
BFH benign familial hematuria
BFHD Beukes familial hip dysplasia
BFHI Baby-Friendly Hospital Initiative [UNICEF]
BFHR basal fetal heart rate
BFIC benign familial infantile convulsions

BFIRM binary formal inference-based recessive modeling
BFL bird fancier's lung; Börjeson-Forssman-Lehman [syndrome]
BFLS Börjeson-Forssman-Lehmann syndrome
BFM benign familial megalocephaly or macrocephaly
BFNC benign familial neonatal convulsions
BFO balanced forearm orthosis; ball-bearing forearm orthosis; blood-forming organ
BFOD binary frames of discernment
BFP biologic false-positive
BFPR biologic false-positive reaction
BFPSTS biologic false-positive serological test for syphilis
BFR biologic false reaction; blood flow rate; bone formation rate; buffered Ringer [solution]
BFS blood fasting sugar
BFT bentonite flocculation test; biofeedback training
BFU burst-forming unit
BFU-E burst-forming unit, erythrocytes
BFU-ME burst-forming unit, myeloid/erythroid
BFU-Meg burst-forming unit, megakaryocyte
BFV Barmah Forest virus; bovine feces virus; bovine foamy virus
BG *Bacillus globigii*; basal ganglion; basic gastrin; basophilic granulocyte; Bender Gestalt [test]; beta-galactosidase; beta-glucuronidase; bicolor guaiac [test]; Birbeck granule; blood glucose; bone graft; brilliant green; buccogingival
B-G Bordet-Gengou [agar, bacillus, phenomenon]
BGA blue-green algae
BGAg blood group antigen
BGAV blue-green algae virus
BGC basal ganglion calcification; blood group class
BGCA bronchogenic carcinoma
BGD blood group degradation
BGE butyl glycidyl ether
BGG bovine gamma-globulin
bGH bovine growth hormone
BGIV Bangui virus
Bg^J beige [mouse]
BGLB brilliant green lactose broth

BGlu blood glucose

BGM bedside glucose monitoring

BGMR basal ganglion disorder-mental retardation [syndrome]

BGMV bean golden mosaic virus

BGNV Bangoran virus

BGO bismuth germanium oxide

BGP beta-glycerophosphatase

BGPS Belgian General Practitioners' Study

BGS balance, gait, and station; Baller-Gerold syndrome; blood group substance; British Geriatrics Society

BGSA blood granulocyte-specific activity

BGTT borderline glucose tolerance test

BGV Bahia Grande virus

BH base hospital; benzalkonium and heparin; bill of health; birth history; Bishop-Harman [instruments]; boarding home; board of health; Bolton-Hunter [reagent]; borderline hypertensive; both hands; brain hormone; Braxton-Hicks [contractions], breathholding; bronchial hyperreactivity; Bryan high titer; bundle of His

BH4 tetrahydrobiopterin

BHA bound hepatitis antibody; butylated hydroxyanisole

BHAT Beta Blocker Heart Attack Trial

BHAV Bhanja virus

BHB beta-hydroxybutyrate

bHb bovine hemoglobin

BHBA beta-hydroxybutyric acid

BHC benzene hexachloride

BHCDA Bureau of Health Care Delivery and Assistance

β-hCG beta human chorionic gonadotropin

BHF Bolivian hemorrhagic fever; British Heart Foundation

BHFS Benzapril Heart Failure Study

BHI biosynthetic human insulin; brain-heart infusion [broth]; British Humanities Index; Bureau of Health Insurance

BHIA brain-heart infusion agar

BHIBA brain-heart infusion blood agar

BHIRS brain-heart infusion and rabbit serum

BHIS beef heart infusion supplemented [broth]

BHK baby hamster kidney [cells]; type-B Hong Kong [influenza virus]

BHL bilateral hilar lymphadenopathy; biological half-life

bHLH basic helix-loop-helix

bHLH-ZIP basic helix-loop-helix-leucine zipper

BHM Bureau of Health Manpower

BHN bephenium hydroxynaphthoate; Brinell hardness number

BHP basic health profile

BHPr Bureau of Health Professions

BHR basal heart rate; benign hypertrophic prostatitis; borderline hypertensive rat; bronchial hyperreactivity

BHS Bachelor of Health Science; Ballarat Health Services [Australia]; Beck Hopelessness Scale; beta-hemolytic streptococcus; Bogalusa Heart Study; breathholding spell; Brisighella Heart Study

BHT beta-hydroxytheophylline; breath hydrogen test; bronchial hygiene therapy; butylated hydroxytoluene

BHTE bioheat transfer equation

BHU basic health unit

Bhu *Bordetella* heme utilization

BhuR *Bordetella* heme utilization receptor

BHV bovine herpes virus

BH/VH body hematocrit-venous hematocrit [ratio]

BHyg Bachelor of Hygiene

BI background interval; bacterial or bactericidal index; base-in [prism]; basilar impression; bifunctional inducer; Billroth I [operation]; biological indicator; biotechnology infomatics; bodily injury; bone injury; bowel impaction; brain injury; burn index

Bi bismuth

BIA biolectric impedance analysis; bioimmunoassay; biomechanical impedance analyses

BIAC Bioinstrumentation Advisory Council

BIAD blind insertion airway device

BIB bibliography; biliointestinal bypass; brought in by

bib, biblio bibliography

BIBRA British Industrial Biological Research Association

B-IBS B-immunoblastic sarcoma

BIC Bayes information criterion; bicoherence; blood isotope clearance; brain imaging center

Bic biceps

BICAO bilateral internal carotid artery occlusion

bicarb bicarbonate
BiCAT bilateral carotid artery traction
BICC Biomedical Information Communications Center
BiCNU 1,3-bis-(2-chloroethyl)-1-nitrosourea [carmustine]
BICS Brigham Integrated Computing System
BICS-OE Brigham Integrated Computing System-order entry
BICST biceps skin tone
BID bibliographic information and documentation; brought in dead
BIDA butyl iminodiacetic acid
BIDLB block in posteroinferior division of left branch
BIDS biological integrated detection system; brittle hair, intellectual impairment, decreased fertility, and short stature [syndrome]
BIE Bayes inference engine; bullous ichthyosiform erythroderma
BIG bone injection gun
BIG 6 analysis of 6 serum components
BIGGY bismuth glycine glucose yeast
BIGMAC Beaumont Interventional Group-Mevacor, ACE Inhibitor, Colchicine Restenosis [trial]; Bidirectional Gantry Multiarray Coil [study]
BIGPRO Biguanides and the Prevention of the Risk of Obesity [study]
BIH benign intracranial hypertension; Beth Israel Hospital
BII beat inclusion index; Billroth II [operation]; butanol-insoluble iodine
BIL basal insulin level; bilirubin
Bil bilirubin
bil bilateral
BILAG British Isles Lupus Assessment Group [Index]
BIL/ALB bilirubin/albumin [rate]
bilat bilateral
bili bilirubin
bili-c conjugated bilirubin
bilirub bilirubin
bili T&D bilirubin total and direct
BIM buffered isolation medium
BIMA bilateral internal mammary artery
BIMV Bimiti virus
BIN butylisonitrile
Bin binary
biochem biochemistry, biochemical
BIOD bony intraorbital distance

bioeng bioengineering
BIOETHICSLINE Bioethical Information Online
BIOF biologic function [UMLS]
biol biology, biological
bioLH bioassay of luteinizing hormone
BIOMACS Biochemical Markers of Acute Coronary Syndromes
biophys biophysics, biophysical
BIOSIS BioScience Information Service
biotyping biochemical typing
BIP bacterial intravenous protein; Bezafibrate Infarction Prevention [study]; biparietal; bismuth iodoform paraffin; Blue Cross interim payment; brief infertility period
Bip binding protein
BIPAP biphasic positive airway pressure
BIPLED bilateral, independent, periodic, lateralized epileptiform discharge
BIPM International Bureau of Weights and Measures [Fr. *Bureau International des Poids et Mesures*]
BIPP bismuth iodoform paraffin paste
BIR basic incidence rate; British Institute of Radiology
BIRADS Breast Imaging Reporting and Data System
BIRD Bolus vs Infusion Rescupase Development
BIRLS Beneficiary Identification and Record Locator Subsystem [Veterans Benefit Administration]
BIRN Biomedical Informatics Research Network
BIRNH Belgian Interuniversity Research on Nutrition and Health [study]
BIRV Birao virus
BIS bioimpedance spectroscopy; bispectral index; bone cement implantation syndrome; Brain Information Service; British Infection Society; building illness syndrome
BIScV blueberry scorch virus
B-ISDN broadband-integrated services digital network
BIShV blueberry shock virus
BiSP between ischial spines
bisp bispinous [diameter]
BISTI Biomedical Information Service Technology Initiative
BIT binary digit; bitrochanteric
bit binary digit

BITE Bulimic Investigatory Test

BITNET Because It's Time Network [mail-only electronic network]

BIU barrier isolation unit; billion international units

BIV Bohle iridovirus; bovine immunodeficiency virus

BIVAS Body Image Visual Analogue Scale

BJ Bence Jones [protein, proteinuria]; biceps jerk; Bielschowsky-Jansky [syndrome]; bones and joints

B&J bones and joints

BJE bones, joints, and examination

BJM bones, joints, and muscles

BJP Bence Jones protein or proteinuria

BK below the knee; bovine kidney [cells]; bradykinin

B-K initials of two patients after whom a multiple cutaneous nevus [mole] was named

B/K below knee [amputation]

Bk berkelium

bk back

BKA below-knee amputation

BK-A basophil kallikrein of anaphylaxis

BK amp below-knee amputation

BKAT Basic Knowledge Assessment Tool for Critical Care

BKD bacterial kidney disease

bkf breakfast

BKG, Bkg background

BKPyV BK polyomavirus

BKS beekeeper serum

BKTT below knee to toe

BKWP below knee walking plaster

BL Barré-Lieou [syndrome]; basal lamina; baseline; Bessey-Lowry [unit]; biosafety level; black light; bladder; bleeding; blind loop; blood loss; bone marrow lymphocyte; borderline lepromatous; bronchial lavage; buccolingual; buffered lidocaine; Bullard laryngoscope; Burkitt lymphoma

Bl black

B-l bursa-equivalent lymphocyte

bl black; blood, bleeding; blue

BLA Biologics License Application

BLAD borderline left axis deviation

blad bladder

BLAS Bronx Longitudinal Aging Study

BLASP Barbados Low-Dose Aspirin Study in Pregnancy

BLAST basic linear alignment and search tool [algorithm]

BLAT Blind Learning Aptitude Test

BLAV Bobia virus

BLB Baker-Lima-Baker [mask]; Bessey-Lowry-Brock [method or unit]; black light bulb; Boothby-Lovelace-Bulbulian [oxygen mask]; bronchoscopic lung biopsy; bulb [syringe]

BL = BS bilateral equal breath sounds

BlC blood culture

BLCL Burkitt lymphoma cell line

B-LCL B-lymphocyte cell line

bl cult blood culture

BLCV beet leaf curly top virus

BLD basal liquefactive degeneration; benign lymphoepithelial disease

bld blood

Bld Bnk blood bank

BLE both lower extremities; buffered lidocaine with epinephrine

BLEL benign lympho-epithelial lesion

BLEO bleomycin

bleph blepharitis

BLEVE boiling liquid expanding vapor explosion

BLFD buccolinguofacial dyskinesia

BLG behavioral leadership group; beta-lactoglobulin

bLH biologically active luteinizing hormone

BLI bombesin-like immunoreactivity

blk black

BLL below lower limit

BLLD British Library Lending Division

BLLV Bloodland Lake virus

BLM basolateral membrane; bilayer lipid membrane; bimolecular liquid membrane; black lipid membrane; bleomycin; Bloom syndrome; buccolinguomasticatory

BLMoV blueberry leaf mottle virus

BLMV Belem virus

BLN bronchial lymph node

BLOB binary large object

BLOBS bladder obstruction

BLOC body location [UMLS]

BLOSUM block substitution matrix [searching algorithm]

BLOT Bimodality Lung Oncology Trial; British Library of Tape

BLP beta-lipoprotein

BlP blood pressure

B-LPH beta-lipoprotein hormone

B-LPN beta-lipotropin

bl pr blood pressure

BLQ both lower quadrants

BLRC Biomedical Library Review Committee

BLROA British Laryngological, Rhinological, and Otological Association

BLRV, blrv bean leafroll virus

BLS bare lymphocyte syndrome; basic life support; B-cell lymphoproliferative syndrome; blind loop syndrome; blood and lymphatic system; blood sugar; Bloom syndrome; Bureau of Labor Statistics

BlS blood sugar

BLSA Baltimore Longitudinal Study of Aging; basic life support ambulance

BLSD bovine lumpy skin disease

BLS-D basic life support-defibrillation; Blessed Scale-Dementia

BLT bleeding time; blood-clot lysis time; blood test

BlT bleeding time; blood test; blood type, blood typing

BLU Bessey-Lowry unit

BluMVd-RNA Blueberry mosaic viroid-like ribonucleic acid

BLV biological limit value; blood volume; bovine leukemia virus

BlV blood viscosity; blood volume

BLVd bent leaf viroid

BLVR biliverdin reductase

Blx bleeding time

BM Bachelor of Medicine; barium meal; basal medium; basal metabolism; basement membrane; basilar membrane; betamethasone; biomedical; black male; blood monitoring; body mass; Bohr magneton; bone marrow; bowel movement; breast milk; buccal mass; buccomesial

B/M black male

B2M beta-2-microglobulin

bm black male

BMA biological movement artifacts; bone marrow arrest; bone mineral area; British Medical Association

BmA *Brugia malayi* adult antigen

BMAD Medicare Part B Annual Data [file]

BMAP bone marrow acid phosphatase

B-MAST Short Michigan Alcoholism Screening Test

BMAV Batama virus

B_{max} maximum amount bound; maximum binding capacity

BMB biomedical belt; bone marrow biopsy

BMBL benign monoclonal B cell lymphocytosis

BMBMA bulk motion biological movement artifacts

BMC blood mononuclear cell; bone marrow cell; bone mineral content

BMCC beta-methylcrotonyl coenzyme A carboxylase

BMCHRD Bureau of Maternal and Child Health and Resources Development

BMD Becker muscular dystrophy; Boehringer Mannheim Diagnostics; bone marrow depression; bone mineral density; bovine mucosal disease

BMDC Biomedical Documentation Center; bone marrow dendritic cell

BMDP biomedical [computer] program

BMDSC bone marrow-derived stem cell

BMDW Bone Marrow Donor Worldwide

BME basal medium Eagle; biundulant meningoencephalitis; brief maximal effort

BMed Bachelor of Medicine

BMedBiol Bachelor of Medical Biology

BMedSci Bachelor of Medical Science

BMEI benign myoclonic epilepsy in childhood

BMES Biomedical Engineering Society

BMET biomedical equipment technician

BMF bone marrow failure

BMG benign monoclonal gammopathy

BMH biomechanical heart

BMI body mass index; brief motivational intervention

BMic Bachelor of Microbiology

BMIPP beta-methyliodophenylpentadecanoic acid

BMJ bones, muscles, joints

bmk birthmark

BML biomedical library; bone marrow lymphocytosis

BMLS billowing mitral leaflet syndrome

BMM bone marrow-derived macrophages

BMMP benign mucous membrane pemphigoid

BMMS [electronic] Better Medical Management System [Australia]; Better Medication Management System [Australia]

BMMV bean mild mosaic virus

BMN bone marrow necrosis

BMNC blood mononuclear cell

BMOC Brinster's medium for ovum culture

Bmod behavior modification

B-mode brightness modulation

BMP bitmap; bone morphogenetic protein

bmp bone morphogenetic protein

BMPI bronchial mucous proteinase inhibitor

BMPP benign mucous membrane pemphigus; beta-methyliodophenylpentadecanoic acid

BMQA Board of Medical Quality Assurance

BMR basal metabolic rate

BMRC British Medical Research Council

BMS Bachelor of Medical Science; Belfast Metoprolol Study; betamethasone; biomedical monitoring system; biomedical science; bleomycin sulfate; broadcast message server; Bureau of Medical Services; Bureau of Medicine and Surgery; burning mouth syndrome

BMSA British Medical Students Association

BMSP biomedical sciences program

BMST Bruce maximum stress test

BMT Bachelor of Medical Technology; basement membrane thickening; benign mesenchymal tumor; bone marrow transplant; bone marrow transplantation

BMT-GVHD bone marrow transplantation-graft versus host disease

BMTU bone marrow transplantation unit

BMU basic metabolic unit; basic multicellular unit

BMYV beet mild yellowing virus

BMZ basement membrane zone

BN Bayesian network; binucleated; bladder neck; branchial neuritis; bronchial node; brown Norway [rat]; bulimia nervosa

BNA Basle Nomina Anatomica; bronchoscopic needle aspiration

BNAML Brown Norway acute myelocytic leukemia

BNC brain sodium channel

BNCT boron neutron capture therapy

BND barely noticeable difference

BNDD Bureau of Narcotics and Dangerous Drugs

BNEd Bachelor of Nursing Education

BNF British National Formulary

BNG Bayesian Network Generation [system]

BNIST National Bureau of Scientific Information [Fr. *Bureau National d'Information Scientifique*]

Bnl branchless

BNML brown Norway rat myelocytic leukemia

BNO bladder neck obstruction; bowels not opened

bNOS brain nitric oxide synthase

BNP brain natriuretic peptide

BNPA binasal pharyngeal airway

BNR beam nonuniformity ratio [ultrasound]

BN/RN baccalaurate registered nurse

BNS Belfast Nifedipine Study; benign nephrosclerosis

BNSc Bachelor of Nursing Science

BNT Boston Naming Test; brain neurotransmitter

BNYV broccoli necrotic yellow virus

BNYVV beet necrotic yellow vein virus

BO Bachelor of Osteopathy; base of prism out; behavior objective; belladonna and opium; body odor; bowel obstruction; bowels opened; bronchiolitis obliterans; bucco-occlusal

Bo Bolton point; constant magnetic field in a magnetic resonance scanner

bo bowels

B&O belladonna and opium

BOA behavioral observation audiometry; born on arrival; British Orthopaedic Association

BOAS Bank of America Study [of retiree population]

BOAT back pain outcome assessment team; Balloon vs Optimal Atherectomy Trial

BOB biorthogonal basis

BOBA beta-oxybutyric acid

BOC blood oxygen capacity; Bureau of Census; butyloxycarbonyl

BOCC biomedical occupation [UMLS]

BoCV bovine enteric calicivirus

BOD biochemical oxygen demand; brachymorphism-onychodysplasia-dysphalangism [syndrome]

Bod Bodansky [unit]

BOE benign occipital epilepsy

BOEA ethyl biscoumacetate

BOEC blood outgrowth epithelial cell
BOF branchio-oculofacial [syndrome]
BOFS branchio-oculofacial syndrome
BOH board of health
BoHV bovine herpesvirus
BoiHV Boid herpesvirus
BOILER Balloon Occlusive Intravascular Lysis Enhanced Recanalization Strategy
BOL beginning of life [pacemaker battery]
BOLD bleomycin, Oncovin, lomustine, dacarbazine; blood oxygenation level dependent
BoIVX Boletus virus X
BOM bilateral otitis media
BOMA bilateral otitis media, acute
BoNT A, B , C, D, E botulinum neurotoxin A, B, C, D, and E
BOOP bronchiolitis obliterans-organizing pneumonia
BOP buffalo orphan prototype [virus]
BOPP boronated protoporphyrin
BOR basal optic root; before time of operation; bowels open regularly; branchio-oto-renal [syndrome]
BORR blood oxygen release rate
BORSA borderline resistant *Staphylococcus aureus*
BoRV *Buthus occitanus* reovirus
BOS Bioethics Online Service
BOSC Board of Scientific Counselors
BoSM Bolivian squirrel monkey
BOSS Balloon Optimization vs Stent Study
BOT botulinum toxin
bot bottle
BOTV Botambi virus
BoTV bovine torovirus
BOU branchio-oto-ureteral [syndrome]
BOUV Bouboui virus
BoV Boolarra virus
BOW bag of waters
BOZOV Bozo virus
BP Bachelor of Pharmacy; backpassage [culture]; back pressure; back projection; back propagation [algorithm]; barometric pressure; basic protein; bathroom privileges; bed pan; before present; behavior pattern; Bell palsy; benzpyrene; beta-protein; binding protein; biotic potential; biparietal; biphenyl; bipolar; birth place; bisphosphonate; blood pressure; body plethysmography; boiling point; Bolton point; borderline personality; bowenoid

papulosis; breech presentation; British Pharmacopoeia; bronchopleural; bronchopulmonary; buccopulpal; bullous pemphigus/pemphigoid; bypass
B/P blood pressure
BP II bipolar type II disorder
BP180 bullous pemphigoid antigen II
BP230 bullous pemphigoid antigen I
bp base pair; bed pan; boiling point
BPA basic probability assignment; bisphenol A; blood pressure assembly; bovine plasma albumin; British Paediatric Association; bronchopulmonary aspergillosis; burst-promoting activity
BPAEC bovine pulmonary artery endothelial cell
BPAG bullous pemphigoid antigen
BPANN back propagation artificial neural network
BPAR body part [UMLS]
BPAS body profile analysis system
BPB bromphenol blue; biliopancreatic bypass
BPC Behavior Problem Checklist; bile phospholipid concentration; blood pressure cuff; British Pharmaceutical Codex
BPCS back pain classification scale
BPD biparental disomy; biparietal diameter; blood pressure decrease; borderline personality disorder; bronchopulmonary dysplasia
BPDE benzo(α)pyrene-diol-epoxide
BPE bacterial phosphatidylethanolamine
BPEAS benign partial epilepsy with affective symptoms
BPEC benign partial epilepsy of childhood; bipolar electrocardiogram
BPEG British Pacing and Electrophysiology Group [study]
BPEI blepharophimosis, ptosis, epicanthus inversus
BPES blepharophimosis-ptosis-epicanthus inversus syndrome
BPF bandpass filter; bradykinin-potentiating factor; Brazilian purpuric fever; bronchopulmonary fistula; burst-promoting factor
BPFC Brazilian purpuric fever clone
BPG benzathine penicillin G; D-2,3-bisphosphoglycerate; blood pressure gauge; bypass graft
BPGM bisphosphoglyceromutase

BPH Bachelor of Public Health; benign prostatic hyperplasia; benign prostatic hypertrophy

BPh British Pharmacopoeia; buccopharyngeal

Bph bacteriopheophytin

BPharm Bachelor of Pharmacy

BPHEng Bachelor of Public Health Engineering

BPheo bacteriopheophytin

BPHN Bachelor of Public Health Nursing

BPI bactericidal/permeability increasing [protein]; Basic Personality Inventory; beef-pork insulin; bipolar type I; blood pressure increase; blood pressure index; Brief Pain Inventory

BPIV bovine parainfluenza virus

BPL Beneficiary Program Liability [data file]; benign proliferative lesion; benzyl penicilloyl-polylysine; beta-propiolactone

BPLA blood pressure, left arm

BPM beats per minute; best partial match [imaging]; biperidyl mustard; block perfusion monitor; body protein monitor; breaths per minute; brompheniramine maleate

bpm beats per minute

BPMF British Postgraduate Medical Federation

BPMS blood plasma measuring system

BPMV bean pod mottle virus

BPN bacitracin, polymyxin B, neomycin sulfate; back propagation neural network [algorithm]; brachial plexus neuropathy

BPO basal pepsin output; benzyl penicilloyl

BPP binding property pair; biophysical profile; bovine pancreatic polypeptide; bradykinin potentiating peptide

BP&P blood pressure and pulse

BPPD Biopesticides and Pollution Prevention Division

BPPN benign paroxysmal positioning nystagmus

BPPV benign paroxysmal positional vertigo; bovine paragenital papillomavirus

BPQ Berne Pain Questionnaire

BPR blood pressure recorder; blood production rate

BPRA blood pressure, right arm

BPROP backpropagation neural network

BPRS Brief Psychiatric Rating Scale; Brief Psychiatric Reacting Scale

BPS Basel Prospective Study; beats per second; Behavioral Pharmacological Society; biophysical profile score; bits per second; bovine papular stomatitis; brain protein solvent; breaths per second; bytes per second; systolic blood pressure

Bps, bps bits per second; bytes per second

BPSA bronchopulmonary segmental artery

BPSD behavioral and psychiatric symptoms of dementia

BPSMC Blood Pressure Study in Mexican Children

BPsTh Bachelor of Psychotherapy

BPSU British Paediatric Surveillance Unit

BPSV bovine papular stomatitis virus

BPT benign paroxysmal torticollis; binding property torsion; bronchial provocation test

BPTI basic pancreatic trypsin inhibitor; basic polyvalent trypsin inhibitor; bovine pancreatic trypsin inhibitor

BPV bat paramyxovirus; bee paralysis virus; benign paroxysmal vertigo; benign positional vertigo; bioprosthetic valve; bovine papillomavirus; bovine parvovirus

BP(Vet) British Pharmacopoeia (Veterinary)

BPXY buffalopox virus

BPYV beet pseudoyellow virus

BPyV baboon polyomavirus; bovine polyomavirus

Bq becquerel

BQA Bureau of Quality Assurance

BQSV Barranqueras virus

BR baroreflex; barrier reared [experimental animals]; baseline recovery; bathroom; bed rest; bedside rounds; bilirubin; biologic response; blink reflex; branchial; breathing rate; breathing training; bronchial, bronchitis, bronchus; *Brucella*; brush cytology

Br brain; breech; bregma; bridge; bromine; bronchitis; brown; *Brucella*; brucellosis

bR bacteriorhodopsin

br boiling range; brachial; branch; branchial; breath; brother

BRA bilateral renal agenesis; bone-resorbing activity; brain; brain-reactive antibody; brainstem auditory [response]

BRAC basic rest-activity cycle

Brach brachial

Brady, brady bradycardia

BRAFE brachial, radial and femoral [approach for elective coronary stent implantation]

BRAGS Bioelectric Repair and Growth Society

BRAINS Biochemical Research and Information Study; Brain Research, Analysis of Images, Networks, and Systems

BRAMS Bech-Rafaelson Melancholia Scale

BRAO branch retinal artery occlusion

BRAP burst of rapid atrial pacing

BrAP brachial artery pressure

BRAT Baylor rapid autologous transfusion [system]

BRATT bananas, rice, applesauce, tea and toast

BRAV black currant reversion-associated virus

BRAVE biosense revascularization approach for viable endocardium

BRB bright red blood

BRBC bovine red blood cell

BRBN blue rubber bleb nevus

BRBNS blue rubber bleb nevus syndrome

BRBPR bright red blood per rectum

BRbx breast biopsy

BRC brain reserve capacity

Brc bromocriptine

BRCA breast cancer

BRCA1, BRCA2 breast cancer susceptibility genes

BRCD breast cancer, ductal

BRCM below right costal margin

BRCS British Red Cross Society

BRCT Brain Resuscitation Clinical Trial

BRD bladder retraining drill; bovine respiratory disease

BrdU bromodeoxyuridine

BrdUrd bromodeoxyuridine

BRDV Broadhaven virus

BRE benign rolandic epilepsy

BREASTS bronchopulmonary aspergillosis, radiotherapy, extrinsic allergic alveolitis, ankylosing spondylitis, sarcoidosis, tuberculosis, silicosis [x-ray findings in fibrotic pulmonary changes]

BRESEK brain anomalies-retardation of mentality-ectodermal dysplasia-kidney dysplasia/hypoplasia [syndrome]

BRESHECK brain anomalies-retardation of mentality and growth-ectodermal hypoplasia-Hirschsprung disease-ear deformity and deafness-eye hypoplasia-cleft palate-cryptorchidism-kidney dysplasia/hypoplasia [syndrome]

BRESUS British Hospital Resuscitation Study

BRF bone-resorbing factor

BRFSS Behavioral Risk Factor Surveillance System

BRH benign recurrent hematuria; British Regional Heart [study]; Bureau of Radiological Health

BRHS British Regional Heart Study

BRIC benign recurrent intrahepatic cholestasis

BRILLIANT Blood Pressure, Renal Effects, Insulin Control, Lipids, Lisinopril and Nifedipine Trial

BRIME brief repetitive isometric maximal exercise

BRIN Biomedical Research Infrastructure Networks

Brkf breakfast

BRM biological response modifier; biuret reactive material

BRMS Bannayan-Riley-Myhre-Smith [syndrome]; Bech-Rafaelsen Melancholia Scale

BRMV bean rugose mosaic virus; Berrimah virus

BRN Board of Registered Nursing

brn brown

BRNV black raspberry necrosis virus

BRO bronchiolitis obliterans; bronchoscopy

bro brother

brom bromide

Bron, Bronch bronchi, bronchial; bronchoscopy

Broncho bronchoscopy

BRP bathroom privileges; bilirubin production; biological reference preparation; bronchophony

Brph bronchophony

BRR Bannayan-Riley-Ruvalcaba [syndrome]; baroreceptor reflex response; breathing reserve ratio

BRRV blueberry red ringspot virus

BRS baroreflex sensitivity; behavior rating scale; battered root syndrome; Bibliographic Retrieval Services; British Roentgen Society

BrSM Brazilian squirrel monkey

BRSV beet ringspot virus; bovine respiratory syncytial virus
BRT Brook reaction test
brth breath
5-BrU 5-bromouracil
BRU bone remodeling unit
BrU bromouracil
Bruc *Brucella*
BRUV Bruconha virus
BRV baboon orthoreovirus; bovine rhinovirus; Breda virus
BRVO branch retinal vein occlusion
BRW Brown-Robert-Wells [stereotactic system]
BS Bachelor of Science; Bachelor of Surgery; *Bacillus subtilis*; Bartter syndrome; base strap; bedside; before sleep; Behçet syndrome; bilateral symmetrical; bile salt; Binet-Simon [test]; bismuth sulfite; blood sugar; Bloom syndrome; Blue Shield [plan]; body system; borderline schizophrenia; bowel sound; breaking strength; breath sound; British Standard; buffered saline; Bureau of Standards; byte structure
B-S Bjork-Shiley [valve]
B&S Brown and Sharp [sutures]
B/s, b/s bytes per second
bs bedside; bowel sound; breath sound
b × s brother × sister inbreeding
BSA benzenesulfonic acid; Biofeedback Society of America; bismuth-sulfite agar; bis-trimethylsilyl-acetamide; Blind Service Association; Blue Shield Association; body surface area; bovine serum albumin; bowel sounds active
bsa bovine serum albumin
BSAG Bristol Social Adjustment Guides
BSAM basic sequential access method
BSA-NO nitrosated bovine serum albumin
BSAP brief short-action potential; brief, small, abundant potentials
BSB body surface burned
BS = BL breath sounds equal bilaterally
BSBMV beet soil-borne mosaic virus
BSBV beet soil-borne virus; bushbush virus
BSC bedside care; bedside commode; bench scale calorimeter; best supportive care; bile salt concentration; Biological Stain Commission; biologic safety cabinet; Biomedical Science Corps
BSc Bachelor of Science

BSC-1, BS-C-1 *Cercopithecus* monkey kidney cells
BSCC Björk-Shiley convexo-concave [heart valve]; British Society for Clinical Cytology
BSCP bovine spinal cord protein
BSD bedside drainage
BSDAC Biological Sciences Division [office] of Academic Computing
BSDLB block in the superior division of left branch
BSE behavior summarized evaluation; bilateral intranasal sphenoethmoidectomy; bilaterally symmetrical and equal; bovine spongiform encephalopathy; brain surface extractor; breast self-examination; bystander effect [ability of genetically modified cells to survive cytotoxic effects]
BSEP brain stem evoked potential
BSER brain stem evoked response [audiometry]
BSF back scatter factor; B-cell stimulatory factor; benign senescent forgetfulness; busulfan
BSG basigin; biotin-streptavidin-gold; branchio-skeleto-genital [syndrome]
BSG-DNA biotin-streptavidin-gold-deoxyribonucleic acid
BSH benign sexual headache
BSI behavior status inventory; blood stream infection; body substance isolation; borderline syndrome index; bound serum iron; brainstem injury; brief symptom inventory; British Standards Institution
BSID Bayley Scale of Infant Development
BSIF bile salt independent fraction
BSL benign symmetric lipomatosis; biosafety level; blood sugar level
BSM Bachelor of Science in Medicine; Björk-Shiley monostrut [prosthetic heart valve]; body surface mapping
BSMC bronchial smooth muscle cell
BSMV barley stripe mosaic virus
BSN baccalaureate of science in nursing; Bachelor of Science in Nursing; bowel sounds normal
BSNA bowel sounds normal and active
BSO bilateral sagittal osteotomy; bilateral salpingo-oophorectomy; butathione sulfoximine
BSOFP blood spotted on filter paper
BSOP blood spot on filter paper

BSP bone sialoprotein; bromosulphthalein

BSp bronchospasm

BSPA body space [UMLS]

BSPh bachelor of science in pharmacy

BSPM body surface potential mapping

BSQ behavior style questionnaire

BSQV Bussuquara virus

BSR basal skin resistance; blood sedimentation rate; bowel sounds regular; brain stimulation reinforcement; burst suppression ratio; Buschke selective reminding [test]

BSS Bachelor of Sanitary Science; balanced salt solution; Bernard-Soulier syndrome; black silk suture; buffered salt solution; buffered single substrate

B-SS Bernard-Soulier syndrome

BSSE bile salt-stimulated esterase

BSSG sitogluside

BSSL bile salt-stimulated lipase

BSSV blueberry shoestring virus

BST bacteriuria screening test; bed nucleus of the striae terminalis; blood serologic test; bovine somatotropin; brief stimulus therapy

BSTFA bis-trimethylsilyltrifluoroacetamide

BSU Bartholin, Skene, urethral [glands]; basic structural unit; British standard unit

BSUB body substance [UMLS]

BSV banana streak virus; binocular single vision

BS-VLC byte structure variable length coding

BT base of tongue; bedtime; biomedical technology; bitemporal; bitrochanteric; bladder tumor; Blalock-Taussig [shunt]; bleeding time; blood type, blood typing; blue tetrazolium; blue tongue; body temperature; borderline tuberculoid; bovine turbinate [cells]; brain tumor; breast tumor

Bt *Bacillus thuringiensis*

BTA Blood Transfusion Association

BTB breakthrough bleeding; bromthymol blue

BTBL bromothymol blue lactose

BTC basal temperature chart; body temperature chart; butylcholinesterase

BTCG Brain Tumor Cooperative Group

BTD biliary tract disease

BTDG Biological Therapeutics Development Group

BTDS benzoylthiamine disulfide

BTE behind the ear [hearing aid]; biphasic truncated exponential; bovine thymus extract

BTFS breast tumor frozen section

BTG beta-thromboglobulin

BTg bovine trypsinogen

BThU British thermal unit

Bti *Bacillus thuringiensis* var. *israelensis*

Btk Bruton's tyrosine kinase

BTKV Boteke virus

BTL bilateral tubal ligation

Btl breathless

BTLS basic trauma life support

BTM benign tertian malaria; blood temperature monitor; body temperature monitor

BTMSA bis-trimethylsilacetylene

BTMV beet mosaic virus

BTP biliary tract pain; biological treatment planning; broad terminal phalanges

BTPABA *N*-benzoyl-L-tyrosyl-*p*-aminobenzoic acid

BTPS at body temperature and ambient pressure, and saturated with water vapor [gas]

BTR Bezold-type reflex; biceps tendon reflex

BTr bovine trypsin

BTRID binomial transform reduced interference distribution

BTRS Belgian Ticlodipine Retinopathy Study

BTS Batten syndrome; blood transfusion service; blue toe syndrome; bradycardia-tachycardia syndrome; British Thoracic Society

BTSG Brain Tumor Study Group

bTSH bovine thyroid-stimulating hormone

BTU British thermal unit

BTV blue tongue virus; bushy top virus

BTW biological and toxin weapon

BTWC Biological and Toxin Weapons Convention

BTX botulinum toxin; brevetoxin; bungarotoxin

BTx blood transfusion

BTX-B brevetoxin-B

BTZ benzothiazepine

BU base of prism up; Bethesda unit; blood urea; Bodansky unit; bromouracil; burn unit

Bu butyl
bu bushel
BUA blood uric acid; broadband ultrasonic attenuation
BUB budding uninhibited by benzimidazole
Buc, Bucc buccal
BuChE butyrocholinesterase
BUD budesonide
BUDR bromodeoxyuridine
BUDS bilateral upper dorsal sympathectomy
BUE both upper extremities
BUEV Buenaventura virus
BUF buffalo [rat]
BUFUL bumetanide and furosemide on lipid [profile]
BUG buccal ganglion
BUGT bilirubin-uridine diphosphate glucuronysyltransferase
BuHV bubaline herpesvirus
BUI brain uptake index
BUJV Bujaru virus
BULIT bulimia test
BULL buccal or upper lingual of lower
BuMed Bureau of Medicine and Surgery
BUMP behavioral regression or upset in hospitalized medical patients [scale]
BUN blood urea nitrogen
bun br bundle branch
BUN/CR blood urea nitrogen/creatine ratio
BUNV Bunyamwera virus
BUO bleeding of undetermined origin, bruising of undetermined origin
BUQ both upper quadrants
BUR bilateral ureteral occlusion
Burd Burdick suction
BUS Bartholin, urethral, and Skene glands; busulfan
BuSVd Burdock stunt viroid
But, but butyrate, butyric
BV bacilliform virus; bacitracin V; bacterial vaginosis; balloon valvuloplasty; biologic value; blood vessel; blood volume; bracovirus; bronchovesicular
Bv Bracovirus, bracovirus
BVA Blind Veterans Association; British Veterinary Association
BVAD biventricular assist device
BVC British Veterinary Codex
BVD bovine viral diarrhea
BVDT brief vestibular disorientation test

BVDU bromovinyldeoxyuridine
BVDV bovine viral diarrhea virus
BVE binocular visual efficiency; blood vessel endothelium; blood volume expander
BVEC bovine valve endothelial cell
BVF bone volume fraction
BVH biventricular hypertrophy
BVI blood vessel invasion
BVL bilateral vas ligation
BVM bag-valve-mask; bronchovascular markings; Bureau of Veterinary Medicine
BVMGT Bender Visual-Motor Gestalt Test
BVMOT Bender Visual-Motor Gestalt Test
BVMS Bachelor of Veterinary Medicine and Science
BVO black vinyl overboot; branch vein occlusion
BVP blood vessel prosthesis; blood volume pulse; burst of ventricular pacing
BVQ beet virus Q
BVR baboon virus replication; Balloon Valvuloplasty Registry
BVS biventricular support; blanked ventricular sense
BVSc Bachelor of Veterinary Science
BV/TV bone volume/trabecular volume [ratio]
BVU bromoisovalerylurea
BVV bovine vaginitis virus
BW bacteriological warfare; Beckwith-Wiedemann [syndrome]; bed wetting; below waist; biological warfare; biological weapon; birth weight; bladder washout; blood Wasserman [reaction]; body water; body weight
B&W black and white [milk of magnesia and cascara extract]
bw body weight
BWAV Bwamba virus
BWC bladder wash cytology
BWD bacillary white diarrhea
BWFCM bladder wash flow cytometry
BWFI bacteriostatic water for injection
BWG Bland-White-Garland syndrome
BWIS Baltimore-Washington Infant Study
BWS battered woman (or wife) syndrome; Beckwith-Wiedemann syndrome
BWSpV Brazilian wheat spike virus
BWST black widow spider toxin

BWSV black widow spider venom
BWt birth weight
Bwt body weight
BWYV, bwyv beet western yellow virus
BX, bx bacitracin X; biopsy
Bx biopsy
BXO balanitis xerotica obliterans
BXV Bee virus X
ByCPR bystander cardiac pulmonary resuscitation
BYDV barley yellow dwarf virus
BYE Barila-Yaguchi-Eveland [medium]
BYMV bean yellow mosaic virus

BYP Baeza-Yates-Perleberg [algorithm]
BYSMV barley yellow striate mosaic virus
BYSV beet yellow stunt virus
BYV bee virus Y; beet yellow virus
BYVBV bean yellow vein–banding virus
BZ benzodiazepine
Bz, Bzl benzoyl
BZD benzodiazepine
BZQ benzquinamide
BZRP benzodiazepine receptor peripheral [type]
BZS Bannayan-Zonana syndrome

C

C about [Lat. *circa*]; ascorbic acid; bruised [Lat. *contusus*]; calcitonin-forming [cell]; calculus; calorie [large]; *Campylobacter*; *Candida*; canine tooth; capability [list]; capacitance; capsid protein; carbohydrate; carbon; cardiac; cardiovascular disease; carrier; cast; cathode; Caucasian; cell; Celsius; centigrade; central; central electrode placement in electroencephalography; centromeric or constitutive heterochromatic chromosome [banding]; cerebrospinal; certified; cervical; cesarean [section]; chest (precordial) lead in electrocardiography; chicken; *Chlamydia*; chloramphenicol; cholesterol; class; clearance; clonus; *Clostridium*; closure; clubbing; coarse [bacterial colonies]; cocaine; coefficient; colorectal tumor with metastases to lymph nodes [Dukes classification]; color sense; colored [guinea pig]; communicating [pacemaker]; complement; complex; compliance; component; compound [Lat. *compositus*]; concentration; concept [UMLS]; conditioned, conditioning; condyle; constant; consultation; contamination; contraction; control; conventionally reared [experimental animal]; convergence; correct; cortex; coulomb; count; criteria; *Cryptococcus*; cubic; cubitus; cyanosis; cylinder; cysteine; cytidine; cytochrome; cytosine; gallon [Lat. *congius*]; horn [Lat. *cornu*]; hundred [Lat. *centum*]; large calorie; molar heat capacity; rib [Lat. *costa*]; total capacitance; velocity of light; with [Lat. *cum*]

C⁰ concentration zero

C1 first cervical nerve; first cervical vertebra; first component of complement

C₁ first rib

C̄1 activated first component of complement

C1–9 complement proteins 1 to 9

CI first concept [UMLS]; first cranial nerve; prostatic tumor with extracapsular extension and negative margins [Jewett staging system]; tumor with metastases to lymph nodes without involvement of perirectal adipose tissue [Astler-Coller classification]

2C 2-component

C2 prostatic tumor with extracapsular extension and positive margins [Jewett staging system]; second cervical nerve; second cervical vertebra; second component of complement; second concept [UMLS]; tumor with metastases to lymph nodes and extension into perirectal adipose tissue

C² community capacity [AIDS prevention]

C₂ second rib

C̄2 activated second component of complement

CII second cranial nerve

3C 3-component; cranio-cerebello-cardiac syndrome

C3 prostatic tumor with seminal vesical involvement [Jewett staging system]; third cervical nerve; third cervical vertebra; third component of complement

C₃ Collins' solution; third rib

C̄3 activated third component of complement

CIII third cranial nerve

C4 controlled collapse chip connection; fourth cervical nerve; fourth cervical vertebra; fourth component of complement

C̄4 activated fourth component of complement

CIV fourth cranial nerve

C5 fifth cervical nerve; fifth cervical vertebra; fifth component of complement

C̄5 activated fifth component of complement

CV fifth cranial nerve

C6 sixth cervical nerve; sixth cervical vertebra; sixth component of complement

C̄6 activated sixth component of complement

CVI sixth cranial nerve

C7 seventh cervical nerve; seventh cervical vertebra; seventh component of complement

C̄7 activated seventh component of complement

CVII seventh cranial nerve

C8 eighth component of complement

C̄8 activated eighth component of complement

CVIII eighth cranial nerve

C9 ninth component of complement

C̄9 activated ninth component of complement

CIX–CXII ninth to twelfth cranial nerves

°C degree Celsius

C′ complement

c about [Lat. *circa*]; calorie [small]; candle; canine tooth; capacity; capillary; carat; centi-; clinical; complementary [strand]; concentration; contact; cup; curie; cyclic; meal [Lat. *cibus*]; specific heat capacity; with [Lat. *cum*]

c′ coefficient of partage

c- centi- [10^{-1}]

χ see *chi*

CA anterior commissure [Lat. *commissura anterior*]; calcium antagonist; California [rabbit]; cancer; cancer antigen; *Candida albicans*; caproic acid; capsid; capsid protein; carbohydrate antagonist; carbonic anhydrase; carcinoma; cardiac angiography; cardiac apnea; cardiac arrest; cardiac arrhythmia; carotid artery; cast; catecholamine, catecholaminergic; cathode; Caucasian adult; celiac axis; cell automation; cellulose acetate; cerebral aqueduct; cerebral atrophy; certification authority; cervicoaxial; Chemical Abstracts; chemotactic activity; child abuse; chloroamphetamine; cholic acid; chorio-amniotic; chromosomal aberration; chronic anovulation; chronological age; citric acid; clotting assay; coagglutination; coarctation of the aorta; Cocaine Anonymous; coefficient of absorption; cold agglutinin; colloid antigen; common antigen; compressed air; computer-assisted; conceptional age; condyloma acuminatum; coracoacromial; coronary angioplasty; coronary artery; corpora allata; corpora amylacea; corpus albicans; corrected [echo] area; cortisone acetate; cricoarytenoid; cricoid arch; croup-associated [virus]; cytosine arabinoside; cytotoxic antibody

C&A Clinitest and Acetest

CA1 carbonic anhydrase I

CA-2 second colloid antigen

CA 15.3 marker for breast carcinoma

CA 19.9 marker for colorectal and pancreatic carcinomas

CA 27.29 marker for breast carcinoma

CA 50 marker for pancreatic or colorectal carcinomas

CA 72.4 marker for gastrointestinal and ovarian carcinomas

CA 125 marker for ovarian and endometrial carcinomas

CA 242 marker for pancreatic and colorectal carcinomas

CA 549 marker for breast carcinoma

Ca calcium; cancer, carcinoma; *Candida albicans*; cathode

ca about [Lat. *circa*]; candle; carcinoma

CAA carotid audiofrequency analysis; cerebral amyloid angiopathy; circulating anodic antigen; Clean Air Act; computer-assisted assessment; constitutional aplastic anemia; coronary artery aneurysm; crystalline amino acids

CAADAC California Association of Alcohol and Drug Abuse Counselors

CAAH chronic active autoimmune hepatitis

CAAS cardiovascular angiographic analysis system; Commission on Accreditation of Ambulance Services

CAASET Canadian Amlodipine and Atenolol Stress Echo [trial]

CAAT computer-assisted axial tomography

CAAV canine adeno-associated virus

CAAX [box] protein segment in which C is cysteine, A is usually but not always an aliphatic amino acid, and X is methionine or serine

CAB captive air bubble; cellulose acetate butyrate; coronary artery bypass

CABADAS [prevention of] Coronary Artery Bypass Graft Occlusion by Aspirin, Dipyridamole and Acenocoumarol Study

CABBS computer-assisted blood background subtraction

CABF coronary artery blood flow

CABG coronary artery bypass grafting

CABG-PATCH Coronary Artery Bypass Graft [trial with/without epicardial] Patch [for automatic implantable cardioverter-defibrillator]

CABGS coronary artery bypass graft surgery

CaBI calcium bone index

Ca^{2+}-blocker calcium channel blocker

CABM Center for Advanced Biotechnology and Medicine

CABMET Colorado Association of Biomedical Engineering Technicians

CaBP calcium-binding protein

CABRI Coronary Angioplasty versus Bypass Revascularization Investigation; Coronary Artery Bypass Revascularization Investigation

CABS citric acid-buffered saline [solution]; continuous ambulatory blood sampler; coronary artery bypass surgery

CABV Cabassou virus

cabyv cucurbit aphid-borne yellow virus

CAC Carcinogeneity Assessment Committee [FDA]; cardiac-accelerator center; cardiac arrest code; children's asthma center; circulating anticoagulant; clinical application coordinator

CaCC calcium-sensitive chloride channel; cathodal closure contraction

CAC/CIC chronic active/inactive cirrhosis

CACCN Canadian Association of Critical Care Nurses

CACHET Comparison of Abciximab Complications with Hirulog for Ischemic Events Trial

CACP cisplatin

CaCTe cathodal closure tetanus

CACTIS Comparison of Aspirin with Clopidogrel or Ticlopidine in Stents [trial]

CACV cacao virus

CaCV canine calicivirus

CaCX cancer of cervix

CACY calcyclin

CAD cadaver, cadaveric; central appointment desk [computer-based coordination]; chronic actinic dermatitis; coenzyme A dehydrogenase; cold agglutinin disease; collisionally activated dissociation; compressed air disease; computer-aided design; computer-aided dispatch; computer-assisted design; computer-assisted diagnosis; congenital abduction deficiency; coronary artery disease; coronoradiographic documentation

Cad cadaver, cadaveric

CADA Council on Alcohol and Drug Abuse

CADASIL cerebral autosomal dominant arteriopathy with subcortical infarcts and leukoencephalopathy

CAD/CAM computer-aided design/computer-aided manufacturing

CADCCC Central Australia Disease Control Coordinating Committee

CADD computer-aided drug design

CADHYP Coronary Artery Disease in Hypertension [study]

CADI coronary artery disease index

CADILLAC Controlled Abciximab and Device Investigation to Lower Late Angioplasty Complications [study]

CADL Communicative Abilities in Daily Living

CADMIO computer-assisted design for medical information objectives

cADPR cyclic adenosinephosphate-ribose

CADR coronary artery descriptors and restenosis

CADRES Coronary Artery Descriptors and Restenosis [project]

CADS Captopril and Digoxin Study

CaDTe cathodal-duration tetanus

CADV Cano Delgadito virus

CAdV canine adenovirus; caprine adenovirus

CADx computer-aided diagnosis

CAE caprine arthritis-encephalitis; cellulose acetate electrophoresis; childhood absence epilepsy; contingent after-effects; coronary artery embolism

CaE calcium excretion

CaEDTA calcium disodium ethylene-diaminetetraacetate

CAE-IEF cellulose acetate-isoelectric focusing [electrophoresis]

CAEP Canadian Association of Emergency Physicians; cortical auditory evoked potential

CAER community awareness and emergency response

CAESA computer-assisted estimation of synthetic accessibility

CAESAR Canada, Australia, Europe and South Africa Republic [trial]; computer-assisted ear nose and throat surgery using augmented reality; Computer-Assisted Evaluation of Stenosis and Restenosis [system]

CAEV caprine arthritis-encephalitis virus; *Chironomus attenuatus* entomopoxvirus

CAF cell adhesion factor; citric acid fermentation; combined acetabular and femoral [navigation in computer-assisted surgery]; common assembly format [genome sequencing]; cortical activation function

Caf caffeine

CAFA Canadian Atrial Fibrillation Anticoagulation [study]

CAFE Coronary Artery Flow Evaluation

CAFS Canadian Atrial Fibrillation Study

CAG cholangiogram, cholangiography; chronic atrophic gastritis; coronary angiography

CAGA calgranulin A

CAGB calgranulin B

CAGC Canadian Association of Genetic Counsellors

CAGE capillary affinity gel electrophoresis; *c*ut down, *a*nnoyed by criticism, guilty about drinking, *e*ye-opener drinks (a test for alcoholism)

CAH CAS [Chemical Abstracts] Surveyor Hazardous Materials; chronic active hepatitis; chronic aggressive hepatitis; combined atrial hypertrophy; congenital adrenal hyperplasia; cyanacetic acid hydrazide

CAHD coronary arteriosclerotic heart disease

CAHEA Committee on Allied Health Education and Accreditation

CAHMR cataract-hypertrichosis-mental retardation [syndrome]

CAHPS Consumer Assessment of Health Plans Survey

CAHS central alveolar hypoventilation syndrome

CAHV central alveolar hypoventilation

CaHV canid herpesvirus

CAI celiac artery infusion; cellular adaptive immunotherapy; chemical accident or incident; complete androgen insensitivity; computer-assisted instruction; computer-assisted interview; confluence of informatics

CAID computer-aided implant dentistry

CAIRA chemical accident or incident response and assistance

CAIS complete androgen insensitivity syndrome

CAIUS Carotid Atherosclerosis Italian Ultrasound Study

CAIV Caimito virus

CaIV *Campoletis aprilis* ichnovirus

C(a-jb)O$_2$ arterial-jugular bulb venous oxygen ratio

CAK cyclin-dependent kinase-activating kinase

cAK cyclic adenosine monophosphate [cAMP] dependent protein kinase

CAL café au lait; calcium test; calculated average life; calories; chronic airflow limitation; computer-assisted learning; coracoacromial ligament

Cal caliber; large calorie

cal small calorie

C$_{alb}$ albumin clearance

Calc calcium

CALC calcitonin

calc calculation

calcif calcification

CALCR calcitonin receptor

CALD chronic active liver disease

CALGB cancer and leukemia group B

CALH chronic active lupoid hepatitis

CalHV callitrichine herpesvirus

cALL common null cell acute lymphocytic leukemia

CALLA, cALLA common acute lymphoblastic leukemia antigen

CALM café-au-lait macules

CALP congenital absence of left pericardium

CALS café-au-lait spots

CaLV cardamine latent virus

CALYPSO Cylexin as an Adjunct to Lytic Therapy to Prevent Superoxide Reflow Injury

CAM calf aortic microsome; cell adhesion molecule; cell-associating molecule; chemical agent monitor; chorioallantoic membrane; complementary and alternative medicine(s); compressed adjacency matrix; computer assisted myelography; confusion assessment method [rating for delirium]; content-addressable memory; contralateral axillary metastasis; cystic adenomatoid malformation

CaM calmodulin

C$_{am}$ amylase clearance

CaM-A calmodulin-agarose

CAMAC computer automated measurement and control

CAMAK cataract-microcephaly-arthrogryposis-kyphosis [syndrome]

CAMAT Canadian Amiodarone Myocardial Infarction Arrhythmia Trial

CAMC camera augmented mobile C-arm; computer application in medical care; computer analysis of mammography phantom images

CAMCAM Center for Assessment and Management of Changes in Academic Medicine

CAMCAT Canadian Multicenter Clentiazem Angina Trial

CAMCOG Cambridge cognitive capacity scale

CAMD computer-aided molecular design

CAMDEX Cambridge mental disorders of the elderly examination

CAMF cyclophosphamide, Adriamycin, methotrexate, fluorouracil

CAMFAK cataract-microcephaly-failure to thrive-kyphoscoliosis [syndrome]

CAMH Center for Addiction and Mental Health

CAMI Canadian Assessment of Myocardial Infarction [study]; computer-assisted medical intervention

CAMIAT Canadian Amiodarone Myocardial Infarction Arrhythmia Trial; Canadian Myocardial Infarction Amiodarone Trial

CAMIS Center for Applied Medical Information Systems Research

CAMK calmodulin-dependent protein kinase

CaMK calcium-mediated kinase

CAML cystic adenomatoid malformation of the lung

CAMP Christie-Atkins-Munch-Petersen [test]; computer-assisted management protocol; computer-assisted menu planning; concentration of adenosine monophosphate; cyclic adenosine monophosphate; cyclophosphamide, Adriamycin, methotrexate, and procarbazine

cAMP cyclic adenosine monophosphate

CAMPASS Cambridge Database on Protein Alignments Organized as Structural Superfamilies

CAMRT Canadian Association of Medical Radiation Technologists

CAMS computer-assisted monitoring system

CAMT Center for Advanced Medical Technology

CAMTS Commission for Accreditation of Medical Transport Services

CAMV congenital anomaly of mitral valve

CaMV cauliflower mosaic virus

CAMVA chorioallantoic membrane vascular assay

CAN cardiac autonomic neuropathy

Can cancer; *Candida*; *Cannabis*

CA/N child abuse and neglect

CANA circulating antineuronal antibody

CaNaEDTA calcium-disodium ethylenediamine tetraacetic acid

CANAHOP Canadian Ambulatory, Home and Office Pressure Study

CANARIE Canadian Network for the Advancement of Research, Industry, and Education

canc cancelled

c-ANCA antineutrophil antibodies against protease 3 in cytoplasmic granules

C-ANCA cytoplasmic anti-neutrophilic cytoplasmic antibody

CANCERLIT Cancer Literature [NLM database]

CANCERPROJ Cancer Research Projects

CANDA computer-assisted new drug application

CANDELA computer-assisted notification of drug effects on laboratory animals [test]

CANDY Communication Aids Negating Disabilities of Youth [laboratory]

CA*Net Canada's High Performance Network

CANOST autoCANOnization system for organic STructures

CANP calcium-activated neutral protease

CANS central auditory nervous system

CAN'T LEAP cyclosporine, alcohol, nicotinic acid, thiazides, lasix, ethambutanol, aspirin, pyrazinamide [substances causing hyperuricemia]

CANV Caninde virus

CANX calnexin

CAO chronic airway obstruction; coronary artery obstruction

CAO$_2$ arterial oxygen content

C$_a$O$_2$ arterial oxygen content

CaOC cathodal opening contraction

CaOCL cathodal opening clonus

CAOD coronary artery occlusive disease

CAOHC Council for Accreditation of Occupational Hearing Conservation

CAOM chronic adhesive otitis media

CAOS computer-assisted orthopedic surgery

CAOT Canadian Association of Occupational Therapy

CaOTe cathodal opening tetanus

CAP camptodactyly-arthropathy-pericarditis [syndrome]; Canada Assistance Plan; capsule; captopril; Caribbean Association of Pharmacists; catabolite gene activator protein; cell attachment protein; cellular acetate propionate; cellulose acetate phthalate; central apical part; chloramphenicol; chronic alcoholic pancreatitis; clinical access program; College of American Pathologists; community-acquired pneumonia; complement-activated plasma; compound action potential; coupled atrial pacing; cyclophosphamide, Adriamycin, and Platinol [cisplatin]; cystine aminopeptidase

C_{AP} cationic antimicrobial protein; circumference of apex

CaP carcinoma of the prostate

cap capacity; capsule

CAPA cancer-associated polypeptide antigen

CAPARES Coronary Angioplasty Amlodipine in Restenosis Trial

CAPAS Cutting Balloon Angioplasty vs Plain Old Balloon Angioplasty Randomized Study

CAPBL computer-assisted problem-based learning

CAPCC Canadian Association of Poison Control Centers

CAPD continuous ambulatory peritoneal dialysis

CAPE Circadian Anti-Ischemia Program in Europe; Clifton assessment procedures for the elderly; computer-assisted patient emulator

CAPERS Computer Assisted Psychiatric Evaluation and Review System

CAPHIS Consumer and Patient Health Information Section [American Library Association]

CAPI computer-assisted personal interview; cryptographic applications programming interface

CAP-IT Client Adherence Profiling-Intervention Tailoring [model]

CAPITOL Captopril Postinfarction Tolerance [trial]

CapLV caper latent virus

CAPM continuous airway pressure monitoring

CAPP Captopril Prevention Project [study]; computer-assisted preoperative planning; Concerted Action Polyp Prevention

CAPPHY Captopril Primary Prevention in Hypertension [study]

CAPPP Captopril Prevention Project

CAPPS Current and Past Psychopathology Scale

CAPRCA chronic, acquired, pure red cell aplasia

CAPRI Cardiopulmonary Research Institute

CAPRICORN Carvedilol Postinfarct Survival Controlled Evaluation

CAPRIE Clopidogrel vs Aspirin in Patients at Risk of Ischemic Events

CAPS Cardiac Arrhythmia Pilot Study; care profile system; community adjustment profile system; computer-aided prototyping system

caps capsule

CAPTIN Captopril Before Reperfusion in Acute Myocardial Infarction; Captopril Plus Tissue Plasminogen Activator Following Acute Myocardial Infarction

CAPTISM Captopril Insulin Sensitivity Multicenter [study]

CAPTURE Chimeric 7E3 Antiplatelet Therapy in Unstable Refractory Angina [trial]

CAPV Capim virus

CAR Canadian Association of Radiologists; cancer-associated retinopathy; Cardiac Ablation Registry; cardiac ambulation routine; carvedilol; cell adhesion regulator; chronic articular rheumatism; computer-assisted radiology; computer-assisted research; conditioned avoidance response; congenital articular rigidity

car carotid

CARA chronic aspecific respiratory ailment

CARAF Canadian Registry of Atrial Fibrillation

CARAFE Cocktail Attenuation of Rotational Ablation Flow Effects [study]

CAR AMP carotid pulse amplitude

CARAT Coronary Angioplasty and Rotablator Atherectomy Trial; coronary artery risk assessment and treatment

CARB carbohydrate; coronary artery bypass graft

carb carbohydrate; carbonate

carbo carbohydrate

CARC chemical agent resistant coating

CARD cardiac automatic resuscitative device; caspase activating and recruiting domain

card cardiac

CARDIA Coronary Artery Risk Development in Young Adults [study]

CARDIAC Cardiovascular Disease and Alimentary Comparison [study]

card insuff cardiac insufficiency

cardiol cardiology

CARDIS Cardiology Information System

CARD PORT Cardiac Arrhythmia and Risk of Death Patient Outcome Research Team

CARE calcium antagonist in reperfusion; cardiac arrhythmias research and education; Carvedilol Atherectomy Restenosis [trial]; Cholesterol and Recurrent Events [study]; comprehensive assessment and referral evaluation; computerized adult and records evaluation [system]; computerized clinical assessment, research and education; cyclic adenosine monophosphate response element

CAREC Caribbean Epidemiology Centre

CARES cancer rehabilitation evaluation system

CARET Beta-Carotene and Retinol Efficacy Trial

CARF Commission on Accreditation and Rehabilitation Facilities

CARG coronary artery bypass grafting

CAR$_{hd}$ high-dose carvedilol

CarIV *Casinaria arjuna* ichnovirus

CARMEN Carvedilol Angiotensin Converting Enzyme Inhibitors Remodelling Mild Heart Failure Evaluation

CARP carbonic anhydrase-related polypeptide

CARPORT Coronary Artery Restenosis Prevention on Repeated Thromboxane A$_2$-Receptor Antagonism Study

CARS Childhood Autism Rating Scale; Children's Affective Rating Scale; Coronary Artery Regression Study; Coumadin Aspirin Reinfarction Study; cysteinyl-transfer ribonucleic acid synthetase

CART classification and regression tree; cocaine-related transcript; Colchicine Angioplasty Restenosis Trial; computer-assisted radiotherapy; constrained access robotic therapy

cart cartilage

CARV Caraparu virus

CAS calcarine sulcus; calcific aortic stenosis; Cancer Attitude Survey; carbohydrate-active steroid; Cardiac Adjustment Scale; cardiac surgery; carotid artery stenting; Celite-activated normal serum; Center for Alcohol Studies; central anticholinergic syndrome; cerebral atherosclerosis; Chemical Abstract Service; clinical application suite; clinical assessment score; clinical asthma score; Cognitive Assessment Scale; cold agglutinin syndrome; computer-assisted surgery; congenital alcoholic syndrome; contralateral acoustic stimulation; control adjustment strap; coronary artery spasm; Council of Academic Societies

Cas casualty

cas castration, castrated

CASA cancer-associated serum antigen; Center for Addiction and Substance Abuse; clinical assessment software application; computer-assisted self-assessment; computer-assisted semen analysis

CASANOVA Coronary Artery Stenosis with Asymptomatic Narrowing: Operation vs Aspirin [study]

CASCADE Cardiac Arrest in Seattle: Conventional vs Amiodarone Drug Evaluation; Conventional Arrhythmic vs Amiodarone in Survivors of Cardiac Arrest Drug Evaluation

CASCO Calcium Sensitization in Congestive Heart Failure

CASD computer-assisted synthesis design

CASE Community, Attachment, Structures and Epidemic [study]; computer-aided simulation of clinical encounter; computer-aided systems engineering; Coordinated Activities, Services, and Encounters [data]

CASET Carotid Artery Stenting vs Endarterectomy Trial; computer-aided systems engineering

CASH Cancer and Steroid Hormone [study]; Cardiac Arrest Study, Hamburg; Caring About Seniors' Health [study]; Commission for Administrative Services in Hospitals; Consensus Action on Salt and Hypertension; corticoadrenal stimulating hormone; cruciform anterior spinal hyper-extension

CASHD coronary arteriosclerotic heart disease

CASI cognitive abilities screening instrument; computer-assisted self-interviewing

CASIS Canadian Amlodipine/Atenolol in Silent Ischemia Study; Coronary Artery Stent Implantation Study

CASMD congenital atonic sclerotic muscular dystrophy

CASP Critical Appraisal Skills Programme [UK]

CASPER computer-assisted pericardial puncture; computer-assisted pericardial surgery

CaspIV *Casinaria* sp. ichnovirus

CASPR contactin-associated protein

CASQ calsequestrin

CASR calcium-sensing receptor

CAS-REGN Chemical Abstracts Service Registry Number

CASRN Chemical Abstract Service Registry Number

CASRT corrected adjusted sinus node recovery time

CASS cataract-alopecia-sclerodactyly syndrome; coding accuracy support system [software]; Coronary Artery Surgery Study

CASSIS Classification and Search Support Information System [Patent Office]; Czech and Slovak Spirapril Intervention Study

CAST calpastatin; CAnonical representation of STereochemistry [coding]; Cardiac Arrhythmia Suppression Trial; Carotid Artery Stenting Trial; Children of Alcoholism Screening Test; Chinese Acute Stroke Trial; computer-adaptive sequential testing; cyclic amplification and selection of targets

CASTEL Cardiovascular Study in the Elderly

CASTOR Coronary Angioscopic Study of Restenosis

CAT California Achievement Test; cancer after transplantation; capillary agglutination test; Cardiomyopathy Trial; care support terminal; catalase; cataract; catecholamine; Children's Apperception Test; Chinese Angiotensin Converting Enzyme Inhibitor in Acute Myocardial Infarction Trial; chloramphenicol acetyltransferase; chlormerodrin accumulation test; choline acetyltransferase; chronic abdominal tympany; Cognitive Abilities Test; Columbia Center for Advanced Technology; computed abdominal tomography; computed axial tomography; computer-assisted

tomography; computer of average transients; coronary angioplasty trial; critically appraised topic

cat catalysis, catalyst; cataract

CAT'ase catalase

CATB catalase B

CAT-CAM contoured adduction trochanteric-controlled alignment method

CATCEC Computer-Supported Assessment and Treatment Consultation for Emotional Crises

CATCH Canadian Association of Teachers of Community Health; Child and Adolescent Trial for Cardiovascular Health; Community Action to Control High Blood Pressure; comprehensive assessment for tracking community health

CATCH 22 cardiac defects-abnormal facies-thymic hypoplasia-cleft palate-hypocalcemia [syndrome]

Cath cathartic; catheter, catheterize

cath catheterization

CATI computer-assisted telephone interview

CATIPO Computer-Aided Therapy Planning in Pediatric Oncology

CATLINE Catalog Online [NLM database]

CATS Canadian American Ticlopidine Study; Captopril and Thrombolysis Study

CAT-S Children's Apperception Test, Supplemental

CAT scan computed axial tomography scan

CATSIM computer case simulation

CATT calcium tolerance test

CATUV Catu virus

Cauc Caucasian

caud caudal

caut cauterization

CAV cardiac allograft vasculopathy; *Chara australis* virus; chicken anemia virus; congenital absence of vagina; congenital adrenal virilism; constant angular velocity; croup-associated virus

cav cavity

CAVA Coronary Atherectomy vs Angioplasty [study]

CAVATAS Carotid and Vertebral Artery Transluminal Angioplasty Study

CAVB complete atrioventricular block

CAVD complete atrioventricular dissociation; completion, arithmetic problems, vocabulary, following directions [test]; congenital aplasia of vas deferens

CAVE cerebroacrovisceral-early lethality [phenotype]

CAVEAT Coronary Angioplasty vs Excisional Atherectomy Trial

CAVEAT-I Comparison of Directional Atherectomy vs Coronary Angioplasty Trial

CAVEAT-II Coronary Angioplasty vs Directional Atherectomy for Patients with Saphenous Vein Bypass Graft Lesions [trial]

CAVG coronary artery vein graft

CAVH continuous arteriovenous hemofiltration

CAVHD continuous arteriovenous hemodialysis

CAVHDF continuous arteriovenous hemodiafiltration

CavHV caviid herpesvirus

CAVLT Children's Auditory Verbal Learning Test

CAVO common atrioventricular orifice

C(a-v)$_{O_2}$ arteriovenous oxygen tension difference

C[a&v̄]O$_2$ arteriovenous gradient of oxygen content

CAVR continuous arteriovenous rewarming

CAVS Conformance Assessment to Voluntary Standards

CAVSD complete atrioventricular septal defect

CAVU continuous arteriovenous ultrafiltration

CAW central airways

C$_{AW}$ airway conductance

CawLV caraway latent virus

CAX central axis [radiotherapy]

CaYMV canine yellow mottle virus

CB Bachelor of Surgery [Lat. *Chirurgiae Baccalaureus*]; calcium blocker; carbenicillin; carotid body; chocolate blood [agar]; chromatin body; chronic bronchitis; circumflex branch; code blue; color blind; compensated base; consensus band [genome computing]; conus branch; Coomassie blue; coprocessor board; coracobrachial

8CB octylcyanobiphenyl

Cb cerebellum; niobium [columbium]

C3b complement component 3b

CBA chronic bronchitis and asthma; Columbia blood agar [test]; cost-benefit analysis

CBAB complement-binding antibody

CBADAA Certifying Board of the American Dental Assistants Association

CBAS carotid bifurcation angioplasty and stenting

CBAVD congenital bilateral absence of vas deferens

CBBEST cutting balloon before stent

CBBM color blindness, blue mono-cone-monochromatic type

CBC carbenicillin; child behavior characteristics; compensatory base change; complete blood cell count

cbc complete blood cell count

CBCL Child Behavior Checklist; cutaneous B-cell lymphoma

CBCL/2–3 Child Behavior Checklist for ages 2–3

CBCN carbenicillin

CBCT cone-beam computed tomography

CbCtx cerebellar cortex

CBD carotid body denervation; closed bladder drainage; color blindness, deutan type; common bile duct; Convention on Biological Diversity

CBDC chronic bullous disease of children

CBDE Chemical and Biological Defense Establishment [Canada]; common bile duct exploration

CBDMP California Birth Defects Monitoring Program

CBDPR computer-based dental patient record

CBDV *Colocasia bobone* disease virus

CBE clinical breast examination

CBER Center for Biologic Evaluation and Research

CBET certified biomedical equipment technician

CBEV *Choristoneura biennis* entomopoxvirus

CBF capillary blood flow; cerebral blood flow; ciliary beat frequency; collagen-binding factor; core-binding factor; coronary blood flow; cortical blood flow

CBFB core-binding factor, beta

CBFb beta subunit of core-binding factor

CBFV coronary blood flow velocity

CBG capillary blood gases; coronary bypass graft; corticosteroid-binding globulin; cortisol-binding globulin

CBGv corticosteroid-binding globulin variant

CBH chronic benign hepatitis; cutaneous basophilic hypersensitivity

CbHV cebine herpesvirus

CBI chemical binding index; children's behavior inventory; continuous bladder irrigation; convergent beam irradiation

CBIC Certification Board in Infection Control

CBL circulating blood lymphocytes; chronic blood loss; cord blood leukocytes

Cbl cobalamin

CBLVd Citrus bent leaf viroid

CBM capillary basement membrane

CBMMP chronic benign mucous membrane pemphigus

CBN cannabinol; central benign neoplasm; Commission on Biological Nomenclature

CBNB Chemical Business News Database

CBNV Colony B North virus

CBO community-based organization; Congressional Budget Office

CBOC completion bed occupancy care

CBOD chemical and biological oxygen demand

CBOD5 5-day chemical and biological oxygen

CBP calcium-binding protein; cAMP-binding protein; carbohydrate-binding protein; cardiopulmonary bypass; chlorobiphenyl; cobalamin-binding protein; color blindness, protan type; convolution back projection; cruciform binding protein; cyclic adenosine monophosphate [cAMP] binding protein

C4BP complement 4 binding protein

CBPR computer-based patient record

CBPS chemical and biological protected shelter; congenital bilateral perisylvian syndrome

CBPV chronic bee paralysis virus

CBR carbonyl reductase; case-based reasoning; chemical, biological, and radiological [warfare]; chemically-bound residue; chronic bed rest; complete bed rest; crude birth rate

CBRL contextual Bayesian relaxation labeling technique

CBS cervicobrachial syndrome; chronic brain syndrome; clinical behavioral science; conjugated bile salts; culture-bound syndrome; cystathionine beta-synthase

CB3S Coxsackie B3 virus susceptibility

CBSD component-based software development

CBT carotid body tumor; code blue team; cognitive behavioral treatment/therapy; computed body tomography; computer-based testing; computer-based training instruction; cord blood transplant; corticobulbar tract

CBV capillary blood cell velocity; carnation bacilliform virus; catheter balloon valvuloplasty; central blood volume; cerebral blood volume; circulating blood volume; corrected blood volume; cortical blood volume; Coxsackie B virus

CBVD cerebrovascular disease

CbVd Coleus blumei viroid

CBVI computer-based video instruction

CBW chemical and biological warfare

CBX computer-based examination

CBZ carbamazepine

CC calcaneal-cuboid; calcium cyclamate; cardiac catheterization; cardiac center; cardiac contusion; cardiac cycle; cardiovascular clinic; cascade correlation; cell culture; central compartment; cerebral commissure; cerebral cortex; cervical cancer; chest circumference; chief complaint; cholecalciferol; choledochocholedochostomy; chondrocalcinosis; choriocarcinoma; chronic complainer; circulatory collapse; classical conditioning; clean catch [of urine]; Clinical Center [NIH]; clinical course; clomiphene citrate; closed cup; closing capacity; coefficient of consistency; collagenous colitis; colony count; colorectal cancer; columnar cells; commission certified; common cold; communication-client; complicating condition; complications and co-morbidity; compound cathartic; computation constant; computer calculated; computer center; concordance; congenital cardiopathy; congenital cataract; consumptive coagulopathy; contrast cystogram; conversion complete; coracoclavicular; cord compression; coronary care; corpus callosum; correlation coefficient; costochondral; Coulter counter; craniocaudal; craniocervical; creatinine clearance; critical care; critical condition; Crohn colitis; Cronkhite-Canada [syndrome]; cross correlation; crus cerebri; cubic centimeter [JCAHO unapproved abbreviation]; current complaint; Current Contents

C-C convexo-concave

C&C cold and clammy

Cc concave

cc clean catch [urine]; concave; corrected; cubic centimeter [JCAHO unapproved abbreviation]

CCA canonical correlation; cephalin cholesterol antigen; chick cell agglutination; chimpanzee coryza agent; choriocarcinoma; chromated copper arsenate; circulating cathodic antigen; circumflex coronary artery; common carotid artery; congenital contractural arachnodactyly; constitutional chromosome abnormality

CCAB complex cognitive assessment battery

CCABOT Cornell Coronary Artery Bypass Outcomes Trial

CCAg corpus callosum agenesis

CCAIT Canadian Coronary Atherosclerosis Intervention Trial

CCAM congenital cystic adenomatoid malformation; General Classification of Medical Procedures [Classification Commune des Actes Medicaux]

CCAP Cancer Chromosomal Aberration Project [database]; client-centered accreditation program

CCAT Canadian Coronary Atherectomy Trial; chick cell agglutination test; conglutinating complement absorption test

CCB calcium channel blocker

CCBD central cell-binding domain

CCBV central circulating blood volume

CCC calcium cyanamide; Canadian Cardiovascular Coalition [study]; care-cure coordination; cathodal closure contraction; center for clinical computing; child care center; Children's Communication Checklist; chlorcholine chloride; chronic calculus cholecystitis; chronic catarrhal colitis; comprehensive cancer center; comprehensive care clinic; concentration, clustering and continuity; concurrent care concern; consecutive case conference; continuous curvilinear capsulotomy;

Council on Clinical Classification; craniocerebello-cardiac [dysplasia or syndrome]; critical care complex; cylindrical confronting cisternae

CC&C colony count and culture

CCCC centrifugal countercurrent chromatography

CCCCP Comprehensive Cardiovascular Community Control Program

CCCD cooled charge-coupled device

cccDNA covalently closed circular deoxyribonucleic acid

CCCE cross-cultural cognitive examination

CCCl cathodal closure clonus

CC/CM Current Contents/Clinical Medicine

CCCN community care coordination network

CCCP carbonyl cyanide m-chloro-phenylhydrazone

CCCR closed chest cardiac resuscitation

CCCS condom catheter collecting system; critical care computer system

CCCT closed craniocerebral trauma

CCCU comprehensive cardiac care unit

CCCV *Callistephus chinensis chlorosis* virus

CCCVd Coconut cadang-cadang viroid

CCD calibration curve data; central collodiaphyseal; central core disease; charge-coupled device; childhood celiac disease; cleidocranial dysplasia; clinical cardiovascular disease; cortical collecting duct; countercurrent distribution; cumulative cardiotoxic dose

CCDC Canadian Communicable Disease Center; consultant in communicable disease control

CCD-CAMPI charge coupled device-computer analysis of mammography phantom images

CCDN Central Council for District Nursing

ccDNA closed circle deoxyribonucleic acid

CCDS case cart delivery system; color-coded duplex sonography

CCE capacitative calcium entry; carboline carboxylic acid ester; chamois contagious ecthyma; cholesterol crystal emboli; clear-cell endothelioma; clubbing, cyanosis, and edema; cornified cell envelope; countercurrent electrophoresis; cruciform cutting endonuclease

CCEHRP Committee to Coordinate Environmental Health and Related Programs

CCEI Crown-Crisp Experimental Index

CCEV cardamine chlorotic fleck virus; *Choristoneura conflicta* entomopoxvirus

CCF cancer coagulation factor; cardiolipin complement fixation; carotid-cavernous fistula; centrifuged culture fluid; cephalin-cholesterol flocculation; chronic cardiac failure; compound comminuted fracture; congestive heart failure; cross-correlation function; crystal-induced chemotactic factor

CCFA cefotoxin-cycloserine fructose agar

CCFAS compact colony-forming active substance

CCFE cyclophosphamide, cisplatin, fluorouracil, and extramustine

CCFMG Cooperating Committee on Foreign Medical Graduates

CCFV cardamine chlorotic fleck virus

CCG Children's Cancer Study Group; cholecystogram, cholecystography; clinically coherent group

CCGC capillary column gas chromatography

CCGS cell cycle G and S

CCH C-cell hyperplasia; central clinical hospital; chronic chloride hemagglutination; chronic cholestatic hepatitis; cross-correlation histogram

CCHA Canadian Council on Hospital Accreditation

CCHAT Canadian Cozaar, Hyzaar and Amlodipine Trial

CC-HC coordinated collective homecare [France]

CCHD Caephilly Collaborative Heart Disease [study]; cyanotic congenital heart disease

CCHE Central Council for Health Education

CCHF, C-CHF Crimean-Congo hemorrhagic fever

CCHFA Canadian Council on Health Facilities Accreditation

CCHMS Central Committee for Hospital Medical Services

CChMVd Chrysanthemum chlorotic mottle viroid

CCHP Consumer Choice Health Plan; Corpus Christi Heart Project

CCHPR Canadian Consortium for Health Promotion Research; clinical classification of health policy research

CCHS congenital central hypoventilation syndrome; Copenhagen City Heart Study

CCHSA Canadian Council on Health Services Accreditation

CCI Canadian Classification of Health Interventions; Cancer Care International; Cardiovascular Credentialing International; cholesterol crystallization inhibitor; chronic coronary insufficiency; common client interface; component communication interface; correct coding initiative; corrected count increment; Cronqvist cranial index; crowded cell index

CCI/F cortico-cortical inhibition and facilitation

CC-IMED California Consortium of Information in Medical Education and Development

CCK cholecystokinin

CCK-8 cholecystokinin octapeptide

CCKLI cholecystokinin-like immunoreactivity

CCK-OP cholecystokinin octapeptide

CCK-PZ cholecystokinin-pancreozymin

CCKRB cholecystokinin receptor B

CCL carcinoma cell line; certified cell line; Charcot-Leyden crystal; continuing care level; continuous cell line; costoclavicular ligament; critical carbohydrate level

CCLE chronic cutaneous lupus erythematosus

CCLI composite clinical and laboratory index

CC/LS Current Contents/Life Sciences

CCM cerebrocostomandibular [syndrome]; chemical cleavage of mismatch; complicated case management; congestive cardiomyopathy; craniocervical malformation; critical care medicine

c cm cubic centimeter

CCMC Committee on the Costs of Medical Care

CCMDS Core Community Minimum Data Set [Scotland]

CCME Coordinating Council on Medical Education

CCMG Canadian College of Medical Geneticists

CCML Comprehensive Core Medical Library

CCMoV cereal chlorotic mottle virus

CCMS cerebrocostomandibular syndrome; clean catch midstream [urine]; clinical care management system

CCMSU clean catch midstream urine

CCMT catechol methyltransferase

CCMV cowpea chlorotic mottle virus

CCMU critical care medical unit

CCN cancer center network; caudal central nucleus; community care network; coronary care nursing; critical care nursing

CCNHP community college nursing home project

CCNU N-(2-chloroethyl)-N'-cyclo-hexyl-N-nitrosourea [lomustine]

CCO cytochrome C oxidase

CcO$_2$ capillary oxygen content

CCORP Cornell-China-Oxford Research Project

CCOT cervical compression overloading test

CCoV canine coronavirus

CCP Canadian Classification of Diagnostic, Therapeutic, and Surgical Interventions; cephalin-cholesterol flocculation; charge class pair; chronic calcifying pancreatitis; ciliocytophthoria; columnar cell papilloma; community care plan; comprehensive care plan; cooperative cardiovascular project; coordinated care program; critical control point [food safety]; cytidine cyclic phosphate

CCPD continuous cycling (cyclical) peritoneal dialysis

CCPDS Centralized Cancer Patient Data System

C-CPE C terminal half of *Clostridium perfringens* enterotoxin

CCPMS Cancer Centre Patient Management System [Australia]; computer-assisted clinical pathway management system

CCPR closed-chest cardiopulmonary resuscitation; crypt cell production rate

CCPT Chinese Cancer Prevention Trial

CCR Canadian Cancer Registry; complete continuous remission; complex chromosome rearrangement; consistency and concurrency reporting; Coriell Cell Repositories; correct classification rate; creatinine clearance

C-CR Computing-Communications Research Division [National Science Foundation (NSF)]

Ccr, C$_{cr}$ creatinine clearance

CCRC comprehensive care retirement community; continuing care retirement community

CCRG Cooperative Cataract Research Group

CCRIS Chemical Carcinogenesis Research Information System [NLM database]

CCRN Critical Care Registered Nurse

CCRS Chemical Carcinogenesis Research Information System; computer-controlled radiotherapy system

CCRS/SP computer-controlled radiotherapy system sequence processor

CCRT Cardiac Catheter Reuse Trial; computer-controlled conformal radiotherapy; computer-controlled radiation therapy

CcRV-W2 *Carcinus mediterraneus* W2 virus

CCS Canadian Cardiovascular Society; cardiac care system; case-control study; casualty clearing station; cell cycle specific; certified coding specialist; Chinese Cardiac Study; cholecystosonography; chronic cerebellar stimulation; chronic compartment syndrome; clear cell sarcoma; cloudy cornea syndrome; composite cultured skin; concentration camp syndrome; costoclavicular syndrome; crippled children's service

CCSCS central cervical spinal cord syndrome

CCSE Cognitive Capacity Screening Examination

CCSG Canadian Cooperative Study Group; Children's Cancer Study Group

CCSK clear cell sarcoma of the kidney

CCSM cervical cancer-specific mortality

CCSP Clara cell-specific protein

CCSRG Cochrane Collaboration Stroke Review Group

CCST chemical casualty site team

CCT carotid compression tomography; central conduction time; cerebrocranial trauma; charge class torsion; Chinese Captopril Trial; chocolate-coated tablet; coated compressed tablet; combined cortical thickness; composite cyclic therapy; computerized cranial tomography; continuum charge transfer; contrast-enhanced computed tomography; controlled cord traction; conventional computed tomography; coronary care team; cortical collecting tubule; cranial computed tomography; critical care technician; cyclocarbothiamine

CCTA coronal computed tomographic arthrography

CCTe cathodal closure tetanus

CCTG California Cooperative Treatment Group

CC-TGA congenitally corrected transposition of great vessels

CC-TOE continuum of care trauma outcome evaluation

CCTP coronary care training program

CCTR Cochrane Controlled Trials Register [UK]; common clinical term reference

CCTV closed circuit television

CCU cardiac care unit; Cherry-Crandall unit; Consulting Committee on Units [Comité Consultatif des Unités]; coronary care unit; critical care unit

ccua clean catch urinalysis

CCUP colpocystourethropexy

CCV carnation cryptic virus; channel catfish virus; closed circuit voltage; conductivity cell volume

CCVD chronic cerebrovascular disease

CCVM congenital cardiovascular malformation

CCW critical care workstation; counterclockwise

CCWISB Canadian Chemical Warfare Inter-Service Board

CCX cyclo-oxygenase

CD cadaver donor; caldesmon; canine distemper; canine dose; carbohydrate dehydratase; carbon dioxide; cardiac disease; cardiac dullness; cardiac dysrhythmia; cardiovascular disease; Carrel-Dakin [fluid]; Castleman disease; cation-dependent; caudad, caudal; celiac disease; cell dissociation; cervicodorsal; cesarean delivery; chemical dependency; chlordecone; circular dichroism; *cis*-dioxolane; cluster of differentiation [antigens]; color Doppler; combination drug; common [bile] duct; communicable disease; compact disk; completely denaturated; conduct disorder; conduction disorder; conjugata diagonalis; consanguineous donor; conserved domain; contact dermatitis; contagious disease; contrast-detail [imaging]; control diet; controlled drug; conventional dialysis; convulsive disorder; convulsive dose; corneal dystrophy; cortical dysplasia; Cotrel-Dubousset [rod]; Crohn disease; crossed diagonal; curative dose; cutdown; cystic duct; cytochalasin D; cytoplasmic domain

2CD two-cycle duration

CD4 HIV helper cell count

CD8 HIV suppressor cell count

CD₅₀ median curative dose

C/D cigarettes per day; cup to disc ratio

C&D cystoscopy and dilatation

Cd cadmium; caudal; coccygeal; condylion

cd candela; caudal

c/d cigarettes per day

CDA Canadian Dental Association; Certified Dental Assistant; chenodeoxycholic acid; ciliary dyskinesia activity; clinical document architecture; complement-dependent antibody; completely denatured alcohol; compound document architecture; computer diagnostic assistant; congenital dyserythropoietic anemia

CdA chlorodeoxyadenosine

CDAC Clinical Data Abstraction Center

CDAD Clostridium difficile-associated disease

CDAE chemical defense aircrew ensemble

CDAI Crohn disease activity index

CDAL clinical data analysis laboratory

CDAP continuous distending airway pressure

CDB communication-database

C&DB cough and deep breath

CDC calculated date of confinement; cancer diagnosis center; capillary diffusion capacity; casualty decontamination center; cell division control; cell division cycle; Centers for Disease Control and Prevention; chenodeoxycholate; children's diagnostic classification; Communicable Disease Center; complement-dependent cytotoxicity; Crohn disease of colon

CD-C controlled drinker-control

CDCA chenodeoxycholic acid

CDC-BRFS Centers for Disease Control Behavioral Risk Factor Survey

CDCC complement-dependent cellular cytotoxicity

CDCE constant denaturant capillary electrophoresis

cDCIS comedo-type ductal carcinoma in situ

CDC NAC Centers for Disease Control and Prevention of National AIDS Clearinghouse

CDCV Caddo Canyon virus

CDD certificate of disability for discharge; choledochoduodenostomy; chronic degenerative disease; chronic disabling dermatosis; congenital diaphragmatic defect; conserved domain database; contrast-detail-dose [imaging]; craniodiaphyseal dysplasia; current disease descriptions; [poly]chlorinated dibenzo-*p*-dioxin

CDDP cis-diaminedichloroplatinum

CDE canine distemper encephalitis; chlordiazepoxide; color Doppler energy [imaging]; common data element; common duct exploration

CDEC Comprehensive Developmental Evaluation Chart

CDER Center for Drug Evaluation and Research

CDEV *Choristoneura diversuma* entomopoxvirus

CDF chondrodystrophia foetalis; class conditional density function; clinical data field; clinical data framework; common data format; cumulative distribution function; [poly]chlorinated dibenzofuran

CDG carbohydrate-deficient glycoprotein syndrome; central developmental groove

CDGE constant denaturant gel electrophoresis

CDGG corneal dystrophy Groenouw type, granular

CDGS carbohydrate-deficient glycoprotein syndrome

cDGS complete form of DiGeorge syndrome

CDH ceramide dihexoside; congenital diaphragmatic hernia; congenital dislocation of hip; congenital dysplasia of hip

CDHAp calcium-deficient hydroxyapatite

CDI cell-directed inhibitor; central or chronic diabetes insipidus; Children's Depression Inventory; clinical data interchange; color Doppler imaging; communicable disease intelligence; cranial diabetes insipidus; cyclin-dependent kinase interactor

CDILD chronic diffuse interstitial lung disease

CDK caldesmon kinase; cell division kinase; climatic droplet keratopathy; cyclin-dependent kinase

CDL chlordeoxylincomycin; Cornelia de Lange [syndrome]

CDLE chronic discoid lupus erythematosus

CDLS Cornelia de Lange syndrome

CDM chemically defined medium; clinical decision making; common data model

CDMMS chorioretinal dysplasia-microcephaly-mental retardation syndrome

CDMNS clinical decision making in nursing scale

CD-MPR cation-dependent mannose-6-phosphate receptor

CdMV cardamom mosaic virus

cDNA circular deoxyribonucleic acid; complementary deoxyribonucleic acid

CDNANZ Communicable Disease Network of Australia and New Zealand

CDNB 1-chloro-2,4-dinitrobenzene

CDP chondrodysplasia punctata; chronic destructive periodontitis; collagenase-digestible protein; continuous distending pressure; coronary drug project; Council on Dental Practice; cytidine diphosphate; cytosine diphosphate

CDPAS Coronary Disease Prevention with Aspirin Study; Coronary Drug Project Aspirin Study

CDPC cytidine diphosphate choline

CDPR chondrodysplasia punctata, rhizomelic

CDPS calcium-dependent protease small subunit

CDPX X-linked chondrodysplasia punctata

CDR calcium-dependent regulator; clinical data repository; clinical dementia rating; close delay ratio; common data repository; complementarity-determining region; complementary-determining region; computerized digital radiography; cup/disk ratio

CDRH Center for Devices and Radiological Health

CD-ROM compact disk-read only memory

CDRP clinical database research program

CDRS Children's Depression Rating Scale

CDS cardiovascular surgery; Care Dependency Scale; catechol-3, 5-disulfonate; caudal dysplasia syndrome; Chemical Data System; Children's Diagnostic Scale; Christian Dental Society; clean data set; clinical decision-support; cumulative duration of survival

CdS cadmium sulfide; [gene] coding sequence

CDSA common data security architecture

CDSC Communicable Diseases Surveillance Centre [UK]

CDSM Committee on Dental and Surgical Materials

CDSR Cochrane Database of Systematic Reviews

cd-sr candela-steradian

CDSRF chronic disease and sociodemographic risk factors

CDSS [computer-assisted] clinical decision support system

CD(S)U Communicable Diseases (Scotland) Unit

CDT carbohydrate-deficient transferrin; carbon dioxide therapy; Certified Dental Technician; children's day treatment; *Clostridium difficile* toxin; color discrimination test; combined diphtheria-tetanus [vaccine]

CDTA cyclohexanediaminetetraacetic acid

CDTe cathode duration tetanus

CDTF chemical decontamination training facility

CdTV chino del tomate virus

CDU cardiac diagnostic unit; clinical decision unit; color Doppler ultrasound; complete dependence unit

CDUV Candiru virus

CDV canine distemper virus; chlorotic dwarf virus; clinical diagnostic validity; Colombian datura virus

cDVH cumulative dose-volume histogram

Cdyn, C$_{dyn}$ dynamic compliance

Cdyn, rs dynamic compliance of the respiratory system

CDYS cell dysfunction [UMLS]

CDZ chlordiazepoxide; conduction delay zone

CE California encephalitis; capillary electrophoresis; carboxylesterase; cardiac enlargement; cardioesophageal; carotid endarterectomy; catamenial epilepsy; cataract extraction; cell extract; center-edge [angle]; central episiotomy; chemical energy; chick embryo; chloroform ether; cholesterol esters; cholesteryl ester; chorioepithelioma; chromatoelectrophoresis; ciliated epithelium; cloning efficiency; coded element; coefficient of error; columnar epithelium; conical elevation; conjugated estrogens; constant error; continuing education; contractile element; contrast-enhancement [imaging]; converting enzyme; cornified epithelium; crude extract; cytoplasmic extract; cytopathic effect

C-E chloroform-ether

Ce cerium

C$_e$ effect [compartment] concentration

CEA carcinoembryonic antigen; carotid endarterectomy; cholesterol-esterifying activity; cost-effectiveness analysis; cranial epidural abscess; crystalline egg albumin; cultured epithelial autograft

CEAC clinical education and assessment center; cost-effectiveness acceptability curve

CEAF cost-effectiveness acceptability frontier

CEAL carcinoembryonic antigen-like [protein]

CEAP class, etiology, anatomy, pathophysiology [classification of venous diseases]; Clinical Efficacy Assessment Project

CEARP Continuing Education Approval and Recognition Program

CEASE Collaborative European Anti-Smoking Evaluation

CEAT chronic ectopic atrial tachycardia

CEB calcium entry blocker

cEBV chronic Epstein-Barr virus [infection]

CEC central echo complex; ciliated epithelial cell; Commission of the European Community

CECCC confidential enquiry into cardiac catheterization complications

CECR cat eye syndrome chromosome region

CECT contrast-enhanced computed tomography

CED chondroectodermal dysplasia; clinical engineering department

CEDARS Comprehensive Evaluation of Defibrillators and Resuscitative Shock Study

CeDNV *Casphalia externa* densovirus

CEE Central European encephalitis; chick embryo extract; component execution environment

CEEA curved end-to-end anastomosis [stapler]

CEEF clinical evaluation encounter form

CEEG computer-analyzed electroencephalography

CEES chloroethyl ethyl sulfide

CEET chicken enucleated eye test

CEEV Central European encephalitis virus

CEF centrifugation extractable fluid; chick embryo fibroblast; constant electric field

CEFA continuous epidural fentanyl anesthesia

CE-FAST contrast enhanced-fast acquisition in a steady state

CEFMG Council on Education for Foreign Medical Graduates

CEG chronic erosive gastritis

CEH cholesterol ester hydrolase

CEHC calf embryonic heart cell; cost-effective healthcare

CEHN Children's Environmental Health Network

CEHO Chief Environmental Health Officer [UK]

CeHV cercopithecine herpesvirus

CEI character education inquiry; converting enzyme inhibitor

CEI-AMI converting enzyme inhibitor in the treatment of acute myocardial infarction

CEID crossed electroimmunodiffusion

CEJ cement-enamel junction

CEJA Council on Ethical and Judicial Affairs [American Medical Association]

CEK chick embryo kidney

CEL carboxyl-ester lipase

CelCer1V *Caenorhabditis elegans* Cer1 virus

CELDIC Commission on Emotional and Learning Disorders in Children

CELL Cost Effectiveness of Lipid Lowering [study]

Cell celluloid

CELO chick embryonal lethal orphan [virus]

CELP code excited linear prediction [ECG]

Cels Celsius

CEM care environment management; central extensor mechanism; clinical event monitor; computerized electroencephalographic map; conventional transmission electron microscope

CEMIA Center for Engineering and Medical Image Analysis

CEMIS community-based environmental management information system

CE-MRA contrast enhanced magnetic resonance angiography

CE-MRI contrast-enhanced magnetic resonance imaging

CeMV celery mosaic virus; cetacean morbillivirus

CEN Certificate for Emergency Nursing; Clinical Experience Network [study]; Comité European de Normalisation (standards); continuous enteral nutrition

cen centromere; central

CENMR capillary electrophoresis nuclear magnetic resonance

CENOG computerized electro-neuro-ophthalmography

CENP centromere protein

CENPA centromeric protein A

CENPB centromeric protein B

CENPC centromeric protein C

CENPD centromeric protein D

CENPE centromeric protein E

CENT Committee for European Normalisation

cent centigrade; central

CEO chick embryo origin; Chief Executive Officer

CEOEECP Clinical Evaluation of Enhanced External Counterpulsation

CEOT calcifying epithelial odontogenic tumor

CEP care evaluation program; centromere evaluation probe; chronic eosinophilic pneumonia; chronic erythropoietic porphyria; clinical evaluation protocol; congenital erythropoietic porphyria; continuing education program; cortical evoked potential; counter-electrophoresis

CEPA chloroethane phosphoric acid

CEPH cephalic; cephalosporin; Council on Education for Public Health

ceph cephalin

CEPH FLOC cephalin flocculation

CEPU cerebellar Purkinje [cell]

CEQ Council on Environmental Quality

CER capital expenditure review; ceramide; ceruloplasmin; conditioned emotional response; control electrical rhythm; cortical evoked response

CERAD Consortium to Establish a Registry for Alzheimer disease

CERCLA Comprehensive Environmental Response, Compensation, and Liability Act

CERCLIS Comprehensive Environmental Response, Communication, and Liability Information System

CERD chronic end-stage renal disease

CERP complex event-related potential; Continuing Education Recognition Program

CERT Cardiovascular Event Reduction Trial; Center for Education and Research on Therapeutics; computer emergency response team

Cert, cert certified

Cer1V Cer1 virus

cerv cervix, cervical

CES carboxylesterase; cauda equina syndrome; cat's eye syndrome; Center for Epidemiological Study; central excitatory state; chronic electrophysiological study; clinical engineering services; conditioned escape response; Corpus Encoding Standard

CESAR Centralised European Studies in Angina Research

CESARZ Clinical European Studies in Angina and Revascularization

CESD cholesterol ester storage disease

CES-D Center for Epidemiological Studies of Depression [scale]

CESG Cerebral Embolism Study Group [trial]

CESNA Comparative Efficacy and Safety of Nisoldipine and Amlodipine [in hypertension]

CESNA II Comparative Efficacy and Safety of Nisoldipine and Amlodipine [in hypertension with ischemic heart disease]

CESS Cooperative Ewing's Sarcoma Study

CET capital expenditure threshold; cholesterol-ester transfer; Collaborative Eclampsia Trial; congenital eyelid tetrad

CETE Central European tick-borne encephalitis

CETP cholesteryl ester transfer protein

CEU congenital ectropion uveae; continuing education unit

CEV California encephalitis virus; *Citrus exocortis* viroid

CEVd *Citrus exocortis* viroid

CEVd-III *Citrus exocortis* III viroid

CEVd-IV *Citrus exocortis* IV viroid

CEX clinical evaluation exercise

CeYMB celery yellow mosaic virus

CeYMV celery yellow mosaic virus

CEZ cefazolin

CF calcaneal fibular [ligament]; calcium leucovorin; calf blood flow; calibration factor; cancer-free; carbol-fuchsin; carbon filtered; carboxyfluorescein; cardiac failure; cardiac fibroblast; carotid foramen; carrier-free; cascade filtration; case file; Caucasian female; centrifugal force; characteristic frequency; chemotactic factor; chest and left leg [lead in electrocardiography]; Chiari-Frommel [syndrome]; chick fibroblast; Christmas factor; chronicity factor; circumflex; citrovorum factor; clotting factor; colicin factor; collected fluid; colonization factor; colony forming; complementary feeding; complement fixation; computed fluoroscopy; constant frequency; contractile force; cord factor; coronary flow; correction factor; cough frequency; count fingers; counting finger; coupling factor; cycling fibroblast; cystic fibrosis; folinic acid [citrovorum factor]

Cf californium

cf centrifugal force; bring together, compare [Lat. *confer*]; confidence factor

CFA cerebello-facio-articular [syndrome]; 2-chloro-4-fluoroaniline; colonization factor antigen; colony-forming assay; common femoral artery; complement-fixing antibody; complete Freund's adjuvant; configuration frequency analysis; cryptogenic fibrosing alveolitis

CFAG cystic fibrosis antigen

CFAV cell fusing agent virus

CFB central fibrous body

CFC capillary filtration coefficient; cardiofaciocutaneous [syndrome]; chlorofluorocarbon; colony-forming capacity; colony-forming cell; continuous flow centrifugation

CfCPV *Choristoneura fumiferana* cypovirus

CFD cephalofacial deformity; color flow Doppler; computational fluid dynamics; craniofacial dysostosis

CF-DA carboxyfluorescein diacetate

CFDS craniofacial dyssynostosis

CFDU color-flow Doppler ultrasonography; color flow Doppler ultrasound

CFEV *Choristoneura fumiferana* entomopoxvirus

CFF critical flicker fusion [test]; critical fusion frequency; cystic fibrosis factor; Cystic Fibrosis Foundation

cff critical flicker fusion; critical fusion frequency

CFFA cystic fibrosis factor activity

CFH complement factor H; Council on Family Health

CFHL complement factor H-like [protein]

CFHP Council on Federal Health Programs

CFI chemotactic-factor inactivator; closed-clenched fist injury; color flow imaging; community fluorosis index; complement fixation inhibition

CfIV *Campoletis flavicincta* ichnovirus

CFM cerebral function monitor; chlorofluoromethane; close-fitting mask; composite filling material; craniofacial microsomia

CFMA Council for Medical Affairs

CFMDB Cystic Fibrosis Mutation Database

CFMG Commission on Foreign Medical Graduates

CfMNPV *Choristoneura fumiferana* multiple nucleopolyhedrovirus

CfMS careflow management system

CFMV constant flow mechanical ventilation

CFND craniofrontonasal dysostosis; craniofrontonasal dysplasia

CFNS chills, fever, night sweats; craniofrontonasal syndrome

CFO chief financial officer

CfoIV *Casinaria forcipata* ichnovirus

CFOS constrained fast orthogonal search

CFP chronic false positive; ciguatera fish poisoning; Clinical Fellowship Program; culture filtrate protein; cyclophosphamide, fluorouracil, prednisone; cystic fibrosis of pancreas; cystic fibrosis protein

CFPC College of Family Physicians of Canada

CFPP craniofacial pattern profile

CFPR Canadian Familial Polyposis Registry

CFR case-fatality ratio; citrovorum-factor rescue; Code of Federal Regulations; complement-fixation reaction; coronary flow reserve; correct fast reaction; cyclic flow reduction

CFS cancer family syndrome; Chiari-Frommel syndrome; chronic fatigue syndrome; craniofacial stenosis; crush fracture syndrome; culture fluid supernatant; Cystic Fibrosis Society

CFSAN Center for Safety and Applied Nutrition

CFSE crystal field stabilization energy

CFSTI Clearinghouse for Federal Scientific and Technical Information

CFT cardiolipin flocculation test; clinical full time; complement-fixation test; crystal field theory

CFTC complication-free tumor control

CFTR cystic fibrosis transmembrane conductance regulator

CFU colony-forming unit; coupling factor unit

cfu colony-forming unit

CFU-C, CFU$_C$ colony-forming unit, culture

CFU-E, CFU$_E$ colony-forming unit, erythrocyte

CFU-EOS, CFU$_{EOS}$ colony-forming unit, eosinophil

CFU-F, CFU$_F$ colony-forming unit-fibroblastoid

CFU-G, CFU$_G$ colony-forming unit, granulocyte

CFU-GEMM, CFU$_{GEMM}$ colony forming unit, granulocyte, erythrocyte, macrophage, megakaryocyte

CFU-GM, CFU$_{GM}$ colony-forming unit, granulocyte macrophage

CFU-L, CFU$_L$ colony-forming unit, lymphocyte

CFU$_M$ colony-forming unit-megakaryocyte

CFU-MEG, CFU$_{MEG}$ colony-forming unit, megakaryocyte

CFUN cell function [UMLS]

CFU-NM, CFU$_{NM}$ colony-forming unit, neutrophil-monocyte

CFU-S, CFU$_S$ colony-forming unit, spleen; colony-forming unit, stem cells

CFUSA Cystic Fibrosis Foundation USA

CfuT1V *Cladosporium fulvum* T-1 virus

CFUV Corfu virus

CFV chimpanzee foamy virus; chlorotic fleck virus; *Chrysanthemum frutescens* virus; continuous flow ventilation

CFV/HU chimpanzee foamy virus/human

CFVS cerebrospinal fluid flow void sign

CFW Carworth farm [mouse] Webster strain

CFWM cancer-free white mouse

CFX cefoxitin; circumflex coronary artery

CFX-MARG marginal branch of the circumflex [coronary] artery

CFZ capillary free zone

CFz clofazimine

CFZC continuous-flow zonal centrifugation

CG calcium gluconate; cardiography; Cardio-Green; caregiver; central gray matter; choking gas; cholecystogram; cholecystography; choriogenic gynecomastia; chorionic gonadotropin; chromogranin; chronic glomerulonephritis; cingulate gyrus; colloidal gold; continuous flow ventilation; control group; cryoglobulin; cystine guanine; cytosine-guanine-guanine; phosgene [choking gas]

cg center of gravity; centigram; chemoglobulin

Cγ gamma chain constant region [immunoglobulins]

CGA catabolite gene activator; color graphics adapter; comprehensive geriatric assessment

CGAB congenital abnormality [UMLS]

CGAS Children's Global Assessment Scale

CGAP Cancer Genome Anatomy Project

CGAT Canadian Genome and Technology [program]; chromatin granule amine transformer

CGB chronic gonadotropin, beta-unit

CGC cumulus-granulosa cell

CGD Cattle Genome Database; chronic granulomatous disease

CGDE contact glow discharge electrolysis

CGE capillary gel electrophoresis

CGF cell generating factor

CGFH congenital fibrous histiocytoma

CGFNS Commission on Graduates of Foreign Nursing Schools

CGGE constant gradient gel electrophoresis

CGH chorionic gonadotropic hormone; comparative genome hybridization; congenital generalized hypertrichosis

CGI chronic granulomatous inflammation; Clinical Global Impression [scale]; combustible gas indicator; common gateway interface [of the NCSA]; computer-generated imagery

cGK cyclic guanosine monophosphate [cGMP] dependent protein kinase

CGKD complex glycerol kinase deficiency

CGL chronic granulocytic leukemia; clinical guidelines

c gl correction with glasses

CGLV Changuinola virus

CGM Center for Genetics in Medicine; central gray matter

cgm centigram

CGMC Center for Graphic Medical Communication

CGMMV cucumber green mottle mosaic virus

CGMP current good manufacturing practices

cGMP cyclic guanosine monophosphate; cyclic guanosyl monophosphate

CGN chronic glomerulonephritis

CGNB composite ganglioneuroblastoma

CG/OQ cerebral glucose-oxygen quotient

CGP *N*-carbobenzoxy-glycyl-L-phenylalanine; choline glycerophosphatide; chorionic growth hormone-prolactin; circulating granulocyte pool; circulatory gene pool

CGPM Conférence Générale de Poids et Mesures [General Conference of Weights and Measures]

CGRMV cherry green ring mottle virus

CGRP, cGRP calcitonin gene-related peptide

CGRPR calcitonin gene-related peptide receptor

CGS cardiogenic shock; catgut suture; causal genesis syndrome

CGS, cgs centimeter-gram-second [system]

CGT chorionic gonadotropin; cyclodextrin glucanotransferase

CGTT cortisone glucose tolerance test

CGV Chobar Gorge virus

CGVHD chronic graft-versus-host disease

CGW caregiver workstation

cGy centigray (1 rad)

CH case history; Chédiak-Higashi [syndrome]; chiasma; *Chinese hamster*; chloral hydrate; cholesterol; Christchurch chromosome; chronic hepatitis; chronic hypertension; common hepatic [duct]; communicating hydrocele; community health; community hospital; completely healed; congenital hypothyroidism; Conradi-Hünermann [syndrome]; continuous heparin [infusion]; cortical hamartoma; crown-heel [length]; cycloheximide; cystic hygroma; wheelchair

C$_H$1, C$_H$2, C$_H$3, C$_H$4 1st to 4th constant regions in heavy chains of immunoglobulin molecules

CH$_{50}$ 50% hemolyzing dose of complement

C_H constant region in heavy chain of immunoglobulin molecule

C&H cocaine and heroin; coarse and harsh [breathing]

Ch chest; Chido [antibody]; chief; child; choline; Christchurch [syndrome]; chromosome

Ch⁺ hydrogen ion concentration

ch chest; child; chronic

CHA Canadian Hospital Association; Catholic Health Association; *Chinese hamster*; chronic hemolytic anemia; common hepatic artery; congenital hypoplasia of adrenal glands; congenital hypoplastic anemia; continuously heated aerosol; cyclohexyladenosine; cyclohexylamine

ChA choline acetylase

ChAC choline acetyltransferase

CHAD Cholesterol, Hypertension and Diabetes [study]; cold hemagglutinin disease; cyclophosphamide, hexamethylmelamine, Adriamycin (doxorubicin), and cisplatin

ChAdV chimpanzee adenovirus

CHAF central hyperalimentation nutrition

CHAID chi-squared automatic interaction detection; chi-squared automatic interaction detector

CHAIN Contact Health Advice Information Network for Effective Health Care [UK]

CHAMP Cardiac Hospitalization Atherosclerosis Management Program; chemically hardened air-management plant; Children with HIV and Acquired AIDS Model Program; Children's Hospital Automated Medical Program; Combination Hemotherapy and Mortality Prevention [study]

CHAMPUS Civilian Health and Medical Program of Uniformed Services

CHAMPVA Civilian Health and Medical Program of Veterans Administration

CHANDS curly hair-ankyloblepharon-nail dysplasia syndrome

Chang C Chang conjunctiva cells

CHANGE Chronic Heart Failure and Graded Exercise [study]

Chang L Chang liver cells

CHAOS Cambridge Heart Antioxidant Study; Cardiovascular Disease, Hypertension and Hyperlipidemia, Adult-onset Diabetes, Obesity, and Stroke [study]

CHAP Certified Hospital Admission Program; child health assessment program; Community Health Accreditation Program

CHAPS Carvedilol Heart Attack Pilot Study; 3[3-cholaminopropyl diethylammonio]-1-propane sulfonate

CHAR continuous hyperfractionated accelerated radiotherapy

CHARGE coloboma, heart disease, atresia choanae, retarded growth and retarded development and/or CNS anomalies, genital hypoplasia, and ear anomalies and/or deafness [syndrome]

CHARM Candesartan in Heart Failure Assessment in Reduction of Mortality

CHARMM Chemistry at Harvard Molecular Mechanics

CHART Continuous Hormones as Replacement Therapy [study]; Continuous Hyperfractionated Accelerated Radiotherapy Trial

CHAS Center for Health Administration Studies; Community Health Assessment Study

CHASE cut holes and sink 'em [operation]

CHAT conversational hypertext access technology

ChAT choline acetyltransferase

CHATH chemically hardened air transportable hospital

CHB chronic hepatitis B; complete heart block; congenital heart block

ChB Bachelor of Surgery [Lat. *Chirurgiae Baccalaureus*]

CHBA congenital Heinz body hemolytic anemia

CHBHA congenital Heinz body hemolytic anemia

CHC chromosome condensation; community health center; community health computing; community health council

CH₃ CCNU semustine

CHCIS community health care information system

CHCL congenital healed cleft lip

CHCP correctional health care program

CHCS composite health care system

CHCT caffeine/halothane contracture test

CHD Chédiak-Higashi disease; childhood disease; child in semantic hierarchy [UMLS]; chronic hemodialysis; common hepatic duct; congenital or congestive heart disease; congenital hip dislocation;

constitutional hepatic dysfunction; coronary heart disease; cyanotic heart disease

ChD Doctor of Surgery [Lat. *Chirurgiae Doctor*]

CHDM comprehensive hospital drug monitoring

CHDP Child Health and Disability Prevention [program]

ChE cholinesterase

che a gene involved in chemotaxis

CHEAPER Confirmation that Heparin Is an Alternative to Promote Early Reperfusion in Acute Myocardial Infarction [study]

CHEC clearinghouse for emergency aid to the community; community hypertension evaluation clinic

CHED congenital hereditary endothelial dystrophy

CHEER Chest Pain Evaluation in Emergency Room [trial]

CHEF Chinese hamster embryo fibroblast; contour-clamped homologous electric field

CHEM chemical [UMLS]

chem chemistry, chemical; chemotherapy

ChemID Chemical Identification; Chemical Identification File [NLM database]

CHEMLINE Chemical Dictionary On-Line

Chemo chemotherapy

CHEMTREC Chemical Transportation Emergency Center

CHEP cricohyoidoepiglottopexy

CHEPER Chest Pain Evaluation Registry [study]

CHERSS continuous high-amplitude EEG rhythmical synchronous slowing

CHESS chemical shift selective; Comprehensive Health-Enhancement Support System

CHEST chick embryotoxicity screening test; Combined Higher Education Software Team

CHF chick embryo fibroblast; chronic heart failure; congenital hepatic fibrosis; congestive heart failure; Crimean hemorrhagic fever

CHFD controlled high flux dialysis

CHFDT congestive heart failure data tool

CHF-IES Congestive Heart Failure-Italian Epidemiological Study

CHF-STAT Congestive Heart Failure-Survival Trial of Antiarrhythmic Therapy

CHFV combined high-frequency ventilation

chg change, changed

CHGA chromogranin A

CHGB chromogranin B

CHH cartilage-hair hypoplasia

CHHS congenital hypothalamic hamartoma syndrome

ChHV chelonid herpesvirus

CHI clinical health informatics; closed head injury; consumer health information; creatinine height index

chi chimera

χ Greek letter *chi*

χ^2 chi-squared [test, measure goodness of fit]; chi-squared statistic

χ_m magnetic susceptibility

χ_s electric susceptibility

Chi-A chimpanzee leukocyte antigen

CHIC Cardiovascular Health In Children [study]

CHID Combined Health Information [NIH] Database

CHIKV Chikungunya virus

CHILD congenital hemidysplasia with ichthyosiform erythroderma and limb defects [syndrome]

CHILI Consumer Health Information Literature [database, UK]

CHIM Center for Healthcare Information Management

CHIME Center for Health Information Management and Evaluation; College of Healthcare Information Management Executives; coloboma, heart anomaly, ichthyosis, mental retardation, ear abnormality

CHIMR Centre for Health Information Management Research [UK]

CHIMS community-based health information system

CHIMV Chim virus

CHIN community health information network

CHINA chronic infectious neurotropic agent

CHIP child health improvement program; Children's Health Insurance Program; comprehensive health insurance plan; Coronary Health Improvement Project

CHIPA community health planning agency

CHIPASAT Children's Paced Auditory Serial Addition Task

CHIPS catastrophic health insurance plans

CHiQ Centre for Health Information Quality [UK]

Chir Doct Doctor of Surgery [Lat. *Chirurgiae Doctor*]

chirug surgical [Lat. *chirurgicalis*]

CHIS community health information system; Consumer Health Information Systems

CHIV Chilibre virus

CHL Chinese hamster lung; chlorambucil; chloramphenicol

Chl chloroform; chlorophyll

CHLA cyclohexyl linoleic acid

Chlb chlorobutanol

CHLD chronic hypoxic lung disease

chlor chloride

CHLS combined heart and lung surgery

ChlVPP chlorambucil, vinblastine, procarbazine, prednisone

ChM Master of Surgery [Lat. *Chirurgiae Magister*]

CHMD clinical hyaline membrane disease

CHMIS community health management information system

CHMR Centre for Health Information Management Research [UK]

ChmVd chlorotic mottle viroid

CHN carbon, hydrogen, and nitrogen; child health nurse; child neurology; Chinese [hamster]; community health nurse

CHNS China Health and Nutrition Survey

CHO carbohydrate; Chinese hamster ovary; chorea; comprehensive health organization

Cho choline

C$_{H_2O}$ water clearance

choc chocolate

CHOICE Caring for Hypertension on Initiation: Cost and Effectiveness [study]; Congestive Heart Failure Mortality: Investigation on Carvedilol's Efficacy

CHOICES Cancer, Heart Disease, Osteoporosis Interventions, and Community Evaluation Studies

CHOIR Center for Health Outcomes Improvement Research

CHOL, chol cholesterol

c hold withhold

CHOP cyclophosphamide, hydroxydaunomycin, Oncovin, and prednisone

ChoP cell-surface phosphocholine

CHORUS Collaborative Hypertext in Radiology

CHOV Chaco virus

CHP calcineurin homologue protein; capillary hydrostatic pressure; charcoal hemoperfusion; Chemical Hygiene Plan; child psychiatry; Children's Health Project; community health plan; comprehensive health planning; coordinating hospital physician; cricohyoidopexy; cutaneous hepatic porphyria

ChP chest physician

CHPA community health planning agency; community health purchasing alliance

CHPV Chandipura virus; chicken parvovirus

ChPV chipmunk parvovirus

chpx chickenpox

CHQ chloroquinol

CHQCP Cleveland Health Quality Choice Project

CHR cerebrohepatorenal [syndrome]; chemical hazards regulations

Chr *Chromobacterium*

chr chromosome; chronic

c hr candle hour

c-hr curie-hour

ChRBC chicken red blood cell

CHREF Connecticut Healthcare Research and Education Foundation

CHRIS Cancer Hazards Ranking and Information System; Chemical Hazard Response Information System

CHRISTMAS Carvedilol Hibernation Reversible Ischemia Trial: Marker of Success

CHROMINFO chromosome information [database]

chron chronic

CHRONIC chronic disease, rheumatoid arthritis, neoplasms, infections, cryoglobulinemia [conditions in which rheumatoid factor is produced]

CHRPE congenital hypertrophy of the retinal pigment epithelium

CHRS cerebrohepatorenal syndrome; Christian syndrome

CHRV Chub reovirus

CHS Canada Health Survey; cardiovascular health study; Center for Health Statistics; central hypoventilation syndrome; Charleston Heart Study; Chédiak-Higashi syndrome; Chinese Health Study; cholinesterase; chondroitin sulfate; citizen health system [Greece]; community health study; compression hip screw; Congenital Heart Surgeons Society [study]; congenital hypoventilation syndrome; contact hypersensitivity; Copenhagen City Heart Study; coronary heart study

CHSD Children's Health Services Division

CHSO total hemolytic serum C activity

CHSP Child Health Surveillance Programme [Scotland]; Clinton Health Security Plan

CHSS cooperative health statistics system

CHT chemotherapy; combined hormone therapy; contralateral head turning

ChTg chymotrypsinogen

ChTK chicken thymidine kinase

ChTX charybdotoxin

CHU centigrade heat unit; closed head unit

CHUSPAN [treatment of] Churg-Strauss Syndrome and Polyarteritis Nodosa [study]

CHV canine herpes virus; Cryphonectria hypovirus

CHVF chemically viewed functionally [UMLS]

CHVS chemically viewed structurally [UMLS]

CHVV Charleville virus

ChYNMV Chinese yam necrotic mosaic virus

CI calcium ionophore; cardiac index; cardiac insufficiency; cation-independent; cell immunity; cell inhibition; cephalic index; cerebral infarction; cervical incompetence; chemical ionization; chemically induced; chemo-immunotherapy; chemotactic index; chemotherapeutic index; chromatid interchange; chronic infection; chronic inflammation; clinical investigator; clomipramine; clonus index; cochlear implant; coefficient of intelligence; colloidal iron; color index; Colour Index; competitive index [microbial]; complete iridectomy; confidence index; confidence interval [statistics]; conformity index [imaging]; contamination index; contextual inquiry; continued insomnia; continuous imaging; continuous improvement; continuous infusion; contraindication or contraindicated; convergence insufficiency; coronary insufficiency; corrected count increment; covering index; crystalline insulin; cumulative incidence; cytotoxic index

Ci curie

C^i intercept on concentration

CIA chemiluminescent immunoassay; chymotrypsin inhibitor activity; colony-inhibiting activity; congenital intestinal aganglionosis

CIAC central independent adjudication committee

CIAIT Chinese Infarction Angiotensin Converting Enzyme Inhibitor Trial

CIBD chronic inflammatory bowel disease

CiBER Centre for Information Behaviour and Analysis Research [UK]

CIBHA congenital inclusion-body hemolytic anemia

CIBIS Cardiac Insufficiency Bisoprolol Study

CIBP chronic intractable benign pain

CIBPS chronic intractable benign pain syndrome

CIC cardioinhibitor center; care improvement council; certification in infection control; circulating immune complex; clean intermittent catheterization; completely in the canal [hearing aid]; computers in cardiology; computing, information, and communication; constant initial concentration; crisis intervention center

Cic cicletanine

CICA cervical internal carotid artery

CICR calcium-induced-calcium release process [calcium channel]

CICU cardiac intensive care unit; cardiovascular inpatient care unit; coronary intensive care unit

CID cellular immunodeficiency; Center for Infectious Diseases; charge injection device; chick infective dose; combined immunodeficiency disease; Cosmetic Ingredient Dictionary; cytomegalic inclusion disease

CID$_{50}$ median chimpanzee infective dose

CI$_d$ inter-compartmental diffusion

CIDEMS Center for Information and Documentation

CIDEP chemically induced dynamic electron polarization

CIDI composite international diagnostic interview

CIDI-SAM Composite International Diagnostic Interview-Substance Abuse Module

CIDM computerized infectious disease monitor

CIDNP chemically induced dynamic nuclear polarization

CIDP chronic idiopathic polyradiculopathy; chronic inflammatory demyelinating polyradiculoneuropathy; Clinical Initiatives Development Program

CIDS Canadian Implantable Defibrillator Study; Canadian Internal Defibrillator Study; cellular immunity deficiency syndrome; circular intensity differential scattering; continuous insulin delivery system

CIE Canberra Interview for the Elderly; cellulose ion exchange; congenital ichthyosiform erythroderma; counter-current immunoelectrophoresis; counterimmunoelectrophoresis; crossed immunoelectrophoresis

CIEBOV Côte d'Ivoire Ebola virus

CIEP counterimmunoelectrophoresis; crossed immunoelectrophoresis

CIF cartilage induction factor; cloning inhibitory factor; congenital infantile fibrosarcoma

CIFC Council for the Investigation of Fertility Control

CIG cardiointegram; cold-insoluble globulin; computer-interpretable guidelines

CIg intracytoplasmic immunoglobulin

cIgM cytoplasmic immunoglobulin M

CIGTS Comparison of Initial Glaucoma Treatment Study

CIH carbohydrate-induced hyperglyceridemia; Certificate in Industrial Health; children in hospital

CIHI Canadian Institute for Health Information

CIHR Canadian Institutes of Health Research

ci-hr curie-hour

CIHS central infantile hypotonic syndrome

CiHV ciconiid herpesvirus

CII cancer informatics infrastructure; Carnegie Interest Inventory; continuous intravenous infusion

CIIA common internal iliac artery

CIIP chronic idiopathic intestinal pseudo-obstruction

CIIPX [X-linked] chronic idiopathic intestinal pseudo-obstruction

CIIR Center for Intelligent Information Retrieval

CiIV *Casinaria infesta* ichnovirus

CILIP Chartered Institute of Library and Information Professionals [UK]

CIM cimetidine; cortically induced movement; Cumulated Index Medicus; cytoimmunological monitoring

Ci/ml curies per milliliter

CI-MPR cation-independent mannose-6-phosphate receptor

CIMS chemical ionization mass spectrometry

CIN central inhibition; cervical intraepithelial neoplasia; chronic interstitial nephritis; community information network

CIN 1, CIN I cervical intraepithelial neoplasia, grade 1 (mild dysplasia)

CIN 2, CIN II cervical intraepithelial neoplasia, grade 2 (moderate-severe)

CIN 3, CIN III cervical intraepithelial neoplasia, grade 3 (severe dysplasia and carcinoma in situ)

C_{in} increased concentration [of blood]; insulin clearance

CINAHL Cumulative Index to Nursing and Allied Health Literature

Cinahl Cumulative Index to Nursing and Allied Health [UK]

CINCA chronic infantile neurological cutaneous and auricular [syndrome]

CINDI Countrywide Integrated Noncommunicable Disease Intervention [study]

CINE chemotherapy-induced nausea and emesis

C1 INH complement 1 inhibitor

C_1-INH C_1-esterase inhibitor

CINI Computers in Nursing Interactive

CIO chief information officer; corticoid-induced osteoporosis

CIOMS Council for International Organizations of Medical Sciences

CIP care information provision; chronic idiopathic polyradiculoneuropathy; chronic intestinal pseudo-obstruction; Collection de l'Institut Pasteur

CIPA client interface for professional access; Computer-Aided Identification of Phlebotomine Sandflies of the Americas [leishmaniasis]

CIPC Center for Injury Prevention and Control

CIPD continuous intermittent peritoneal dialysis

CIPF classic interstitial pneumonitis-fibrosis; clinical illness promoting factor

CIPHER Common Information for Public Health Reporting

CIPM International Committee on Weights and Measures [Comité International de Poids et Mesures]

CIPN chronic inflammatory polyneuropathy

CIPRA Comprehensive International Program of Research on AIDS

CIPSO chronic intestinal pseudo-obstruction

CIR constant interval reciprocal

CIRC Ca^{2+}-induced Ca^{2+} release

circ circuit; circular; circumcision; circumference

circ & sens circulation and sensation

CIREN Crash Injury Research and Engineering Network

CIRF clinically insignificant renal fragments; contrast-induced renal failure

CIRSE Cardiovascular and Interventional Radiological Society of Europe

CIRSET Committee on Immunization Registry Standards and Electronic Transactions

CIS capacity information system; carcinoma in situ; catheter-induced spasm; central inhibitory state; Chemical Information Service; clinical information system; computer-integrated surgery; computerized information system; continuous interleaved sampler; Coronary Intervention Study; cumulative impairment score

CI-S calculus index, simplified

CiS cingulate sulcus

CISC complex-instructional-set computing

CISCA$_{II}$B$_{IV}$ Cytoxan, Adriamycin, platinum, vinblastine, bleomycin

cis-**DPP** cisplatin

CISE Computer and Information Science and Engineering [National Science Foundation Directorate]

CISET Committee on International Science, Engineering, and Technology

CISH competitive in situ hybridization

CISMeF Catalog and Index of French-Speaking Resources

CISP chronic intractable shoulder pain

CIS PT cisplatin

13-*cis*-RA 13-*cis*-retinoic acid

CISS chromosome in situ suppression; Common Internet Scheme Syntax; constructive interference in steady state

CISST computer integrated surgical system and technology

CIT citrate; combined intermittent therapy; conjugated-immunoglobulin technique; critical incident technique; crossed intrinsic transfer

cit citrate

CITS Carey Infant Temperament Scale

CITT Chemical Industry Institute for Toxicology

CITTS Central Illinois Thrombolytic Therapy Study

CIV Carey Island virus; ceratitis I virus; continuous intravenous infusion

CIVI continuous intravenous infusion

CIVII continuous intravenous insulin infusion

CIXA constant infusion excretory urogram

CJ conjunctivitis

CJA Creutzfeldt-Jakob agent

CJD Creutzfeldt-Jakob disease

CJS Creutzfeldt-Jakob syndrome

CJSV Carajas virus

CjvO$_2$ jugular venous oxygen content

CK calf kidney; casein kinase; chemokine; chicken kidney; cholecystokinin; choline kinase; contralateral knee; creatine kinase; cyanogen chloride; cytokinin

CKII casein kinase II

ck check, checked

C$_\kappa$ kappa light chain constant region [immunoglobulins]

CKB creatine kinase, brain type

CKC cold-knife conization

CKD cone-kernal distribution

CKG cardiokymography

C/kg coulomb per kilogram

CKI cyclin-dependent kinase inhibitor

CKM creatine kinase, muscle type

CKMB creatine kinase, myocardial bound

CKMM creatine kinase, muscle type

CK-PZ cholecystokinin-pancreozymin

CKR chemokine receptor

CKRM clinical knowledge repository manager

CKS classic form of Kaposi sarcoma

CL capillary lumen; cardiolipin; case library; cell line; central [venous] line;

centralis lateralis; cervical line; chemiluminescence; chest and left arm [lead in electrocardiography]; childhood leukemia; cholelithiasis; cholesterol-lecithin; chronic leukemia; cirrhosis of liver; clavicle; clear liquid; clearance; cleft lip; clinical laboratory; clomipramine; complete linkage; complex loading; composite lymphoma; computational linguistics; confidence limit or level; contact lens; corpus luteum; corrected [echo long axis] length; cricoid lamina; criterion level; critical list; cutaneous leishmaniasis; cutis laxa; cycle length; cytotoxic lymphocyte; lung capacity; lung compliance

C-L consultation-liaison [setting]

C$_L$ constant region of light chain of immunoglobulin molecule; lung compliance

Cl chloride; chlorine; clavicle; clear; clearance; Cl esterase; clinic; *Clostridium*; closure; colistin

cl centiliter; clarified; clean; clear; cleft; clinic; clinical; clonus; clotting; cloudy

Cλ lambda light chain constant region [immunoglobulins]

CLA cerebellar ataxia; Certified Laboratory Assistant; cervicolinguoaxial; closed loop algorithm [for infusion of catecholamine in heart stress test]; contralateral local anesthesia; cutaneous lichen amyloidosis; cutaneous lymphocyte antigen; cyclic lysine anhydride

Cl-a alternative chloride channel

ClAc chloroacetyl

CLAH congenital lipoid adrenal hyperplasia

CLam cervical laminectomy

CLAS Cholesterol-Lowering Atherosclerosis Study; circulating lupus anticoagulant syndrome; classification [UMLS]; computerized laboratory alerting system; congenital localized absence of skin

CLASP Collaborative Low-Dose Aspirin Study in Pregnancy

CLASS Clomethiazole Acute Stroke Study

class, classif classification

CLASSICS Clopidrogrel Aspirin Stent Interventional Cooperative Study

clav clavicle

CLB chlorambucil; clobazam; configurable logic block; curvilinear body

CLBBB complete left bundle branch block

CLBP chronic low back pain

CLC Charcot-Leyden crystal; Clerc-Levy-Critesco [syndrome]

CLCA compact low-chromatin area

CLCD cleidocranial dysostosis

CLCN chloride channel

CL/CP cleft lip/cleft palate

Cl$_{cr}$ creatinine clearance

CLCS colchicine sensitivity

CLD central low density; central lung distance; chloride diarrhea; chronic liver disease; chronic lung disease; command line interface [user-computer interface]; congenital limb deficiency; crystal ligand field

cld closed

CLDH choline dehydrogenase

cldy cloudy

CLE centrilobular emphysema; congenital lobar emphysema; continuous lumbar epidural [anesthesia]

CLED cystine-lactose-electrolyte-deficient [agar]

CLEMANTIS clinical engineering management tool and information system

CLEOPAD Clopidogrel in Peripheral Arterial Disease [study]

CLEV *Chironomus luridus* entomopoxvirus

CLF cardiolipin fluorescent [antibody]; ceroid lipofuscinosis; cholesterol-lecithin flocculation

Clf clumping factor

ClfA clumping factor A

CLH chronic lobular hepatitis; cleft limb-heart [syndrome]; corpus luteum hormone; cutaneous lymphoid hyperplasia

CLI complement lysis inhibitor; corpus luteum insufficiency

CLIA Clinical Laboratories Improvement Act

CLIBS cation and ligand induced binding site

CLIF cloning inhibitory factor; *Crithidia luciliae* immunofluorescence

CLIMS clinical laboratory information management system

clin clinic, clinical

Cl-INH Cl esterase inhibitor

CLINPROT Clinical Cancer Protocols

ClinQuery clinical query

CLINT clinical informatics network

Cl$_{int}$ intrinsic clearance

CLIP capitolunate instability pattern; Cholesterol-Lowering Intervention Program; corticotropin-like intermediate lobe peptide

CLIPS C language integrated production system

CLL cholesterol-lowering lipid; chronic lymphatic leukemia; chronic lymphocytic leukemia; cow lung lavage

CLM capillary-lymphatic malformation

Cl$_M$ metabolic clearance

CLMA Clinical Laboratory Management Association

Cl$_2$MD dichloromethylene diphosphate

CLMF cytotoxic lymphocyte maturation factor

CLML Current List of Medical Literature

CLMS classification or coding system for clinical management system

CLMV cauliflower mosaic virus

CLN ceroid lipofuscinosis

CLO cod liver oil; *Campylobacter*-like organism

clo "clothing" [a unit of thermal insulation]

Cl$_O$ oral clearance

CLOF clofibrate

CLON clonidine

Clon *Clonorchis*

CLOS common list processing language object system

Clostr *Clostridium*

CLOT Clinical Perspectives on Lysis of Thrombi [study]

CLOUT Clinical Outcomes with Ultrasound Trial; Core Laboratory Ultrasound Analysis Study

CLP cardiac laboratory panel; cecal ligation and puncture; chymotrypsin-like protein; cleft lip with cleft palate; common lymphocyte progenitor; constraining logic programming; paced cycle length

CL/P cleft lip with or without cleft palate

CL(P) cleft lip without cleft palate

CIP clinical pathology

Cl$_R$ renal clearance

CLRT continuous lateral rotational therapy

CLRV cherry leaf roll virus; *Cimex lectularius* reovirus

CLS café-au-lait spot; classical least square; Clinical Laboratory Scientist; Coffin-Lowry syndrome; Cornelia de Lange syndrome

CLSC Centres Locaux de Services Communitaires [Quebec]

CLSE calf lung surfactant extract

CLSH corpus luteum stimulating hormone

CLSL chronic lymphosarcoma (cell) leukemia

CLSM confocal laser scanning microscope

CLSV cucumber leaf spot virus

CLT Certified Laboratory Technician; chronic lymphocytic thyroiditis; Clinical Laboratory Technician; clot lysis time; clotting time; lung-thorax compliance

CL$_{TB}$ total body clearance

CLT(NCA) Laboratory Technician Certified by the National Certification Agency for Medical Laboratory Personnel

CLU clusterin

CLV carnation latent virus; cassava latent virus; *Colletotrichum lindemuthianum* virus; common latent virus; constant linear velocity

CLVd Columnea latent viroid

CL VOID clean voided specimen [urine]

CLZ clozapine

CM California mastitis [test]; calmodulin; capreomycin; carboxymethyl; cardiac monitoring; cardiac murmur; cardiac muscle; cardiomyopathy; carpometacarpal; Caroll/Mackie [radiotherapy]; castrated male; Caucasian male; cause of death [Lat. *causa mortis*]; cavernous malformation; cell membrane; center of mass; cerebral malaria; cerebral mantle; cervical mucosa or mucus; Chick-Martin [coefficient]; chloroquine-mepacrine; chondromalacia; chopped meat [medium]; chronic meningitis; chylomicron; circular muscle; circulating monocyte; circumferential measurement; classification-maximization; clindamycin; clinical medicine; clinical modification; coccidioidal meningitis; cochlear microphonic; combined modality; common migraine; complete medium; complications; condition median; conditioned medium; congenital malformation; congestive myocardiopathy; continuous murmur; contrast material; contrast medium; copulatory mechanism; costal margin; cow's milk; cytometry; cytoplasmic membrane; Master of Surgery [Lat. *Chirurgiae Magister*]; narrow-diameter endosseous screw implant [Fr. *crête manche*]

C-M cardiomyopathy

C/M counts per minute

C&M cocaine and morphine

C$_M$ metabolite clearance

Cm curium; minimal concentration

C$_m$ maximum clearance; membrane capacitance

cM centimorgan

cm centimeter

cm^2 square centimeter

cm^3 cubic centimeter

Cμ mu light chain constant region [immunoglobulins]

CMA Canadian Medical Association; Certified Medical Assistant; chronic metabolic acidosis; cingulate motor area; cow's milk allergy; cultured macrophages

CMAC cerebellar model articulation controller

CMAP compound muscle (or motor) action potential

CMAR cell matrix adhesion regulator

Cmax, C$_{max}$ maximum concentration

CMB carbolic methylene blue; Central Midwives' Board; chloromercuribenzoate

CMBC concentration of moving blood cells

CMBES Canadian Medical and Biological Engineering Society

CMBs center for maximally inscribed balls

CMBV citrus mosaic virus

CMC carboxymethylcellulose; care management continuity; carpometacarpal; cell-mediated cytolysis or cytotoxicity; chemical mismatch cleavage; chloramphenicol; chronic mucocutaneous candidiasis; Comprehensive Medicinal Chemistry [database]; critical micellar concentration

cmc critical micelle concentration

CMCC chronic mucocutaneous candidiasis

CMCJ carpometacarpal joint

CMCS computer-mediated communication system

CMCT central motor conduction time

CMCt care management continuity across settings

CMD camptomelic dwarfism; camptomelic dysplasia; cartilage matrix deficiency; cerebromacular degeneration; Certified

Medical Densitometrist; chief medical director; childhood muscular dystrophy; common mental disorder; comparative mean dose; congenital muscular dystrophy; corticomedullary differentiation; count median diameter; craniomandibular disorder

CMDD choline and methionine deficient diet

cmDNA cytoplasmic membrane-associated deoxyribonucleic acid

CMDS computer misuse detection system

CME cervical mediastinal exploration; continuing medical education; Council on Medical Education; crude marijuana extract; cystoid macular edema

CMED central medical emergency dispatch center

CMF calcium-magnesium free; catabolite modular factor; chloromethylfluorescein; chondromyxoid fibroma; Christian Medical Fellowship; cold mitten fraction; cortical magnification factor; craniomandibulofacial; cyclophosphamide, methotrexate, and fluorouracil

CMFDA chloromethylfluorescein diacetate

CMFT cardiolipin microflocculation test

CMFV cyclophosphamide, methotrexate, fluorouracil, and vincristine

CMFVP cyclophosphamide, methotrexate, fluorouracil, vincristine, prednisone

CMG canine or congenital myasthenia gravis; case mix group; chopped meat glucose [medium]; cystometrography, cystometrogram

CMGN chronic membranous glomerulonephritis

CMGS chopped meat-glucose-starch [medium]; Clinical Molecular Genetics Society

CMGT chromosome-mediated gene transfer

CMH cardiomyopathy, hypertrophic; community mental health [services or program]; congenital malformation of the heart

CMHC community mental health center

C/MHC community/migrant health center

CMHIS Community Mental Health Information System [Canada]

cmH$_2$O centimeters of water

CMHS center for mental health services; Continuous Medicare History Sample

CMHT community mental health team

CMI carbohydrate metabolism index; care management integration; case mix index; cell-mediated immunity; cell multiplication inhibition; chronic mesenteric ischemia; circulating microemboli index; colonic motility index; combat medical informatics; combined myocardial infarction; Commonwealth Mycological Institute; computed maxillofacial imaging; computer managed instruction; Cornell Medical Index

CMID cytomegalic inclusion disease

c/min cycles per minute

CMINET Chinese Medical Information Network

CMIO chief medical information officer

CMIR cell-mediated immune response

CMIS common management information services

CMISP common management information standards/protocol

CMIT Current Medical Information and Terminology

CMJ carpometacarpal joint

CMK chloromethyl ketone; congenital multicystic kidney

CML carboxymethyl lysine; cell-mediated lymphocytotoxicity; cell-mediated lympholysis; central motor latency; chronic myelocytic leukemia; chronic myelogenous leukemia; clinical medical librarian; clinical medical library

c/mL copies per milliliter

CMLNP comprehensive multi-level nursing practice [model]

CMLV camelpox virus

CMM cell-mediated mutagenesis; color Doppler M-mode; Columbia Mental Maturity [scale]; coordinate measuring machine [orthopedic surgery]; cross modality matching; cutaneous malignant melanoma

cmm cubic millimeter

CMMC cervical myelomeningocele

CMME chloromethyl methyl ether

CMML chronic myelomonocytic leukemia

CMMoL chronic myelomonocytic leukemia

CMMS Columbia Mental Maturity Scale

CMN canine minute virus; caudal mediastinal node; certification of medical necessity; cystic medial necrosis

CMNA complement-mediated neutrophil activation

CMN-AA cystic medial necrosis of ascending aorta

CMO cardiac minute output; Chief Medical Officer; comfort measures only; competitive medical organization; corticosterone methyloxidase

CMO₂ cerebral metabolic oxygen rate

cMO centimorgan

cMOAT canalicular multispecific organic anion transporter

CMOL chronic monocytic leukemia

CMoMV carrot mottle mosaic virus

CMOS compatible monolithic conductivity sensor; complementary metal-oxide semiconductor

CMoV carrot mottle virus; chlorotic mottle virus

CMP cardiomyopathy; cartilage matrix protein; chondromalacia patellae; competitive medical plan; comprehensive medical plan; cytidine monophosphate

CMPD chronic myeloproliferative disorder

cmpd compound, compounded

CMPGN chronic membranoproliferative glomerulonephritis

cmps centimeters per second

CMR cardiomodulorespirography; cerebral metabolic rate; chief medical resident; child mortality rate [under age 5]; chloroform-methanol residue [vaccine]; chylomicron remnant; common medical record; common mode rejection; computerized medical record; congenital mitral regurgitation; cross-reacting material; crude mortality ratio

CMRG cerebral metabolic rate of glucose

CMRGlc combined metabolic rate of glucose

CMR_Glu, CMRglu cerebral metabolic rate of glucose

CMRI cardiac magnetic resonance imaging

CMRL cerebral metabolic rate of lactate

CMRNG chromosomal control of mechanisms of resistance of *Neisseria gonorrhoeae*

CMRO, CMRO₂ cerebral metabolic rate of oxygen consumption

CMRP cervical magnetic resonance phlebography

CMRR common mode rejection ratio

CMS Centers for Medicare and Medical Services; children's medical services; Christian Medical Society; chromosome modification site; chronic myelodysplastic syndrome; circulation, motion, sensation; clinical management system; clofibrate-induced muscular syndrome; Clyde Mood Scale; complement-mediated solubility; Copenhagen Male Study; cortical magnetic stimulation

cm/s centimeters per second

CMSC computer science

CMSD congenital myocardial sympathetic dysinnervation

cm/sec centimeters per second

CMSS circulation, motor ability, sensation, and swelling; Council of Medical Specialty Societies

CMT California mastitis test; cancer multistep therapy; catechol methyltransferase; certified medical transcriptionist; cervical motion tenderness; Charcot-Marie-Tooth [syndrome]; chemotherapy; circus movement tachycardia; complex motor tic; continuous memory test; controlled medical terminology; convergent medical terminology; Council on Medical Television; Current Medical Terminology

CMT1 Charcot-Marie-Tooth [disease or neuropathy] type 1

CMTC cutis marmorata telangiectatica congenita

CMTD Charcot-Marie-Tooth disease; chronic multiple tic disorder

CMTIA Charcot-Marie-Tooth [disease or neuropathy] type IA

CMTIB Charcot-Marie-Tooth [disease or neuropathy] type IB

CMTL computer-mediated tutorial laboratory

CMTS Charcot-Marie-Tooth syndrome

CMTX Charcot-Marie-Tooth [syndrome], X-linked

CMU chlorophenyldimethylurea

CMUA continuous motor unit activity

CMV canine minute virus; cassava mosaic virus; chlorotic mottle virus; Clo Mor virus; common mosaic virus; continuous mandatory ventilation; controlled mechanical ventilation; controlled medical vocabulary; conventional mechanical ventilation; cool mist vaporizer; cowpea mosaic virus; cucumber mosaic virus; curly mottle virus; cytomegalovirus

CMV-E cytomegalovirus encephalitis

CMV-MN cytomegalovirus mononucleosis

CMV-VE cytomegalovirus ventriculoencephalitis

CMX cefmenoxime

CN caudate nucleus; cellulose nitrate; charge nurse; child nutrition; chloroacetophenone; clinical nursing; cochlear nucleus; condensation nucleus; congenital nystagmus; cranial nerve; Crigler-Najjar [syndrome]; cyanogen; cyanosis neonatorum

C:N calorie:nitrogen [ratio]

C/N carbon/nitrogen [ratio]; carrier/noise [ratio]; contrast to noise [ratio]

CN⁻ cyanide anion

CN I first cranial nerve [olfactory]

CN II second cranial nerve [optic]

CN III third cranial nerve [oculomotor]

CN IV fourth cranial nerve [trochlear]

CNV fifth cranial nerve [trigeminal]

CN VI sixth cranial nerve [abducent]

CN VII seventh cranial nerve [facial]

CNVIII eighth cranial nerve [vestibulocochlear]

CN IX ninth cranial nerve [glossopharyngeal]

CN X tenth cranial nerve [vagus]

CNXI eleventh cranial nerve [accessory]

CN XII twelfth cranial nerve [hypoglossal]

CNA calcium nutrient agar; Canadian Nurses Association; certified nursing assistant

CNAF chronic nonvalvular atrial fibrillation

CNAG chronic narrow angle glaucoma

CNAP career nurse assistants' programs; compound nerve action potential

CNAV Cananeia virus

CNB cutting needle biopsy

CNBP cellular nucleic acid binding protein

CNC community nursing center

CNCbl cyanocobalamin

CNCC certified nurse in critical care

CND care need determination

CNDC chronic nonspecific diarrhea of childhood; chronic nonsuppurative destructive cholangitis

CNDI congenital nephrogenic diabetes insipidus

CNE chief nurse executive; chronic nervous exhaustion; concentric needle electrode

C3NeF C3 nephritic factor

CNEMG concentric needle electrode electromyography

CNES chronic nervous exhaustion syndrome

C$_{NET}$ net compliance

CNF chronic nodular fibrositis; congenital nephrotic syndrome of the Finnish [type]; conjunctive normal form system [Boolean logic]; cytotoxic necrotizing factor

CNFS craniofrontonasal syndrome

CNFV carnation necrotic fleck virus

CNGC cyclic nucleotide gated channel

CNH central neurogenic hyperpnea; community nursing home

CNHD congenital nonspherocytic hemolytic disease

CNI center of nuclear image; chronic nerve irritation; community nutrition institute

CNIDR Clearinghouse for Networked Information Discovery and Retrieval

CNIS computerized or clinical nursing information system

CNK cortical necrosis of kidneys

CNL cardiolipin natural lecithin; chronic neutrophilic leukemia

CNLS complex nonlinear least square

CNM centronuclear myopathy; Certified Nurse-Midwife; combinatorial neural model; computerized nuclear morphometry

CNMDSA community nursing minimum data set, Australia

CNMetHb cyanmethemoglobin

CnMoV *Cynosurus* mottle virus

CNMT Certified Nuclear Medicine Technologist

CNN Canadian National Network; computational neural network

CNO community nursing organization

cNOS constitutive nitric oxide synthase

CNP community nurse practitioner; continuous negative pressure; cranial nerve palsy; C-type natriuretic peptide; 2′,3′-cyclic nucleotide 3′-phosphodiesterase

CNPase 2′,3′-cyclic nucleotide 3′-phosphohydrolase

CNPB continuous negative pressure breathing

CNPV canarypox virus; continuous negative pressure ventilation

CNQX 6-cyano-7-nitroquinoxaline-2,3-dione

CNR cadherin-related neuronal receptor; cannabinoid receptor; Center for Nursing Research; contrast-to-noise ratio; Council of Nurse Researchers

C(N,r) combination of N things taken r at a time

CNRC Children's Nutrition Research Center

CNRT corrected sinus node recovery time

CNS central nervous system; clinical nurse specialist; coagulase-negative staphylococci; congenital nephrotic syndrome; cutaneous nerve stimulator; sulfocyanate

CNSHA congenital nonspherocytic hemolytic anemia

CNS-L central nervous system leukemia

CNSLD chronic nonspecific lung disease

CNST coagulase-negative staphylococci

C$_{NS}$[t] non-specific tracer concentration

CNT *Clostridium* neurotoxin

CNTF ciliary neutrophilic factor

CNTFR ciliary neutrophilic factor receptor

CNTHM conotruncal heart malformation

CNTV Connecticut virus

CNUV Ch nuda virus

CNV choroidal neovascularization; contingent negative variation; cutaneous necrotizing vasculitis

CO carbon monoxide; cardiac output; castor oil; casualty officer; centric occlusion; cervical orthosis; cervicoaxial; choline oxidase; coccygeal; coenzyme; compound; control; corneal opacity; cross over; cyclophosphamide and vincristine

C/O check out; complains of; in care of

CO$_2$ carbon dioxide

Co cobalt

c/o complains of

Co I coenzyme I

Co II coenzyme II

COA Canadian Ophthalmological Association; Canadian Orthopaedic Association; certificate of authority; cervico-oculo-acusticus [syndrome]; condition on admission

CoA coenzyme A

COACH Canadian Organization for the Advancement of Computers in Health; cerebellar vermis hypoplasia/aplasia-oligophrenia-congenital ataxia-ocular colobomata-hepatic fibrosis [syndrome]

COAD chronic obstructive airway disease; clinician-oriented access to data

COAG chronic open angle glaucoma

coag coagulation, coagulated

COAL chronic obstructive airflow limitation

COAP cyclophosphamide, cytosine arabinose, vincristine, prednisone

coarct coarctation

COAS clinical observations access service

CoASH uncombined coenzyme A

CoA-SPC coenzyme A-synthesizing protein complex

COAT Children's Orientation and Amnesia Test; Cooperative Osaka Adenosine Trial

COB chronic obstructive bronchitis; coordination of benefits

COBALT Continuous Infusion vs Bolus Alteplase Trial; Continuous Infusion vs Double-Bolus Administration of Alteplase

coban cohesive bandage

COBOL common business oriented language

COBRA Comparison of Balloon vs Rotational Angioplasty; computer-operated birth defect recognition aid; Consolidated Omnibus Reconciliation Act

COBS cesarean-obtained barrier-sustained; chronic organic brain syndrome

COBT chronic obstruction of the biliary tract

COC cathodal opening contraction; coccygeal; combination oral contraceptive; commission on cancer; cumulus-oocyte complex

COCI Consortium on Chemical Information

COCl cathodal opening clonus

COCM congestive cardiomyopathy

COCP combined oral contraceptive pill

Co-Cr-Mo cobalt-chromium-molybdenum [alloy]

COCS Cornell-Oxford China Study

COCV cocal virus

COD cause of death; cerebro-ocular dysplasia; chemical oxygen demand; codeine; collaborative organization design; computer-assisted optical densitometry; condition on discharge

cod codeine

CODAS cerebro-oculo-dento-auriculo-skeletal [syndrome]

CODATA Committee on Data for Science and Technology

CODEC coder/decoder [device]; compression and decompression

COD-MD cerebro-ocular dysplasia-muscular dystrophy [syndrome]

CODS Charnes Organizational Diagnosis Survey

coeff coefficient

COEPS cortical originating extra-pyramidal system

COER controlled onset, extended release

COF cutoff frequency

CoF cobra factor; cofactor

C of A coarctation of the aorta

COFS cerebro-oculo-facial-skeletal [syndrome]; certificate of free sale

COG center of gravity; cluster of orthologous groups; cognitive function tests

CoGME Council on Graduate Medical Education

COGTT cortisone oral glucose tolerance test

COH carbohydrate; controlled ovarian hyperstimulation

COHb, CoHb carboxyhemoglobin

CoHgb carboxyhemoglobin

COHN Certified Occupational Health Nurse

COHR computer-based oral health record

COHSE Confederation of Health Service Employees

CoHV Columbid herpesvirus

COI Central Obesity Index; certificate of insurance; conflict of interest; cost of illness

COIF congenital onychodysplasia of the index finger

COIN conformal index

COL central object library; colposcopy

col colicin; collagen; collection; colony; colored; column; strain [Lat. *cola*]

COLD chronic obstructive lung disease; computer output on laser disk

COLD A cold agglutinin titer

COLING computational linguistics

coll collateral; collection, collective; college; colloidal

collat collateral

COLTS Coronary Observational Long-Term Study

CoLV Cole latent virus

COM chronic otitis media; College of Osteopathic Medicine; component object model; computer-output microfilm

CoM center of noise

com comminuted; commitment

COMA Committee on Medical Aspects [food and nutrition]

COMAC/HRS/QA Community Concerted Action Programme on Quality Assurance in Health Care [European]

comb combination, combine

COMBIMAN Computerized Biomechanical Man

COMC carboxymethylcellulose

COME chronic otitis media with effusion

COMET Carvedilol or Metoprolol European Trial; Carvedilol or Metoprolol Evaluation Trial

CoMET concept modeling environment for teachers

comf comfortable

CoMFA comparative molecular field analysis

COMLEX Comprehensive Osteopathic Medical Licensing Examination

comm, commun communicable

CoMMA comparative molecular moment analysis

COMMIT Community Intervention Trial [for Smoking Cessation]; Comprehensive Multidisciplinary Interventional Trial [for Regression of Coronary Heart Disease]

COMP cartilage oligomeric matrix protein; cells outside the main population; complication; cyclophosphamide, vincristine, methotrexate, prednisone

comp comparative; compensation, compensated; complaint; complete; composition; compound, compounded; comprehension; compress; computer

COMPACCS Committee on Manpower for the Critical Care Societies

COMPACT computer optimized parametric analysis for chemical toxicity

COMPASS Comparative Trial of Saruplase vs Streptokinase; Computerized Online Medicaid Pharmaceutical Analysis and Surveillance System

compd compound, compounded

compl complaint; complete, completed, completion; complication, complicated

complic complication, complicated

compn composition

compr compression

comp stud comparative study

COMS cerebrooculomuscular syndrome

CoMSIA comparative molecular similarity index analysis

COMT catecholamine *O*-methyl transferase; certified ophthalmic medical technologist

COMTRAC computer-based case tracing

COMUL complement fixation murine leukosis [test]

COMY catechol-*O*-methyltransferase

CON certificate of need; cortisone

Con concanavalin

con against [Lat. *contra*]; continuation, continue

CONA cortisone acetate

CON A, Con A concanavalin A

Con A–HRP concanavalin A–horseradish peroxidase

CONC conceptual entity [UMLS]

conc, concentr concentrate, concentrated, concentration

c-onc cellular oncogene

COND cerebro-osteo-nephrodysplasia

cond condensation, condensed; condition, conditioned; conductivity; conductor

conf conference; confined; confinement; confusion

cong congested, congestion; gallon [Lat. *congius*]

congen congenital

CongHD congenital heart disease

coniz conization

conj conjunctiva, conjunctival

conjug conjugated, conjugation

CONPA-DRI I vincristine, doxorubicin, and melphalan

CONPA-DRI III CONPA-DRI I plus intensified doxorubicin

CONQUEST Computerized Needs-Oriented Quality Measurement Evaluation System

CONS coagulase-negative *Staphylococcus*; consultant, consultation

cons conservation; conservative; consultation

CONSENSUS Cooperative North Scandinavian Enalapril Survival Study

CONSORT Consolidated Standards of Reporting Trials

const constant

constit constituent

consult consultant, consultation

CONSUME Compliance of National Supplements Using Multiform Energy Sources [study]

cont against [Lat. *contra*]; bruised [Lat. *contusus*]; contains, contents; continue, continuation

contag contagion, contagious

contr contracted, contraction

contra contraindicated

contralat contralateral

contrib contributory

CoNV cocoa necrosis virus

conv convalescence, convalescent, convalescing; convergence, convergent; convulsions, convulsive

converg convergence, convergent

CONVINCE Controlled Onset Verapamil Investigation for Cardiovascular Endpoints [study]; Controlled Onset Verapamil Investigation of Clinical Endpoints [study]

COO chief operating officer; cost of ownership [analysis]

COOD chronic obstructive outflow disease

COOH carboxy group; carboxy terminus

COOHTA Canadian Coordinating Office for Health Technology Assessment

COOP charts for primary care practices; cooperative

coord coordination, coordinated

COP capillary osmotic pressure; change of plaster; coefficient of performance; colloid oncotic pressure; colloid osmotic pressure; competitive oligonucleotide priming; cryptogenic organizing pneumonitis; cyclophosphamide, Oncovin, and prednisone

COPA Council on Postsecondary Accreditation

COPAD cyclophosphamide, vincristine, Adriamycin, prednisone, cytarabine, asparagine, intrathecal methotrexate

COPC community oriented primary care

COPD chronic obstructive pulmonary disease

COPE chronic obstructive pulmonary emphysema

COPEM Committee on Pediatric Emergency Medicine

COPERNICUS Carvedilol Prospective Randomized Cumulative Survival [trial]

COP$_i$ colloid osmotic pressure in interstitial fluid

CO/PLL/CG crystal oscillator/phase lock loop/clock generator [telemedicine]

COPMED Council for Postgraduate Medical Deans [UK]

COPP cyclophosphamide, vincristine [Oncovin], procarbazine, prednisone

COP$_p$ colloid osmotic pressure in plasma

COPRO coproporphyrin; coproporphyrinogen

COPS constrained optimal parameter search

COPT circumoval precipitin reaction test; computerized oxygen therapy protocol

COPV canine oral papillomavirus

CoQ coenzyme Q

COR cardiac output recorder; center of rotation; comprehensive outpatient rehabilitation; conditional origin of replication; conditioned orientation reflex; consensual ophthalmotonic reaction; corrosion, corrosive; cortisone; cortex; crude odds ratio; custodian of records

CoR Congo red

cor body [Lat. *corpus*]; coronary; correction, corrected

CORA conditioned orientation reflex audiometry

CORALI coronarography and alimentation

CORAMI Cohort of Rescue Angioplasty in Myocardial Infarction

CORBA Common Object Request Broker Architecture

CORD Commissioned Officer Residency Deferment; Council of [Emergency Medicine] Residency Directors

CORDIS Cardiovascular Occupational Risk Factor Determination in Israel [study]

CORE Center for Organ Recovery and Education; Collaborative Organization for RheothRx Evaluation; comprehensive assessment and referral evaluation; concept reference

CORGENE Coronary Disease and Angiotensin Converting Enzyme I/D Genotype [study]

CORIS Coronary Risk Factor Study

CorPP coronary perfusion pressure

corr correspondence, corresponding

CORRECT Complete vs Restrictive Revascularization by Coronary Angioplasty Trial

CORSICA Chronic Occlusion Revascularization with Stent Implantation vs Coronary Angioplasty [study]

CoRSV coffee ringspot virus

CORT corticosterone

cort bark [Lat. *cortex*]; cortex

CORTES Clivarin Assessment of Regression of Thrombus: Efficacy and Safety [study]; coordinate reduction time encoding system [ECG]

CORV Corriparta virus

COS carbon oxysulfide; cheiro-oral syndrome; chief of staff; clinically observed seizures; Clinical Orthopaedic Society

CoS class of service

CoSA comparative spectra analysis

COSATI Committee on Scientific and Technical Information

COSHH Control of Substances Hazardous to Health Regulations [UK]

COSMIS Computer System for Medical Information Systems

COSSMHO [National] Coalition of Hispanic Health and Human Services Organizations

COST Cardiac Output Study Technology

COSTAR Computer-Stored Ambulatory Record

COSTART Common Standard Thesaurus of Adverse Reaction Terms

COSTED Committee on Science and Technology in Developing Countries

COSTEP Commissioned Officer Student Training and Extern Program

COSY correlated spectroscopy

COT colony overlay test; committee on trauma; content of thought; contralateral optic tectum; critical off-time

COTA Certified Occupational Therapy Assistant; colon-ovary tumor antigen

COTAIM Continuation of Trial Antihypertensive Interventions and Management

COTD cardiac output by thermodilution

COTe cathodal opening tetanus

COTH Council of Teaching Hospitals and Health Systems

COTRANS Coordinated Transfer Application System

COTS commercial off-the-shelf [software or hardware]

COU cardiac observation unit

coul coulomb

COURAGE Clinical Outcomes Using Revascularization vs Aggressive Strategies; Clinical Outcomes Utilization Revascularization and Aggressive Drug Evaluation

COURT Contrast Media Utilization in High-Risk Percutaneous Transluminal Coronary Angioplasty [trial]

C$_{out}$ outgoing concentration [of blood]

COV covariance; cross-over value

CoV coronavirus

COVER Cover of Vaccination Evaluated Rapidly [UK]

COVESDEM costovertebral segmentation defect with mesomelia [syndrome]

CoVF cobra venom factor

COVISE Collaborative Visualization and Simulation Environment [software]

COVRA Computer Vision in Radiology

COWS cold to opposite and warm to same side

COX cytochrome oxidase; cyclooxygenase

COYV colony virus

CP candle power; capillary pressure; capsid protein; cardiac pacing; cardiac performance; cardiopulmonary; caudate putamen; cell passage; center of pressure; central pit; cephalic presentation; cerebellopontine; cerebral palsy; ceruloplasmin; chemically pure; chemical protection; chest pain; child psychiatry; child psychology; *Chlamydia pneumoniae*; chloropurine; chloroquine-primaquine; chondrodysplasia punctata; choroid plexus; chronic pain; chronic pancreatitis; chronic polyarthritis; chronic pyelonephritis; cicatricial pemphigoid; cleft palate; clinical pathology; clock pulse; closing pressure; cochlear potential; code of practice; cold pressor; color perception; combining power; compound; compressed; congenital porphyria; constant predictor; constant pressure; constrictive pericarditis; coproporphyrin; cor pulmonale; coracoid process; cosine packet; counter propagation [algorithm]; coverage probability [radiotherapy]; C peptide; creatine phosphate; creatine phosphokinase; critical pressure; cross-linked protein; crude protein; current practice; cyclophosphamide; cyclophosphamide and prednisone; cytosol protein; [viral] coat protein

C&P compensation and pension; complete and pain free [joint movement]; cystoscopy and pyelography

C/P cholesterol-phospholipid [ratio]

C + P cryotherapy with pressure

4-CP chlorophenoxyacetic acid

Cp ceruloplasmin; chickenpox; *Corynebacterium parvum*; peak concentration

C_p concentration in plasma; constant pressure; phosphate clearance

cP centipoise

cp candle power; centipoise; chemically pure; circular plasmid; compare

c_p constant pressure

CPA Canadian Physiotherapy Association; Canadian Psychiatric Association; carboxypeptidase A; cardiophrenic angle; cardiopulmonary arrest; carotid phonoangiography; cerebellopontine angle; chlorophenoxyacetic acid; chlorophenylalanine; chronic pyrophosphate arthropathy; circulating platelet aggregate; complement proactivator; control, preoccupation, and addiction; costophrenic angle; cyclophosphamide; cyclopiazonic acid; cyproterone acetate

C3PA complement-3 proactivator

C_{pa} cardiac peak amplitude

CPAD chronic peripheral arterial disease

CPAF chlorpropamide-alcohol flushing

C_{pah} para-aminohippurate clearance

CP-ANN counterpropagation artificial neural network

CPAP continuous positive airway pressure

CPAS Canadian Prinivil Atenolol Study

CPB carboxypeptidase B; cardiopulmonary bypass; cetylpyridinium bromide; competitive protein binding

CPBA competitive protein-binding analysis

CpBDV chickpea bushy dwarf virus

CPBV cardiopulmonary blood volume

CPC central posterior curve; cerebellar Purkinje cell; cerebral palsy clinic; cerebral performance category; cetylpyridinium chloride; chemical protective clothing; chest pain center; child protection center; chronic passive congestion; circumferential pneumatic compression; clinicopathological conference

CpCDV chickpea chlorotic dwarf virus

CPCL congenital pulmonary cystic lymphangiectasia

CPCP chronic progressive coccidioidal pneumonitis

CPCR cardiopulmonary cerebral resuscitation; Center for Primary Care Research

CPCS circumferential pneumatic compression suit; computer-based patient case simulation system

CPCV Cacipacore virus

CPD calcium pyrophosphate deposition; cephalopelvic disproportion; cerebelloparenchymal disorder; childhood or congenital polycystic disease; chorioretinopathy and pituitary dysfunction; chronic peritoneal dialysis; chronic protein deprivation; citrate-phosphate-dextrose; contact potential difference; contagious pustular dermatitis; critical point drying; cyclobutane pyrimidine dimer; cyclopentadiene

cpd cigarettes per day; compound; cycles per degree

CPDA citrate-phosphate-dextrose-adenine

CPDD calcium pyrophosphate deposition disease; *cis*-platinum-diamine dichloride

cpd E compound E

CP DEPMEDS chemically protected deployable medical system

cpd F compound F

CPDL cumulative population doubling level

CPDX cefpodoxime

CPDX-PR cefpodoxime proxetil

CPE capillary parenchymal element; carbon paste electrode; cardiac pulmonary edema; chronic pulmonary emphysema;

clinical progress exercise; *Clostridium perfringens* enterotoxin; collective protection equipment; compensation, pension, and education; complete physical examination; complicated pleural effusion; corona-penetrating enzyme; cryptogenic partial epilepsy; cytopathogenic effect

CPEO chronic progressive external ophthalmoplegia

CPEP Chicago Coronary Prevention Evaluation Program; clinical practice enhancement project

CPE-R *Clostridium perfringens* enterotoxin receptor

CPEV *Chironomus plumosus* entomopoxvirus

CPF center point of force; clot-promoting factor; complication probability factor; contraction peak force; current patient file

C$_{pf}$ cardiac peak frequency

CPFC chemically protective footgear cover

CpFV chickpea filiform virus

CPG capillary blood gases; cardiopneumographic recording; carotid phonoangiogram; central pattern generator; clinical practice guidelines; computerized pattern generator

CPGMV cowpea golden mosaic virus

CPGN chronic proliferative glomerulonephritis

CPGs clinical practice guidelines

CPH Certificate in Public Health; chronic paroxysmal hemicrania; chronic persistent hepatitis; chronic primary headache

CPHA Canadian Public Health Association; Commission on Professional and Hospital Activities

CPHA-PAS Commission on Professional and Hospital Activities-Professional Activity Study

CPHL Central Public Health Laboratory [UK]

CPHQ certified professional in healthcare quality

CPHRP Coronary Prevention and Hypertension Research Project

CPHS Centre for Public Health Sciences

CpHV caprine herpesvirus

CPI California Personality Inventory; Cancer Potential Index; common patient index; congenital palatopharyngeal incompetence; constitutional psychopathic inferiority; conventional planar imaging;

coronary prognosis index; cysteine proteinase inhibitor

CPIB chlorophenoxyisobutyrate

CPIJH compass proximal interphalangeal joint hinge

CPIP chronic pulmonary insufficiency of prematurity

CPIR cephalic-phase insulin release

CPK cell population kinetic [model]; creatine phosphokinase

cPK cytosolic protamine kinase

CPK-BB creatine phosphokinase, brain-type

cPKC classical protein kinase C

CPKD childhood polycystic kidney disease

CPL caprine placental lactogen; conditioned pitch level; congenital pulmonary lymphangiectasia

C/PL cholesterol/phospholipid [ratio]

cpl complete, completed

CPLM cysteine-peptone-liver infusion medium

CPLS cleft palate-lateral synechia syndrome

CPM calorie-protein malnutrition; central pontine myelinosis; chlorpheniramine maleate; confidence profile method; confined placental mosaicism; continuous passive motion; critical path method; cyclophosphamide

CP/M control program for microcomputers

C$_{PM}$ circumference of papillary muscle

cpm counts per minute; cycles per minute

CP-MCT chirp pulse microwave computed tomography

CPMG Carr-Purcell-Meiboom-Gill [sequence]

CPMMV cowpea mild mottle virus

CPMoV cowpea mottle virus

CPMP Committee for Proprietary Medicinal Products [EEC]; complete patient management problems

CPMS chronic progressive multiple sclerosis

CPMV cowpea mosaic virus

CPN causal probabilistic network; celiac plexus neurolysis; central parenteral nutrition; chronic polyneuropathy; chronic pyelonephritis; community pediatric nurse; community psychiatric nurse

CPNE clinical performance nursing examination

CPNM corrected perinatal mortality

CPO cleft palate only; contract provider organization; coproporphyrinogen oxidase

CPOE computerized physician order entry

CPOG chemically protective overgarment

CPOPR computerized problem-oriented patient record

C-PORT Cardiovascular Patient Outcomes Research Team [trial]

CPOS chest pain order sheet

CPOTHA chest pain onset to hospital arrival

CPOU chest pain observation unit

CPP cancer proneness phenotype; canine pancreatic polypeptide; cerebral perfusion pressure; chest pain policy; *dl*-2[3-(2′-chlorophenoxy)phenyl] propionic [acid]; chronic pigmented purpura; coronary perfusion pressure; cyclopentenophenanthrene

CPPB continuous positive pressure breathing

CPPD calcium pyrophosphate dihydrate deposition [syndrome]; cisplatin; cost per patient day

CPPT Coronary Primary Prevention Trial

CPPV continuous positive pressure ventilation

CPQA certified professional in quality assurance

CPR cardiopulmonary reserve; cardiopulmonary resuscitation; centripetal rub; cerebral cortex perfusion rate; chlorophenyl red; computerized patient record; cortisol production rate; cumulative patency rate; customary, prevailing and reasonable [rate]

c-PR cyclopropyl

cpr computerized patient record

CPRAM controlled partial rebreathing anesthesia method

CPRCA constitutional pure red cell aplasia

CPRD Committee on Prosthetics Research and Development

CPRG Coronary Prevention Research Group

CPRI Computerized Patient Record Institute

CPRMV cowpea rugose mosaic virus

CPRO coproporphyrinogen oxidase

CPRP chemical personnel reliability program

CPRS Children's Psychiatric Rating Scale; Comprehensive Psychopathological Rating Scale; computerized patient record system

CPS Caerphilly Prospective Study; Cancer Prevention Study; carbamoylphosphate synthetase; cardioplegic perfusion solution; cardiopulmonary support; center for preventive services; centipoise; cervical pain syndrome; characters per second; chest pain syndrome; Child Personality Scale; Child Protective Services; chloroquine, pyrimethamine, and sulfisoxazole; chronic prostatitis syndrome; clinical performance score; Clinical Pharmacy Services; coagulase-positive *Staphylococcus*; complex partial seizures; concurrent planning system; constitutional psychopathic state; contagious pustular stomatitis; coronary perfusate solution; C-polysaccharide; cumulative probability of success; current population survey

cps counts per second; cycles per second

CPSA charged particle surface area

CPSC congenital paucity of secondary synaptic clefts [syndrome]; Consumer Products Safety Commission

CPSD carbamyl phosphate synthetase deficiency

CpSDaV chickpea stunt disease associated virus

CPSE complex partial status epilepticus

CPSF cleavage and polyadenylation specificity factor

CPSM Council for Professions Supplementary to Medicine

CPSMP chronic pain self-management program

CPSMV cowpox severe mosaic virus

CPSO College of Physicians and Surgeons of Ontario

CPSP central poststroke pain

CPSTS Chinese Poststroke Treatment Study

CPsV citrus psorosis virus

CPT camptothecin; carnitine palmityl transferase; carotid pulse tracing; chest physiotherapy; child protection team; ciliary particle transport; cold pressor test; combining power test; complex physical therapy; computer psychometric test; conditional probability table; conjunctival provocation test; continuous performance task; continuous performance test; Current Procedural Terminology

CPT-11 irinotecan

CPTA Center for Practice and Technology Assessment [Agency for Healthcare Research and Quality]

CPTH chronic post-traumatic headache

CPTN culture-positive toxin-negative

CPTP culture-positive toxin-positive

CPTX chronic parathyroidectomy

CPU caudate putamen; central processing unit

CPUE chest pain of unknown etiology

CPV canine parvovirus; cytoplasmic polyhedrosis virus; Coastal Plains virus; Cotia virus; cypovirus

CpV *Calliteara pudibunda* virus; cypovirus

CPVC common pulmonary venous channel

CPVD congenital polyvalvular disease

CPX cleft palate, X-linked; clinical practice examination; complete physical examination

CPXD chondrodysplasia punctata, X-linked dominant

CPXR chondrodysplasia punctata, X-linked recessive

CPXV cowpox virus

CPZ cefoperazone; chlorpromazine; Compazine

CQ chloroquine; chloroquine-quinine; circadian quotient; conceptual quotient

CQI continuous quality improvement

CQIN clinical quality improvement network

CQI/TQM continuous quality improvement/total quality management

CQIV Calchaqui virus

CQM chloroquine mustard

CQMS cost quality management system

CQOLC caregiver quality-of-life index – cancer

CQS central query system

CqV *Callimorpha quadripunctata* virus

CR cadherin-specific repeat; calculation rate; calculus removed; calorie-restricted; cardiac rehabilitation; cardiac resuscitation; cardiac rhythm; cardiorespiratory; cardiorrhexis; caries-resistant; cathode ray; cellular receptor; central ray; centric relation; chemoradiation; chest and right arm [lead in electrocardiography]; chest roentgenogram, chest roentgenography; chief resident; child-resistant [bottle top]; choice reaction; chromium; chronic rejection; chrysene; clinical record; clinical remission; clinical research; clot retraction; coefficient of fat retention; colon resection; colonization rate; colonization resistance; colony reared [animal]; colorectal; complement receptor; complete remission; complete response; compression ratio; computed radiography; computerized record; conditioned reflex, conditioned response; confidence region [radiotherapy]; congenital rubella; Congo red; controlled release; controlled respiration; conversion rate; cooling rate; correlation; correlation ratio; cortico-resistant; creatinine; cremaster reflex; cresyl red; critical ratio; crownrump [measurement]

CR1, 2, 3, 4, 5 complement receptor types 1 to 5

C&R convalescence and rehabilitation

Cr chromium; cranium, cranial; creatinine; crown

CRA central retinal artery; Chinese restaurant asthma; chronic rheumatoid arthritis; clinical research associate; constant relative alkalinity

CRABP cellular retinoic acid-binding protein

CRAC calcium release-activated channel; compliance-related acute complication

CRADA Cooperative Research and Development Agreement [Army and NIH]

CRAFT Catheterization Rescue Angioplasty Following Thrombolysis [trial]; Controlled Randomized Atrial Fibrillation Trial

CRAG *Cryptococcus* antigen

CRAHCA Center for Research in Ambulatory Health Care Administration

CRAM common random access memory

CRAMS circulation, respiration, abdomen, motor, speech

cran cranium, cranial

CRAO central retinal artery occlusion

CRASH corpus callosum hypoplasia-retardation-adducted thumbs-spastic paraplegia-hydrocephalus [syndrome]

CraV Cynara virus

CRAW computed tomography acquisition workstation

CRB chemical, radiological, and biological; congenital retinal blindness; Cramer-Rao bound

CRBBB complete right bundle branch block

CRBC chicken red blood cell

CRBP cellular retinol-binding protein

CRC calcium release channel; cancer research campaign; cardiovascular reflex clinical research center; cardiovascular reflex conditioning; class responsibilities collaboration; colorectal cancer; colorectal carcinoma; concentrated red blood cells; contrast recovery coefficient; corrected reticulocyte count; creatinine clearance; cross-reacting cannabinoids; cyclic redundancy check

CrCl creatinine clearance

CRCS cardiovascular reflex conditioning system

CRD carbohydrate-recognition domain; child restraint device; childhood rheumatic disease; chorioretinal degeneration; chronic renal disease; chronic respiratory disease; complete reaction of degeneration; complex repetitive discharge; cone-rod retinal dystrophy; congenital rubella deafness; crown-rump distance

CRDC Central Research and Development Committee

CRDEC Chemical Research Development & Engineering Center

CR-DIP chronic relapsing demyelinating inflammatory polyneuropathy

CRDS Charles River Data System; client response documentation system

CRE cumulative radiation effect; creatinine; cyclic adenosine monophosphate-response element

creat creatinine

CREATE Cholesterol Research Education and Treatment Evaluation

CREB cyclic adenosine monophosphate responsive element-binding [protein]

CREDO Clopidogrel Reduction of Events During Extended Observation [study]

CREG cross-reactive antigen group

CREM center for rural emergency medicine; cyclic adenosine monophosphate-response element modulator

crem cremaster

CREOG Council on Resident Education in Obstetrics and Gynecology

crep crepitation; crepitus

CREST calcinosis, Raynaud phenomenon, esophageal involvement, sclerodactyly, and telangiectasia [syndrome]; Carotid Revascularization and Endarterectomy vs Stent Trial

CREW Coronary Regression with Estrogen in Women [study]

CRF cardiorespiratory function; case report form; chronic renal failure; chronic respiratory failure; coagulase-reacting factor; complex reduction forceps; continuous reinforcement; coronary reserve flow; corticotropin-releasing factor; cytokine receptor family

CRFK Crandell feline kidney cells

CRFR corticotropin-releasing factor receptor

CRG cardiorespirogram; central respiratory generator; collaborative review group

CRH corticotropin-releasing hormone

CRHBP corticosterone-releasing hormone binding protein

CRHL Collaborative Radiological Health Laboratory

CRHV cottontail rabbit herpesvirus

CrHV cricetid herpesvirus

CRI Cardiac Risk Index; catheter-related infection; chronic renal insufficiency; chronic respiratory insufficiency; Composite Risk Index; congenital rubella infection; contact ratio index; corneal relaxing incision; cross-reaction idiotype

C-RI corecessive inheritance

CRIB clinical risk index for babies

CRIE crossed radioimmunoelectrophoresis

CRIP cysteine-rich intestinal protein

CRIS Calcium Antagonist Reinfarction Italian Study; clinically related information system

CRISP Cholesterol Reduction in Seniors Program [pilot study]; Computer Retrieval of Information on Scientific Projects [NIH database]; Consortium Research in Systems Performance; Consortium Research on Indicators of System Performance

Crit, crit critical; hematocrit

CRIYFS Cardiovascular Risk in Young Finns Study

CRL cell repository line; central right lung; Certified Record Librarian; clinical reasoning learning; complement receptor location; complement receptor lymphocyte; crown-rump length

CRLV cherry rasp leaf virus

CRM Certified Reference Materials; coding recognition module [of gene]; counting rate meter; cross-reacting material; crown-rump measurement

CRM + cross-reacting material-positive

CRMO chronic recurrent multifocal osteomyelitis

CR-MVB Cramer-Rao minimum variance bound

CRN complement requiring neutralization

CRNA Certified Registered Nurse Anesthetist

CRNF chronic rheumatoid nodular fibrositis

Cr Nn, cr nn cranial nerves

CRO cathode ray oscilloscope; centric relation occlusion; contract research organization

CROM cervical range of motion

CROME congenital cataracts-epileptic fitsmental retardation [syndrome]

C-ROMS comprehensive radiation oncology management system

CROP compliance, rate, oxygenation, and pressure

CROS contralateral routing of signals [hearing aid]

CRP chronic relapsing pancreatitis; corneal-retinal potential; coronary rehabilitation program; C-reactive protein; cross-reacting protein; cyclic adenosine monophosphate receptor protein; cysteine-rich protein

CrP creatine phosphate

CRPA C-reactive protein antiserum

CRPD chronic restrictive pulmonary disease

CRPF chloroquine-resistant *Plasmodium falciparum*; closed reduction and percutaneous fixation; contralateral renal plasma flow

CRPG central respiratory pattern generator

CRPS complex regional pain syndrome [types I and II]

CRPV cottontail rabbit papillomavirus; crowpox virus

CRQ-M Chronic Respiratory Questionnaire Mastery Subscale

CRRMP Committee of Radiation from Radioactive Medicinal Products

CRRN certified rehabilitation registered nurse

CRRT continuous renal replacement therapy

CrRT cranial radiotherapy

CRS Carroll rating scale for depression; catheter-related sepsis; caudal regression syndrome; cervical spine radiography; Chinese restaurant syndrome; cis-acting repressive sequence; colon and rectum surgery; compliance of the respiratory system; congenital rubella syndrome; craniosynostosis; cryptidin-related sequence

C$_{RS +}$ respiratory system compliance

CRSM cherry red spot myoclonus

CRSP comprehensive renal scintillation procedure

CRST calcinosis, Raynaud phenomenon, sclerodactyly, telangiectasia [syndrome]; corrected sinus recovery time

CRSV carnation ringspot virus; chlorotic ringspot virus

CRT cadaver renal transplantation; calreticulin; cardiac resuscitation team; cathode-ray tube; central reaction time; certified; Certified Record Techniques; chemoradiation therapy; choice reaction time; chromium release test; complex reaction time; computed renal tomography; conformal radiation therapy; conformal radiotherapy; copper reduction test; corrected; corrected retention time; cortisone resistant thymocyte; cranial radiation therapy

CrT crista terminalis

crt hematocrit

CRTM cartilage matrix protein

CRTP Consciousness Research and Training Project

CRTT Certified Respiratory Therapy Technician

CRU cardiac rehabilitation unit; clinical research unit

CRUISE Can Routine Ultrasound Influence Stent Expansion? [study]

CRUSADE Coronary Reserve Utilization for Stent and Angiography: Doppler Endpoint [study]; Coronary Revascularization Ultrasound Angioplasty Device [trial]

CRV Channel catfish reovirus; central retinal vein; cherry rosette virus; Cowbone Ridge virus; Nile crocodile poxvirus

CRVF congestive right ventricular failure

CRVO central retinal vein occlusion

Cry crystal [protein]

CRYG gamma crystallin gene

CRYM mu-crystallin

cryo cryogenic; cryoglobulin; cryoprecipitate; cryosurgery; cryotherapy

Cryoppt cryoprecipitate

CRYP cryptospiridiosis

crys, cryst crystal, crystalline

CS calf serum; campomelic syndrome; canalicular system; Capgras syndrome; carcinoid syndrome; cardiogenic shock; caries-susceptible; carotid sheath; carotid sinus; cat scratch; celiac sprue; central service; central supply; cerebral scintigraphy; cerebrospinal; cervical spine; cervical stimulation; cesarean section; chest strap; chief of staff; cholesterol stone; cholesterol sulfate; chondroitin sulfate; chorionic somatomammotropin; chronic schizophrenia; cigarette smoke; cigarette smoker; circumsporozoite; citrate synthase; climacteric syndrome; clinical laboratory scientist; clinical stage; clinical status; clinic scheduling; Cockayne syndrome; complete stroke; compression syndrome; concentrated strength; conditioned stimulus; congenital syphilis; conjunctival secretion; connection service; conscious, consciousness; conscious sedation; conservative surgery; constant spring; contact sensitivity; continue same; contrast sensitivity; control serum; control subjects; convalescence, convalescent; coordinate system; coronary sclerosis; coronary sinus; corpus striatum; corticoid-sensitive; corticosteroid; corticosubcortical; countershock; crush syndrome; current smoker; current strength; Cushing syndrome; cyclic somatostatin; cycloserine; cyclosporine

C/S cesarean section; cycles per second

C&S calvarium and scalp; conjunctiva and sclera; culture and sensitivity

CS IV clinical stage 4

C4S chondroitin-4-sulfate

Cs case; cell surface; cyclosporine; static compliance

Cₛ standard clearance; static compliance; static respiratory compliance

cS centistoke

cs catalytic subunit; chromosome; consciousness

CSA Cambridge Scientific Abstracts; Canadian Standards Association; canavaninosuccinic acid; carbonyl salicylamide; cell surface antigen; chemical shift anisotropy; chondroitin sulfate A; chorionic somatomammotropin A; classical simulated annealing; client server architecture; clinical skills assessment; colony-stimulating activity; colony survival array; compressed spectral array; computerized spectral analysis; Controlled Substances Act; cross section area; cyclosporin A

CsA cyclosporin A

CSAA Child Study Association of America

CSAD corporate services administration department

CSAT cell substratum attachment; center for substance abuse treatment

CSAVP cerebral subarachnoid venous pressure

CSB contaminated small bowel; craniosynostosis, Boston type

csb chromosome break

CSBF coronary sinus blood flow

CSBS contaminated small bowel syndrome

CSC blow on blow [Fr. *coup sur coup*]; chondroitin sulfate C; cigarette smoke condensate; collagen sponge contraceptive; corticostriatocerebellar; cryogenic storage container; cytokine-secreting cell

CSCC circuits, systems, communications, and computers; cutaneous squamous cell carcinoma

CSCD Center for Sickle Cell Disease

CSCE Committee on Scientific Conduct and Ethics [NIH]

CSCHDS Caerphilly and Speedwell Collaborative Heart Disease Studies

CSCI corticosterone side-chain isomerase

CSCL computer-supported collaborative learning

CsCMV cassava common mosaic virus

CSCR Central Society for Clinical Research

CSCV critical serum chemistry value

CSCW computer-supported collaborative work

CSD carotid sinus denervation; cat scratch disease; collimator-skin distance; combined system disease; computerized severity index; conditionally streptomycin dependent; conduction system disease; cortical spreading depression; craniospinal defect; critical stimulus duration

CSDB cat scratch disease bacillus

CSDH chronic subdural hematoma

CSDMS Canadian Society of Diagnostic Medical Sonographers

CSE clinical-symptom/self-evaluation [questionnaire]; common standards for quantitative electrocardiography; cone-shaped epiphysis; conventional spin-echo; cross-sectional echocardiography

C sect, C-section cesarean section

CSEP clinical sepsis; conducted somatosensory evoked potential; cortical somatosensory evoked potential

CSEPP Chemical Stockpile Emergency Preparedness Program

CSER cortical somatosensory evoked response

CSERIAC Crew System Ergonomics Information Analysis Center [Canada]

CSES Chronic Obstructive Pulmonary Disease [COPD] Self-Efficacy Scale

CSF cancer family syndrome; cerebrospinal fluid; cold stability factor; colony-stimulating factor; coronary sinus flow; critical success factor

CS-F colony-stimulating factor

CSFH cerebrospinal fluid hypotension

CSFII Continuing Survey of Food Intakes by Individuals

CSF-IR colony-stimulating factor I receptor

CSFP cerebrospinal fluid pressure

CSFQ Changes in Sexual Functioning Questionnaire

CSFR colony-stimulating factor receptor

CSFV cerebrospinal fluid volume; classical swine fever virus

CSF-WR cerebrospinal fluid-Wassermann reaction

CSG cell surface glycoprotein; central sympathetic generator; cholecystography, cholecystogram; clinical study group; collaborative study group

csg chromosome gap

CSGBI Cardiac Society of Great Britain and Ireland

CSGBM collagenase soluble glomerular basement membrane

CSGE conformational sensitive gel electrophoresis

CsGMV cassava green mottle virus

CSGTEI Collaborative Study Group Trial on the Effect of Irbesartan

CSH carotid sinus hypersensitivity; chronic subdural hematoma; combat support hospital; cortical stromal hyperplasia

CSHA Canadian Study of Health and Aging

CSHCN children with special health care needs

CSHE California Society for Hospital Engineering

CSHH congenital self-healing histiocytosis

CSHL Cold Spring Harbor Laboratory

CSHN children with special health needs

CSHS Canadian Smoking Health Survey

CSI calculus surface index; cancer serum index; cavernous sinus infiltration; cervical spine injury; chemical safety inspection; chemical shift imaging; chemical surety inspection; cholesterol saturation index; computerized severity of illness [index]; coronary sinus intervention; cranio-spinal irradiation

CSICU cardiac surgical intensive care unit

CSIF cytokine synthesis inhibitory factor

CSII continuous subcutaneous insulin infusion

CSIIP continuous subcutaneous insulin infusion pump

CSIN Chemical Substances Information Network

CSIRO Commonwealth Scientific and Industrial Research Organisation [Australia]

CSIS clinical supplies and inventory system

CsIV *Campoletis sonorensis* ichnovirus

CSL cardiolipin synthetic lecithin; corticosteroid liposome

CSLM confocal scanning laser microscopy

CSLP cervical spine locking plate

CSLT Canadian Society of Laboratory Technology

CSLU chronic stasis leg ulcer

CSM cardiosynchronous myostimulator; care systems management; carotid sinus massage; cerebrospinal meningitis; circulation, sensation, motion; Committee on Safety of Medicines [UK]; confined space medicine; Consolidated Standards Manual; corn-soy milk

CSMA chronic spinal muscular atrophy

CSMA/CD carrier sense multiple access and collision detection

CSMAP celiac-superior mesenteric artery portography

C-SMART Cardiomyoplasty-Skeletal Muscle Assist Randomized Trial

CSMB Center for the Study of Multiple Births

CSMLS Canadian Society of Medical Laboratory Science

CSMMG Chartered Society of Massage and Medical Gymnastics

CSMP chloramphenicol-sensitive microsomal protein

CSMSS Collaborative Social and Medical Services System

CSMT chorionic somatomammotropin

CSN cardiac sympathetic nerve; carotid sinus nerve; Chemical Safety Newsbase; cycloserine

CSNA congenital sensory neuropathy with anhidrosis [syndrome]

CSNB congenital stationary night blindness

CS(NCA) Clinical Laboratory Scientist Certified by the National Certification Agency for Medical Laboratory Personnel

CSNDB Cell Signaling Network Database

CSNK casein kinase

CSNRT, cSNRT corrected sinus node recovery time

CSNS carotid sinus nerve stimulation

CSNU cystinuria

CSO claims services only; common source outbreak; craniostenosis; craniosynostosis; ostium of coronary sinus

CSOM chronic suppurative otitis media

CSOP coronary sinus occlusion pressure

CSP carotid sinus pressure; cavum septi pellucidi; cell surface protein; central silent period; cerebrospinal protein; Chartered Society of Physiotherapy; chemistry screening panel; chondroitin sulfate protein; circumsporozoite protein; complications screening program; Cooperative Statistical Program; criminal sexual psychopath; cutaneous silent period; cyclosporin

Csp, C-spine cervical spine

CSPAMM complementary spatial modulation of magnetization [imaging]

CSPG chondroitin sulfate proteoglycan

CSPI Center for Science in the Public Interest

CSPINE corticosteroid use, seropositive RA, peripheral joint destruction, involvement of cervical nerves, nodules (rheumatoid), established disease [cervical spine disease risk factors]

CspIV *Campoletis* sp. ichnovirus

CSPS continual skin peeling syndrome

CSpT corticospinal tract

CSQ Coping Strategies Questionnaire

CSR Center for Scientific Review; central supply room; chart-stimulated recall [test]; Cheyne-Stokes respiration; continued stay review; corrected sedimentation rate; corrected survival rate; cortisol secretion rate; cumulative survival rate

CSRA cardio-surgical recovery area

CSRM case specific reference model

CSRP cysteine-rich protein

CSRS cardiac surgery reporting system

CSRT Canadian Society of Respiratory Technology; continuous-speech recognition technology

CSS Canadian Stroke Scale; Cancer Surveillance System; carotid sinus stimulation; carotid sinus syndrome; cavernous sinus syndrome; central sterile section; central sterile supply; chewing, sucking, swallowing; chronic subclinical scurvy; Churg-Strauss syndrome; client satisfaction scale; clinical support system; Copenhagen Stroke Study; cranial sector scan; critical care system

C^{ss} [plasma] concentration at steady state

CSSA Carotid Stent-Supported Angioplasty [trial]

CSSAE Communication Skills Self-Assessment Exam

CSSCD Cooperative Study of Sickle Cell Disease

CSSD central sterile supply department

CSSRD Cooperative Systematic Study of Rheumatic Diseases

CSSU central sterile supply unit

CSSV cacao swollen shoot virus

CST cardiac stress test; cardiovascular self-assessment tool; cavernous sinus thrombosis; certified surgical technologist; chemostatin; Christ-Siemens-Touraine [syndrome]; compliance, static; computer scatter tomography; contraction stress test; conversational speech task; convulsive shock therapy; corticospinal tract; cosyntropin stimulation test; cystatin

cSt centistoke

C$_{st}$, C$_{stat}$ static compliance

CSTB Computer Science and Telecommunications Board [National Academy of Sciences]

CSTD chronic single tic disorder

CSTE Council of State and Territorial Epidemiologists

CstF cleavage stimulation factor

CSTI Clearinghouse for Scientific and Technical Information

CSTM cervical prevertebral soft tissue measurement

c-STM cervical specimen transport medium

CSTP Committee for Scientific and Technological Policy

Cst,rs static compliance of respiratory system

CSTT cold-stimulation time test

CSU casualty staging unit; catheter specimen of urine; central statistical unit; clinical specialty unit

CSUF continuous slow ultrafiltration

CSV chick syncytial virus; chlorotic spot virus; chlorotic streak virus; cocksfoot streak virus

CsVC cassava virus C

CSVd Chrysanthemum stunt viroid

CsVMV cassava vein mosaic virus

CSVT central splanchnic venous thrombosis

CsVX cassava virus X

CSW Certified Social Worker; commercial sex worker; current sleep walker

CSWG Clinical Systems Working Group

CSWSS continuous spike-waves of slow sleep

CT calcitonin; calf testis; carboxyl terminal; cardiac tamponade; cardiothoracic [ratio]; carnitine transporter; carotid tracing; carpal tunnel; cell therapy; cerebral thrombosis; cerebral tumor; cervical traction; cervicothoracic; chemotaxis; chemotherapy; chest tube; chicken tumor; *Chlamydia trachomatis*; chlorothiazide; cholera toxin; cholesterol, total; chordae tendineae; chronic thyroiditis; chymotrypsin; circulation time; classic technique; clinical trial; closed thoracotomy; clotting time; coagulation time; coated tablet; cobra toxin; cognitive therapy; coil test; collecting tubule; colon, transverse;

combined tumor; compressed tablet; computed tomography; connective tissue; continue treatment; continuous-flow tube; contraceptive technique; contraction time; controlled temperature; Coombs test; corneal transplant; coronary thrombosis; corrected transposition; corrective therapy; cortical thickness; corticospinal tract; cough threshold; crest time; crista terminalis; cystine-tellurite; cytotechnologist; cytotoxic therapy; unit of attenuation [number]

C/T compression/traction [ratio]

C&T color and temperature

C$_T$ total compliance

C$_{T-1824}$ T-1824 (Evans blue) clearance

CTI cardiac troponin I

Ct carboxyl terminal; concentration

ct carat; chromatid; count

CTA Canadian Tuberculosis Association; center for total access; chemotactic activity; chromotropic acid; Committee on Thrombolytic Agents; computed tomographic angiography; computed tomography of the abdomen; congenital trigeminal anesthesia; cyanotrimethyl-androsterone; cystine trypticase agar; cytoplasmic tubular aggregate; cytotoxic assay

CTAB cetyltrimethyl-ammonium bromide

CTAC Cancer Treatment Advisory Committee

CTAF Canadian Trial of Atrial Fibrillation; conotruncal anomaly face [syndrome]

CTAFS conotruncal anomaly face syndrome

cTAL cortical thick ascending limb

CTAP computed tomography in arterial portography; connective tissue activating peptide

CTAT computerized transaxial tomography

CTB ceased to breathe; cholera toxin B

ctb chromated break

CTC chlortetracycline; Clinical Trial Certificate; Common Toxicity Criteria [database]; computed tomographic colography; computer-aided tomographic cisternography; consent to continue; cultured T cells

CTCL cutaneous T-cell lymphoma

ctCO$_2$ carbon dioxide concentration

CTD carboxy-terminal domain; chest tube drainage; carpal tunnel decompression;

congenital thymic dysplasia; connective tissue disease; cumulative trauma disorder

CT&DB cough, turn, and deep breathe

CTDI computed tomography dose index

ctDNA chloroplast deoxyribonucleic acid

CTE calf thymus extract; cultured thymic epithelium

CTEM conventional transmission electron microscopy

CTEP Cancer Therapy Evaluation Program

CTEV *Camptochironomus tentans* entomopoxvirus

CTeV carrot temperate virus

CTF cancer therapy facility; certificate; Colorado tick fever; contrast transfer function; cytotoxic factor

ctf certificate

CTFE chlorotrifluoroethylene

CTFS complete testicular feminization syndrome

CTFV Colorado tick fever virus

CTG cardiotocography; cervicothoracic ganglion; chymotrypsinogen; control technique guidelines

C/TG cholesterol-triglyceride [ratio]

ctg chromated gap

CTGA complete transposition of great arteries

CTGF connective tissue growth factor

CTGFN Convergent Terminology Group for Nursing

CTH ceramide trihexoside; chronic tension headache; computer-assisted tomographic holography; cystathionase

CTh carrier-specific T-helper [cell]

C$_{Th}$ thoracic compliance

CTHA computed tomographic hepatic angiography

CTHD chlorthalidone

CTI coffee table injury; computers in teaching initiatives; computer-telephony integration [telemedicine]

CTiVd Coconut tinangaja viroid

CTL cervico-thoraco-lumbar; computational tree logic; control; cytolytic T lymphocyte; cytotoxic T lymphocyte

CTLA cytotoxic T lymphocyte antigen

CTLL cytotoxic lymphoid line

CTLp cytotoxic T lymphocyte precursor

CTLSO cervicothoracolumbosacral orthosis

CTLV carrot thin leaf virus

CtLV carrot latent virus

CTM calibration of test material; cardiotachometer; central tendency measure; Chlortrimeton; computed tomographic myelography; cricothyroid membrane; cricothyroid muscle

CTMC connective tissue mast cell

CTMM computed tomographic metrizamide myelography

CTMM-SF California Test of Mental Maturity-Short Form

CTMR clinical treatment and medical research

CT/MRI computed tomography/magnetic resonance imaging

CtMV carrot mosaic virus

CTN calcitonin; clinical trials notification; computer tomography number; continuous noise

cTn-I cardiac troponin I

cTNM clinical classification of primary tumors, regional nodes and metastases [coding]

CTO cervicothoracic orthosis

CTOPP Canadian Trial of Physiological Pacing

CTP California Test of Personality; citrate transport protein; clinical terms project; comprehensive treatment plan; cytidine triphosphate; cytosine triphosphate

C-TPN cyclic total parenteral nutrition

CTPP cerebral tissue perfusion pressure

CTPVO chronic thrombotic pulmonary vascular obstruction

CTR cardiothoracic ratio; carpal tunnel release; central tumor registry; Connecticut Tumor Registry

ctr central; center; centric

CTRB chymotrypsinogen B

CTRD Cardiac Transplant Research Database

CTRL chymotrypsin-like [protease]

CtRLV carrot red leaf virus

CTRS certified therapeutic recreation specialist

CTRX ceftriaxone

CTS cardiothoracic surgery; cardiotonic steroids; carpal tunnel syndrome; clinical trials support [program]; Collaborative Transplant Study; composite treatment score; computed tomographic scan; conflict tactics scales; contralateral threshold shift; corticosteroid

CTSB cathepsin B
CTSD cathepsin D
CTSE cathepsin E
CTSG cathepsin G
CTSH cathepsin H
CTSI computerized tomography severity index
CTSL cathepsin L
CTSNFR corrected time of sinoatrial node function recovery
CTSP Cooperative Triglyceride Standardization Program
CTSS cathepsin S; closed tracheal suction system
CTT cefotetan; central tegmental tract; central transmission time; classic test theory; colonic transit time; compressed tablet triturate; computed transaxial tomography; critical tracking time
CTTAC clinical trials and treatment advisory committee
CTU cardiac-thoracic unit; centigrade thermal unit; constitutive transcription unit
CTV cervical and thoracic vertebrae; citrus tristeza virus; clinical target volume; clinical tumor volume; curly top virus
CTVDR conformal treatment verification, delivery and recording [system]
CTW central terminal of Wilson; combined testicular weight
CTX cefotaxime; ceftriaxone; cerebrotendinous xanthomatosis; chemotaxis; ciguatoxin; clinical trials exemption scheme; costotendinous xanthomatosis; cytoxan
CTx cardiac transplantation; conotoxin
CTZ cetirizine; chemoreceptor trigger zone; chlorothiazide
CU cardiac unit; casein unit; cause unknown or undetermined; chymotrypsin unit; clinical unit; color unit; contact urticaria; convalescent unit
C$_u$ urea clearance
cu cubic
CUA cost-utility analysis [ratio]
CUAVD congenital unilateral absence of vas deferens
CuB copper band
CUBA Cutting Balloon vs Conventional Balloon Angioplasty [study]
CUC chronic ulcerative colitis
cu cm cubic centimeter
CuCV cucumber cryptic virus

CUD cause undetermined; congenital urinary deformity
CuD copper deficiency
CUE confidential unit exclusion; cumulative urinary excretion
CUG Computer-Stored Ambulatory Record User's Group; cystidine, uridine, and guanidine; cystourethrogram, cystourethrography
CUI character-based interface; concept unique identifier [UMLS]; Cox-Uphoff International [tissue expander]
cu in cubic inch
cult culture
cum cumulative
cu m cubic meter
CUMITECH Cumulative Techniques and Procedures in Clinical Microbiology
cu mm cubic millimeter
CUMULVS collaborative user migration, user library for visualization and steering
CuNV cucumber necrosis virus
CUP carcinoma unknown primary
CUR cystourethrorectal
cur cure, curative; current
CURE Clopidogrel in Unstable Angina to Prevent Recurrent Ischemic Events [trial]; Columbia University Restenosis Elimination [trial]
CURL compartment of uncoupling of receptors and ligands
CURN Conduct and Utilization of Research in Nursing
CurrMIT Curriculum Management and Information Tool
CUS carotid ultrasound examination; catheterized urine specimen; contact urticaria syndrome
CuS copper supplement
CUSA Cavitron ultrasonic aspirator
CuSBV cucumber soilborne virus
CUSSN computer use in social service network
CuTS cubital tunnel syndrome
CV calicivirus; canker virus; cardiac volume; cardiovascular; care vigilance; carotenoid vesicle; cell viability; cell volume; central venous; cephalic vein; cerebrovascular; cervical vertebra; Chikungunya virus; Chlorella virus; chlorosis virus; chorionic villi; circovirus; closing volume; clump virus; coefficient of variation [statistics]; color vision; concentrated

volume; conducting vein; conduction velocity; conjugata vera; contrast ventriculography; conventional ventilation; corpuscular volume; costovertebral; cresyl violet; crinkle virus; cross validation; cryptic virus; crystal violet; cultivar; cutaneous vasculitis; cyclic voltamogram; cyclic voltometry

C/V coulomb per volt

Cv specific heat at constant volume

C$_v$ coefficient of variation; constant volume

cv coefficient of variability; cultivar

CVA cardiovascular accident; cerebrovascular accident; cherry virus A; chronic villous arthritis; common variable agammaglobulinemia; costovertebral angle; cyclophosphamide, vincristine, and Adriamycin

CV-A1 to A22 human coronavirus A 1 to 22

CVAH congenital virilizing adrenal hyperplasia

CVAP cerebrovascular amyloid peptide

CVAT costovertebral angle tenderness

CVB chorionic villi biopsy

CV B1 to B6 human coxsackievirus B1 to B6

CVBS congenital vascular bone syndrome

CVC calcifying vascular cell; central venous catheter

CV cath central venous catheter

CVCT cardiovascular computed tomography

CVD cardiovascular disease; Center for Vaccine Development; chemical vapor deposition; chronic venous disease; collagen vascular disease; color-vision-deviant; common variable immunodeficiency; congenital vascular disorder

CVd crinkle viroid

CVELTP Comox Valley Electronic Lab Transfer Project [Canada]

CVF cardiovascular failure; central visual field; cervicovaginal fluid; cobra venom factor

CVFn cardiovascular function

CVFS computerized visual feedback system

CVG composite valve graft; contrast ventriculography; coronary venous graft; cutis verticis gyrata

CVG/MR cutis verticis gyrata/mental retardation [syndrome]

CVGV Csiro Village virus

CVH cerebroventricular hemorrhage; cervicovaginal hood; combined ventricular hypertrophy; common variable hypogammaglobulinemia

CVHD chronic valvular heart disease

CvHV cervid herpesvirus

CVI cardiovascular incident; cardiovascular insufficiency; cerebrovascular incident; cerebrovascular insufficiency; Children's Vaccine Initiative; chronic venous insufficiency; common variable immunodeficiency; content validity index

CVICU cardiovascular intensive care unit

CVID common variable immunodeficiency

CVIS cardiovascular imaging system

CVK computerized videokeratography

CVL central venous line

CVLM caudal ventrolateral medulla; caudoventrolateral medulla

CVLP chimeric virus-like particle

CVLT California Verbal Learning Test; clinical vascular laboratory

CVM cardiovascular monitor; cerebral venous malformation; congenital vascular malformation; contingent valuation method; cyclophosphamide, vincristine, and methotrexate

CVMoV carnation vein mottle virus

CVMP Committee on Veterans Medical Problems

CVO central vein occlusion; central venous oxygen; Chief Veterinary Officer; circumventricular organ; credentialing verification organization

CVO$_2$ central venous oxygen content or saturation

CVOD cerebrovascular obstructive disease

CVP cardioventricular pacing; cell volume profile; central venous pressure; chlorfenvinphos; cyclophosphamide, vincristine, and prednisone

cvPO$_2$, cvP$_{O_2}$ cerebral venous partial pressure of oxygen

CVPR computer vision and pattern recognition

CVR cardiovascular-renal; cardiovascular-respiratory; cephalic vasomotor response; cerebrovascular resistance

CVRD cardiovascular-renal disease

CVRMED computer vision, virtual reality, and robotics in medicine

CVRR cardiovascular recovery room

CVRS cardiovascular and respiratory elements of trauma score

CVS cardiovascular surgery; cardiovascular system; challenge virus strain; chorionic villi sampling; clean voided specimen; coronavirus susceptibility; current vital signs

CVSMC cultured vascular smooth muscle cells

CVST cerebral venous sinus thrombosis; computerized visual search task

CVST-T Cerebral Venous Sinus Thrombosis Trial

CVT cardiovascular technologist; central venous temperature; cerebral venous thrombosis; congenital vertical talus

CVTR charcoal viral transport medium

CVV Cache Valley virus; ceratitis V virus; citrus variegation virus

CVVH continuous veno-venous hemofiltration

CVVHD continuous veno-venous hemodialysis

CVVHDF continuous venovenous hemodiafiltration

CVX cactus virus X; code for vaccines administered

CW cardiac work; case work; cell wall; chemical warfare; chemical weapon; chest wall; children's ward; clinical workbench; clockwise; continuous wave; crutch walking

Cw crutch walking

C/W compare with; consistent with

CWA cognitive work analysis

CWBTS capillary whole blood true sugar

CWC Chemical Weapons Convention; chest wall compliance

CWD cell wall defect; Choi-Williams distribution; continuous-wave Doppler

CWDF cell wall-deficient form [bacteria]

CWD/NAF cell wall-deficient, non-acid fast [*Mycobacterium tuberculosis*]

CWEQ conditions of work effectiveness scale

CWF Cornell Word Form

CWG Communications Working Group [NLM]

CWH cardiomyopathy and wooly haircoat [syndrome]

CWHB citrated whole human blood

CWI cardiac work index

CWIS campus-wide information system

CWL cutaneous water loss

CWM cardiological workspace manager

CWMI common warehouse metadata interchange

CWMS color, warmth, movement sensation

CWOP childbirth without pain

CWP childbirth without pain; coal worker's pneumoconiosis

CWPEA Childbirth Without Pain Education Association

CWRUNET Case Western Reserve University Network

CWS cell wall skeleton; Chemical Warfare Service; chest wall stimulation; child welfare service; children's clinical workstation; clinician's workstation; cold water-soluble; cotton wool spots

CWT circuit weight training; cold water treatment; continuous wavelet transform

Cwt, cwt hundredweight

CWV Cape Wrath virus

CWW clinic without walls

CWXSP Coal Workers' X-ray Surveillance Program

CX cervix; chest x-ray; connexin; critical experiment; phosgene oxime [war gas]

Cx cervix; circumflex; clearance; complaint; complex; connexin; convex

cx cervix; complex; connexin; culture; cylinder axis

CXB3S Coxsackie B3 virus susceptibility

CxCor circumflex coronary [artery]

CXEV *Chorizagrotis auxiliaris* entomopoxvirus

CXMD canine X-linked muscular dystrophy

CXR, CxR chest x-ray

CY casein-yeast autolysate [medium]; cyclophosphamide

Cy cyanogen; cyclophosphamide; cyst; cytarabine

Cy3 cyanine 3

Cy5 cyanine 5

cy, cyan cyanosis

CyA cyclosporine A

CYC cyclophosphamide; cytochrome C

cyc cyclazocine; cycle; cyclotron

CYCAZAREM Cyclophosphamide vs Azathioprine during Remission of Systemic Vasculitis [trial]

CYCLO, Cyclo cyclophosphamide; cyclopropane

Cyclo C cyclocytidine hydrochloride

CYCLOPS cyclically ordered phase sequence; Cyclophosphamide in Systemic Vasculitis

Cyd cytidine

cydv cereal yellow dwarf virus

CYE charcoal yeast extract [agar]

CYH chymase

CyHV cyprinid herpesvirus

CYL casein yeast lactate

cyl cylinder; cylindrical lens

CYLV carrot yellow leaf virus

CYM chymase, mast cell

CYMP chymosin, pseudogene

CYMV cacao yellow mosaic virus

CYN cyanide

CYP cyclophilin; cyproheptadine; cytochrome P

CYPA cyclophilin A

CYPC cyclophilin C

CypCV *Cypripedium calceolus* virus

CYPH cyclophilin

CYS cystoscopy

Cys cyclosporine; cysteine

Cys-Cys cystine

CysLT1 cysteinyl leukotriene 1

CySNO nitrosated L-cysteine

CYSTO cystogram

cysto cystoscopy

CYSV carnation yellow stripe virus

CYT cytochrome

Cyt cytolytic

Cyt cytoplasm; cytosine

cyt cytochrome; cytology, cytological; cytoplasm; cytosine

Cyto cytotechnologist

cytol cytology, cytological

CY-VA-DIC cyclophosphamide, vincristine, Adriamycin, and dacarbazine

CZ carzinophilin; cefazolin

Cz central midline placement of electrodes in electroencephalography

CZE capillary zone electrophoresis

CZI crystalline zinc insulin

C_{zn} zinc clearance

CZP clonazepam

D

D absorbed dose aspartic acid; cholecalciferol; coefficient of diffusion; dacryon; dalton; date; daughter; day; dead; dead air space; debye; deceased; deciduous; decimal reduction time; degree; density; dental; dermatology, dermatologic; dermatologist; deuterium; deuteron; development; deviation; dextro; dextrose; diabetic; diagnosis; diagonal; diameter; diaphorase; diarrhea; diastole; diathermy; died; difference; diffusion, diffusing; diffusion coefficient; dihydrouridine; dilution [rate]; diopter; diplomate; dipyridamole; disease; dispense; displacement [loop]; distal; distance [focus-object]; diuresis; diurnal; divergence; diversity; diverticulum; divorced; doctor; dog; donor; dorsal; double [pacemaker]; drive; drug; dual; duct; duodenum, duodenal; duration; dwarf; electric displacement; mean dose; right [Lat. *dexter*]; unit of vitamin D potency

1-D one-dimensional

D1 prostatic tumor with microscopic involvement of pelvic lymph nodes [Jewett staging system]

D₁ diagonal one; first dorsal vertebra

2-D two-dimensional

D₂ diagonal two; second dorsal vertebra

2,4-D 2,4-dichlorophenoxyacetic acid

3-D three-dimensional

D/3 distal third

D₃₋₁₂ third to twelfth dorsal vertebrae

4D 4-dimensional [imaging]

4-D four-dimensional

D4 domain 4; fourth digit

D₁₀ decimal reduction time

D50 50% dextrose solution

D̄ mean dose

d atomic orbital with angular momentum quantum number 2; dalton; day [Lat. *dies*]; dead; deceased; deci-; decrease, decreased; degree; density; deoxy; deoxyribose; dextro-; dextrorotatory; diameter; diastasis; died; diopter; distal; distance [between radiographic grids or between subject and film or cassette]; diurnal; dorsal;

dose; doubtful; duration; dyne; right [Lat. *dexter*]

d- deci- $[10^{-1}]$

1/d once a day

2/d twice a day

d̄ mean difference of samples observations [statistics]

Δ see *delta*

δ see *delta*

DA dark adaptation; dark agouti [rat]; daunomycin; decision analysis; decontaminating agent; degenerative arthritis; degree of anisotropy; delayed action; dental assistant; deoxyadenosine; descending aneurysm; descending aorta; detrusor areflexia; developmental age; dextroamphetamine; diabetic acidosis; differential amplifier; differential analyzer; differentiation antigen; digital angiography; digital to analog [converter]; diphenylchlorarsine; Diploma in Anesthetics; direct agglutination; disability assistance; disaggregated; discriminant analysis; dissecting aneurysm; distal arthrogryposis; dopamine; drug addict, drug addiction; drug administration; ductus arteriosus

D-A donor-acceptor

D/A date of accident; date of admission; digital-to-analog [converter]; discharge and advise

D&A dilatation and aspiration; drugs and allergy

DA1 distal arthrogryposis type 1

DA2 distal arthrogryposis type 2

2,4-DA 2,4-diaminoanisole

Da dalton

d(A) primary donor

da daughter; day; deca-

da- deka- $[10^1]$

DAA decompensated autonomous adenoma; dementia associated with alcoholism; dialysis-associated amyloidosis; diaminoanisole

DAAF deoxyoyribonucleic acid amplification fingerprinting; Digoxin in Acute Atrial Fibrillation [study]

DAAO diaminoacid oxidase

D(A-a)O₂ alveolar arterial oxygen gradient

DAB days after birth; 3,3'-diaminobenzidine; dysrhythmic aggressive behavior

DABA 2,4-diaminobutyric acid

DABP D site albumin promoter binding protein

DABV Dabakala virus

DAC derived air concentration; digital acquisition; digital-to-analog converter; disaster assistance center; Division of Ambulatory Care

dac dacryon

DACCM department of anesthesiology and critical care medicine

DACL Depression Adjective Check List

DACM *N*-(7-dimethylamino-4-methyl-3-coumarinyl) maleimide

DACMD deputy associate chief medical director

DACS data acquisition and control system

DACT dactinomycin; daily activity [UMLS]

DAD delayed afterdepolarization; diffuse alveolar damage; Disability Assessment in Dementia; discharge abstract databank; dispense as directed

DADA dichloroacetic acid diisopropyl-ammonium salt

DADDS diacetyldiaminodiphenylsulfone

DADS Director Army Dental Service

DAdV duck adenovirus

DAdV-1 egg drop syndrome virus

DAE differential algebraic equation; diphenylanthracene endoperoxide; diving air embolism; dysbaric air embolism

DA/ES data analysis expert system

DAEV *Dermolepida albohirtum* entomo-poxvirus

DAF decay-accelerating factor; delayed auditory feedback; drug-adulterated food

DAFV Desulfurolobus virus

DAG diacylglycerol; dianhydrogalactitol; directed acyclic graph; dystrophin-associated glycoprotein

DAGK diacylglycerol kinase

DAGL diacylglycerol lipase

DAGT direct antiglobulin test

DAGV D'Aguilar virus

DAH diffuse alveolar hemorrhage; disordered action of the heart

DAHEA Department of Allied Health Education and Accreditation

DAHM Division of Allied Health Manpower

DAI diffuse axonal injury; drug attitude inventory

DAIDS Division of Acquired Immunodeficiency Syndrome (AIDS) [NIH]

DAIS Diabetes Atherosclerosis Intervention Study

DAISY Diabetes Autoimmunity Study in the Young

DAIT Division of Allergy, Immunology and Transplantation [NIH]

DalV *Diadegma acronyctae* ichnovirus

Dal, dal dalton

DALA delta-aminolevulinic acid

DALE disability-adjusted life expectancy; Drug Abuse Law Enforcement

DALM dysplasia with associated lesion or mass

DALT dalton

DALY(s) disability-adjusted life year(s)

DAM data-associated message; database access module; degraded amyloid; diacetyl monoxime; diacetylmorphine

dam decameter

DAMA discharged against medical advice

DAMAD Diabetic Microangiopathy Modification with Aspirin vs Dipyridamole

DAMET Diet and Moderate Exercise Trial

DAMOS drug application methodology with optical storage

dAMP deoxyadenosine monophosphate; deoxyadenylate adenosine monophosphate

DAN data acquisition in neurophysiology; diabetic autonomic neuropathy

DANAMI Danish Multicenter Study of Acute Myocardial Infarction

DANC decontaminating agent, noncorrosive

D and C dilatation and curettage

DANS 1-dimethylaminonaphthalene-5-sulfonyl chloride

DANTE delays altered with nutation for tailored excitation

DAO diamine oxidase

DAo descending aorta

DAOM depressor anguli oris muscle

DAP data acquisition processor; data architecture project; depolarizing afterpotential; diabetes-associated peptide; diaminopimelic acid; diaminopyridine; diastolic aortic pressure; diastolic arterial pressure; dihydroxyacetone phosphate; dipeptidylaminopeptidase; direct latex agglutination pregnancy [test]; dose area product;

Draw-a-Person [test]; Drug Action Programme [WHO]

D-AP5 D-2-amino-5-phosphonovaleric acid

D-AP7 D-2-amino-7-phosphonoheptanoic acid

DAP&E Diploma of Applied Parasitology and Entomology

DAPI 4,6-diamino-2-phenylindole

DAPPAF Dual-Site Atrial Pacing for Prevention of Atrial Fibrillation [trial]

DAPRE daily adjustable progressive resistive exercise

DAPRU Drug Abuse Prevention Resource Unit

DAPs Database Access Project [UK]

DAPT diaminophenylthiazole; direct agglutination pregnancy test

DAQ data acquisition; Diagnostic Assessment Questionnaire; digital acquisition

DAR daily activity record; daily effective rhythm; death after resuscitation; diacereine; differential absorption ratio; dual asthmatic reaction

DA-R dopamine receptor

DARE Database of Abstracts of Reviews of Effectiveness; Drug Abuse Resistance Education

DARP drug abuse rehabilitation program

DARPA Defense Advanced Research Project Agency [Department of Defense]

DART Developmental and Reproductive Toxicology [NLM database]; Diet and Reinfarction Trial; Dilation vs Ablation Revascularization Trial

D/ART Depression, Awareness, Recognition, and Treatment [NIMH hotline]

DARTS Diabetes Audit and Research in Tayside, Scotland; Drug and Alcohol Rehabilitation Testing System

DAS data acquisition system; dead air space; Death Anxiety Scale; delayed anovulatory syndrome; dextroamphetamine sulfate; 4,15-diacetoxyscripenol; Dietary Alternatives Study; digital angiography segmentation; double addition of serum; dyadic adjustment scale

DASA distal articular set angle

DASD direct access storage device

DASH Delay in Accessing Stroke Healthcare [trial]; Dietary Approaches to Stop Hypertension [trial]; Distress Alarm for the Severely Handicapped

DASI Duke activity status index

DASM data acquisition system management

DASS Dilazep Aspirin Stroke Study

DAST diethylaminosulfur trifluoride; drug abuse screening test; drug and alcohol screening test

DAstV duck astrovirus

DAT delayed-action tablet; dementia Alzheimer's type; dental aptitude test; diacetylthiamine; diet as tolerated; differential agglutination titer; Differential Aptitude Test; diphtheria antitoxin; direct agglutination test; direct antiglobulin test; Disaster Action Team; divided attention; dopamine transporter

DATA Diltiazem as Adjunctive Therapy to Activase [study]

DATE dental auxiliary teacher education

DATF Difficult Airway Task Force

DATOS Diet and Antismoking Trial of Oslo Study

DATP deoxyadenosine triphosphate

dATP deoxyadenosine monophosphate

DATTA diagnostic and therapeutic technology assessment

DAU 3-deazauridine; Dental Auxiliary Utilization

dau daughter

DAUs drug abuse testing and urines

DAV data valid; Disabled American Veterans; disease-associated virus; duck adenovirus

DAVF dural arteriovenous fistula

DAVIT Danish Verapamil Infarction Trial

DAVM dural arteriovenous malformation

DAvMED Diploma in Aviation Medicine

DAVP deamino-arginine vasopressin

DAWN Drug Abuse Warning Network

DAZ deleted in azoospermia

DB database; date of birth; deep breath; dense body; dextran blue; diabetes, diabetic; diagonal band; diet beverage; direct bilirubin; disability; distobuccal; double-blind [study]; double buffer [board]; duodenal bulb; Dutch belted [rabbit]

Db diabetes, diabetic

D$_b$ database; body density

dB, db decibel

db database; date of birth; diabetes, diabetic

DBA database administrator; Diamond-Blackfan anemia; dibenzanthracene; *Dolichos biflorus* agglutinin
DBAE dihydroxyborylaminoethyl
DBB diagonal band of Broca
DBC dibencozide; distal balloon catheter; dye-binding capacity
DB&C deep breathing and coughing
DBCL dilute blood clot lysis [method]
DBCP dibromochloropropane
DBD definite brain damage; deoxyribonucleic acid–binding domain; dibromodulcitol; dynamic beam delivery [radiotherapy]
DBDC distal bile duct carcinoma
DBDG distobuccal developmental groove
DBDO decabromodiphenyl oxide; desert battle dress overgarment
DBDS database definition structure
DB/DS database of data sets
dB/dt change of magnetic flux with time
DBE deep breathing exercise; dibromoethane
DBED *N,N′*-bis-dibenzyl ethylenediaminediacetic acid
dbEST database expressed sequence tag; Database of Expressed Sequence Tags [NLM]
DBEV Demodema entomopoxvirus
dbGSS database genome survey sequence; Database on Genome Survey Sequences [NLM]
DBH dopamine beta-hydroxylase
DbH diagnosis by hybridization
DBI development at birth index; phenformin hydrochloride
DBil direct bilirubin
DBIOC database input/output control
DBIR Directory of Biotechnology Information Resources
dBk decibels above 1 kilowatt
DBL desbromoleptophos
DBLE Double Bolus Lytic Efficacy [trial]
DBM database management; dibromomannitol; dobutamine
dBm decibels above 1 milliwatt
dBMAN database manager
DBMS database management system
DBN dynamic Bayesian network
DBNN decision-based neural network
DBO distobucco-occlusal
db/ob diabetic obese [mouse]
DBP deoxyribonucleic acid–binding peptide; diastolic blood pressure; dibutylphthalate; distobuccopulpal; Döhle body panmyelopathy; vitamin D-binding protein
DBPOFC double-blind placebo-controlled oral food challenge
DBP-PEG/DNA deoxyribonucleic acid–binding peptide-polyethylene glycol/deoxyribonucleic acid
DBR distorted breathing rate
DBRI dysfunctional behavior rating instrument
DBRPC double-blind randomized placebo-controlled
DBS deep brain stimulation; Denis Browne splint; despeciated bovine serum; Diamond-Blackfan syndrome; dibromosalicil; diminished breath sounds; direct bonding system; Division of Biological Standards; double blind study; double-burst stimulus; dysgenesis of corpus callosum
dbSNP Database of Single Nucleotide Polymorphism [NLM]
DBSP dibromosulphthalein
dbSTS database of Sequence Tagged Sites [NLM]; database sequence target site
DBSV deconvolution based on shape variation
DBT dry bulb temperature
DBV Dakar bat virus; *Dioscorea* bacilliform virus
DBW desirable body weight
dBW decibels above 1 watt
DC daily census; data communication; data conversion; decrease; deep compartment; defining characteristic; dendritic cell; dendritic core; Dental Corps; deoxycholate; descending colon; dextran charcoal; diagonal conjugate; diagnostic center; diagnostic cluster; diagnostic code; differentiated cell; diffusion capacity; digit copying; digital computer; dilatation and curettage; dilation catheter; diphenylcyanoarsine; direct Coombs' [test]; direct current; discharge, discharged; discontinue, discontinued; distal colon; distocervical; Doctor of Chiropractic; donor cells; dopachrome; dorsal column; dressing change; duodenal cap; Dupuytren contracture; duty cycle; dyskeratosis congenita; electric defibrillator using DC discharge
D/C discharge [JCAHO unapproved abbreviation]; discontinue

D&C dilatation and curettage; drugs and cosmetics

Dc critical dilution rate

D/c discontinue; discharge

DC65 Darvon compound 65

dC deoxycytidine

dc decrease; direct current; discharge; discontinue

DCA deoxycholate-citrate agar; deoxycholic acid; desoxycorticosterone acetate; dichloroacetate; directional color angiography; directional coronary atherectomy

DCa deoxycortisone acetate

DCABG double coronary artery bypass graft

DCAF dilated cardiomyopathy and atrial fibrillation

2D-CAG 2-dimensional coronary angiography

DCAld dichloroacetaldehyde

DCB 3,4-dichlorobenzamil

DCBE double contrast barium enema

DCBF dyamic cardiac blood flow

DCbN deep cerebellar nucleus

DCC day care center; deleted in colorectal cancer; desquamated cornified cells; device communication controller; dextran-coated charcoal; diameter of cylindrical collimator; N,N'-dicyclohexylcarbodiimide; digital compact cassette; disaster control center; dorsal cell column; double concave; dysgenesis of corpus callosum

2DCC 2-dimensional cross-correlation

DCCMP daunomycin, cyclocytidine, 6-mercaptopurine, and prednisolone

DC$_{CO_2}$ diffusing capacity for carbon dioxide

DCCT Diabetes Control and Complications Trial

DCCV direct current cardioversion

DCD differential current density; Diploma in Chest Diseases; disorders of cortical development; dynamic cooling device

D/c'd, dc'd discontinued

D/CDK D-type cyclin-dependent kinase

DCE desmosterol-to-cholesterol enzyme; distributed computing environment

DCE-MRI dynamic contrast enhanced magnetic resonance imaging

DCET dicarboxyethoxythiamine

DCF 2'-deoxycoformycin; dichlorofluorescein; direct centrifugal flotation; dopachrome conversion factor

DCFDA 2',7'-dichlorofluorescein diacetate

DCFH dichlorofluorescein

DCFH-DA dichlorofluorescein diacetate

DCG dacryocystography; deoxycorticosterone glucoside; diagnosis cost-related group; disodium cromoglycate; dynamic electrocardiography

DCGE denaturation gradient gel electrophoresis

DCH delayed cutaneous hypersensitivity; Diploma in Child Health

DCh Doctor of Surgery [Lat. *Doctor Chirurgiae*]

DCHA docosahexaenoic acid

DCHEB dichlorohexafluorobutane

DCHN dicyclohexylamine nitrite

DChO Doctor of Ophthalmic Surgery

DCI dichloroisoprenaline; dichloroisoproterenol; digital cardiac imaging; Doppler color imaging; duplicate coverage inquiry

DCIA deep circumflex iliac artery

DCIEM Defense and Civil Institute for Environmental Medicine [Canada]

DCIP dichlorophenolindophenol

DCIS ductal carcinoma in situ

DCK, dCK deoxycytidine kinase

DCL data control language; dicloxacillin; diffuse or disseminated cutaneous leishmaniasis; digital case library

DCLHb diaspirin cross-linked hemoglobin

DCLS deoxycholate citrate lactose saccharose

DCM dichloromethane; dichloromethotrexate; dilated cardiomyopathy; Doctor of Comparative Medicine; dyssynergia cerebellaris myoclonica

DCMADS [Washington] DC Metropolitan Area Drug Study

DCML dorsal column medial lemniscus

3D-CMM 3-dimensional coordinate measuring machine [orthopedic surgery]

DCMP daunomycin, cytosine arabinoside, 6-mercaptopurine, and prednisolone

dCMP deoxycytidine monophosphate

DCMS data creation and maintenance system

DCMT Doctor of Clinical Medicine of the Tropics

3D-CMT three-dimensional computed x-ray microtomography

DCMX 2,4-dichloro-*m*-xylenol

DCN data collection network; deep cerebral nucleus; delayed conditioned necrosis;

depressed, cognitively normal; dorsal cochlear nucleus; dorsal column nucleus; dorsal cutaneous nerve

DCNB 1,2-dichloro-4-nitrobenzene

DCNU chlorozotocin

DCO death certificate only; Diploma of the College of Optics

D$_{CO}$ diffusing capacity for carbon monoxide

dCO$_2$ dissolved carbon dioxide

DCOG Diploma of the College of Obstetricians and Gynaecologists

DCOM [Microsoft] distributed component object model

DCOP distal coronary occlusion pressure

DCOR dopachrome oxidoreductase

DCP des-γ-carboxy prothrombin; dicalcium phosphate; Diploma in Clinical Pathology; Diploma in Clinical Psychology; District Community Physician; dual chamber pacemaker; dynamic compression plate

DCPA chlorthal-dimethyl

DCPP Disease Control Priorities Project [WHO]

DCR dacryocystorhinostomy; data conversion receiver; digitally composited radiograph; direct cortical response

DCRT Division of Computer Research and Technology [NIH]

3DCRT, 3D CRT three-dimensional conformal radiation therapy; three-dimensional conformal radiotherapy

DCS decompression sickness; dense canalicular system; diffuse cortical sclerosis; discharge summary; distal coronary sinus; dorsal column stimulation, dorsal column stimulator; dynamic condylar screw; dynamic contrast-enhanced subtraction; dynamic contrast-enhanced tomography; dynamic control system; dyskinetic cilia syndrome

dcSSc diffuse cutaneous systemic sclerosis

DCSWS dementia with continuing spike-wave during slow-wave sleep

DCT detached ciliary tuft; direct Coombs' test; discrete cosine transform; distal convoluted tubule; diurnal cortisol test; dynamic computed tomography

3DCT, 3D-CT 3-dimensional computed tomography

DCTMA desoxycorticosterone trimethylacetate

dCTP deoxycytidine triphosphate

DCTPA desoxycorticosterone triphenylacetate

DCTS dynamic carpal tunnel syndrome

DCV diagnostic content validity; distribution of conduction velocities

D$_{2CV}$ Doppler 2-chamber view

D$_{4CV}$ Doppler 4-chamber view

DCVC dichlorovinyl cystine

DCVMN Developing Country Vaccine Manufacturers' Network

DCX double charge exchange

DCx double convex

DD dangerous drug; Darier disease; data definition; data dictionary; day of delivery; D-dimer; death domain; degenerated disk; degenerative disease; delusional disorder; depth dose [x-ray]; detrusor dyssynergia; developmental disability; diastrophic dysplasia; died of the disease; differential diagnosis; differential display; digest and discharge; digestive disorder; Di Guglielmo disease; disc diameter; discharge diagnosis; discharged dead; dog dander; double diffusion; double dummy; drug dependence; dry dressing; Duchenne dystrophy; Dupuytren disease

D&D design and development

D6D delta-6-desaturase

dd dideoxy

DDA Dangerous Drugs Act; dideoxyadenosine; digital differential analysis

ddA 2′,3′-dideoxyadenosine

DDase deoxyuridine diphosphatase

ddATP dideoxyadenosine triphosphate

DDAVP, dDAVP 1-deamino-8-D-arginine vasopressin; 1-desamino-8-D-arginine vasopressin

DDB dosimetric databank [radiotherapy]

DDBJ Deoxyribonucleic acid [DNA] Data Bank of Japan

DDC dangerous drug cabinet; dideoxycytidine; 3,5-diethoxycarbonyl-1,4-dihydrocollidine; diethyl-dithiocarbamate; dihydroxyphenylalanine decarboxylase; direct display console; diverticular disease of the colon

DDc double concave

ddC dideoxycytidine

DDD AV universal [pacemaker]; Dali domain dictionary; defined daily dose; degenerative disk disease; dehydroxydinaphthyl disulfide; dense deposit disease;

Denver dialysis disease; dichlorodiphenyl-dichloroethane; dihydroxydinaphthyl disulfide; dorsal dural deficiency; double dose delay; Dowling-Degos disease; dual mode, dual pacing, dual sensing

DDD CT double-dose-delay computed tomography

DDDD-CAT Drug Delivery Device Dispatch in Coronary Angioplasty Trial

DDDi infant defined daily dose

DDE dichlorodiphenyldichloroethylene; dynamic data exchange

DDEB dominantly inherited dystrophic epidermolysis bullosa

DDF demographic data form

ddF dideoxy fingerprinting

DDFP dodecafluoropentane

DDG deoxy-D-glucose

ddGTP dideoxyguanidine triphosphate

DDH developmental dysplasia of the hip; dihydrodiol dehydrogenase; Diploma in Dental Health; dissociated double hypertropia

ddH₂O double-distilled water

DDI dideoxyinosine; dynamic data icon

ddI didanoside; dideoxyinosine

DDIB Disease Detection Information Bureau

DDKase deoxynucleoside diphosphate kinase

DDL data definition language

DDM differential diagnosis manager; Diploma in Dermatological Medicine; Doctor in Dental Medicine; Dyke-Davidoff-Masson [syndrome]

DDMR Dam-directed DNA mismatch repair

dDNA denatured deoxyribonucleic acid

DDNTP, ddNTP dideoxynucleotide triphosphate

DDO Diploma in Dental Orthopaedics

DDP cisplatin; density-dependent phosphoprotein; difficult denture patient; digital data processing; distributed data processing

DDPA Delta Dental Plans Association

DD-PCR, DDPCR differential display polymerase chain reaction

DDQ database directed query

2D DQFC NMR 2-dimensional double quantum filtered correction nuclear magnetic resonance spectroscopy

DDR diastolic descent rate; Diploma in Diagnostic Radiology; DNA damage response

DDRB Doctors' and Dentists' Review Body

DDRP DNA damage responsive protein

DDRT diseases, disorders and related topics

DDS damaged disk syndrome; dapsone; data definition structure; dendrodendritic synaptosome; dental distress syndrome; depressed DNA synthesis; dialysis disequilibrium syndrome; diaminodiphenylsulfone; directional Doppler sonography; dirty data set; Director of Dental Services; disability determination service; Disease-Disability Scale; Doctor of Dental Surgery; dodecyl sulfate; double decidual sac; dystrophy-dystocia syndrome

DDSc Doctor of Dental Science

DDSI digital damage severity index

DDSO diaminodiphenylsulfoxide

DDSS Defense Dental Standard System; Diagnostic Decision Support System [software]

DDST Denver Developmental Screening Test

DDST-R Denver Developmental Screening Test-Revised

DDT dichlorodiphenyltrichloroethane; ductus deferens tumor; dynamic data table

Ddt deceleration time

DDTC diethyldithiocarbamate

DDTN dideoxy-didehydrothymidine

ddTTP dideoxythymidine triphosphate

DDU data deficit unit; data definition unit; dermo-distortive urticaria; duplex Doppler ultrasound

dDVH differential dose-volume histogram

DDW Digestive Diseases Week

D/DW dextrose in distilled water

D 5% DW 5% dextrose in distilled water

DDx differential diagnosis

DE data encoder; dendritic expansion; deprived eye; design effect; diagnostic error; dialysis encephalopathy; diesel exhaust; digestive energy; direct excitation; dose equivalent; dream elements; drug evaluation; duodenal exclusion; duration of ejection

D&E diet and elimination; dilation or dilatation and evacuation

D=E dates equal to examination

2DE two-dimensional echocardiography
3DE 3-dimensional echocardiography
dE differential in energy
DEA dehydroepiandrosterone; diethanolamine; Drug Enforcement Administration
DEAD Dying Experience at Dartmouth
DEAE diethylaminoethyl [cellulose]
DEAE-D diethylaminoethyl dextran
DEAFF detection of early antigen fluorescent foci
DEALE declining exponential approximation of life expectancy [method]
DEATH Dying Experience at the Hitchcock
DEB diepoxybutane; diethylbutanediol; Division of Environmental Biology; dystrophic epidermolysis bullosa
deb debridement
DEBA diethylbarbituric acid
DEBATE Doppler Endpoints Balloon Angioplasty Trial, Europe
debil debilitation
DEBRA Dystrophic Epidermolysis Bullosa Research Association
DEBS dominant epidermolysis bullosa simplex
DEC decrease; deoxycholate citrate; diagnostic episode cluster; diethylcarbamazine; dynamic environmental conditioning
Dec, dec decant
dec deceased; deciduous; decimal; decompose, decomposition; decrease, decreased
DECA Demographic and Economic Characteristics of the Aged [database]
decd deceased
DECG differentiated ECG
decoct decoction
DECODE Diabetes Epidemiology, Collaborative Analysis of Diagnostic Criteria in Europe
DECOMP decomposition [EMG into separate channels]
decomp decompensation; decompose, decomposition
decr decrease, decreased
D-ECST Dutch-European Cerebral Sinus Thrombosis [trial]
DECU decubitus [ulcer]
decub lying down [Lat. *decubitus*]
DED date of expected delivery; death effector domain [cell]; defined exposure dose; delayed erythema dose

DEEDS Data Elements for Emergency Department Systems
DEEG depth electroencephalogram, depth electroencephalography
DEER Diet and Exercise in Elevated Risk [trial]
DEET N,N-diethyl-m-toluamide
DEF decayed primary teeth requiring filling, decayed primary teeth requiring extraction, and primary teeth successfully filled; dose-effect factor
def defecation; deferred; deficiency, deficient
DEFIANT Doppler Flow and Echocardiography in Functional Cardiac Insufficiency Assessment of Nisoldipine Therapy [trial]
defib defibrillation
DEFIBRILAT Defibrillator as Bridge to Later Transplantation [study]
defic deficiency, deficient
DEFN Danubian endemic familial nephropathy
DEF$_{NT}$ dose-effect factor for normal tissue
deform deformed, deformity
DEFT direct epifluorescent filter technique
DEF$_T$ dose-effect factor for tumor
DEFV deceleration of early flow velocity
DEG degenerin; diagnostic evaluation group; diethylene glycol
Deg, deg degeneration, degenerative; degree
degen degeneration, degenerative
DEH dysplasia epiphysealis hemimelica
DEHP di(2-ethylhexyl)phthalate
DEHR distributed electronic health record
DEHS Division of Emergency Health Services
DEHT developmental hand function test
dehyd dehydration, dehydrated
DEJ, dej dentino-enamel junction; dermoepidermal junction
del deletion; delivery; delusion
DELFIA dissociated enhanced lanthanide fluoroimmunoassay
deliq deliquescence, deliquescent
DELIRIUM drugs-electrolytes-low temperature and lunacy-intoxication and intracranial processes-retention of urine or feces-infection-unfamiliar surroundings-myocardial infarction [causes of delirium]
Delt deltoid

DELTA Descriptive Language for Taxonomy [program]; dietary effects on lipoproteins and thrombogenic activity

Δ Greek capital letter *delta*

δ Greek lower case letter *delta*; immunoglobulin D

Δ df differences between degrees of freedom

ΔP change in pressure

ΔR additional resistance

ΔR,L additional resistance, lung

ΔR,rs additional resistance, respiratory system

ΔR,w additional resistance, chest wall

ΔV change in volume

DEM demerol; diethylmaleate; diffusion equation method

Dem Demerol

DEMO dynamic essential modeling

DEN denervation; dengue; dermatitis exfoliativa neonatorum; Device Experience Network [of the CDRH]; diethylnitrosamine

denat denatured

DENT Dental Exposure Normalization Technique

Dent, dent dental; dentist; dentistry; dentition

DENTALPROJ Dental Research Projects

DENV dengue virus

DEP depression emulation program [computer simulation]; dielectrophoresis; diethylpropanediol; dilution end point

dep dependent; deposit

DEPA diethylene phosphoramide

DEPC diethyl pyrocarbonate

depr depression, depressed

DEPS distal effective potassium secretion

DEP ST SEG depressed ST segment

DEPT distortionless enhancement by polarization transfer

dept department

DEQ Depression Experiences Questionnaire

DER disulfiram-ethanol reaction; dual energy radiography

DeR degeneration reaction

der derivative [chromosome]

DERI Diabetes Epidemiology Research International [study]

deriv derivative, derived

Derm, derm dermatitis; dermatological, dermatologist, dermatology; dermatome

DERS dependent error regression smoothing

DES Danish Enoxaparin Study; data encryption standard; dementia rating scale; dermal-epidermal separation; descendant [UMLS]; desmin; dialysis encephalopathy syndrome; diethylstilbestrol; diffuse esophageal spasm; disequilibrium syndrome; dissociative experience scale; doctor's emergency service

DES₁ descendant, first level in hierarchy [UMLS]

desat desaturated

desc descendant; descending

Desc Ao descending aorta

desq desquamation

DESIRE Debulking and Stenting in Restenosis Elimination [trial]

DESS double-echo steady state

DEST Denver Eye Screening Test; dichotic environmental sounds test; differentially expressed sequence tag

DESTINI Doppler Endpoint Stent International Investigation; Duke University Clinical Cardiology Study Elective Stent Trial: A Cost Containment Initiative

DeSyGNER Decision Systems Group Nucleus of Extensible Resources

DET diethyltryptamine; dipyridamole echocardiography test

DETC diethyldithiocarbamate

Det-6 detroid-6 [human sternal marrow cells]

determ determination, determined

detn detention

detox detoxification

DEUC direct electronic urethrocystometry

DEV deviant, deviation; duck embryo vaccine; duck embryo virus

dev development; deviation

devel development

DevPd developmental pediatrics

DEW diagnostic encyclopedia workstation

DEX dexamethasone

Dex dextrose

dex dexterity; dextrorotatory; right [Lat. *dexter*]

DEXA dual-energy x-ray absorptiometry

DF decapacitation factor; decontamination factor; deferoxamine; defibrillation; deficiency factor; defined flora [animal]; degree of freedom; diabetic father; dietary fibers; digital fluoroscopy; diphase fix;

discriminant function; disseminated foci; distribution factor; dominant frequency; dorsiflexion; dysgonic fermenter

D&F Diamond and Forrester [analysis of probability]

Df *Dermatophagoides farinae*; discrimination factor; duodenal fluid

df degrees of freedom [statistics]

DF-2 dysgonic fermenter 2

DFA detrended fluctuation analysis; direct fluorescent antibody; discriminant function analysis; dorsiflexion angle; dorsiflexion assistance

DFB dinitrofluorobenzene; dysfunctional bleeding

DFC developmental field complex; dry-filled capsule

DFD data flow diagram; defined formula diets; developmental field defect; diisopropyl phosphorofluoridate

DFDB demineralized freeze-dried bone

dFdCTP difluorodeoxycytidine triphosphate

DFDT difluoro-diphenyl-trichloroethane

df/dx differential diagnosis

DFE diffuse fasciitis with eosinophilia; distal femoral epiphysis

DFECT dense fibroelastic connective tissue

3DFEM three-dimensional finite element method

2D-FFT 2-dimensional fast Fourier transform

DFG direct forward gaze

DFHom Diploma of the Faculty of Homeopathy

DFHS Department of Family and Health Services [Australia]

DFI disease-free interval; dye fluorescence index

DFIB defibrillation

DFL digital film library

DFM decreased fetal movement

DFMC daily fetal movement count

DFMO difluoromethylornithine

DFMR daily fetal movement record

DFN distal femoral nail

DFO, DFOM deferoxamine

DFP diastolic filling period; diisopropylfluorophosphate

DF³²P radiolabeled diisopropylfluorophosphate

DFPP double filtration plasmapheresis

DFR designated family respondent; diabetic floor routine; digital fluororadiography

DFS disease-free survival; distraction-flexion staging; distributed file system

DFSP dermatofibrosarcoma protuberans

DFT defibrillation threshold; dementia of frontal type; diagnostic function test; discrete Fourier transform

DFT₃ dialyzable fraction of triiodothyronine

DFT₄ dialyzable fraction of thryoxine

2DFT two-dimensional Fourier transform

3DFT three-dimensional Fourier transform

DFTS digital flashing tomosynthesis

DFU dead fetus in utero; dideoxyfluorouridine

DFV diarrhea with fever and vomiting

DG data gathering; dentate gyrus; deoxyglucose; desmoglein; diacylglycerol; diagnosis; diastolic gallop; DiGeorge [anomaly or syndrome]; diglyceride; distogingival

2DG 2-deoxy-D-glucose

Dg dentate gyrus

dg decigram; diagnosis

DGA DiGeorge anomaly

DGAP deoxyribonucleic acid [DNA] guided assembly of proteins

DGAT diacylglycerol transferase

DGAVP desglycinamide-9-[Arg-8]-vasopressin

DGBG dimethylglyoxal bisguanyl-hydrazone

DGCR DiGeorge chromosome region; DiGeorge critical region

DGE delayed gastric emptying; diglycidyl ether

dge drainage

2D-GEMS 2-dimensional gel electrophoresis mass spectrometry

DGF duct growth factor

DGGE denaturing gradient gel electrophoresis

DGI dentinogenesis imperfecta; disseminated gonococcal infection

dGI dorsal giant interneuron

DGIM Division of General Internal Medicine

DGKV Dera Ghazi Khan virus

DGLA dihomogamma-linolenic acid

dGMP deoxyguanosine monophosphate

DGMS Division of General Medical Sciences

DGN diffuse glomerulonephritis

DGNA delayed gamma neutron activation

DGO Diploma in Gynaecology and Obstetrics

DGP 2,3-diglycerophosphate; Dutch General Practices Study

DGPG diffuse proliferative glomerulonephritis

DGR duodenogastric reflux

DGS developmental Gerstmann syndrome; diabetic glomerulosclerosis; DiGeorge sequence; DiGeorge syndrome; disease guidance systems; dysplasia-gigantism syndrome

DGSCR DiGeorge syndrome critical region

DGSX X-linked dysplasia gigantism syndrome

dGTP deoxyguanosine triphosphate

DGU uracil deoxyribonucleic acid glycosylase

DGV dextrose-gelatin-Veronal [buffer]

DG/VCF DiGeorge/velocardiofacial [syndrome]

DH daily habits; day hospital; dehydrocholate; dehydrogenase; delayed hypersensitivity; department of health; dermatitis herpetiformis; developmental history; diaphragmatic hernia; disseminated histoplasmosis; dominant hand; dorsal horn; drug history; ductal hyperplasia; Dunkin-Hartley [guinea pig]

D&H distributed and heterogeneous [information sources]

D/H deuterium/hydrogen [ratio]

DHA dehydroacetic acid; dehydroascorbic acid; dehydroepiandrosterone; dihydroacetic acid; dihydroxyacetone; district health authority

DHAD mitoxantrone hydrochloride

DHAOS Dutch Hypertension and Offspring Study

DHAP dihydroxyacetone phosphate

DHAP-AT dihydroxyacetone phosphate acyltransferase

DHAS dehydroandrostenedione

DHB dihydroxybenzoate; duck hepatitis B

DHBE dihydroxybutyl ether

DHBG dihydroxybutyl guanine

DHBS dihydrobiopterin synthetase

DHBV duck hepatitis B virus

DHC dehydrocholate; dehydrocholesterol; delivery of health care

DHCA deep hypothermia and circulatory arrest; dihydroxycholestanoic acid

DHCC dehydroxycholecalciferol

DHCCP Department of Health and Social Security Hypertension Care Computing Project

DHCP decentralized or distributed hospital computer program; dental health care provider; dynamic host control protocol

DHCS Department of Health and Community Services [Australia]

DHD district health department

DH-DATA Department of Health Library Database [UK]

DHE dihematoporphyrin ether; dihydroergocryptine; dihydroergotamine; distributed healthcare environment

DHEA dehydroepiandrosterone

DHEAS dehydroepiandrosterone sulfate

DHEC dihydroergocryptine

DHES Division of Health Examination Statistics

DHESN dihydroergosine

DHEW Department of Health, Education, and Welfare

DHF dengue hemorrhagic fever; dihydrofolate; dorsihyperflexion

DHF/DSS dengue hemorrhagic fever/dengue shock syndrome

DHFR dihydrofolate reductase

DHFRase dihydrofolate reductase

DHFRP dihydrofolate reductase pseudogene

DHFS Diet-Heart Feasibility Study

DHg Doctor of Hygiene

DHGG deaggregated human gammaglobulin

DHHS Department of Health and Human Services

DHI Dental Health International; dihydroxyindole

DHIA dehydroisoandrosterol

DHIAP Defense Healthcare Information Assurance Program

DHIC dihydroisocodeine

DHICA 5,6-dihydroxyindole-2-carboxylic acid

DHIS distributed healthcare information system; district health information system; Duke Hospital Information System

DHL diffuse histiocytic lymphoma

DHLA haloalkane dehalogenase

DHLD dihydrolipoamide dehydrogenase

DHM dihydromorphine

DHMA 3,4-dihydroxymandelic acid

DHMO dental health maintenance organization

DHO dihydro-orotate

dH₂O distilled water

DHODH dihydro-orotate dehydrogenase

DHOV Dhori virus

DHP dehydrogenated polymer; dihydroprogesterone; 1,4-dihydropyridine; dual heuristic programming

DHPA dihydroxypropyl adenine

DHPCCB dihydropyrimidine calcium channel blocker

DHPDH dihydropyrimidine dehydrogenase

DHPG dihydroxyphenylglycol; dihydroxypropoxymethylguanine

DHPR dihydropteridine reductase

DHR delayed hypersensitivity reaction; Department of Human Resources; disclarge homologous region

DHS delayed hypersensitivity; demographic and health survey; diabetic hyperosmolar state; document handling system; duration of hospital stay; dynamic hip screw

D-5-HS 5% dextrose in Harman's solution

DHSM dihydrostreptomycin

DHSS Department of Health and Social Security; dihydrostreptomycin sulfate

DHT dehydrotestosterone; dihydroergotoxine; dihydrotachysterol; dihydrotestosterone; dihydrothymine; dihydroxytryptamine; discrete Hartley transform

5,7-DHT 5,7-dihydroxytryptamine

DHTP dihydrotestosterone propionate

DHTR dihydrotestosterone receptor

DHU dihydroxyuracil

DHUA Division of Health and Utilization Analysis

DHV duck hepatitis virus

DHy, DHyg Doctor of Hygiene

DHZ dihydralazine

DI date of injury; date interviewed; defective interfering [particle]; dental index; dental informatics; dentinogenesis imperfecta; deoxyribonucleic acid index; depression inventory; desorption ionization; deterioration index; detrusor instability; diabetes insipidus; diagnostic imaging; dialyzed iron; diastolic interval; disability insurance; dispensing information; distoincisal; document index; donor insemination; dorso-iliac; dose intensity; double indemnity; drug information; drug injection; drug interactions; duct injection; dyskaryosis index

3DI three-dimensional imaging

5′DI 5′-deiodinase

DIA depolarization-induced automaticity; diabetes; diaphorase; diazepam; Drug Information Association

DiA Diego antigen

dia diakinesis; diathermy

diab diabetes, diabetic

DIACOMP Diabetes Complications [study]

DiaComp diabetes computer-aided [management]

DIAG diagnostic procedure [UMLS]

Diag diagnosis

diag diagonal; diagnosis; diagram

diam diameter

DIAMOND Danish Investigation of Arrhythmia and Mortality on Dofetilide

DIAMOND-CHF Danish Investigation of Arrhythmia and Mortality on Dofetilide in Congestive Heart Failure

DIAMOND-MI Danish Investigation of Arrhythmia and Mortality on Dofetilide in Myocardial Infarction

diaph diaphragm

dias diastole, diastolic

diath diathermy

DIB diagnostic interview for borderlines; difficulty in breathing; disability insurance benefits; dot immunobinding; duodenoileal bypass

DIBAL diisobutylaluminum

diBr-HQ 5,7-dibromo-8-hydroxy-quinidine

DIC dicarbazine; differential interference contrast microscopy; diffuse intravascular coagulation; direct isotope cystography; disseminated intravascular coagulation; drip infusion cholangiography; drug information center

dic dicentric [chromosome]

DICA diagnostic interview of children and adolescents

DICD dispersion-induced circular dichroism

DICO diffusing capacity of carbon monoxide

DICOM digital imaging and communication in medicine

DICOM-RT digital image communications in medicine-radiation therapy

DICPM distributed information, computation, and process management

DID dead of intercurrent disease; Dictionary of Drugs [database]; dissociative identity disorder; double immunodiffusion

DIDA diethyl iminodiacetic acid

DIDD dense intramembranous deposit disease

DiDi Diltiazem in Dilated Cardiomyopathy [trial]

DIDMOA diabetes insipidus-diabetes mellitus-optic atrophy [syndrome]

DIDMOAD diabetes insipidus, diabetes mellitus, optic atrophy, deafness [syndrome]

DIDS 4,4'diisothiocyanostilbene-2,2-disulfonate

DIE died in emergency department; difference in electronegativity

DIEA diisopropylethylamine

diEMG diaphragmatic electromyography

DIEP deep inferior epigastric perforator

DIET Dietary Intervention: Evaluation of Technology [study]

DIEV *Dicentrarchus labrax* encephalitis virus

DIF diffuse interstitial fibrosis; direct immunofluorescence; dose increase factor

DIFF, diff difference, differential; diffusion

diff diagn differential diagnosis

DIFP diffuse interstitial fibrosing pneumonitis; diisopropyl fluorophosphonate

dif-PIPE diffuse persistent interstitial pulmonary emphysema

DIG digitalis; Digitalis Investigation Group; digoxigenin; digoxin; drug-induced galactorrhea

dig digitalis; digoxigenin; digoxin

DIGAF Digoxin in Atrial Fibrillation [study]

DIGAMI Diabetes Mellitus, Insulin Glucose Infusion in Acute Myocardial Infarction [study]

DIH digoxin-induced hyperkalemia; Diploma in Industrial Health

DIHE drug-induced hepatic encephalopathy

diHETE dihydroxyeicosatetraenoic acid

DIHPPA di-iodohydroxyphenylpyruvic acid

DII dynamic invocation interface [computer-assisted surgery]

D$_{ii}$ input delay

DiIV *Diadegma interruptum* ichnovirus

D$_{ij}$ transfer delay

DIL Dilantin; drug-induced lupus [erythematosus]

Dil Dilantin; dilatation, dilated; drug-induced lupus [erythematosus]

dil dilute, diluted, dilution

dilat dilatation

DILCACOMP Diltiazem Captopril Comparative Study

DILD diffuse infiltrative lung disease; diffuse interstitial lung disease

DILDURANG Diltiazem Duration in Angina [study]

DILE drug-induced lupus erythematosus

DILPLACOMP Diltiazem Placebo Comparative Trial

DILS diffuse infiltrative lymphocytosis syndrome

DIM divalent ion metabolism; domain information model; median infective dose [Lat. *dosis infectionis media*]

dim dimension; diminished

DiMe [childhood] Diabetes Mellitus [in Finland]

DIMFP differential inverse mean free path

DIMIT 3,5-dimethyl-3'-isopropyl-L-thyronine

DIMOAD diabetes insipidus, diabetes mellitus, optic atrophy, deafness

DIMS disorder in initiating and maintaining sleep

DIMSE DICOM message service element

DIMT Dutch Ibopamine Multicenter Trial

DIN damage inducible [gene]; digital imaging network; ductal intraepithelial neoplasia

din damage inducible [gene]

DIN/PACS digital imaging network/picture archiving communications system

DIP desquamative interstitial pneumonitis; diffuse interstitial pneumonitis; digital imaging processing; diisopropylamine; diisopropyl phosphate; diphtheria; distal interphalangeal; drip infusion pyelogram;

dual-in-line package; dynamic integral proctography

Dip diplomate

dip diploid; diplotene

DIPA diisopropylamine

DIPAP Dipyridamole in Peripheral Arteriopathy [study]

DipBact Diploma in Bacteriology

DIPC diffuse interstitial pulmonary calcification

DipChem Diploma in Chemistry

DipClinPath Diploma in Clinical Pathology

DIPF diffuse interstitial pulmonary fibrosis; diisopropylphosphofluoridate

diph diphtheria

diph-tet diphtheria-tetanus [toxoid]

diph-tox AP alum precipitated diphtheria toxoid

DIPI defective interfering particle induction

DIPJ distal interphalangeal joint

DIPPER distributed Internet protocol performance [test system]

DIPS-PCR detection of integrated papillomavirus sequences by polymerase chain reaction

Dipy dipyridamole

DIR double isomorphous replacement

Dir, dir direction, directions; director

DIRD drug-induced renal disease

DIRECT Diabetes Intervention: Reaching and Educating Communities Together; Direct Myocardial Revascularization in Regeneration of Endomyocardial Channels Trial

DIRLINE Directory of Information Resources Online [NLM database]

DIRS Dutch Invasive Reperfusion Study

DIS Department of Information Services; departmental information system; Diagnostic Interview Schedule; Diagnostic Interview Survey; draft international standard; drug information system

DI-S debris index, simplified

dis disability, disabled; disease; dislocation; distal; distance

DISC Diagnostic Interview Schedule for Children; Dietary Intervention Study in Children; digital interchange standards for cardiology

disc discontinue

disch discharge, discharged

DISC-HSV disabled infectious single-cycle herpes simplex virus

dis eval disability evaluation

DISF-SR Derogatis Interview for Sexual Functioning - Short Report

DISH Dietary Intervention Study of Hypertension; diffuse idiopathic skeletal hyperostosis; disseminated idiopathic skeletal hyperostosis

DISI dorsal intercalated segment instability

DISIDA diisopropyl iminodiacetic acid

disinfect disinfection

disl, disloc dislocation, dislocated

disod disodium

disp dispensary, dispense

DISS disease or syndrome [UMLS]; distributed image spreadsheet

diss dissolve, dissolved

dissem disseminated, dissemination

DIST Dutch Iliac Stent Trial

dist distal; distance; distill, distillation, distilled; distribution; disturbance, disturbed

DISTRESS Dispatch Stent Restenosis Study

DIT deferoxamine infusion test; defining issues test; diet-induced thermogenesis; diiodotyrosine; drug-induced thrombocytopenia

dit dictyate

dITP deoxyinosine triphosphate

D$_{iv}$ intravenous dose

div divergence, divergent; divide, divided, division

DIVBC disseminated intravascular blood coagulation

DIVC disseminated intravascular coagulation

DJ duodenal juice

DJD degenerative joint disease

DJJ duodenojejunal junction

DJOA dominant juvenile optic atrophy

DJS Dubin-Johnson syndrome

DK dark; decay; diabetic ketoacidosis; diet kitchen; diseased kidney; dog kidney [cells]

dk deka

dk- deka- [10^1]

DKA diabetic ketoacidosis

DKB deep knee bends

DKC dyskeratosis congenita

dkg dekagram

DKI dextrose potassium insulin

DKIE decontaminating kit, individual equipment

dkl decaliter

dkm dekameter

DKP dikalium phosphate

DKS Damus-Kaye-Stansel [anastomosis]

DKTC dog kidney tissue culture

DKV deer kidney virus

DL danger list; data language; deep lobe; De Lee [catheter]; description language; description logic; developmental level; diagnostic laparoscopy; difference limen; digital library; dipole layer; direct laryngoscopy; disabled list; dissimilarity level; distolingual; equimolecular mixture of the dextrorotatory and levorotatory enantiomorphs; lethal dose [L. *dosis lethalis*]; lung diffusion [capacity]

DL, D-L Donath-Landsteiner [antibody]

D$_L$ diffusing capacity of the lungs

dl deciliter

D$_{LA}$ diameter of left atrium

DLa distolabial

DLaI distolabioincisal

DLaP distolabiopulpal

DL&B direct laryngoscopy and bronchoscopy

DLBD diffuse Lewy body disease

DLC Dental Laboratory Conference; differential leukocyte count; dual-lumen catheter

DLCL diffuse large cell lymphoma

DLCO, DL$_{CO}$ carbon monoxide diffusion in the lung

DL$_{CO_2}$ carbon dioxide diffusion in the lungs

DL$_{CO}$^{SB} single-breath carbon monoxide diffusing capacity of the lungs

DL$_{CO}$^{SS} steady-state carbon monoxide diffusing capacity of the lungs

DLD dihydrolipoamide dehydrogenase

dld D-lactate dehydrogenase [gene]

D-LDH D-lactate dehydrogenase

DLE delayed light emission; dialyzable leukocyte extract; discoid lupus erythematosus; disseminated lupus erythematosus

D$_1$LE diagonal 1 lower extremity

D$_2$LE diagonal 2 lower extremity

DLF Disabled Living Foundation; dorsolateral funiculus

DLG distolingual groove

Dlg, dlg disc large

Dlg-R disc large related

DLI Digital Libraries Initiative; distolinguoincisal; donor lymphocyte infusion; double label index

DLIS digoxin-like immunoreactive substance

DLK diffuse lamellar keratitis

DLL dihomo-gammalinoleic acid; dynamic link library

DLLI dulcitol lysine lactose iron

DLMD Duchenne-like muscular dystrophy

DLMP date of last menstrual period

DLN draining lymph nodes

DLNMP date of last normal menstrual period

DLO Diploma in Laryngology and Otology; distolinguo-occlusal

DL$_{O_2}$ diffusing capacity of the lungs for oxygen

DLP delipidized serum protein; direct linear plotting; dislocation of patella; distolinguopulpal; dysharmonic luteal phase

DLPFC dorsolateral prefrontal cortex

DLR digital luminescence radiography

D/LR dextrose in lactated Ringer solution

D$_5$LR dextrose in 5% lactated Ringer solution

DLST dihydrolipoamide *S*-succinyltransferase

DLT digital library technology; dihydroepiandrosterone loading test; direct linear transformation; dose-limiting toxicity; double-lumen endotracheal tube; double lung transplantation

DLV defective leukemia virus; delavirdine

DLW dry lung weight

DM defined medium; dermatomyositis; Descemet's membrane; design manager [database module]; dextromaltose; dextromethorphan; diabetes mellitus; diabetic mother; diastolic murmur; differentiation medium; diphenylaminearsine; distal metastases; dopamine; dorsomedial; double minute [chromosome]; duodenal mucosa; dry matter; dystrophia myotonica

D$_M$ membrane component of diffusion

dm decimeter; diabetes mellitus; dorsomedial

dm^2 square decimeter

dm^3 cubic decimeter

DMA department of medical assistance; dimethylamine; dimethylaniline; dimethylarginine; dimethylarsinic acid; direct memory access; director of medical affairs; distributed multiple analysis

dMA dominant motor area

DMAA dimethylarsinic acid

DMAB dimethylaminobenzaldehyde

DMAC *N,N*-dimethylacetamide; disseminated *Mycobacterium avium* complex

DMAD dimethylaminodiphosphate

DMAE dimethylaminoethanol

DMAEM, DMAEMA *N,N'*-dimethylaminoethyl methacrylate

DMAP dimethylaminophenol; dimethylaminopyridine

DMAPN dimethylaminopropionitrile

DMARD disease-modifying anti-rheumatic drug

D$_{max}$ maximum denaturation; maximum diameter; maximum dose

DMB diffuse microvascular bleeding; diffusional microburet

DMBA 7,12-dimethylbenz[a]anthracene

DMC demeclocycline; di(*p*-chlorophenyl) methylcarbinol; direct microscopic count; duration of muscle contraction; Dyggve-Melchior-Clausen [syndrome]

DMCC direct microscopic clump count

DMCL dimethylclomipramine

DMCO Disease Management and Clinical Outcomes

DMCS Diagnostic Marker Cooperative Study

DMCT, DMCTC dimethylchlortetracycline

DMD disease-modifying drug; Doctor of Dental Medicine; Duchenne muscular dystrophy; dystonia musculorum deformans

DMD/BMD Duchenne/Becker muscular dystrophy

DMDC 2'-deoxy-2'-methylidenecytidine; dimethyldithiocarbamate

DMDT dimethoxydiphenyl trichloroethane

DMDZ desmethyldiazepam

DME degenerative myoclonus epilepsy; dimethyl diester; dimethyl ether; diphasic meningoencephalitis; direct medical education; director of medical education; Division of Medical Education [AAMC]; dropping mercury electrode; drug-metabolizing enzyme; Dulbecco modified Eagle [medium]; durable medical equipment

DMEM Dulbecco modified Eagle medium

DMF decayed, missing, and filled [teeth]; dimethyl fluoride; *N,N*-dimethylformamide; diphasic milk fever

DmFb dermal fibroblast

DMFT decayed, missing, and filled teeth

DMG dimethylglycine

DMGBL dimethyl-gammabutyrolactone

DMGT deoxyribonucleic acid-mediated gene transfer

DMH diffuse mesangial hypercellularity; 1,2-dimethylhydrazine; dorsal medial hypothalamic [nucleus]

DMHD dimenhydrinate

DMI Defense Mechanism Inventory; Diagnostic Medical Instruments; diaphragmatic myocardial infarction; direct migration inhibition

DMID Division of Microbiology and Infectious Diseases [NIH]

DMIM Defense Medical Information Management

D$_{min}$ minimum diameter

dmin double minute

DMIS Defense Medical Information System

DMJ Diploma in Medical Jurisprudence

DMKA diabetes mellitus ketoacidosis

DMKase deoxynucleoside monophosphate kinase

DML data manipulation language; distal motor latency

DMLP Dutch Medical Language Processor

DMM dimethylmyleran; disproportionate micromelia

DMN desmuslin; dimethylnitrosamine; dorsal motor nucleus; dysplastic melanocytic nevus

DMNA dimethylnitrosamine

DMNL dorsomedial hypothalamic nucleus lesion

DMNX dorsal motor nucleus of the vagus nerve

DMO 5,5-dimethyl-2,4-oxazolidinedione (dimethadione)

D$_{mo2}$ membrane diffusing capacity for oxygen

DMOA diabetes mellitus-optic atrophy [syndrome]

DMOD disease model

DMOOC diabetes mellitus out of control

DMP data map publication; diabetes mellitus program; diffuse mesangial proliferation; dimercaprol; dimethylphthalate

DMPA depot medroxyprogesterone acetate

DMPC dimyristyl phosphatidyl choline

DMPE, DMPEA 3,4-dimethoxyphenyl-ethylamine

DMPP dimethylphenylpiperazinium

DMPS dysmyelopoietic syndrome

DMPTU dimethylphenylthiourea

DMR depolarizing muscle relaxant; differentially methylated region; Diploma in Medical Radiology; direct myocardial revascularization; distributed medical record; dose monitoring rate

DM-R decayed plus missing teeth, minus replaced teeth

DMRD Diploma in Medical RadioDiagnosis

DMRE Diploma in Medical Radiology and Electrology

DMRF dorsal medullary reticular formation

dMRI diffusion tensor magnetic resonance imaging

3D-MRI 3-dimensional magnetic resonance imaging

DMRT Diploma in Medical Radio Therapy

DMS delayed match-to-sample; delayed microembolism syndrome; demarcation membrane system; department of medicine and surgery; dermatomyositis; diagnostic medical sonographer; diffuse mesangial sclerosis; dimethylsulfate; dimethylsulfoxide; Doctor of Medical Science; drug misuse statistics; dysmyelopoietic syndrome

DMSA dimercaptosuccinic acid; dimethylsuccinic acid; disodium monomethanearsonate

DMSO dimethyl sulfoxide

DMSS data mining surveillance system

DMT dermatophytosis; [3-(2-dimethylamino)ethyl]indole; *N,N*-dimethyltryptamine; District Management Team; Doctor of Medical Technology; dynamometer muscle testing

DMTU dimethylthiourea

DMU dimethanolurea; dual method of use

DMV diurnal mood variations; Doctor of Veterinary Medicine; dorsal motor nucleus of the vagus nerve; dwarf mosaic virus

DMWP distal mean wave pressure

DN Deiter's nucleus; dextrose-nitrogen; diabetic neuropathy; dibucaine number; dicrotic notch; DiFrancesco-Noble [equation]; dinitrocresol; Diploma in Nursing;

Diploma in Nutrition; District Nurse; Doctor of Nursing; dominant-negative; do not [resuscitate]; duodenum

D/N dextrose/nitrogen [ratio]

D&N distance and near [vision]

Dn dekanem

dn decinem

DNA deoxyribonucleic acid; did not answer

DNA DSB DNA double-strand break

DNAP DNA phosphorus

DNA-PK DNA-protein kinase

DNAR do not attempt resuscitation

DNASE, DNAse, DNase deoxyribonuclease

DNB dinitrobenzene; Diplomate of the National Board [of Medical Examiners]; dorsal nonadrenergic bundle

DNBP dinitrobutylphenol

DNBS 2,4-dinitrobenzene sulfonate

DNC did not come; dinitrocarbanilide; dinitrocresol; Disaster Nursing Chairman

DNCB dinitrochlorobenzene

DNCM cytoplasmic membrane-associated deoxyribonucleic acid

DND died a natural death; Drugs for Neglected Diseases [*Médicins Sans Frontières*]

DNE Director of Nursing Education; Doctor of Nursing Education

DNET dysembryoplastic neuroepithelial tumor

DNF distinctive normal form system [Boolean logic]

DNFB dinitrofluorobenzene

DNH do-not-hospitalize [order]

DNIC diffuse noxious inhibitory control

DNK did not keep [appointment]

DNKA did not keep appointment

DNLL dorsal nucleus of lateral lemniscus

dNMP deoxynucleotide monophosphate

1D NMR one-dimensional nuclear magnetic resonance

2D NMR two-dimensional nuclear magnetic resonance

DNMS delayed nonmatch-to-sample; Director of Naval Medical Services

DNMT deoxyribonucleic acid methyltransferase

Dnmt DNA methyltransferase gene

DNO District Nursing Officer

DNOC dinitroorthocresol

DNP deoxyribonucleoprotein; dinitrophenol; dinitropyrene; dynamic nuclear polarization

2,4-DNP 2,4-dinitrophenol

DNPH dinitrophenylhydrazine

DNPM dinitrophenol-morphine

DNQX 6,7-dinitroquinoxaline-2,3-dione

DNR daunorubicin; do not resuscitate; dorsal nerve root

DNS deviated nasal septum; diaphragmatic nerve stimulation; did not show [for appointment]; Dietitians in Nutrition Support; Doctor of Nursing Services; domain name system [electronic mail addressing system]; dysplastic nevus syndrome

D/NS dextrose in normal saline [solution]

D5NS 5% dextrose in normal saline [solution]

D₅NSS 5% dextrose in normal saline solution

DNT dermonecrotic toxin; did not test; 2,4-dinitrotoluene; dysembryoplastic neuroepithelial tumor

DNTM disseminated nontuberculous mycobacterial [infection]

dNTP deoxyribonucleoside triphosphate

DNTT terminal deoxynucleotidyltransferase

DNV densovirus; dorsal nucleus of vagus nerve; double-normalized value

DO diamine oxidase; digoxin; Diploma in Ophthalmology; Diploma in Osteopathy; directly observed; dissolved oxygen; disto-occlusal; distraction osteogenesis; Doctor of Ophthalmology; Doctor of Optometry; Doctor of Osteopathy; doctor's orders; drugs only

D_O oxygen diffusion

D_{O₂} oxygen delivery

DOA date of admission; dead on arrival; Department of Agriculture; depth of anesthesia; differential optical absorption; dominant optic atrophy

DOAC Dubois oleic albumin complex

DOB date of birth; 1-(2,5-dimethoxy-4-bromophenyl)-2-aminopropane; doctor's order book

Dob dobutamine

DObstRCOG Diploma of the Royal College of Obstetricians and Gynaecologists

DOBV Dobrava-Belgrade virus; double outlet both ventricles

DOC date of conception; deoxycholate; deoxycorticosterone; diagnostically operative causal [graph]; died of other causes; disorders of cornification; dissolved organic carbon; distributed object computing; doctor on call; Doctors Ought to Care [project]

doc doctor; document, documentation

DOCA deoxycorticosterone acetate

DOCG deoxycorticosterone glucoside

DOCLINE Documents On-Line

DO₂crit critical oxygen delivery

DOCS deoxycorticosteroids

DOcSc Doctor of Ocular Science

DOCUSER Document Delivery User [NLM database]

DOD date of death; dementia syndrome of depression; depth of discharge; Dictionary of Organic Compounds [database]; died of disease; dissolved oxygen deficit

DoD Department of Defense

DoDCPR Department of Defense computerized patient record

DOE date of examination; desoxyephedrine; direct observation evaluation; dyspnea on exertion

DOES disorders of excessive sleepiness

DOF, dof degree of freedom

DOFCOSY double-quantum filtered correlated spectroscopy

DOFISK Dose Finding of Streptokinase [trial]

DOFOS disturbance of function occlusion syndrome

DOG deoxyglucose; derivative of gaussian [function]; difference of gaussians; distraction osteogenesis

DoG difference of gaussians

DOH, DoH department of health

DOHyg Diploma in Occupational Hygiene

DOI date of injury; died of injuries; digital object identifier; document object identifier

DO₂I oxygen delivery index

DOIA Dermatological Online Atlas

Dol dolichol

dol pain [Lat. *dolor*]

DOLLS [Lee] double-loop locking suture

DOLV double outlet left ventricle

DOM deaminated *O*-methyl metabolite; department of medicine; dimethoxymethylamphetamine; dissolved organic matter; document object model; dominance, dominant

dom dominant

DOMA dihydroxymandelic acid

DOMBL distal, occlusal, mesial, buccal, lingual

DOMF 2′,7′-dibromo-4′-(hydroxymercuri)fluorescein

DOMIOS Determinants of Myocardial Infarction Onset [study]

DOMS Diploma in Ophthalmic Medicine and Surgery

DON deoxynivalenol; diazooxonorleucine; Director of Nursing

DONALD dissection of neck arteries: long-term follow-up determination

DOOR deafness, onycho-osteodystrophy, mental retardation [syndrome]

DOP dioctyl phthalate; Directory of Physicians

DOPA, dopa dihydroxyphenylalanine

DOPAC dihydrophenylacetic acid

dopamine dihydroxyphenylethylamine

dopase dihydroxyphenylalanine oxidase

DOPC determined osteogenic precursor cell; dioleoyl-phosphatidyl choline

DOPE dioleoyl-phosphatidyl ethanolamine

DOph Doctor of Ophthalmology

DOPP dihydroxyphenylpyruvate

DOPS diffuse obstructive pulmonary syndrome; dihydroxyphenylserine; dioleoylphosphatidyl serine

DO-PT directly observed preventive therapy

dor dorsal

DORNA desoxyribonucleic acid

Dors dorsal

DOrth Diploma in Orthodontics; Diploma in Orthoptics

DORV double outlet right ventricle

DoRV *Dacus oleae* reovirus

DOS day of surgery; deoxystreptamine; disk operating system; Doctor of Ocular Science; Doctor of Optical Science; dysosteosclerosis

dos dosage, dose

DOSC Dubois oleic serum complex

DOSPO documentation system for pediatric oncology

DOSS dioctyl sodium sulfosuccinate; distal over-shoulder strap; docusate sodium

DOT date of transfer; Dictionary of Occupational Titles; directly observed therapy

DOTA tetraazacyclododecanetetraacetic acid

DOTC Dameshek's oval target cell

DOTES dosage record and treatment emergent symptoms

DOTF Document Oncology Task Force

DOTMA di-oleoyloxopropyl-trimethylammonium chloride

DOTS directly observed therapies; directly observed treatment, short course

DOUBLE Double Bolus Lytic Efficacy [trial]

DOUBTFUL double quantum transition for finding unresolved lines

DOUBTLESS Doppler and Ultrasound-Guided Balloon Therapeutics for Coronary Lesions [study]

DOUV Douglas virus

DOV dolphin poxvirus

DOVE deoxyverrucarol

DOX doxorubicin

Dox doxorubicin

dOxo 2′-deoxyaxanosine

DOX-SL stealth ribosomal doxorubicin

DP data processing; deep pulse; definitive procedure; degradation product; degree of polymerization; dementia praecox; dementia pugillistica; dendritic peptide; dental prosthodontics, dental prosthesis; *Dermatophagoides pteronyssimus*; desmoplakin; dexamethasone pretreatment; diabetic patient; diastolic pressure; diazepam; diffuse precipitation; diffusion pressure; digestible protein; diphosgene; diphosphate; dipropionate; directional preponderance; disability pension; discrimination power; distal pancreatectomy; distal phalanx; distal pit; distopulpal; docking protein; Doctor of Pharmacy; Doctor of Podiatry; donor's plasma; dorsalis pedis

D/P dialysate-to-plasma [ratio]

Dp duplication; dyspnea

D$_p$ pattern difference

3DP three-dimensional printing

DPA Department of Public Assistance; D-penicillamine; diphenylalanine; diphenylamine; dipicolinic acid; dipropylacetic acid; direct provider agreement; dual photon absorptiometry; dynamic physical activity

DPAHC durable power of attorney for health care

DpAV *Diadromus pulchellus* ascovirus

DPB days post-burn; differential pencil beam [radiotherapy]; diffuse panbronchiolitis

DPBP diphenylbutylpiperidine

DPC delayed primary closure; deoxyribonucleic acid [DNA] probe chromatography; deoxyribonucleic acid [DNA] protein crosslinks; desaturated phosphatidylcholine; diethylpyrocarbonate; direct patient care; discharge planning coordinator; distal palmar crease

dpc days post coitum

DPCM differential pulse code modulation

DpCPV *Danaus plexippus* cypovirus; *Dasychira pudibunda* cypovirus

DPCRT double-blind placebo-controlled randomized clinical trial

DPD Department of Public Dispensary; depression pure disease; desoxypyridoxine; diffuse pulmonary disease; diffusion pressure deficit; diphenamid; Diploma in Public Dentistry; direct patient dose [monitor]

DPDCH dedicated physical data channel [telemedicine]

DPDL diffuse poorly differentiated lymphocytic lymphoma

dP/dt first derivative of pressure measured over time

dpdt double-pole double-throw [switch]

dP/dV pressure per unit change in volume

DPE dipalmitoyl phosphatidyl ethanolamine; dipiperidinoethane; downstream promoter element [RNA processing]

DPEP dipeptidase

DPF Dental Practitioners' Formulary; diisopropyl fluorophosphate; probability density function [implantable cardioverter-defibrillator]

DPFC distal palmar flexion crease

DPFR diastolic pressure-flow relationship

DPG 2,3-diphosphoglycerate; displacement placentogram

2,3-DPG 2,3-diphosphoglycerate

2,3-DPGM 2,3-diphosphoglycerate mutase

DPGN diffuse proliferative glomerulonephritis

DPGP diphosphoglycerate phosphatase

DPH Department of Public Health; diphenhydramine; diphenylhexatriene; diphenylhydantoin; Diploma in Public Health; Doctor of Public Health; Doctor

of Public Hygiene; dopamine beta-hydrolase; ductal papillary hyperplasia

DPhC Doctor of Pharmaceutical Chemistry

DPhc Doctor of Pharmacology

DPHN Doctor of Public Health Nursing

DPhys Diploma in Physiotherapy

DPhysMed Diploma in Physical Medicine

DPI daily permissible intake; days post inoculation; dietary protein intake; diphtheria-pertussis immunization; disposable personal income; drug prescription index; dry powder inhaler; Dynamic Personality Inventory

DPJ dementia paralytica juvenilis

DPKC diagnostic problem-knowledge coupler

DPL diagnostic peritoneal lavage; dipalmitoyl lecithin; distopulpolingual

DPLa distopulpolabial

DPLN diffuse proliferative lupus nephritis

DPLS differentially polarized light scattering

DPM Diploma in Psychological Medicine; discontinue previous medication; Doctor of Physical Medicine; Doctor of Podiatric Medicine; Doctor of Preventive Medicine; Doctor of Psychiatric Medicine; dopamine

dpm disintegrations per minute

DPN dermatosis papulosa nigra; diabetic polyneuropathy; diphosphopyridine nucleotide; disabling pansclerotic morphea; dorsal parabrachial nucleus

DPNB dorsal penile nerve block

DPNH reduced diphosphopyridine nucleotide

DPO dimethoxyphenyl penicillin

D$_{po}$ oral [per os] dose

DPP Diabetes Prevention Program; differential pulse polarography; digital pulse plethysmography; dimethylphenylpenicillin; dipeptidylpeptidase; distal photoplethysmography; document pattern processing

dpp decapentaplegic

DPPC dipalmitoylphosphatidylcholine; double-blind placebo-controlled trial

DPPD diphenylphenylenediamine

DpPHR duodenum-preserving pancreatic head resection

DPPITC diphenyl diphosphoro-isothiocyanate

DPR dietary prevention of recurrent myocardial infarction; drug price review; dynamic perception resolution; dynamic planar reconstructor

DpRV *Diadromus pulchellus* reovirus

DPS delayed primary suture; descending perineum syndrome; dimethylpolysiloxane; Division of Provider Studies [database]; dysesthetic pain syndrome

dps decay per second

dpst double-pole single-throw [switch]

DPSWF discrete prolate spheroidal wave function

DPT Demerol, Phenergan, and Thorazine; dermatopontin; Diabetes Prevention Trial; dichotic pitch discrimination test; diphtheria-pertussis-tetanus [vaccine]; diphtheritic pseudotabes; dipropyltryptamine; dual platform technique; dumping provocation test

Dpt house dust mite

DPTA diethylenetriamine penta-acetic acid

DPTI diastolic pressure time index

DPTP domain protein tyrosine phosphatase

DPTPM diphtheria-pertussis-tetanus-poliomyelitis-measles [vaccine]

Dptr diopter

DPTU diphenylthiourea

DPUF Doppler ultrasound flowmeter

DPV *Dasychira pudibunda* virus; deer papillomavirus; disabling positional vertigo; mule deer poxvirus

DPVS Denver peritoneovenous shunt

DPW Department of Public Welfare; distal phalangeal width

DQ deterioration quotient; developmental quotient

D$_q$ quasithreshold dose [radiation]

3DQCT 3-dimensional quantitative computed tomography

DQE degradation of image quality; detective quantum efficiency

DQFC double quantum filtered correlation spectroscopy

DQFC NMR double quantum filtered correlation nuclear magnetic resonance spectroscopy

DQO data quality objective

DQP data quality probe

3D-QSAR 3-dimensional quantitative structure-activity relationship [dataset]

DR death receptor [cell]; degeneration reaction; delayed rectifier; delivery room; deoxyribose; diabetic retinopathy; diagnostic radiology; dietary recall; digital radiography; direct repeat; distal recurrence; distribution ratio; doctor; dopamine receptor; dorsal raphe; dorsal root; dose ratio; drug receptor; dynamic range; dynamic resistance

Dr doctor

dR dextroribose; deoxyriboside

dr dorsal root; drain; dram; dressing

DRA dextran-reactive antibody; digital rotational angiography; distal rectal adenocarcinoma; distal reference axis [imaging]

3d-RA 3-dimensional rotational angiography

DRACOG Diploma of Royal Australian College of Obstetricians and Gynaecologists

DRACR Diploma of Royal Australasian College of Radiologists

DRAM dynamic random access memory

DRAP dorsal root action potential

dr ap dram, apothecary

DRASIC dorsal root ganglion [DRG] cells acid-sensing ion channel

DRASTIC Dutch Renal Artery Stenosis Intervention Cooperative Study

DRAT differential rheumatoid agglutination test

DRB daunorubicin; dynamic reference basis [computer-assisted surgery]

DRBC denaturated red blood cell; dog red blood cell; donkey red blood cell

DRC damage risk criterion; daunorubicin; dendritic reticulum cell; deoxyribonucleic acid [DNA] repair capacity; diagnostic reporting console; digitorenocerebral [syndrome]; dorsal root, cervical; dose-response curve; dynamic range compression; dynamic range control [algorithm]

DRCOG Diploma of Royal College of Obstetricians and Gynaecologists

DRCPath Diploma of Royal College of Pathologists

DRD dihydroxyphenylalanine-responsive dystonia; dorsal root dilator; dystrophia retinae pigmentosa-dysostosis [syndrome]

DRD$_2$ dopamine D$_2$ receptor

DRD$_3$ dopamine D$_3$ receptor

DRD$_4$ dopamine D$_4$ receptor

DRE damage response element [DNA]; digital rectal examination; dioxin-responsive elements; dioxin-responsive enhancer; direct response element

DREF dose rate effectiveness factor

DREN Department of Defense Research and Engineering Network

DRES dynamic random element stimuli

DRESS depth-resolved surface-coil spectroscopy

DREZ dorsal root entry zone

DRF Daily Rating Form; daily replacement factor; Deafness Research Foundation; digestive-respiratory fistula; dose reduction factor; dynamic reference frame [computer-assisted surgery]

DR-FFP donor-retested fresh frozen plasma

DRFS Dundee Rank Factor Score [risk factors in coronary heart disease]

DRG diagnosis-related group; Division of Research Grants [NIH]; dorsal respiratory group; dorsal root ganglion; duodenal-gastric reflux gastropathy

drg drainage

DrHyg Doctor of Hygiene

DRI defibrillation response interval; discharge readiness inventory; Doppler resistive index; dynamic response index

dRib deoxyribose

DRID double radial immunodiffusion; double radioisotope derivative

DRIN direct reconstructor interface

DRIP delirium and drugs-restricted mobility and retention-infection, inflammation and impaction-polyuria [causes of urinary incontinence]

DRL dorsal root, lumbar; drug-related lupus

D5RL 5% dextrose in Ringer lactate [solution]

DRME Division of Research in Medical Education

Dr Med Doctor of Medicine

DRMF directional recursive median filtering

DRMS drug reaction monitoring system

DrMT Doctor of Mechanotherapy

DRN dorsal raphe nucleus

DRNDP diribonucleoside-3′,3′-diphosphate

DRnt diagnostic roentgenology

DRO differential reinforcement of other behavior; Disablement Resettlement Officer

DRP digoxin reduction product; dorsal root potential; drug-related problems; dystrophin-related protein

dRp deoxyribose-phosphate

dRPase, dRpase deoxyribophosphodiesterase

DrPH Doctor of Public Health; Doctor of Public Hygiene

DRPLA dentorubral-pallidoluysian atrophy

DRQ discomfort relief quotient

DRR digitally reconstructed radiograph; dorsal root reflex; dysjunction regulator region

DRS descending rectal septum; diagnostic review station; diffuse reflectance spectroscopy; Diltiazem Reinfarction Study; disability rating scale; drowsiness; Duane retraction syndrome; dynamic renal scintigraphy; Dyskinesia Rating Scale

drsg dressing

DRSP drug-resistant *Streptococcus pneumoniae*

DRST Delayed Recognition Span Test

DRT dorsal root, thoracic

3DRT three-dimensional radiotherapy

3-DRTP three dimensional radiation treatment planning

DRUGS Doctor, Recreational User, Gynaecological Sensitivities [study]

DRUJ distal radioulnar joint

DrV *Diplocarpon rosae* virus

dRVVT dilute Russell viper venom time

DRY donryu [rat]

DS Dahl strain [rat]; data set; dead air space; dead space; decontaminating solution; deep sedative; deep sleep; defined substrate; dehydroepiandrosterone sulfate; delayed sensitivity; dendritic spine; density standard; dental surgery; dermatan sulfate; dermatology and syphilology; desmosome; desynchronized sleep; Devic syndrome; dexamethasone-spermine; dextran sulfate; dextrose-saline; diameter stenosis; diaphragm stimulation; diastolic murmur; differential stimulus; diffuse scleroderma; dilute strength; dioptric strength; direct sequencing; disaster services; discrimination score; disoriented; disseminated sclerosis; dissolved solids; Doctor of

Science; donor's serum; Doppler sonography; double-stranded; double strength; double stringency; Down syndrome; drug store; dry swallow; dumping syndrome; duplex scan; duration of systole

D&S dermatology and syphilology

D/S dextrose/saline

ds double stranded [DNA]

D1S first year dental student

D2S second year dental student

DS2 decontaminating solution 2

D3S third year dental student

D4S fourth year dental student

D-5-S 5% dextrose in saline solution

%DS percent diameter stenosis

DSA Defense Security Agency; density spectral array; destructive spondyloarthropathy; digital subtraction angiography; dynamic scalable architecture

DSACT, D-SACT direct sinoatrial conduction time

DSAF Decision Support Access Facility [Bureau of Data Management and Strategy Facilities, BDMS]

DSAP disseminated superficial actinic porokeratosis

DSAS discrete subaortic stenosis

DSB, dsb double-strand break [DNA]

Dsb single-breath diffusion capacity

DSBL disabled

DSBR double-strand break repair

DSBT donor-specific blood transfusion

DSC de Sanctis-Cacchione [syndrome]; desmocollin; differential scanning calorimetry; digital scan converter; disodium chromoglycate; Doctor of Surgical Chiropody; Down syndrome child; dynamic susceptibility contrast [imaging]

DSc Doctor of Science

Dsc desmocollin

DSCA double-strand conformation analysis

DSCF Doppler-shifted constant frequency

DSCG disodium chromoglycate

DSC-MRI dynamic susceptibility contrast magnetic resonance imaging

DsCPV *Dendrolimus spectabilis* cypovirus

DSCR developmental self-care requisites

DSCT dorsal spinocerebellar tract

DSCU dementia special care unit

DSD Déjerine-Sottas disease; depression spectrum disease; discharge summary dictated; dry sterile dressing

DS-DAT Discomfort Scale for Dementia of the Alzheimer Type

DSDDT double sampling dye dilution technique

dsDNA double-stranded deoxyribonucleic acid

DsDNV *Diatraea saccharalis* densovirus

DSE dobutamine stress echocardiography; Doctor of Sanitary Engineering

DSG decision system group; desmoglein; dry sterile gauze

Dsg desmoglein

DSH deliberate self harm; dexamethasone suppressible hyperaldosteronism; disproportionate share hospital

DSHEA Dietary Supplements Health and Education Act

DSHEFS Division of Surveillance, Hazard Evaluation and Field Studies

DSHR delayed skin hypersensitivity reaction

DSI deep shock insulin; Depression Status Inventory; desmocollin-specific insertion; disulfide isomerase; Down Syndrome International; dynamic skeleton interface [computer-assisted surgery]

DSIM Doctor of Science in Industrial Medicine

DSIP delta sleep-inducing peptide

DSL distal sensory latency

DSL MU distal sensory latency-median-ulnar

dslv dissolve

DSM dextrose solution mixture; Diagnostic and Statistical Manual [of Mental Disorders]; digital standard MUMPS [Massachusetts General Hospital Utility Multi-Programming System]; Diploma in Social Medicine; drink skim milk

DSM, dsm disease-specific mortality

DSM-III-R Diagnostic and Statistical Manual [of Mental Disorders], Third Edition, Revised

DSM-IV Diagnostic and Statistical Manual [of Mental Disorders], Fourth Edition

DSMA diet and stress management in angina; disodium monomethanearsonate

DSMB Data Safety Monitoring Board [FDA]

DSMC data and safety monitoring committee

DSN data source name

DSNI deep space neck infection

DSO digital storage oscilloscope; distal subungual onychomycosis

DSORT discrete stochastic optimization of radiation therapy [algorithm]

DSP decreased sensory perception; delayed sleep phase; desmoplakin; diarrheic shellfish poisoning; dibasic sodium phosphate; digital signal processing; digital subtraction phlebography; display; distal sensory polyneuropathy; Doppler signal processor

DSPC disaturated phosphatidylcholine

DSPCR, DS-PCR double stringency polymerase chain reaction

DspIV *Dusona* spp. ichnovirus

DSPN distal sensory polyneuropathy; distal symmetrical polyneuropathy

DSR digital subtraction analysis; distal spleno-renal; double simultaneous recording; dynamic spatial reconstructor

DSRCT desmoplastic small round cell tumor

dsRNA double-stranded ribonucleic acid

DSRS distal splenorenal shunt

DSS [computer-aided] decision support system; [computer-based] decision support system; Dejerine-Sottas syndrome; demographic surveillance site; dengue shock syndrome; digital signature standard; digital storage system; dioctyl sodium sulfosuccinate; Disability Status Scale; discrete subaortic stenosis; docusate sodium; dosage-sensitive sex [reversal]; double simultaneous stimulation

DSSc Diploma in Sanitary Science

DSS/DH digital signature standard/Differ-Hellman

DSSEP dermatomal somatosensory evoked potential

DSSI Duke social support index

DSST digital symbol substitution test [sedation scoring]

DST desensitization test; desiccate, sequester, and transport; dexamethasone suppression test; dihydrostreptomycin; disproportionate septal thickening; donor-specific transfusion

D$_{st+}$ Dice's similarity coefficient

DS-TRIEL Decision Support [cancer clinical] Trial Eligibility

DSTY derived semantic type [UMLS]

DSUH directed suggestion under hypnosis

DSur Doctor of Surgery

DSV dermal sarcoma virus; Desert Shield virus

DSVP downstream venous pressure

DSWI deep surgical wound infection

DT database tomography; deceleration time; decision table [hierarchical structures]; decision tree [hierarchical structures]; defibrillation threshold; definitive type; delirium tremens; dental technician; depression of transmission; dietetic [services]; dietetic technician; differential technique; digitoxin; diphtheria-tetanus [toxoid]; discharge tomorrow; dispensing tablet; distance test; dorsalis tibialis; double tachycardia; duration of tetany; dye test

D/T date of treatment; total ratio of deaths

dT deoxythymidine

dt due to; dystonic

d/t due to

D3T 1,2-dithiole-3-thione

d4T stavudine

DTA decision to abort; differential thermal analysis; diphtheria toxin A

DTaP diphtheria and tetanus toxoids and acellular pertussis vaccine

DTB dedicated time block

DTBC D-tubocurarrine

DTBM demineralized trabecular bone matrix

DTBN di-*tert*-butyl nitroxide

DTC day treatment center; differential thyroid carcinoma; dithiocarb sodium

dTc D-tubocurarrine

DTCD Diploma in Tuberculosis and Chest Diseases

DTCH Diploma in Tropical Child Health

DTD delivered total dose; desmoglein terminal domain; diastrophic dysplasia; document type definition

DTDase deoxyuridine triphosphate diphosphohydrolase

DTDES dynamic template driven data entry system

dTDP deoxythymidine diphosphate

DTE desiccated thyroid extract

DTF deep temporal fascia; detector transfer function

D-TGA dextraposed transposition of great arteries

DTH delayed-type hypersensitivity; Diploma in Tropical Hygiene

DTH-T delayed -type hypersensitivity T-cell
DTI diffusion tensor imaging; dipyridamole-thallium′ imaging; direct thrombin inhibitor; Doppler tissue imaging
DTIA Doppler tissue imaging acceleration
DTIC dacarbazine; dimethyltriazenyl imidazole carboxamide
DTICH delayed traumatic intracerebral hematoma; delayed traumatic intracerebral hemorrhage
DTIE Doppler tissue imaging energy
D time dream time
DTIV Doppler tissue imaging velocity
DtIV *Diadegma terebrans* ichnovirus
DTLA Detroit Test of Learning Aptitudes
DTM dermatophyte test medium; Diploma in Tropical Medicine
DTM&H Diplomate of Tropical Medicine and Hygiene
DTMP deoxythymidine monophosphate
DTMS Drug Therapy Monitoring System
dTMS double-pulse transcranial magnetic stimulation
DTN diphtheria toxin, normal
DTNB 5,5′-dithiobis-(2-nitrobenzoic) acid
DTO data terminal operator; deodorized tincture of opium
DtoA digital-to-analog [converter]
DTP Demerol, Thorazine, Phenergan [analgesic cocktail]; diphtheria-tetanus-pertussis [vaccine]; distal tingling on percussion [Tinel's sign]
DTPA diethylenetriaminepentaacetic acid
DTPa diphtheria-tetanus-acellular pertussis [vaccine]
DTPBw diphtheria-tetanus whole-cell pertussis [vaccine]
DTPH Diploma in Tropical Public Health
dTPM deoxythymidine monophosphate
DTR deep tendon reflex; dietetic technician registered
DTRTT digital temperature recovery time test
DTS dense tubular system; diphtheria toxin sensitivity; distributed time service; donor transfusion, specific; Duke treadmill score
DT's delirium tremens
DTT diagnostic and therapeutic team; diphtheria tetanus toxoid; direct transverse traction; dithiothreitol
DTTCI 3,3-diethylthiatricarbocyanamide iodide

dTTP deoxythymidine triphosphate
DTUS diathermy, traction, and ultrasound
DTV desktop videoconferencing [telemedicine]; *Dioscorea trifida* virus
DtV *Darna trima* virus
DT-VAC diphtheria-tetanus vaccine
DTVM Diploma in Tropical Veterinary Medicine
DTVMI developmental test of visual motor integration
DTVP developmental test of visual perception
DTwP diphtheria and tetanus toxoids and whole-cell pertussis vaccine
DTX dendrotoxin; detoxification; dinophysitoxin
DTZ diatrizoate
DU decubitus ulcer; density unknown; deoxyuridine; dermal ulcer; diagnosis undetermined; diagnostic unit; diazouracil; dog unit; duodenal ulcer; duplex ultrasound; duroxide uptake; Dutch [rabbit]
dU deoxyuridine
du dial unit; duplication [chromosome]
DUA dorsal uterine artery
DUB dysfunctional uterine bleeding
DUCCS Duke University Clinical Cardiology Study
DUDP Drug Use and Drug Prevention [study]
dUDP deoxyuridine diphosphate
DUE drug use evaluation
D₁UE diagonal 1 upper extremity
D₂UE diagonal 2 upper extremity
DUET Dispatch Urokinase Efficacy Trial
DUF Doppler ultrasonic flowmeter; drug use forecast
DUFSS Duke-University of North Carolina Functional Social Support [questionnaire]
DUGV Dugbe virus
DUHP Duke-University Health Profile
DUI driving under the influence
DUL diffuse undifferentiated lymphoma
dulc sweet [Lat. *dulcis*]
dUMP deoxyuridine monophosphate
duod duodenum, duodenal
dup duplication
DU-PAN-2 marker for pancreatic cancer
DUQUES Duke University quantitative/qualitative evaluation system
DUR drug use review; drug utilization review

Dur during, duration
dur during
DURAC duration of anticoagulation
DUS diagnostic ultrasonography; Doppler flow ultrasound; dynamic ultrasound of shoulder
3D-US three-dimensional ultrasonography
DUSN diffuse unilateral subacute neuroretinitis
DUSOCS Duke social support and stress scale
DUSOI Duke University severity of illness [index]
dut deoxyuridine triphosphatase [gene]
DUTCH-TIA Dutch Transient Ischemic Attack Study
dUTP deoxyuridine triphosphate
dUTPase deoxyuridine triphosphatase
DUV damaging ultraviolet [radiation]
DUVV Duvenhage virus
DV *Datura* virus; dependent variable; diagnostic variable; difference in volume; digital vibration; dilute volume; distemper virus; domestic violence; domiciliary visit; dorsoventral; double vibration; double vision; ductus venosus; dwarf virus
3-DV three dimensional visualization
D&V diarrhea and vomiting
dv double vibrations
DVA Department of Veterans' Affairs; developmental venous anomaly; distance visual acuity; duration of voluntary apnea; vindesine
DVB divinylbenzene
DVC divanillylcyclohexane; dorsal vagal complex
DVCC Disease Vector Control Center
DVCV Diodia vein chlorosis virus
DVD digital videodisk; dissociated vertical deviation
DV&D Diploma in Venereology and Dermatology
dVDAVP 1-deamine-4-valine-D-arginine vasopressin
DVE duck virus enteritis
DVH Diploma in Veterinary Hygiene; Division for the Visually Handicapped; dose volume histogram
DVI AV sequential [pacemaker]; deep venous insufficiency; device-independent; diastolic velocity integral; digital vascular imaging; Doppler velocity index
DVIS digital vascular imaging system

DVIU direct-vision internal urethrotomy
DVL deep vastus lateralis
DVM digital voltmeter; Doctor of Veterinary Medicine
DVMS Doctor of Veterinary Medicine and Surgery
DVN dorsal vagal nucleus
2D-VNQ 2-dimensional N-Quoit filter [imaging]
3D-VNQ 3-dimensional N-Quoit filter [imaging]
DVNV Dendrobium vein necrosis virus
DVP deep venous pressure; Doppler velocity profile
DVR digital vascular reactivity; direct volume rendering; Doctor of Veterinary Radiology; double valve replacement; double ventricular response
DVS Doctor of Veterinary Science; Doctor of Veterinary Surgery
DVSc Doctor of Veterinary Science
DVT Danish Verapamil Trial; deep venous thrombosis
DVT/PE deep venous thrombosis/pulmonary embolism
DW daily weight; data warehouse; deionized water; dextrose in water; diffusion-weighted [magnetic resonance] imaging; distilled water; doing well; dry weight
D/W dextrose in water
D5W, D₅W 5% dextrose in water
D10W 10% aqueous dextrose solution
dw dwarf [mouse]
DWA died from wounds by the action of the enemy
DWCE density-weighted contrast enhancement
DWD died with disease
DWDL diffuse well-differentiated lymphocytic lymphoma
DWDM dense wave division multiplexing
DWECNP Dr. Welford's Electronic Chart Notes Program
DWI diffusion-weighted [magnetic resonance] imaging; driving while impaired; driving while intoxicated
DWM Dandy-Walker malformation
DWML deep white matter lesion
DWS Dandy-Walker syndrome; demonstrator workstation; disaster warning system
DWT dichotic word test; discrete wavelet transform; dyadic wavelet transform

dwt pennyweight
DWV Dandy-Walker variant
DX dextran; dicloxacillin; DNA region X chromosome
Dx, dx diagnosis
D&X dilation and extraction
DXA dual [energy] x-ray absorptiometry
dx cath diagnostic catheterization
DXD discontinued
DxDx differential diagnosis
DXM, DXMS dexamethasone
DXP digital x-ray prototype
DxPLAIN Massachusetts General Hospital's expert diagnostic system
DXPNET Digital X-Ray Prototype Network
DXR deep x-ray
DXRT deep x-ray therapy
DXT deep x-ray therapy; dextrose
dXTP deoxyxanthine triphosphate

D$_{xx}$ input delay
D$_{xy}$ transfer delay
DY dense parenchyma
Dy dysprosium
dy dystrophia muscularis [mouse]
DYLOMMS dynamic lattice-oriented molecular modeling system
dyn dynamic; dynamometer; dyne
DYNAMO dynamic decision modeling [system]
dyne/cm dyne per centimeter
DYS dysautonomia
dysp dyspnea
DZ diazepam; dizygotic; dizziness
dZ impedance change
dz disease; dozen
dZ/dt time-dependent impedance change
DZM dorsal zone of membranelle
DZP diazepam

E

E air dose; cortisone [compound E]; each; eating; edema; effects variable; elastance; electric charge; electric field vector; electrode potential; electromotive force; electron; embyro; emmetropia; encephalitis; endangered [animal]; endogenous; endoplasm; enema; energy; *Entamoeba*; enterococcus; enzyme; eosinophil; epicondyle; epinephrine; epithelium/epithelial; error; erythrocyte; erythroid; erythromycin; *Escherichia*; esophagus; ester; estradiol; ethanol; ethyl; examination; exhalation; expectancy [wave]; expected frequency in a cell of a contingency table; experiment, experimenter; expiration; expired air; exposure; external control [pacemaker]; extract, extracted, extraction; extraction fraction; extralymphatic; eye; glutamic acid; internal energy; kinetic energy; mathematical expectation; redox potential; unit [Ger. *Einheit*]

E- exa- [10^{18}]

E- stereodescriptor to indicate the configuration at a double bond [Ger. *entgegen* opposite]

E* lesion on the erythrocyte cell membrane at the site of complement fixation

E° standard electrode potential

Ē average beta energy

E$_0$ baseline effect; electric affinity

E$_1$ estrone

E-1 to 33 Human echovirus 1 to 33

E$_2$ 17β-estradiol

E$_3$ estriol

E$_4$ estetrol

4E four-plus edema

e base of natural logarithms, approximately 2.7182818285; egg transfer; ejection; electric charge; electron; elementary charge; exchange

e$^+$ positron

e$^-$ negative electron

ε see *epsilon*

η see *eta*

EA early antigen; educational age; egg albumin; electric affinity; electrical activity; electroacupuncture; electroanesthesia;

electronic patient record [EPR] attributes; electrophysiological abnormality; embryonic antibody; endocardiographic amplifier; Endometriosis Association; enteral alimentation; enteroanastomosis; enzymatically active; epiandrosterone; episodic ataxia; erythrocyte antibody; erythrocyte antiserum; esophageal atresia; estivo-autumnal; ethacrynic acid

E/A early to late diastolic filling ratio; emergency admission

E&A evaluate and advise

E$_a$ energy of aggregation

ea each

Ea kinetic energy of alpha particles

EAA electroacupuncture analgesia; Epilepsy Association of America; essential amino acid; excitatory amino acid; extra-alveolar air; extrinsic allergic alveolitis

EAAC excitatory amino acid carrier

EAAV equine adeno-associated virus

EAB elective abortion; Ethics Advisory Board

EABV effective arterial blood volume

EAC Ehrlich ascites carcinoma; electroacupuncture; endocrine-active compound; epithelioma adenoides cysticum; erythema annulare centrifugum; erythrocyte, antibody, complement; external auditory canal

EACA epsilon-aminocaproic acid

EACD eczematous allergic contact dermatitis

EACH essential access community hospital

EACL European Chapter of the Association for Computational Linguistics

EACSS European and Australian Cooperative Stroke Study

EACT educational activity [UMLS]

EAD early afterdepolarization; Enterprise Access Directory; extracranial arterial disease

EA-D early antigen, diffuse

E-ADD epileptic attentional deficit disorder

EaDNV *Euxoa auxiliaris* densovirus

EADS early amnion deficit spectrum or syndrome

EAdV equine adenovirus

EAdV-B equine adenovirus B

EAE ethylaminoethanol; experimental allergic encephalomyelitis; experimental autoimmune encephalitis

EAEC enteroadherent *Escherichia coli*; enteroaggregative *Escherichia coli*

EAFT European Atrial Fibrillation Trial

EAG electroarteriography

EAGAR Estrogen and Graft Atherosclerosis Research Trial

EAggEC enteroaggregative *Escherichia coli*

EAGLES Expert Advisory Group on Language Engineering Standards

EAHF eczema, asthma, and hay fever

EAHIL European Association for Health Information and Libraries

EAHLG equine antihuman lymphoblast globulin

EAHLS equine antihuman lymphoblast serum

EAI Emphysema Anonymous, Inc.; erythrocyte antibody inhibition

EAK ethyl amyl ketone

EAM episodic ataxia with myokymia; external acoustic meatus

EAMG experimental autoimmune myasthenia gravis

EAMI exercise training in anterior myocardial infarction

EAN experimental allergic neuritis

EAO experimental allergic orchiitis

EAP electric acupuncture; electroactive polymer; employee assistance program; epiallopregnanolone; Epstein-Barr associated protein; erythrocyte acid phosphatase; evoked action potential

EAPV early to atrial peak velocity [ratio]

EAQ eudismic affinity quotient

EAR European Association of Radiology

EA-R early antigen, restricted

Ea R reaction of degeneration [Ger. *Entartungs-Reaktion*]

EARHA East Anglian Regional Health Authority

EARR extended aortic root replacement

EARS European Atherosclerosis Research Study

EAS Edinburgh Artery Study; emergency ambulance service; endarterectomized aortic segment; European Atherosclerosis Society

EASI eczema area and severity index; European Antiplatelet Stent Investigation; European applications in surgical interventions; extra-amniotic saline infusion

EAST Eastern Association for the Surgery of Trauma; elevated-arm stress test; Emory angioplasty vs. surgery trial; external rotation, abduction stress test

EASY European Prototype for Integrated Care [EPIC] assessment system

EAT Eating Attitudes Test; Ehrlich ascites tumor; electro-aerosol therapy; epidermolysis acuta toxica; experimental autoimmune thymitis; experimental autoimmune thyroiditis

EATB European Association of Tissue Banks

EATC Ehrlich ascites tumor cell

EAV entity-attribute-value [data organization]; equine abortion virus; equine arteritis virus

EAVC enhanced atrioventricular conduction

EAVM extramedullary arteriovenous malformation

EAVN enhanced atrioventricular nodal [conduction]

EB elective abortion; electron beam; elementary body; embryoid body; emotional behavior; endometrial biopsy; epidermolysis bullosa; Epstein-Barr [virus]; esophageal body; estradiol benzoate; Evans blue

E_b binding energy

EBA early bacterial activity; epidermolysis bullosa acquisita; epidermolysis bullosa atrophicans; extrahepatic biliary atresia; orthoethoxybenzoic acid

EBC esophageal balloon catheter

EBCDIC Extended Binary Coded Decimal Interchange Code

EBCP evidence-based clinical practice

EBCT electron-beam computed tomography

EBD epidermolysis bullosa dystrophica

EBDA effective balloon dilated area

EBDC ethylene bisdithiocarbamate; evidence-based healthcare

EBDCT Cockayne-Touraine type of epidermolysis bullosa dystrophica

EBDD epidermolysis bullosa dystrophica dominant

EBDR epidermolysis bullosa dystrophica recessiva

EBE Excluder Bifurcated Endoprosthesis

EBER Epstein-Barr encoded RNA

EBF erythroblastosis fetalis; exclusive breast feeding

E-BFU erythroid blood-forming unit

EBG electroblepharogram, electroblepharography

EBH epidermolysis bullosa hereditaria; evidence-based healthcare

EBHC evidence-based healthcare

EBI emetine bismuth iodide; erythroblastic island; estradiol binding index; European Bioinformatics Institute; external beam irradiation

EBIF emotional behavioral index form

EBIORT, EB-IORT electron beam intraoperative radiotherapy

EBK embryonic bovine kidney

EBL erythroblastic leukemia; estimated blood loss

eBL endemic Burkitt lymphoma

EBL/S estimated blood loss during surgery

EBLV European bat lyssavirus

EBM electrophysiologic behavior modification; epidermal basement membrane; epidermolysis bullosa, macular type; evidence-based medicine; expressed breast milk

EBMS Engineering and Biology in Medicine Society

EBMT European Group for Blood and Marrow Transplantation

EBMTR European Bone Marrow Transplantation Registry

EBMWG evidence-based medicine working group

EBN evidence-based nursing

EBNA Epstein-Barr virus-associated nuclear antigen

EBO Ebola [disease or virus]

EBOB 4′-ethynyl-4-*n*-propyl-bicycloorthobenzoate

E/BOD electrolyte biochemical oxygen demand

EBO-R Ebola Reston virus

EBOV Ebola virus

EBP error-back propagation; estradiolbinding protein

EbpS elastin-binding protein of *Staphylococcus aureus*

EBRI Employee Benefits Research Institute

EBRT electron beam radiotherapy; external beam radiation therapy

EBS elastic back strap; electric brain stimulation; Emergency Bed Service; epidermolysis bullosa simplex

EBSS Earle's balanced salt solution

EBT electron beam tomography; external beam therapy

EBV effective blood volume; Egypt bee virus; Epstein-Barr virus; estimated blood volume

EBv Epstein-Barr virus

EBVS Epstein-Barr virus susceptibility

EBZ epidermal basement zone

EC effective concentration; ejection click; electrochemical; electron capture; embryonal carcinoma; emergency center; emergency contraception; endemic cretinism; endocrine cells; endothelial cell; energy charge; enteric coating; entering complaint; enterochromaffin; entorhinal cortex; Enzyme Commission; epidermal cell; epirubicin/cyclophosphamide; epithelial cell; epithelial component; equalization-cancellation; error correction; *Escherichia coli*; esophageal carcinoma; ethyl chloride; excitation-contraction; experimental control; expiratory center; extended care; exterior coat; external carotid [artery]; external conjugate; extracellular; extracellular concentration; extracorporeal; extracranial; eye care; eyes closed

E-C ether-chloroform [mixture]

EC$_{50}$ median effective concentration

E/C endocystoscopy; enteric-coated; estrogen/creatinine ratio

Ec ectoconchion; entorhinal cortex

e/c enteric coated [pills]

ECA electrical control activity; electrocardioanalyzer; endothelial cell antibody; endothelial cytotoxic activity; enterobacterial common antigen; epidemiological catchment area; esophageal carcinoma; ethacrynic acid; ethylcarboxylate adenosine; external carotid artery

E$_{Ca}$ calcium reversal potential

ECAA European Concerted Action on Anticoagulation [study]

E-CABG endarterectomy and coronary artery bypass graft

ECAC European Collection of Animal Cell Cultures

ECaC epithelial calcium channel

E-CAD E-cadherin

ECAF extension corner avulsion fracture

ECAO enteric cytopathogenic avian orphan [virus]

ECAP European Concerted Action Project

ECAQ elderly cognitive assessment questionnaire

ECASS European Cooperative Acute Stroke Study

ECAT emission computer-assisted tomography; European Concerted Action on Thrombosis and Disabilities [study]

ECAT AP European Concerted Action on Thrombosis: Angina Pectoris [study]

ECBD exploration of common bile duct

ECBO enteric cytopathogenic bovine orphan [virus]

ECBS Expert Committee on Biological Standardization [WHO]

ECBV effective circulating blood volume

ECC electrocorticogram, electrocorticography; electronic claim capture; embryonal cell carcinoma; emergency cardiac care; emergency care center; encoding combinatorial chemistry; endocervical cone; endocervical curettage; Erlangen Cancer Center [Germany]; estimated creatinine clearance; external cardiac compression; extracorporeal circulation

ECCE Effects of Captopril on Cardiopulmonary Exercise [study]; extracapsular cataract extraction

ECCI electronic clinical communication implementation

ECCL encephalocraniocutaneous lipomatosis

ECCLS European Committee for Clinical Laboratory Standards

ECCO enteric cytopathogenic cat orphan [virus]; European Culture Collection Organisation

ECCO$_2$ extracorporeal carbon dioxide

ECCOMAC European Concerted Community Action Programmes

ECCO$_2$R extracorporeal carbon dioxide removal

ECD early child development; ectrodactyly; electrochemical detection, electrochemical detector; electron capture detector; emergency call device; endocardial cushion defect; enzymatic cell dispersion; equivalent current dipole; Erdheim-Chester disease; ethylcysteinate dimer; extended criteria donor; external cardioverter-defibrillator; extracellular domain; extracranial Doppler sonography

ECDC *Escherichia coli* Database Collection

E/CDK cyclin E dependent kinase

ECDO enteric cytopathic dog orphan [virus]

ECE equine conjugated estrogen; extracapsular extension

ECEO enteric cytopathogenic equine orphan [virus]

ECETOC European Centre for Ecotoxicity and Toxicology of Chemicals

ECF effective capillary flow; eosinophilic chemotactic factor; erythroid colony formation; *Escherichia coli* filtrate; ethyl chloroformate; extended care facility; extracellular fluid; extracytoplasmic function

ECFA, ECF-A eosinophilic chemotactic factor of anaphylaxis

ECFC eosinophilic chemotactic factor complement

ECFMG Educational Commission on Foreign Medical Graduates; Educational Council for Foreign Medical Graduates

ECFMS Educational Council for Foreign Medical Students

E-CFU erythroid colony-forming unit

ECFV extracellular fluid volume

ECFVD extracellular fluid volume depletion

ECG electrocardiogram, electrocardiography

ECGF endothelial cell growth factor

ECGS endothelial cell growth supplement

ECH educator contact hour

ECHO echocardiography; enteric cytopathic human orphan [virus]; Etoposide, cyclophosphamide, Adriamycin, and vincristine

EchoCG echocardiography

Echo-Eg echoencephalography

Echo-VM echoventriculometry

ECHRA electronic healthcare record architecture

ECHSCP Exeter Community Health Services Computer Project

ECI electrocerebral inactivity; eosinophil chemotaxis index; eosinophilic cytoplasmic inclusions; extracorporeal irradiation

ECIB extracorporeal irradiation of blood

EC/IC extracranial/intracranial

ECICD European Consortium for Intensive Care Data

ECIL extracorporeal irradiation of lymph

ECIS equipment control information system

ECK extracellular potassium

ECL electrochemoluminescent; emitter-coupled logic; enterochromaffin-like [type]; euglobin clot lysis

ECLAP European Collaboration on Low-Dose Aspirin in Polycythemia Vera

ECLAT European Community and Latin American Network on Biology and Control of Triatomines [Chagas disease]

ECLiPS encoded combinatorial libraries in polymeric support

ECLRS electronic clinical laboratory reporting system

ECLS extracorporeal life support

ECM electronic claims management; embryonic chick muscle; erythema chronicum migrans; experimental cerebral malaria; external cardiac massage; extracellular material; extracellular matrix

ECML extracellular membrane layer

ECMO enteric cytopathic monkey orphan [virus]; extracorporeal membrane oxygenation

ECN equipment control number

ecNOS endothelial cell nitric oxide synthase

ECO Pan-American Center for Human Ecology and Health

E co *Escherichia coli*

ECochG electrocochleography

ECOG Eastern Cooperative Oncology Group

ECoG electrocorticogram, electrocorticography

E COLI eighth nerve action potential, cochlear nucleus, olivary complex (superior), lateral lemniscus, inferior colliculus [hearing test]

E coli *Escherichia coli*

ECP ectrodactyly-cleft palate [syndrome]; effective conduction period; effector cell precursor; electronic claims processing; endocardial potential; emergency care provider; entry control point [contamination control]; eosinophil cationic protein; erythrocyte coproporphyrin; erythroid committed precursor; *Escherichia coli* polypeptide; estradiol cyclopentane propionate; external cardiac pressure; external counterpulsation; extracellular protein; extracorporeal photochemotherapy; free cytoporphyrin of erythrocytes

ECPA Electronic Communication Privacy Act

ECPO enteric cytopathic porcine orphan [virus]

ECPOG electrochemical potential gradient

ECPR external cardiopulmonary resuscitation

ECR effectiveness-cost ratio; electrocardiographic response; emergency care research; emergency chemical restraint; European Congress of Radiology; extensor carpi radialis

ECRB extensor carpi radialis brevis

ECRHS European Community Respiratory Health Survey

ECRI Emergency Care Research Institute

ECRL extensor carpi radialis longus

ECRO enteric cytopathogenic rodent orphan [virus]

ECR-SCSI European Committee for Recommendation-Standard on Computer Aspects of Diagnostic Imaging

ECS elective cosmetic surgery; electrocerebral silence; electroconvulsive shock, electroshock; endocervical swab; endothelial cells; extracapsular spread; extracellular solids; extracellular space

ECSG European Cooperative Study Group

ECSO enteric cytopathic swine orphan [virus]

ECSP epidermal cell surface protein

ECSS European Coronary Surgery Study

ECST European carotid surgery trial

ECSURF economic evaluation of surfactant

ECSYSVAS European Community Systemic Vasculitis [trials]

ECT electroconvulsive therapy; emission computed tomography; enteric coated tablet; euglobulin clot test; European compression technique

ect ectopic, ectopy

ECTA esophageal gastric tube airway; Everyman's Contingency Table Analysis

EC-TEOLA epichlorohydrin-triethanolamine

ECTR endoscopic carpal tunnel release

ECTV ectromelia virus

ECU environmental control unit; extended care unit; extensor carpi ulnaris

ECV enteric calicivirus; epithelial cell vacuolization; extracellular volume; extracorporeal volume

EcV *Euploea corea* virus
ECVA extracranial vertebral artery
ECVAM European Centre for the Validation of Alternative Methods
ECVD extracellular volume of distribution
ECW extracellular water
ED early-decision [applicant]; early differentiation; ectodermal dysplasia; ectopic depolarization; effective dose; Ehlers-Danlos [syndrome]; elbow disarticulation; electrodialysis; electron density; electron diffraction; embedding dimension; embryonic death; emergency department; emotional disorder, emotionally disturbed; end-diastole; endocrine disruptor; energy diversive [x-ray analysis]; enteric drainage; entering diagnosis; Entner-Doudoroff [pathway]; enzyme deficiency; epidural; epileptiform discharge; equine dermis [cells]; erectile dysfunction; erythema dose; ethyl dichlorarsine; ethynodiol; event definition; evidence of disease; exertional dyspnea; exponential distribution; extensive disease; extensor digitorum; external diameter; extra-low dispersion
E-D ego-defense; Ehlers-Danlos [syndrome]
ED$_{01}$ effective dose, 1% response
ED$_{50}$ median effective dose
ED$_{99}$ effective dose, 99% response
E$_d$ depth dose
ed edema
EDA ectodermal dysplasia, anhidrotic; electrodermal activity; electrodermal audiometry; electrolyte-deficient agar; electron donor acceptor; electronic design automation; end-diastolic area; exploratory data analysis
EDAC 1-ethyl-3-diethylaminopropyl carbodiimide
EDAM electron-dense amorphous material
EDAP emergency department approved for pediatrics
EDAX energy dispersive x-ray analysis
EDB early dry breakfast; electron-dense body; Enrollment Database [Medicare]; ethylene dibromide; expert database; extended definition beta; extensor digitorum brevis
EDBP erect diastolic blood pressure
EDC emergency decontamination center; end-diastolic count; endocrine-disrupting chemical; endocrine-disrupting compound;

estimated date of conception; ethylene dichloride; expected date of confinement; expected delivery, cesarean; extensor digitorum communis
ED&C electrodesiccation and curettage
EDCF endothelium-derived contracting factor
EDCI energetic dynamic cardiac insufficiency
EDCP eccentric dynamic compression plate [osteosynthesis]
EDCS end-diastolic chamber stiffness; end-diastolic circumferential stress
EDc(V) extrapolated dose converted (volume) [radiotherapy]
EDD effective drug duration; electron dense deposit; end-diastolic dimension; esophageal detection device; estimated due date; expected date of delivery
EDDA expanded duty dental auxiliary
EDDS electronic development delivery system
EDE effective dose equivalent
EDECS emergency department expert charting system
edent edentia, edentulous
EDF edge response function; eosinophil differentiation factor; erythroid differentiation factor; extradural fluid
EDG electrodermography
EDGE Evaluation of Dispatch Catheter for Vein Graft Revascularization
EDH epidural hematoma
EDHEP European Donor Hospital Education Program
EDHF endothelium-derived hyperpolarizing factor
EDI eating disorder inventory; electronic data interchange; estimated daily intake
EDIC Echocardiography Dobutamine International Cooperative Study; Epidemiology of Diabetes Intervention and Complications
EDIM epizootic diarrhea of infant mice
E-diol estradiol
EDIT Early Defibrillator Implantation Trial; Early Diabetes Intervention Trial
EDK energy deposition kernel
EDL end-diastolic length; end-diastolic load; Essential Drug List [WHO]; estimated date of labor; extensor digitorum longus

ED/LD emotionally disturbed and learning disabled

ED LOS emergency department length of stay

EDM early diastolic murmur; electro-discharge machining; electron density map; esophageal Doppler monitoring; Essential Drugs and Medicines [WHO]; extramucosal duodenal myotomy

EDMA ethylene glycol dimethacrylate; Euclidean distance matrix analysis [computer-assisted surgery]

EDMD emergency physician; Emery-Dreifuss muscular dystrophy

EDN electrodesiccation; eosinophil-derived neurotoxin

EDNA Emergency Department Nurses Association

EDNF endogenous digitalis-like natriuretic factor

EDOC estimated date of confinement

EDOU emergency department observation unit

EDP electron dense particle; electronic data processing; end-diastolic pressure

EDQ extensor digiti quinti

EDR early diastolic relaxation; effective direct radiation; electrodermal response; electronic death reporting; endothelium-dependent relaxation

EDRES Effects of Debulking on Restenosis [trial]

EDRF endothelium-derived relaxing factor

EDRM emergency department readmission monitor

EDS edema disease of swine; egg drop syndrome; Ehlers-Danlos syndrome; electronic decision support; Emery-Dreifuss syndrome; energy-dispersive spectrometry; epigastric distress syndrome; essential data set; excessive daytime sleepiness; extra-dimensional shift

EDSR electronic document storage and retrieval

EDSS expanded disability status scale

EDT end-diastolic thickness; erythrocyte density test

EDTA ethylenediamine tetraacetic acid

EDTMP ethylenediamine tetramethylene phosphoric acid

EDTR emergency department-based trauma response

EDTU emergency diagnostic and treatment unit

Educ education

EDV end-diastolic volume; epidermodysplasia verruciformis

ED(V) extrapolated dose (volume) [radiotherapy]

EDVI end-diastolic volume index

EDVX X-linked epidermodysplasia verruciformis

EDWTH end-diastolic wall thickness

EDX, EDx electrodiagnosis

EDXA energy-dispersive x-ray analysis

Edyn,l dynamic elastance, lung

Edyn,rs dynamic elastance, respiratory system

Edyn,w dynamic elastance, chest wall

EE electronic encyclopedia; embryo extract; end-to-end; end expiration; energy expenditure; *Enterobacteriaceae* enrichment [broth]; equine encephalitis; ethinyl estradiol; expressed emotion; external ear; eye and ear

E-E erythema-edema [reaction]

E&E eye and ear

EEA electroencephalic audiometry; end-to-end anastomosis

EE$_{act}$ energy expenditure due to physical activity

EEC ectrodactyly-ectodermal dysplasia-clefting [syndrome]; enteropathogenic *Escherichia coli*

EECD endothelial-epithelial corneal dystrophy

EECG electroencephalography

EED experimental emergency department

EEE eastern equine encephalitis; eastern equine encephalomyelitis; experimental enterococcal endocarditis; external eye examination

EEEP end-expiratory esophageal pressure

EEEV eastern equine encephalitis virus

EEG electroencephalogram, electroencephalography

EEGA electroencephalographic audiometry

EEG-CSA electroencephalography with computerized spectral analysis

EEGL emergency exposure guidance level; low-voltage electroencephalography

EEGV1 electroencephalographic variant pattern 1

EEHS emergency evacuation hyperbaric stretcher

EEL environmental exposure limit

EELS electron energy loss spectroscopy

EELV end-expiratory lung volume

EEM ectodermal dysplasia, ectrodactyly, macular dystrophy [syndrome]; erythema exudativum multiforme

EEMCO European Group for Efficacy Measurements on Cosmetics and Other Tropical Products

EEME, EE3ME ethinylestradiol-3-methyl ether

EEMG evoked electromyogram

EENT eye, ear, nose, and throat

EEP end-expiratory pressure; equivalent effective photon

EEPI extraretinal eye position information

EER electroencephalographic response; extended entity-relationship

EES erythromycin ethylsuccinate; ethyl ethanesulfate

EESG evoked electrospinogram

EET epoxyeicosatrienoic [acid]

EEV endocardial ventriculotomy; equine encephalitis virus; equine encephalosis virus; extracellular enveloped virus

EEV 1–7 equine encephalosis virus 1 to 7

EF ectopic focus; edema factor; ejection fraction; elastic fibril; electric field; elongation factor; embryo-fetal; embryo fibroblasts; emergency facility; encephalitogenic factor; endothoracic fascia; endurance factor; eosinophilic fasciitis; epithelial focus; equivalent focus; erythroblastosis fetalis; erythrocyte fragmentation; escalation factor [radiotherapy]; exposure factor; extrafine; extended field [radiotherapy]; extrinsic factor

E$_f$ free enzyme

EF-1α elongation factor 1-alpha

EFA Epilepsy Foundation of America; essential fatty acid; extrafamily adoptee

EFAD essential fatty acid deficiency

EFAP employee and family assistance program

EFAS embryofetal alcohol syndrome

EFC elastin fragment concentration; endogenous fecal calcium; ephemeral fever of cattle

EFCC European Federation of Coding Centres

EFD estimated fluid deficit

EFDA expanded function dental assistant

EFE endocardial fibroelastosis

EFERF Enalapril Felodipine Extended Release Factorial Study

EFF electromagnetic field focusing

eff effect; efferent; efficiency; effusion

effect effective

effer efferent

EFFU epithelial focus-forming unit

EF-G [prokaryotic] elongation factor G

EFH explosive follicular hyperplasia

EFICAT Ejection Fraction in Carvedilol-treated Transplant Candidates [study]

EFL effective focal length

EFM elderly fibromyalgia; electronic fetal monitoring; electrostatic force microscopy; external fetal monitor

EF/M electrostatic force microscopy

EFMI European Federation of Medical Informatics

EFP early follicular phase; effective filtration pressure; endoneural fluid pressure

EFPO Educating Future Physicians for Ontario

EFR effective filtration rate

EFRT extended field radiotherapy

EFS earliest finishing shift; electric field stimulation; European Fraxiparin Study; event-free survival

EFT Embedded Figures Test

EF-Tu [prokaryotic] elongation factor Tu

EFV extracellular fluid volume

EFVC expiratory flow-volume curve

EFW estimated fetal weight

EFZ efavirenz

EG electrogram; enteroglucagon; eosinophilic granuloma; Erb-Goldflam [syndrome]; esophagogastrectomy; esophagogastric; ethylene glycol; external genitalia

eg for example [Lat. *exempli gratia*]

EGA enhanced graphics adaptation; estimated gestational age

EGAD Expressed Gene Anatomy Database

EGALITÉ Ensuring Global Access to Links, Information and Technology to Promote Equity in Health

EGBUS external genitalia, Bartholin, urethral, Skene glands

EGC early gastric cancer; epithelioid-globoid cell

EGD esophagogastroduodenoscopy

EGDF embryonic growth and development factor

EGDT early goal-directed therapy

EGF early graft failure; endothelial growth factor; epidermal growth factor

EGFP enhanced green fluorescent protein

EGFR, EGF-R epidermal growth factor receptor

EGF-URO epidermal growth factor, urogastrone

EGG electrogastrogram; electroglottogram

EGH equine growth hormone

EGHIN Ellen Gartenfeld Health Information Network

EGIR European Group for the Study of Insulin Resistance

EGL eosinophilic granuloma of the lung

EGLT euglobin lysis time

EGM electrogram; extracellular granular material

EGME ethylene glycol monomethyl ether

EGMV eggplant green mosaic virus

EGN experimental glomerulonephritis

EGNB enteric gamma-negative bacteria

EGOT erythrocytic glutamic oxaloacetic transaminase

EGR early growth response; erythema gyratum repens

E-GR erythrocyte glutathione reductase

EGR-2 early growth response [protein]

EGRA equilibrium-gated radionuclide angiography

EGRAC erythrocyte glutathione reductase activity coefficient

EGS electrogalvanic stimulation; electron gamma shower; external guide sequence

EGT ethanol gelation test

EGTA esophageal gastric tube airway; ethyleneglycol-bis-(β-aminoethylether)-N,N,N',N'-tetraacetic acid

EGTCSA epilepsy with generalized tonic-clonic seizures on awakening

EGTM European Group on Tumor Markers

EH enlarged heart; epidermal hyperplasia; epidermolytic hyperkeratosis; epidural hematoma; epoxide hydratase; esophageal hiatus; essential hypertension; external hyperalimentation

E/H environment and heredity

E&H environment and heredity

E$_h$ redox potential

eh enlarged heart

EHA Emotional Health Anonymous; Environmental Health Agency

EHAA epidemic hepatitis-associated antigen

EHB elevate head of bed

EHBA extrahepatic biliary atresia

EHBD extrahepatic bile duct

EHBF estimated hepatic blood flow; exercise hyperemia blood flow; extrahepatic blood flow

EHC enterohepatic circulation; enterohepatic clearance; essential hypercholesterolemia; ethylhydrocupreine hydrochloride; extended health care; extrahepatic cholestasis

EHCR electronic health care record

EHCW emergency health care worker

EHD electrohemodynamics; epizootic hemorrhagic disease

EHDP ethane-1-hydroxy-1,1-diphosphate

EHDV epizootic hemorrhagic disease virus

EHEC enterohemorrhagic *Escherichia coli*

EHF epidemic hemorrhagic fever; exophthalmos-hyperthyroid factor; extremely high frequency

EHG electrohysterogram, electrohysterography

EHH esophageal hiatal hernia

EHI employer's health insurance; environmental health indicator

EHIA environmental health impact assessment

EHIBCC European Health Industry Business Communications Council

EHIV exposure to human immunodeficiency virus

EHK epidermolytic hyperkeratosis

EHL effective half-life; electrohydraulic lithotripsy; endogenous hyperlipidemia; Environmental Health Laboratory; essential hyperlipemia; extensor hallucis longus

EHM extrahepatic metastases

EHME employee health maintenance examination

EHMS electrohemodynamic ionization mass spectometry

EHNA 9-erythro-2-(hydroxy-3-nonyl) adenine

EHNV epizootic hematopoietic necrosis virus

EHO environmental health officer; extrahepatic obstruction

EHP di-(20-ethylhexyl) hydrogen phosphate; electron hole pair; Environmental Health Perspectives; excessive heat production; extrahigh potency

EHPAC Emergency Health Preparedness Advisory Committee

EHPH extrahepatic portal hypertension

EHPT Eddy hot plate test

EHQ Eating Habits Questionnaire

EHR electronic healthcare record; extended-high rate

EHS environmental health and safety

EHSDS experimental health services delivery system

EHT electrohydrothermoelectrode; essential hypertension

EHV Edge Hill virus; electric heart vector; epidermal hyperplasia virus; equid herpesvirus

EHVT Edinburgh Heart Valve Trial

EI earliness index; Edmonton injector; electrical injury; electrolyte imbalance; electron impact; electron ionization; emotionally impaired; energy index; energy intake; enzyme inhibitor; eosinophilic index; Evans index; excretory index; exercise-induced

E/I expiration/inspiration [ratio]

E$_I$ ionic reversal potential

e-I early inspiratory

EIA electroimmunoassay; enzyme immunoassay; enzyme-linked immunosorbent assay; equine infectious anemia; erythroimmunoassay; excessive inappropriate aggression; exercise-induced anaphylaxis; exercise-induced asthma; external iliac artery; an interface between a computer and a system for transmitting digital information

EIAB extracranial-intracranial arterial bypass

EIAV equine infectious anemia virus

EIB electrophoretic immunoblotting; eosinophilic intracytoplasmic inclusion body; exercise-induced bronchospasm

EIC elastase inhibition capacity; enzyme inhibition complex; extensive intraductal carcinoma; extensive intraductal component

EICESS European Intergroup Cooperative Ewing's Sarcoma Study

EID ecological interface design; egg infectious dose; electroimmunodiffusion; emergency infusion device

EIEC enteroinvasive *Escherichia coli*

EIEE early infantile epileptic encephalopathy

EIES Electronic Information Exchange System

EIF erythrocyte initiation factor; eukaryotic initiation factor

eIF erythrocyte initiation factor; eukaryotic initiation factor

eIF4E eukaryotic initiation factor 4E

EIHDW Evaluation of Ischemic Heart Disease in Women [study]

EII electrical impedance imaging

EIM elastic image matching; equity implementation model; excitability-inducing material

EIMS electron ionization mass spectrometry

EINECS European Inventory of Existing Commercial Chemical Substances

EINet Emerging Infections Network

EIO European Institute of Oncology

EIP end-expiratory pause; ethylisopropylamiloride; extensor indicis proprius

EIPS endogenous inhibitor of prostaglandin synthase

eIPV enhanced inactivated poliomyelitis vaccine

EIRnv extra incidence rate of non-vaccinated groups

EIRP effective isotropic radiated power

EIRv extra incidence in vaccinated groups

EIS Environmental Impact Statement; Epidemic Intelligence Service; European Infarction Study

EIT electrical impedance tomography; erythroid iron turnover

EIU enzyme immunoassay unit

EIV equine influenza virus; external iliac vein

EIW electronic information warehouse

EJ elbow jerk; external jugular

EJB ectopic junctional beat

EJM epilepsy juvenile myoclonic

EJP excitation junction potential

EJV external jugular vein

EK enterokinase; erythrokinase

E$_K$ potassium equilibrium potential; potassium reversal potential

E$_k$ kinetic energy

EKC epidemic keratoconjunctivitis
EKF extended Kalman filtering
EKG electrocardiogram, electrocardiography
EKLF erythroid Krüppel-like factor
EKS epidemic Kaposi sarcoma
EKV erythrokeratodermia variabilis
EKY electrokymogram, electrokymography
EL early latent; elbow; electroluminescence; erythroleukemia; exercise limit; external lamina
El elastase; explanation library
el elixir
ELA elastase; elastomer-lubricating agent; endotoxin-like activity
ELAD extracorporeal liver assist device
ELAM endothelial leukocyte adhesion molecule
ELAS extended lymphadenopathy syndrome
ELAT Embolism in Left Atrial Thrombi [study]
ELAV embryonic lethal, abnormal vision
ELB early light breakfast; elbow
elb elbow
ELBW extremely low birth weight
ELCA Excimer Laser Coronary Angioplasty [registry]
ElCPV *Eriogaster lanestris* cypovirus
ELD egg lethal dose
elec electricity, electric
elect elective; electuary
ELECTZ electrosurgical loop excision of the cervical transformation zone
ELEM equine leukoencephalomalacia
elem elementary
elev elevation, elevated, elevator
ELF elective low forceps; extremely low frequency
ELG eligibility [database]
ELH egg-laying hormone
ELHE Evaluation of Losartan in Hemodialysis [study]
ElHV elephantid herpesvirus
ELI exercise lability index
ELIA enzyme-linked immunoassay
eLib electronic library
ELICT enzyme-linked immunocytochemical technique
ELIEDA enzyme-linked immunoelectron diffusion assay

ELIRA enzyme-linked immunoreceptor assay
ELISA enzyme-linked immunosorbent assay
ELISK excimer laser intrastromal keratomileusis
ELITE Evaluation of Losartan in the Elderly [study]
ELIV Ellidaey virus
elix elixir
ELL elongation factor homologous to mixed lineage leukemia
ELLV Ellidaey virus
ElLV elderberry latent virus
ELM external limiting membrane; extravascular lung mass
ELMCV El Moro Canyon virus
ELMP expertise-led medical protocol
ELN elastin; electronic noise
ELND elective lymph node dissection
ELOD expected average lod [score]
ELOP estimated length of program
ELOS estimated length of stay
ELP elastase-like protein; endogenous limbic potential; exogenous lipoid pneumonia
ELPS excessive lateral pressure syndrome
ELR electronic laboratory-based reporting
ELRA European Language Resources Agency
ELS Eaton-Lambert syndrome; electron loss spectroscopy; emergency life support; enzymatic labile site; extended least squares; extralobar sequestration; extremely low frequency
ELSA European Lacidipine Study on Atherosclerosis; European Longitudinal Study on Aging
ELSI ethical, legal, and social issues
ELSS emergency life support system
ELT endless loop tachycardia; euglobulin lysis time
ELV entero-like virus; environmental limit value; erythroid leukemia virus
ELVD Exercise in Left Ventricular Dysfunction [trial]
ELVd eggplant latent viroid
ELVD-CHF Exercise in Left Ventricular Dysfunction and Chronic Heart Failure [trial]
elx elixir
EM early memory; ejection murmur; electromagnetic; electron micrograph;

electron microscopy, electron microscope; electrophoretic mobility; Embden-Meyerhof [pathway]; emergency management; emergency medicine; emmetropia; emotional disorder, emotionally disturbed; end of memory; ergonovine maleate; erythema migrans; erythema multiforme; erythrocyte mass; erythromycin; esophageal manometry; esophageal motility; estramusine; expectation-maximization [algorithm]; extensive metabolizer; extracellular matrix

E-M expectation-maximization

E/M electron microscope, electron microscopy; evaluation and management

E&M endocrine and metabolic; evaluation and management [coding]

Em emmetropia

E_m mid-point redox potential

EMA electronic microanalyzer; emergency management agency; emergency medical assistance; emergency medical assistant; emergency medical attendant; endothelial monocyte antigen; epithelial membrane antigen; extramural absorber

EMAB endothelial monocyte antigen B

E-mail electronic mail

EMAP Environmental Monitoring and Assessment Program [Environmental Protection Agency]; evoked muscle action potential

E_{max} maximum effect; maximum energy

EMB embryology; endomyocardial biopsy; engineering in medicine and biology; eosin-methylene blue; ethambutol; explosive mental behavior

emb embolism; embryo; embryology

EMBASE Excerpta Medica Database

EMBL European Molecular Biology Laboratory

EMBO European Molecular Biology Organization

embryol embryology

EMBS Engineering in Medicine and Biology Society

EMC electromagnetic compatibility; electron microscopy; emergency medical care; emergency medical condition; emergency medical coordinator; encephalomyocarditis; enzyme mismatch cleavage; essential mixed cryoglobulinemia

EMCR electronic medical care record

EMC&R emergency medical care and rescue

EMCRO Experimental Medical Care Review Organization

EMCV eggplant mottled crinkle virus; encephalomyocarditis virus

EMD electromechanical dissociation; emergency medical dispatcher; emergency medical doctor; Emery-Dreifuss muscular dystrophy; esophageal mobility disorder

EMDIS European Marrow Donor Information System

EMDR eggplant mottled dwarf [virus]; eye movement desensitization and reprocessing

EME electromechanical energy

EMEA European Agency for the Evaluation of Medicinal Products

EMEDI European Medical Electronic Data Interchange [group]

EMEM Eagle minimal essential medium

EMER electromagnetic molecular electron resonance

emer emergency

EMF electromagnetic field; electromagnetic flow; electromagnetic flowmeter; electromotive force; Emergency Medicine Foundation; endomyocardial fibrosis; equivalent molecules of immunofluorescence; erythrocyte maturation factor; evaporated milk formula

emf electromotive force

EMG electromyogram, electromyography; eye movement gauge; exomphalos-macroglossia-gigantism [syndrome]

EMGBF electromyographic biofeedback

EMG(int) integrated electromyographic [value]

EMGN extramembranous glomerulonephritis

EMG/NCV electromyography/nerve conduction velocity [test]

EMI electromagnetic immunity; electromagnetic interference; emergency medical information

EMIAT European Myocardial Infarction Amiodarone Trial; European Myocardial Infarction Arrhythmia Trial

EMIC emergency maternal and infant care; Environmental Mutagen Information Center [NLM]

EMICBACK Environmental Mutagen Information Center Backfile [NLM database]

EMIP European Myocardial Infarction Project

EMIP-FR European Myocardial Infarction Project-Free Radicals

EMIT enzyme multiplied immunoassay technique; European Mivazerol Trial

EmIV *Enytus montanus* ichnovirus

EMJH Ellinghausen-McCullough-Johnson-Harris [medium]

EML erythema nodosum leprosum

EMLA eutectic mixture of local anesthetics

EMM erythema multiforme major

EMMA eye movement measuring apparatus

EMMV eggplant mild mottle virus

EMO Epstein-Macintosh-Oxford [inhaler]; exophthalmos, myxedema circumscriptum praetibiale, and osteoarthropathia hypertrophicans [syndrome]

emot emotion, emotional

EMP electric membrane property; electromagnetic pulse; Embden-Meyerhof pathway; European Myocardial Infarction Project; external membrane potential or protein; extramedullary plasmacytoma; malignant proliferation of eosinophils

EMPAR Enoxaparin MaxEPA Prevention of Angioplasty Restenosis [study]

EMPIRE Economics of Myocardial Perfusion Imaging in Europe [study]

EMPS exertional muscle pain syndrome

EMQ exercise motivation questionnaire

EMR educable mentally retarded; electromagnetic radiation; electronic medical record; emergency mechanical restraint; emergency medicine resident; essential metabolism ratio; eye movement record

EMRA Emergency Medicine Residents Association

EMRC European Medical Research Council

EMRD emergency medicine residency director

E-MRI extremity magnetic resonance imaging

EMRS electronic medical record system

EMRSA epidemic strain of methicillin-resistant *Staphylococcus aureus*

EMS early morning specimen; early morning stiffness; electrical muscle stimulation; Electronic Medical Service; emergency management of stroke; emergency medical services; endometriosis; environmental management system; eosinophilia myalgia syndrome; ethyl methane-sulfonate; European Multicenter Study

EMSA electrophoretic mobility shift assay; Emergency Medical Services Agency

EMSC emergency medical services for children

EMSS emergency medical services system

EMT electronic medical textbook; emergency medical tag; emergency medical team; emergency medical technician; emergency medical treatment; endocardial mapping technique

EMTA endomethylene tetrahydrophthalic acid

EMT-A emergency medical technician-ambulance; emergency medical technician providing basic life support or cardiopulmonary resuscitation

EMTALA Emergency Medical Treatment and Active Labor Act

EMT-B basic emergency medical technician

EMTD estimated maximum tolerated dose

EMT-D emergency medical technician providing basic life support or defibrillation

EMT-I emergency medical technician-intermediate

EMT-M, EMT-MAST emergency medical technician-military antishock trousers

EMT-P emergency medical technician-paramedic

EMTS electromagnetic tracking system

EMT-W emergency medical technician-wilderness

EMU early morning urine; energy-mode ultrasound

emu electromagnetic unit

emul emulsion

EMV eggplant mosaic virus; equine morbillivirus; eye, motor, voice [Glasgow coma scale]

EmV *Eucocytis meeki* virus

EMVC early mitral valve closure

EMWAC European Microsoft Windows NT Academic Centre

EMY emergency medicine resident year

EN endoscopy; enrolled nurse; enteral nutrition; epidemic nephritis; erythema nodosum

En, en enema

ENA Emergency Nurses' Association; epithelial neutrophil-activating [protein]; extractable nuclear antigen

E_Na sodium reversal potential

ENaC epithelial sodium channel

ENACT enzyme activity in chemical toxicity

ENASA Enoxaparin and/or Aspirin in Unstable Angina [trial]

ENC encounter; encryption; endotoxin neutralizing capacity; environmental control

ENCORE Evaluation of Nifedipine and Cerivastatin on Recovery of Endothelial Function [trial]

END early neonatal death; elective neck dissection; endocrinology; endorphin; endothelin; endurance

end endoreduplication

ENDIT European Nicotinamide Diabetes Intervention Trial

Endo endocardial, endocardium; endocrine, endocrinology; endodontics; endonuclease; endotracheal

endo endoscopy

EndoCAM endothelial cell adhesion molecule

Endo-M endocardium and M region

ENDOR electron nuclear double resonance

Endo X endonuclease X

ENDPT end-point of flow velocity after angioplasty; evaluation of Doppler parameters during percutaneous transluminal coronary angioplasty

ENDR endothelin receptor

ENDRB endothelin receptor B

ENDT electroneurodiagnostic technologist

ENE ethylnorepinephrine

ENeG electroneurography

enem enema

ENG electroneurogram, electroneurography; electronystagmogram, electronystagmography

Eng English

ENHR Essential National Health Research [South Africa]

ENI elective neck irradiation; elective nodal irradiation

ENIAC Electronic Numerical Integrator and Computer

ENK enkephalin

ENL equivalent number of looks [echocardiography]; erythema nodosum leproticum

ENMG electroneuromyography

ENMV endive necrotic mosaic virus

ENN environmental noise

ENO, Eno enolase

ENOG, ENoG electroneuronography

eNOS endothelial nitric oxide synthase

ENOXART enoxaparin in arterial surgery

ENP ethyl-p-nitrophenylthiobenzene phosphate; excellence for nursing practice; extractable nucleoprotein

E-NPI end nuclear polymorphism index

ENR eosinophilic nonallergic rhinitis; extrathyroid neck radioactivity

ENRICAD Enhancing Recovery in Coronary Heart Disease [trial]

ENRICHD Enchancing Recovery in Coronary Heart Disease Patients [trial]

ENS enteral nutritional support; enteric nervous system; epidermal nevus syndrome; ethylnorsuprarenin

ENSV Enseada virus

ENT ear, nose, and throat; enzootic nasal tumor; extranodular tissue

ent enterotoxin

ent A enterotoxin A

ENTICES Enoxaparin and Ticlopidine after Elective Stenting [study]

Entom entomology

ENTV *Entamoeba* virus; Entebbe virus

ENTY entity [UMLS]

ENU N-ethyl-nitrosourea

Env envelope [protein]

env, environ environment, environmental

ENVR environmental effect [UMLS]

ENX endonexin

enz enzyme, enzymatic

EO early-onset; eosinophil; ethylene oxide; eyes open

E_o skin dose

EOA effective orifice area; erosive osteoarthritis; esophageal obturator airway; examination, opinion, and advice

EOAD early-onset Alzheimer disease

EOB emergency observation bed; explanation of benefits

EOC emergency observation center; emergency operations center

EoC episode of care

EOCA early-onset cerebellar ataxia

EO-CFC eosinophil-leukocyte colony forming cell

EOD entry on duty; every other day; explosive ordnance disposal

EOF end of file

E of M error of measurement

EOG electro-oculogram, electro-oculography; electro-olfactogram, electro-olfactography; eosinophilic gastroenteritis; ethylene oxide gas

EOGBS early-onset group B streptococcal [infection]

EOJ extrahepatic obstructive jaundice

EOL end of life [pacemaker]

EOM electro-optic modulator; end of message; equal ocular movement; external otitis media; extraocular movement; extraocular muscle

EoM equation of motion

EOMA emergency oxygen mask assembly

EOMB explanation of Medicare benefits

EOMI extraocular muscles intact

EOM NL extraocular eye movements normal

EOP efficiency of plating; emergency outpatient

EOR European Organization for Research; exclusive operating room

EORTC European Organization for Research and Treatment of Cancer

EOS end of saturated bombardment; end of service [pacemaker]; end of study; eosinophil; European Orthodontic Society

eos, eosin eosinophil

Eosm effective osmolarity

EOT effective oxygen transport

EOU epidemic observation unit

EOx eye oximeter

EP echo planar; ectopic pregnancy; edible portion; electronic palpation; electrophoresis; electrophysiologic; electroprecipitin; emergency physician; emergency procedure; endocochlear potential; endogenous pyrogen; endoperoxide; endorphin; endplate; end point; enteropeptidase; environmental protection; enzyme product; eosinophilic pneumonia; epicardial electrogram; epirubicin; epithelium, epithelial; epoxide; erythrocyte protoporphyrin; erythrophagocytosis; erythropoietic porphyria; erythropoietin; esophageal pressure; estramustine phosphate; European Pharmacopoeia; evoked potential; evolutionary programming; excretory phase; exophytic papilloma; expert panel; extreme pressure

E$_p$ primary etiology [of vascular diseases]; proton energy

EPA eicosapentaenoic acid; empiric phrase association; Environmental Protection Agency; erect posterior-anterior; erythroid potentiating activity; extrinsic plasminogen activator

EPAP expiratory positive airway pressure

EPAQ Extended Personal Attitudes Questionnaire

EPA/RCRA Environmental Protection Agency Resource Conservation and Recovery Act

EPAS evolution of physiological analysis systems

EPB extensor pollicis brevis

EPBF effective pulmonary blood flow

EPC endothelial progenitor cell; end-plate current; epilepsia partialis continua; evidence-based practice center; external pneumatic compression

EPCA external pressure circulatory assistance

EPCG endoscopic pancreatocholangiography

EPCOT European Prospective Cohort on Thrombophilia

EPCRLS European Pancreatic Cancer Reference Library System

EPCS emergency portacaval shunt

EPCV *Epirus* cherry virus

EPD embolic protection device; energy-protein deficit; etiological potentials display

EPDML epidemiology, epidemiologic

EPE erythropoietin-producing enzyme

EPEC enteropathogenic *Escherichia coli*

EPEG etoposide

EPESE Established Populations for Epidemiologic Studies of the Elderly

EPF early pregnancy factor; endocarditis parietalis fibroplastica; endothelial proliferating factor; established program financing; estrogenic positive feedback; exophthalmos-producing factor

EPG eggs per gram [count]; electropalatography; electropneumography, electropneumogram; ethanolamine phosphoglyceride

EPH edema-proteinuria-hypertension; episodic paroxysmal hemicrania; extensor proprius hallucis

EPHIP education program for health informatics professionals

EPhMrA European Pharmaceutical Marketing Association

EpHV elapid herpesvirus

EPHX epoxide hydrolase

EPI echo planar imaging; electronic portal imaging; Emotion Profile Index; epilepsy; epinephrine; epirubicin; epithelium, epithelial; Estes Park Institute; evoked potential index; Expanded Programme of Immunization [WHO]; extrapyramidal involvement; extrinsic pathway inhibitor

epi epinephrine

EPIC Echocardiography Persantine International Cooperative Study; Echo Persantine Italian Cooperative Study; European Prevalence of Infection in Intensive Care Study; European Prospective Investigation into Cancer and Nutrition Study; European Prototype for Integrated Care; Evaluation of 7E3 for the Prevention of Ischemic Complications

EPICORE Epidemiology Coordinating Research Centre

EPICS Early Postmenopausal Intervention Cohort Study

EPID electronic portal imaging device

EPIDS Early Post-Myocardial Infarction Intravenous Dipyridamole Study

epid epidemic

epil epilepsy, epileptic

EPILOG Evaluation of Percutaneous Transluminal Coronary Angioplasty to Improve Long-Term Outcome with Abciximab Glycoprotein IIb/IIIa Blockade [trial]

epineph epinephrine

epis episiotomy

EPISODE Evaluation of Peripheral Intramuscular Sonography on Doppler Effect

EPI/STAR echo planar imaging with signal targeting and alternating radiofrequency

EPISTENT EPILOG STENT Trial; Evaluation of IIb/IIIa Platelet Inhibitor for Stenting

epith epithelium

EPIV enhanced potency inactivated polio vaccine

EPIX Emergency Preparedness Information Exchange [Canada]

EPL effective pathlength; effective patient's life; equivalent path length; essential phospholipid; extensor pollicis longus; extracorporeal piezoelectric lithotriptor

EPM electron probe microanalysis; electrophoretic mobility; energy-protein malnutrition

EPMR progressive epilepsy with mental retardation

EPN emphysematous pyelonephritis

EPNP 1,2-epoxy-3(4'-nitrophenoxy)propane

EPO eosinophil peroxidase; erythropoiesis; erythropoietin; evening primrose oil; exclusive provider organization; expiratory port occlusion

Epo erythropoietin

EPOB employee per occupied bed

EPOC excess post-exercise oxygen consumption

EPOCH Erythropoietin in Chinese Hamster Ovary [study]

EPOR erythropoietin receptor

EPOX epoxygenase

EPP end-plate potential; equal pressure point; erythropoietic protoporphyria

epp end-plate potential

EPPB end positive-pressure breathing

EPPS Edwards Personal Preference Schedule

EPQ Eysenck Personality Questionnaire

EPR early phase reaction; early progressive resistance; effective poor radius; electron paramagnetic resonance; electronic patient record; electrophrenic respiration; emergency physical restraint; enhanced permeability and retention; epitympanic recess; estimated protein requirement; estradiol production rate; evoked potential response; extraparenchymal resistance; extrapyramidal reaction

EPRCSS European Prospective Randomized Coronary Surgery Study

EpRE/ARE electrophile/antioxidant response element

EPROM erasable programmable read-only memory

EPROU Electronic Patient Record System at Osaka University Hospital

EPRS electronic patient record system; European Prospective Randomized Study

EPS ear-patella-short stature [syndrome]; early progressing stroke; elastosis perforans serpiginosa; electrophysiologic study; endoscopic pancreatic sphincterectomy; enzyme pancreatic secretion; exhaustion syndrome; exophthalmos-producing substance; expressed prostatic secretions; extracellular polysaccharide; extracellular protein secretion; extrapyramidal side effects; extrapyramidal symptom; extrapyramidal syndrome

ep's epithelial cells

EPSC excitatory postsynaptic current

EPSDT early and periodic screening diagnosis and treatment program

EPSE extrapyramidal side effects

EPSEM equal probability of selection method

EPSI echo planar spectroscopic imaging

ε Greek letter *epsilon*; heavy chain of IgE; permittivity; specific absorptivity

EPSP excitatory postsynaptic potential

EPSS E point to septal separation

EPT early pregnancy test

EPTE existed prior to enlistment

EPTFE, ePTFE expanded polytetrafluoroethylene

EPTS existed prior to service

EPV encephaloclastic proliferative vasculopathy; entomopoxvirus

EPXMA electron probe x-ray microanalyzer

EQ educational quotient; encephalization quotient; energy quotient; equal to

Eq, eq equation; equivalent

EQA external quality assessment

EQAM Ervin quality assessment measure

EQLIPSE Evaluation and Quality in Library Performance-System for Europe

EQOL economics and quality of life

EQP extensor quinti proprius

EqPV equine picornavirus

EQS electroquasistatic

EqTV equine torovirus

EQuIP Evaluation and Quality Improvement Program

equip equipment

EQUIPP Evaluation of Quinapril in Primary Practice [trial]

equiv equivalency, equivalent

ER efficiency ratio; epigastric region; ejection rate; electroresection; emergency room; endoplasmic reticulum; enhanced reactivation; enhancement ratio; entity-relationship [model]; environmental resistance; enzyme reactor; equine rhinopneumonia; equivalent roentgen [unit]; erythrocyte receptor; estradiol receptor; estrogen receptor; etretinate; evoked response; expiratory reserve; extended release; extended resistance; external resistance; external rotation

E-R entity-relationship [model]

E/R entity/relationship

ER⁺ increased estrogen receptor

ER⁻ decreased estrogen receptor

Er erbium; erythrocyte

E_r repulsive energy

er endoplasmic reticulum

ERA early [electronic] referrals application; echo record access study; electrical response activity; electroencephalic response audiometry; Electroshock Research Association; energy return ability; Enoxaparin Restenosis after Angioplasty [study]; entity relationship attribute; estradiol receptor assay; estrogen receptor assay; Estrogen Replacement in Atherosclerosis [study]; evoked response audiometry; extended relational algebra

ERA-ICA estradiol receptor assay immunocytochemical analysis

ERAS electronic residency application service

ERASME Efficacy of Renal Artery Stent Multicentre Evaluation

ERAV equine rhinitis A virus

ERBAC Excimer Laser, Rotablator and Balloon Angioplasty Comparison [study]

ERBF effective renal blood flow

ERBV equine rhinitis B virus

ERC endoscopic retrograde cholangiography; enteric cytopathic human orphan-rhino-coryza [virus]; erythropoietin-responsive cell; ethical review committee; European Resuscitation Council

Erc erythrocyte

ERCC excision repair cross-complementing

ERCoh event related coherence

ERCP endoscopic retrograde cholangio-pancreatography

Ercs erythrocytes

ERD event related desynchronization; evoked response detector

ERDA Energy Research and Development Administration

ERDIP electronic records development and implementation

ERE external rotation in extension

EREP event-related evoked potential

ERF edge response function; Education and Research Foundation; end response function; esophago-respiratory fistula; external rotation in flexion; Eye Research Foundation

eRF eukaryotic release factor

E-RFC E-rosette forming cell

ERFS electrophysiological ring finger splinting

ERG electron radiography; electroretinogram, electroretinography; emergency response guidebook

ErgTX ergotoxin

ERHD exposure-related hypothermic death

ErHV erinaceid herpesvirus

ERI elective replacement indicator [pacemaker]; environmental response inventory; E-rosette or erythrocyte rosette inhibitor

ERIA electroradioimmunoassay

ERIC Educational Resource Information Center; Educational Resource Information Clearinghouse

ERICA European Risk and Incidence: A Coordinated Analysis

ERISA Employee Retirement Income Security Act

ERK extracellular signal-regulated kinase

ErLV *Erysimum* latent virus

ERM electrochemical relaxation method; extended radical mastectomy; ezrin, radixin, and moesin

ERMSa embryonal rhabdomyosarcoma

ERNA early return to normal activities [after acute myocardial infarction]; efferent renal nerve activity; equilibrium radionuclide angiocardiography

ERNST European Resuscitation Nimodipine Study

ERO effective regurgitant orifice [tricuspid regurgitation]; Eugenics Record Office

ERO$_2$ oxygen extraction ratio

EROD 7-ethoxyresorufin-*O*-deethylase

EROS elaboration of reactions for organic synthesis [system]

ERP early receptor potential; effective refractory period; elodoisin-related peptide; emergency response team; endoscopic retrograde pancreatography; enzyme-releasing peptide; equine rhinopneumonitis; estrogen receptor protein; event-related potential

Er-PBMC E-rosette-negative peripheral blood mononuclear cell

ERPC evacuation of retained products of conception

ERPF effective renal plasma flow

ERPG emergency response planning guidelines

ERPLV effective refractory period of left ventricle

ERR excess relative risk

ERS enamel-renal syndrome; endoscopic retrograde sphincterectomy

E$_{rs}$ respiratory system elastance

ERSP event-related slow potential

ERSPC European Randomized Study of Screening for Prostatic Cancer

ERT electronic textbook of radiology; emergency room thoracotomy, emergent resuscitative thoracotomy; esophageal radionuclide transit; estrogen replacement therapy; examination room terminal; external radiation therapy

ERTAS extended reticulo-thalamic activating system

ERTOCS, ERTOS European Randomised Trial of Ovarian Cancer Screening

ERU endorectal ultrasound

ERV Embu virus; entero-like virus; equine rhinopneumonitis virus; Estero Real virus; etched ringspot virus; expiratory reserve volume

ERVEV Erve virus

ERY erysipelas

Ery *Erysipelothrix*

ES ejection sound; elastic stocking; elastic support; electrical stimulus, electrical stimulation; electroshock; electrospray; electrotherapy system; Elejalde syndrome; embryonic stem; emergency service; emission spectrometry; end of systole; endometritis-salpingitis; endoscopic sclerosis; endoscopic sclerotherapy; endoscopic sphincterotomy; end stage [disease]; end-systole; end-to-side; English-speaking; enzyme substrate; epileptic seizures; epileptic syndrome; erythromycin stearate; esophageal, esophagus; esophageal scintigraphy; esterase; evoking strength; Ewing sarcoma; exfoliation syndrome; Expectation Score; experimental study; expert system; exterior surface; extra stimulus; extrasystole

Es einsteinium; estrid

E$_s$ secondary etiology [vascular diseases]; shear energy

ESA Electrolysis Society of America; electronic signature authentication; endocardial surface area; epidermal surface antigen; epididymal sperm aneuploidy; esterase; esterase A

ESAC extra structurally abnormal chromosome

ESADDI estimated safe and adequate daily dietary intake

ESAT esterase activator

ESB electrical stimulation of the brain; enhanced skill building [program]; environmental specimen banking; esterase B

ESBL extended spectrum beta-lactamase

ESBY Electrical Stimulation vs Coronary Artery Bypass [study]

ESC electromechanical slope computer; endosystolic count; environmental stress cracking; epidural spinal cord; erythropoietin-sensitive stem cell; esterase C

ESCA electron spectroscopy for chemical analysis

ESCALAT, ESCALATE Efegatran and Streptokinase to Canalize Arteries Like Accelerated Tissue Plasminogen Activator [study]

ESCAPE Evaluation Study of Congestive Heart Failure and Pulmonary Artery Catheterization Effectiveness

ESCAT Early Self-Controlled Anticoagulation Trial

ESCC epidural spinal cord compression; esophageal squamous cell carcinoma

ESCH European Study Group on Cytogenetic Biomarkers and Health

Esch *Escherichia*

ESCN electrolyte and steroid cardiopathy with necrosis

ESCOBAR Emergency Stenting Compared to Conventional Balloon Angioplasty Randomized Trial

ESCODD European Standards Committee on Oxidative DNA Damage

EsCPS *Euxoa scandens* cypovirus

ESCS epidural spinal cord stimulation

ESD electronic submission document; electronic summation device; electrostatic discharge; emission spectrometric device; end-systolic dimension; esterase-D; exoskeletal device

ESDI enhanced small device interface

ESE electrostatic unit [Ger. *electrostatische Einheit*]; evolutionary stable energy; exercise stress echocardiography

ESEM European Society for Engineering and Medicine

ESETCID European Study of Epidemiology and Treatment of Cardiac Inflammatory Diseases

ESF edge spread function; electron scatter function; electrosurgical filter; erythropoietic stimulating factor

ESFH European Society for Hemapheresis

ESFL end-systolic force-length relationship

ESG electrospinogram; endovascular stent graft; estrogen; exfoliation syndrome glaucoma

ESGE European Society for Gastrointestinal Endoscopy

ESHEL Association for Planning and Development of Services for the Aged in Israel

ESHG European Society of Human Genetics

ESHR elder spontaneously hypertensive rat

EsHV esocid herpesvirus

ESI elastase-specific inhibitor; electrospray ionization; emergency safety information; emergency severity index; enzyme substrate inhibitor; epidural steroid injection

ESIC electrical stimulation-induced contractions

ESIC-LCE electric stimulation-induced contractions leg cycle ergometry

ESI-MS electrospray ionization mass spectrometry

ESIMV expiratory synchronized intermittent mandatory ventilation

ESIN elastic stable intramedullary nailing

ESIPT excited state intermolecular proton transfer

ESL end-systolic length; E-selectin ligand; extracorporeal shockwave lithotripsy

ESLD end-stage liver disease

ESLF end-stage liver failure

ESLV elderberry symptomless virus

ESM ejection systolic murmur; endolymphatic stromal myosis; endoscopic specular microscope; ethosuximide

ESMC entropy sampling Monte Carlo

ESMIR Echocardiographic Selection of Patients for Mitral Regurgitation [study]

ESMIS Emergency Medical Services Management Information System

ESMoV eggplant severe mottle virus

ESMS electrospray mass spectrometry

ESN educationally subnormal; estrogen-stimulated neurophysin

ESnet Energy Sciences Network [Department of Energy]

ESN(M) educationally subnormal-moderate

ESN(S) educationally subnormal-severe

ESO electrospinal orthosis; embolic signal onset

eso esophagoscopy; esophagus

ESOCAP European Study of Community Acquired Pneumonia

ESP early systolic paradox; echo spacing; effective sensory projection; effective systolic pressure; endometritis-salpingitis-peritonitis; end-systolic pressure; eosinophil stimulation promoter; epidermal soluble protein; especially; evoked synaptic potential; extrasensory perception

ESPA electrical stimulation-produced analgesia; extended sib pair analysis

ESPAC European Study Group of Pancreatic Cancer

ESPC enhanced spectral pathology component

EsPeR personalized risk estimation

ESPRIM European Study Prevention Research of Infarct with Molsidomine

ESPRIT Efficacy Safety Prospective Randomized Ibopamine Trial; European and Australian Stroke Prevention in Reversible Ischemia Trial; European Study of the Prevention of Reocclusion after Initial Thrombolysis; European Study Programme for the Relevance of Immunology in Liver Transplantation

ESPS European Secondary Prevention Study; European Stroke Prevention Study

ESPVR end-systolic pressure-volume relationship

ESQ early signs questionnaire

ESR Einstein stroke radius; electric skin resistance; electron spin resonance; equipment service report; erythrocyte sedimentation rate; estrogen receptor; extracytoplasmic stress response

ESRD end-stage renal disease

ESRF end-stage renal failure; European Synchrotron Radiation Facility

ESRI Environmental Systems Research Institute

ESS earliest starting shift; earth and space sciences; elementary sulcal surface; empty sella syndrome; endostreptosin; erythrocyte-sensitizing substance; euthyroid sick syndrome; excited skin syndrome; exonic splicing silencer or suppressor; squamous self-healing epithelioma

ess essential

ESSENCE Efficacy Safety Subcutaneous Enoxaparin in Non-Q-Wave Coronary Events [study]

ESSEX European Scimed Stent Experience

ESSF external spinal skeletal fixation

ESSV Essaouira virus

EST Early Stroke Trial; electric shock threshold; electroshock therapy; endodermal sinus tumor; endometrial sinus tumor; endoscopic sphincterectomy; esterase; exercise stress test; expressed sequence tag

Est estradiol

est ester; estimation, estimated

ESTEEM European Standardised Telematic Tool to Evaluate EMG

esth esthetics, esthetic

Est,l elastance, lung

ESTR Estrogens [dataset]

Est,rs elastance, respiratory system

Est,w elastance, chest wall

ESU electrosurgical unit; electrostatic unit

E-sub excitor substance

ESUE emergency screening ultrasound examination

ESV end-systolic volume; esophageal valve

ESVEM Electrophysiologic Study vs Electrocardiographic Monitoring

ESVH endoscopic saphenous vein harvesting

ESVI end-systolic volume index

ESVS endoscopic vascular surgery; epiurethral suprapubic vaginal suspension

ESWL extracorporeal shock wave lithotripsy

ESWS end-systolic wall stress

E$_{syn}$ reversal potential

ET educational therapy; effective temperature; ejection time; embryo transfer; endothelin; endotoxin; endotracheal; endotracheal tube; end-tidal; endurance time; enterotoxin; epidermolytic toxin; epithelial tumor; esophageal temperature; esotropia; essential thrombocythemia; essential tremor; ethanol; etiocholanolone test; etiology; eustachian tube; examination terminal; exchange transfusion; exercise test; exercise treadmill; exfoliative toxin; expiration time; exploratory thoracoscopy

E:T, E/T effect to target [ratio]

ET-1 endothelin-1

ET$_3$ erythrocyte triiodothyronine

ET$_4$ effective thyroxine [test]

Et ethyl; etiology

et and [Lat. *et*]; end-tidal

ETA electron transfer agent; endotracheal airways; endotracheal aspiration; ethionamide; exfoliative toxin A

ET-A, ET$_A$ endothelin A

η Greek letter *eta*; absolute viscosity

ETAB extrathoracic assisted breathing

ETAC early treatment of the atopic child

ETAF epidermal thrombocyte activating factor; epithelial thymus-activating factor

et al and others [Lat. *et alii*]

ETAR equivalent tissue air ratio

ET-B, ET$_B$ endothelin B

ETC electron transport chain; emergency trauma care; enterotoxigenic *Escherichia coli*; esophageal tracheal combitube; estimated time of conception

ET$_c$ corrected ejection time

ETCC emergency team coordination course

ETCO$_2$, $_{et}$CO$_2$ end-tidal carbon dioxide [concentration]

ETD eustachian tube dysfunction

ETDRS Early Treatment Diabetic Retinopathy Study

ETD(V) extrapolated tolerance dose (volume) [radiotherapy]

ETE end-to-end [anastomosis]

ETEC enterotoxic or enterotoxigenic *Escherichia coli*

ETF electron-transferring flavoprotein; eustachian tube function; extensions teardrop fracture

ETFB electron transfer flavoprotein, beta polypeptide

ETG episode treatment group

ETH elixir terpin hydrate; ethanol; ethmoid

ETh excitability threshold

eth ether

ETHC elixir terpin hydrate with codeine

ETHR education, training, and human resources

ETI endotracheal intubation

ETIC Environmental Teratology Information Center

ETICBACK Environmental Teratology Information Center Backfile [NLM database]

ETIO etiocholanolone

etiol etiology

EtIV *Eriborus terebrans* ichnovirus

ETK erythrocyte transketolase

ETKTM every test known to man

ETL echo train length; expiratory threshold load

ETM erythromycin

ETNet Educational Technology Network

EtNU ethyl nitrosourea

ETO estimated time of ovulation; ethylene oxide

Eto ethylene oxide

E-TOF electron time of flight

ETOH, EtOH ethyl alcohol

ETOX ethylene oxide

ETP electron transport particle; entire treatment period; ephedrine, theophylline, phenobarbital; eustachian tube pressure

ETPCO$_2$ end-tidal partial carbon dioxide [concentration]

ETR effective thyroxine ratio; electronic textbook of radiology; endothelin receptor

ETS educational testing service; electrical transcranial stimulation; electronic trans-impedance scanning; electron transport system; electrosleep therapy; endoscopic transthoracic sympathectomy; environmental tobacco smoke; erythromycin topical solution; event timing system; expiration time signal; extracellular transport system

ET-ST endotracheal tube-stylet unit

ETT endotracheal tube; epinephrine tolerance test; exercise tolerance test; exercise treadmill test; extrathyroidal thyroxine

ET-TL endotracheal tube-Trachlight unit

ETTP enhanced trusted third party

ETU emergency and trauma unit; emergency treatment unit; ethylene thiourea

ETV extravascular thermal volume

ETX etiology

EU Ehrlich unit; elementary unit; emergency unit; endotoxin unit; entropy unit; enzyme unit; esterase unit; etiology unknown; excretory urography; expected utility

Eu europium; euryon

EUA examination under anesthesia

EUBV Eubenangee virus

EUCLID European Diabetes Controlled Trial of Lisinopril in Insulin-Dependent Diabetes Mellitus

EUCROMIC European Collaborative Research on Mosaicism in Chorionic Virus Sample

EUCS end-user computing satisfaction scale

EUDB end-user database

EUFOS European Federation of Oto-Rhino-Laryngological Societies

EUHID encrypted universal health care identifier

EUL expected upper limit

EUM external urethral meatus

EUP extrauterine pregnancy

EURAGE European Community Concerted Action on Aging

EURALIM European Alimentation Study

EURAMIC European Community Multi-center Study on Antioxidants, Myocardial Infarction and Breast Cancer

EURID European Registry for Implantable Cardioverter Defibrillators

EURO-ART European Angiojet Rapid Thrombectomy [study]

EUROASPIRE European Action on Secondary Prevention by Intervention to Reduce Events

EUROCARDI European Concerted Action for the Rapid Diagnosis of Myocardial Infarction

EUROCARE European Carvedilol Restenosis Trial

EURO-CAT European Cancer After Transplant [project]; European Register of Congenital Anomalies and Twins

EURODIAB ACE European Diabetes: Aetiology of Childhood Diabetes on an Epidemiological Basis

EURODIAB IDDM European Diabetes Centers Study of Complications in Patients with Insulin-dependent Diabetes Mellitus

EURODIAB TIGER European Diabetes: Type I Genetic Epidemiology Resources

EURO-DIRECT European Direct Myocardial Revascularization in Regeneration of Endomyocardial Channels Trial

EUROHAZCON Congenital Anomalies Near Hazardous Waste Landfill Sites in Europe [study]

EURO-ISDN European Integrated Services Digital Network

EURONET European On-Line Network

EUROPA European Trial of Reduction of Cardiac Events with Perindopril in Stable Coronary Artery Disease

EuroQol European quality of life [scale]

EUROSCOP European Registry Society Study of Chronic Obstructive Pulmonary Diseases

EUROSTROKE European Collaborative Study of Incidence and Risk Factors for Ischemic and Hemorrhagic Stroke

EUROTOX European Committee on Chronic Toxicity Hazards

EUROWINTER European Study on Cold Exposure and Winter Mortality from Ischemic Heart Disease

EUS endorectal ultrasonography or ultrasound; endoscopic ultrasonography or ultrasound; external urethral sphincter

EUS-CPN endosonography-guided celiac plexus neurolysis

EUS-FNA endoscopic ultrasound fine-needle aspiration

Eust eustachian

EUV extreme ultraviolet laser

EV Ebola virus; eczema vaccinatum; ejected volume; electric vehicle; electronic patient record [EPR] values; emergency vehicle; encephalitis or encephalomyelitis virus; enteritis virus; enterovirus; entomopoxvirus; epidermodysplasia verruciformis; estradiol valerate; eustachian valve; evoked potential [response]; excessive ventilation; expected value; extravascular

Ev, ev eversion

eV, ev electron volt

EV-69, 70, 71 human enterovirus 69, 70, and 71

EVA Epidemiological Study on Vascular and Cognitive Aging; ethyl violet azide; ethylene vinyl acetate; European Vascular Agency [study]

evac evacuate, evacuated, evacuation

EVADE Experience with Left Ventricular Assist Device with Exercise [trial]

eval evaluate, evaluated, evaluation

eval stud evaluation study

evap evaporation, evaporated

EVAR endovascular aneurysm repair

EVB electronic view box; esophageal variceal bleeding

EVC, EvC Ellis-van Creveld [syndrome]

EVCI expected value of clinical information

EVD external ventricular drain; extravascular [lung] density

ever eversion, everted

EVF ethanol volume fraction

EVFMG exchange visitor foreign medical graduate

EVG electroventriculography

EVGLI European Working Group on *Legionella* Surveillance Centre

EVIL exposure to selected viruses in research laboratories

EVL electronic visualization laboratory

EVLW extravascular lung water

EVM electronic voltmeter; extravascular mass

EVNT event [UMLS]

EVOC emergency vehicle operator course

EVP episcleral venous pressure; evoked visual potential

EVPI expected value of perfect information

EVR evoked visual response; exudative vitreoretinopathy

EVRS early ventricular repolarization syndrome

EVS eligibility verification system; endovaginal sonography

EVT endovascular technology

EVTV extravascular thermal volume

EVV Everglades virus

EVXX exudative vitreoretinopathy, X-linked

EW emergency ward; estrogen withdrawal

E-W Edinger-Westphal [nucleus]

EWA estrogen replacement for women with coronary artery disease; exponentially weighted average

EWAs erythrocytes without antigens

EWB estrogen withdrawal bleeding

EWGCP European Working Group on Cardiac Pacing

EWGLP European Workshop for Computer-based Support for Clinical Guidelines and Protocols

EWHO elbow-wrist-hand orthosis

EWKY elder Wistar-Kyoto rat

EWL egg-white lysozyme; evaporation water loss

EWPHE European Working Party on Hypertension in the Elderly

EWR European Wallstent Registry

EWS Ewing sarcoma

EWSMV European wheat striate mosaic virus

EWSR Ewing sarcoma breakpoint region

EX exfoliation; exsmoker

E(X) expected value of the random variable X

ex exacerbation; examination, examined; examiner; example; excision; exercise; exophthalmos; exposure; extraction

EXA electronic x-ray archives

exac exacerbation

EXACT Extended Release Adalat Canadian Trial

EXACTO Excimer Laser Angioplasty in Coronary Total Occlusion

EXAFS extended x-ray absorption fine structure

exam examination, examine, examined

EXBF exercise hyperemia blood flow

ExBRT external beam irradiation or radiation therapy

exc excision

EXCEED excellence center for eliminating ethnic/racial disparities

EXCEL Expanded Clinical Evaluation of Lovastatin [trial]

exch exchange

EXE exemestane

EXCITE Evaluation of Oral Xemilofiban in Controlling Thrombotic Events

excr excretion

ExEF ejection fraction during exercise

EXELFS extended electron-loss line fine structure

exer exercise
EXERT Exercise Rehabilitation Trial
exg exogenous
EXO exonuclease; exophoria
exog exogenous
exoph exophthalmia
EXoS exoenzyme S
exos exostosis
EXP expiration
exp expansion; expectorant; experiment, experimental; expiration, expired; exponential function; exposure
EXPAPS Exeter Primary Angioplasty Pilot Study
exp lap exploratory laparotomy
expect expectorant
exper experiment, experimental
ExPGN extracapillary proliferative glomerulonephritis
expir expiration, expiratory, expired
expl exploratory
Expl Lap exploratory laparotomy
ExpNET Expert Network
exptl experimental
EXREM external radiation-emission man [dose]

EXS external support
EXT exercise testing
Ext extraction, extract
ext extension; extensive; extensor; exterior; external; extract; extreme, extremity
extr extract
EXTRA Evaluation of XT Stent for Restenosis of Native Arteries
extrav extravasation
ext rot external rotation
extub extubation
EXU excretory urogram
exud exudate, exudation
EY egg yolk; epidemiological year
EYA egg yolk agar
EYAV Eyach virus
EYAV-FR578 Eyach virus-France 578
EYAV-GER Eyach virus-Germany
EYMV eggplant yellow mosaic virus
EZ epileptogenic zone
Ez eczema
EZW embedded zero tree wavelet [picture archiving and communication algorithm]

F bioavailability; a cell that donates F factor in bacterial conjugation; coefficient of inbreeding; a conjugative plasmid in F⁺ bacterial cells; degree of fineness of abrasive particles; facies; factor; Fahrenheit; failure; false; family; farad; Faraday constant; fascia; fasting; fat; father; feces; fellow; female; fermentation; fertility; fetal; fiat; fibroblast; fibrous; field of vision; filament; *Filaria*; fine; finger; flexion; flow; fluorine; flux; focal [spot]; focus; foil; fontanel; foramen; force; form, forma; formula; fornix; fossa; fraction, fractional; fracture; fragment; free; French [catheter]; frequency; frontal; frontal electrode placement in electroencephalography; function; fundus; *Fusiformis*; fusion; *Fusobacterium*; gilbert; Helmholz free energy; hydrocortisone [compound F]; inbreeding coefficient; left foot electrode in vectorcardiography; phenylalanine; variance ratio

F₀, F₁ coupling factor

F₁, F₂, etc. first, second, etc., filial generation; years of fellowship study

FI, FII, etc. factors I, II, etc.

F344 Fischer 344 [rat]

°F degree on the Fahrenheit scale

F′ a hybrid F plasmid

F⁻ a bacterial cell lacking an F plasmid

F⁺ a bacterial cell having an F plasmid

f atomic orbital with angular momentum quantum number 3; farad; fasting; father; female; femto; fiber, fibrous; fingerbreadth; fission; flexion; fluid; focal; foot; form, forma; formula; fostered [experimental animal]; fraction; fracture; fragment; frequency [statistics]; frontal; function; fundus; numerical expression of the relative aperture of a camera lens

f- femto- [10⁻¹⁵]

FA factor analysis; false aneurysm; Families Anonymous; Fanconi anemia; far advanced; fatty acid; febrile antigen; femoral artery; fetal age; fibrinolytic activity; fibroadenoma; fibrosing alveolitis; field ambulance; field assessment; filterable agent; filtered air; first aid; flip angle;

fluorescent antibody; fluorescent assay; fluoroalanine; folic acid; follicular area; food allergy; forearm; fortified aqueous [solution]; fractional anisotropy; free acid; Freund adjuvant; Friedreich ataxia; functional activity; functional administration

F/A fetus active

fa fatty [rat]

FAA folic acid antagonist; formaldehyde, acetic acid, alcohol; fumarylacetoacetic acid

FA-A Fanconi anemia A [gene]

FAAN Fellow of the American Academy of Nursing

FAB fast atom bombardment; formalin ammonium bromide; fragment, antigen-binding [of immunoglobulins]; French-American-British [leukemia staging]; functional arm brace

FA-B Fanconi anemia B [gene]

Fab fragment, antigen-binding [of immunoglobulins]

F(ab')₂ fragment, antigen-binding [of immunoglobulins, obtained by pepsin cleavage]

Fabc fragment, antigen and complement binding [of immunoglobulins]

FABER flexion in abduction and external rotation

FABF femoral artery blood flow

FAB-MS fast atom bombardment-mass spectrometry

FABP fatty acid-binding protein; folate-binding protein

FAC familial adenomatosis coli; femoral arterial cannulation; ferric ammonium citrate; fetal abdominal circumference; fluorescent aromatic compound; 5-fluorouracil, Adriamycin, and cyclophosphamide; foamy alveolar cast; fractional area changes; free available chlorine; functional aerobic capacity

FA-C Fanconi anemia C [gene]

Fac factor

fac facility; to make [Lat. *facere*]

FACA Fanconi anemia complementation group A; Fellow of the American College of Anesthetists; Fellow of the American College of Angiology; Fellow of the American College of Apothecaries

FACAI Fellow of the American College of Allergy and Immunology

FACAS Fellow of the American College of Abdominal Surgeons

FACB Fanconi anemia complementation group B

Facb fragment, antigen, and complement binding

FACC Fanconi anemia complementation group C; Fellow of the American College of Cardiologists

FACCT Foundation for Accountability

FACD Fanconi anemia complementation group D; Fellow of the American College of Dentists

FACE fluorophore assisted carbohydrate electrophoresis

FACEP Fellow of the American College of Emergency Physicians

FACES Family Adaptability and Cohesion Evaluation Scale; unique facies, anorexia, cachexia, and eye and skin lesions [syndrome]

FACET Flosequinan Angiotensin Converting Enzyme-Inhibitor [ACEI] Trial; Fosinopril Amlodipine Cardiovascular Events Trial

FACFP Fellow of the American College of Family Physicians

FACFS Fellow of the American College of Foot Surgeons

FACG Fellow of the American College of Gastroenterology

FACH forceps to after-coming head

FACHA Fellow of the American College of Health Administrators; Fellow of the American College of Hospital Administrators

FACHE Fellow of the American College of Healthcare Executives

FACIT fibril-associated collagen with interrupted triple helices

FACL fatty acid coenzyme ligase

FACLM Fellow of the American College of Legal Medicine

FACMTA Federal Advisory Council on Medical Training Aids

FACN Fellow of the American College of Nutrition

FACNHA Foundation of American College of Nursing Home Administrators

FACNM Fellow of the American College of Nuclear Medicine

FACNP Fellow of the American College of Nuclear Physicians

FACO Fellow of the American College of Otolaryngology

FACOG Fellow of the American College of Obstetricians and Gynecologists

FACOS Fellow of the American College of Orthopaedic Surgeons

FACOSH Federal Advisory Committee on Occupational Safety and Health

FACP Fellow of the American College of Physicians

FACPE Fellow of the American College of Physician Executives

FACPM Fellow of the American College of Preventive Medicine

FACR Fellow of the American College of Radiology

FACS Fellow of the American College of Surgeons; fluorescence-activated cell sorter

FACScan fluorescence associated cell sorter scan

FACSM Fellow of the American College of Sports Medicine

FACT Flannagan Aptitude Classification Test; focused appendix computed tomography; functional assessment of cancer therapy

FACT-B functional assessment of cancer therapy-breast

FACTS Functional Angiometric Correlation with Thallium Scintigraphy [trial]

FACWA familial amyotrophic chorea with acanthocytosis

FAD familial Alzheimer dementia; familial autonomic dysfunction; fetal activity-acceleration determination; flash-induced afterdischarge; flavin adenine dinucleotide

FA-D Fanconi anemia D [gene]

FADF fluorescent antibody dark field

FADH₂ reduced form of flavin adenine dinucleotide

FADIR flexion in adduction and internal rotation

FADN flavin adenine dinucleotide

FADS fetal akinesia deformation sequence

FAdV fowl adenovirus

FAE fetal alcohol effect; follicle-associated epithelium

FA-E Fanconi anemia E [gene]

FAEE fatty acid ethyl ester

FAEES fatty acid ethyl ester synthase

FAES Foundation for Advanced Education in the Sciences

FAF fatty acid free; fibroblast-activating factor

FAH Federation of American Hospitals

FAHIS Florida Abuse Hotline Information System

Fahr Fahrenheit

FaHV falconid herpesvirus

FAI first aid instruction; free androgen index; functional aerobic impairment; functional assessment inventory

FAJ fused apophyseal joint

FAK focal adhesion kinase

FALG fowl antimouse lymphocyte globulin

FALP fluoro-assisted lumbar puncture

FALS familial amyotrophic lateral sclerosis; forward angle light scatter

FAM 5-fluorouracil, Adriamycin, and mitomycin C; fuzzy associative memory

Fam, fam family, familial

FAMA Fellow of the American Medical Association; fluorescence-assisted mismatch analysis; fluorescent antibody to membrane antigen

FAM-A functional area model-activity

FAM-D functional area model of data

FAME fatty acid methyl ester

FAMG family group [UMLS]

fam hist family history

FAMIS Fosinopril in Acute Myocardial Infarction Study

FAMMM familial atypical multiple mole-melanoma [syndrome]

FAMOUS Fragmin Advanced Malignancy Outcome Study

FAMP fludarabine

FAN fuchsin, amido black, and naphthol yellow

FANA fluorescent antinuclear antibody

F and R force and rhythm [of pulse]

FANEL Federation for Accessible Nursing Education and Licensure

FANPT Freeman Anxiety Neurosis and Psychosomatic Test

FANTASTIC Full Anticoagulation vs Aspirin and Ticlopidine After Stent Implantation [study]

FAO Food and Agriculture Organization [of United Nations]

FAO$_2$ fractional alveolar oxygen

FAOF family assessment of occupational functioning

FAP familial adenomatous polyposis; familial amyloid polyneuropathy; fatty acid polyunsaturated; fatty acid poor; femoral artery pressure; fibrillating action potential; Fibrinolytics vs Primary Angioplasty [trial]; fixed action potential; frozen animal procedure; functional ambulation profile

FAPA Fellow of the American Psychiatric Association; Fellow of the American Psychoanalytical Association

FAPHA Fellow of the American Public Health Association

FAPIS Flecainide and Propafenone Italian Study

FAPS Felodipine Atherosclerosis Prevention Study; French Aortic Plaque Study

FAPY formamidopyrimidine

FAQ frequently asked question; functional asessment questionnaire

FAR fatal accident rate; Federal acquisitions regulation; fractional albumin rate

far faradic

FARE Federation of Alcoholic Rehabilitation Establishments

FARS Fatality Analysis Reporting System

FARV Farallon virus

FAS Family Attitude Scale; fatty acid synthetase; Federation of American Scientists; fetal akinesia sequence; fetal alcohol syndrome

FASA Federated Ambulatory Surgery Association

FASB Financial Accounting Standards Board

FASC free-standing ambulatory surgical center

fasc fasciculus, fascicular

FASEB Federation of American Societies for Experimental Biology

FASHP Federation of Associations of Schools of the Health Professions

FAST ferment active solution therapy; Fitness, Arthritis and Seniors Trial; flow-assisted, short-term [balloon catheter]; fluorescent antibody staining technique; fluoro-allergosorbent test; focused abdominal sonography for trauma; Fourier acquired steady state; Frenchay Aphasia Screening Test; functional assessment stages

FASTEST Femoral Artery Stent Study

FAST-MI Field Ambulance Study of Thrombolysis in Myocardial Infarction

FAstV feline astrovirus

FAT family attitudes test; fluorescent antibody technique; fluorescent antibody test

FAT$_{DPA}$ fat dual photon absorptiometry

FATIMA Fraxiparin Anticoagulant Therapy in Myocardial Infarction Study in Amsterdam

Fat$_{IVNA}$ fat in vitro neutron activation analysis

FATS face and thigh squeeze [position for bag mask ventilation]; Familial Atherosclerosis Treatment Study; fast adiabatic trajectory in steady state

FAT$_{UWW}$ fat underwater weighing

FAV facio-auriculovertebral [sequence]; feline ataxia virus; floppy aortic valve; fowl adenovirus

FAVS facio-auriculo-vertebral spectrum

F$_{AW}$ airway flow

FAX, fax facsimile

FAZ Fanconi-Albertini-Zellweger [syndrome]; foveal avascular zone; fragmented atrial activity zone

FB factor B; fascicular block; fasting blood [test]; feedback; fiberoptic bronchoscopy; fingerbreadth; flexible bronchoscope; flexible bronchoscopy; foreign body; *Fusobacterium*

FBA fecal bile acid

FBAO foreign-body airway obstruction

F-BAR forward and backward autoregressive [algorithm]

FBC full blood count

FBCOD foreign body of the cornea, oculus dexter (right eye)

FBCOS foreign body of the cornea, oculus sinister (left eye)

FBCP familial benign chronic pemphigus

FBD forward/backward bending; functional bowel disorder

fBDE fractional balanced differential expression [microarray analysis]

FbDP fibrin degradation products

FBE full blood examination

FBEC fetal bovine endothelial cell

FBF forearm blood flow; full breast feeding

FBG fasting blood glucose; fibrinogen; foreign body granulomatosis

fbg fibrinogen

FBH familial benign hypercalcemia

FBHH familial benign hypocalciuric hypercalcemia

FBI flossing, brushing, and irrigation

FBJMSV Finkel-Biskis-Jinkins murine sarcoma virus

FBL follicular basal lamina

FBLN fibulin

FBM felbamate; fetal breathing movements; fractional or fractal brownian motion; fresh bone marrow

FBN Federal Bureau of Narcotics; fibrillin

FBP femoral blood pressure; fibrin breakdown product; filtered back projection [algorithm]; folate-binding protein; fructose-1,6-biphosphatase

FBPM forward-backward Prony method [spectral analysis of heart sounds]

FBPsS Fellow of the British Psychological Society

FBR fetal breathing rate

FBS fasting blood sugar; feedback system; fetal bovine serum; film-based system

FBSC Frederick Biomedical Supercomputing Center [NIH]

FBSS failed back surgery syndrome; field-based similarity searching

FC family coping; fasciculus cuneatus; fast component [of a neuron]; febrile convulsions; feline conjunctivitis; ferric chloride; ferric citrate; fibrocyte; finger clubbing; finger counting; flow compensation; fluorocarbon; fluorocytosine; Foley catheter; follicle culture; foster care; fowl cholera; free cholesterol; frontal cortex; functional castration

5-FC flucytosine; 5-fluorocytosine

F + C flare and cells

Fc centroid frequency; fraction/centrifuge; fragment, crystallizable [of immunoglobulin]

Fc' a fragment of an immunoglobulin molecule produced by papain digestion

fc cutoff frequency; foot candles

FCA ferritin-conjugated antibodies; Freund's complete adjuvant; functional capacity assessment

FCAH familial cytomegaly adrenocortical hypoplasia [syndrome]

FCAP Fellow of the College of American Pathologists

FCAT Federative Committee on Anatomical Terminology

F cath Foley catheter

FCC Federal Communications Commission; follicular center cells; Food Chemicals Codex

fcc face-centered-cubic

f/cc fibers per cubic centimeter of air

FCCA familial congenital cardiac abnormality

FCCH family child care home

FCCL follicular center cell lymphoma

FCCSET Federal Coordinating Committee for Science, Engineering and Technology

FCD feces collection device; fibrocystic disease; fibrocystic dysplasia; focal cytoplasmic degradation

FCE fibrocartilaginous embolism

FceR fragment receptor for immunoglobulin E

FCF fetal cardiac frequency; fibroblast chemotactic factor

FCFC fibroblast colony-forming cell

FcγR fragment receptor for immunoglobulin G

FCH faculty contact hour; family care home; fetal cystic hygroma

FCHL familial combined hyperlipidemia

FChS Fellow of the Society of Chiropodists

FCHSP flight crew health stabilization program [NASA]

FCI fixed-cell immunofluorescence; folded cell index; food chemical intolerance

FCIM Federated Council for Internal Medicine

fCJD familial Creutzfeldt-Jakob disease

FCL fibroblast cell line

fcly face lying

FCM flow cytometry; fuzzy cognitive map [algorithm]

FCMC familial chronic mucocutaneous candidiasis; family centered maternity care

FCMD Fukuyama congenital muscular dystrophy

FCMS Fellow of the College of Medicine and Surgery; Foix-Chavany-Marie syndrome

FCMW Foundation for Child Mental Welfare

FCO Fellow of the College of Osteopathy

FCoV feline coronavirus

FCP F-cell production; femoral hole coronal positioning; final common pathway; Functional Communication Profile

FCPN fuzzy coloured Petri net

FCPR fatigue crack propagation rate

FCPS Fellow of the College of Physicians and Surgeons

FCR flexor carpi radialis; fractional catabolic rate; Fuji computed radiography

FcR Fc receptor; fragment receptor [immunoglobulin]

FCRA fecal collection receptacle assembly; Fellow of the College of Radiologists of Australasia

FCRC Frederick Cancer Research Center

FcRγ fragment receptor gamma chain

FCS faciocutaneoskeletal syndrome; fecal containment system; feedback control system; fetal calf serum; foot compartment syndrome

FCSP Fellow of the Chartered Society of Physiotherapy

FCST Fellow of the College of Speech Therapists

FCSW female commercial sex worker

FCT food composition table; fucosyl transferase

FCU flexor carpi ulnaris

FCV feline calicivirus; fowl calicivirus

FCx frontal cortex

FCXM flow cytometric cross-matching

FD familial dysautonomia; family doctor; fan douche; fatal dose; fetal danger; fibrin derivative; fibrous dysplasia; floppy disk; focal distance; Folin-Denis [assay]; follicular diameter; foot drop; forceps delivery; Fourier descriptor; fractal dimension; fracture-dislocation; freeze drying

FD1 from day 1

FD2 from day 2

FD$_{50}$ median fatal dose

Fd the amino-terminal portion of the heavy chain of an immunoglobulin molecule; ferredoxin

fd fundus

FDA Fisher discriminant analysis; fluorescein diacetate; Food and Drug Administration; right frontoanterior [fetal position]

FDA-CBER Food and Drug Administration, Center for Biologics Evaluation and Research

FDAM fuzzy logic based decision analysis module

FDAMA Food and Drug Administration Modernization Act

FDAW film digitizer acquisition workstation

FDB familial defective apolipoprotein B

FDBL fecal daily blood loss

FDC factor-dependent cell [line]; follicular dendritic cell

FD&C Food, Drug and Cosmetic Act; food, drugs, and cosmetics

FDCA Food, Drug, and Cosmetic Act

FDCPA Food, Drug, and Consumer Product Agency

FDD fluorescent differential display; Food and Drugs Directorate; frequency division duplex [telemedicine]

FDDC ferric dimethyldithiocarbonate

FDDI fiber distributed data interface; film distribution data interface

FDDS Family Drawing Depression Scale

FDE female day-equivalent; final drug evaluation

FDECU field employable environmental control unit

FDF fast death factor; fractional dimension filtering

FDFQ Food/Drink Frequency Questionnaire

FDFT farnesyldiphosphate farnesyltransferase

FDG [clinical] features of differential diagnosis; fluorine 18-labeled deoxyglucose; fluorodeoxyglucose [scan]

fdg feeding

FDGF fibroblast-derived growth factor

FDG-PET fluorodeoxyglucose positron emission tomography

FDH familial dysalbuminemic hyperthyroxinemia; focal dermal hypoplasia; formaldehyde dehydrogenase

FDI facial disability index; fibrillation detection interval; first dorsal interosseous [muscle]; frequency domain imaging; functional disability index; International Dental Federation [Fédération Dentaire Internationale]

FDIU fetal death in utero

FDK Feldkamp [algorithm]

FDL flexor digitorum longus

FDLMP first day of last menstrual period

FDLO fluorescent dye-labeled oligonucleotide

FDLV fer de lance virus

FDM fetus of diabetic mother; fibrous dysplasia of the mandible; finite differentiation method; fluorodeoxymannose

FDMP fluid depth at Morison's pouch

FDNB fluorodinitrobenzene

FDO Fleet Dental Officer

FDOPA fluorodihydroxyphenylalanine

FDP family doctor practice; fibrin degradation product; fibrinogen degradation product; flexor digitorum profundus; fructose-1,6-diphosphate; left frontoposterior [position of fetus]

FDPase fructose-1,6-diphosphatase

FDPM frequency domain photon migration

FDPS farnesyl diphosphate synthetase

FDPSL farnesyl diphosphate synthetase-like

FDQB flexor digiti quinti brevis

FDR first-degree relative; fractional disappearance rate

FDS Fellow in Dental Surgery; fiber duodenoscope; flexor digitorum superficialis

FDSRCSEng Fellow in Dental Surgery of the Royal College of Surgeons of England

FDT right frontotransverse [position of fetus]

FDTD finite difference time domain [method]

FdUrd fluorodeoxyuridine

(F)dUTP fluorescent deoxyuridine triphosphate

FDV Fiji disease virus; foliar decay virus; Friend disease virus

FDWT fast dyadic wavelet transform

FDXD flat dynamic x-ray image detector

FDZ fetal danger zone

FE fatty ester; fecal emesis; fetal erythroblastosis; fetal erythrocyte; figure eight [Doppler signal kernel]; finite element; fluid extract; fluorescent erythrocyte; forced expiration; formaldehyde-ethanol; frequency-encoded; frozen embryo

Fe female; ferret

F$_e$ fraction excreted [of dose]

fe female

FEA finite element analysis

feb fever [Lat. *febris*]

FEBP fetal estrogen-binding protein

FEBS Federation of European Biochemical Societies

FEB SZ febrile seizures

FEC fixed excitation codebook; forced expiratory capacity; free erythrocyte coproporphyrin; freestanding emergency center; Friend erythroleukemia cell

FECH ferrochelatase

FECG fetal electrocardiogram

F$_{ECO_2}$ fractional concentration of carbon dioxide in expired gas

FECP free erythrocyte coproporphyrin

FECSR flexion-extension cervical spine radiography

FECT fibroelastic connective tissue

FECU factor [VIII] correctional unit

FECV feline enteric coronavirus

FECVC functional extracellular fluid volume

FED field emission display; figure eight distribution; fish eye disease

FeD iron deficiency

Fed federal

FedNets Federal agency networks

FEDRIP Federal Research in Progress [database]

FedStats Federal statistics

FEE forced equilibrating expiration

FEEG fetal electroencephalography

FEER field echo with even echo rephasing

FEESST flexible endoscopic evaluation of swallowing with sensory testing

FEF forced expiratory flow

FEF$_{25-75}$ forced expiratory flow at 25–75% of forced vital capacity

FEF$_{50}$ forced expiratory flow at 50% of forced vital capacity

FEF$_{50}$/FIF$_{50}$ ratio of expiratory flow to inspiratory flow at 50% of forced vital capacity

FEFV forced expiratory flow volume

fEGG fast electrogastrogram

FEH focal epithelial hyperplasia

FEHBARS Federal Employee Health Benefit Acquisition Regulations

FEHBP Federal Employee Health Benefits Program

FEHBP-MSA Federal Employees Health Benefits Program-Medical Savings Account

Fe^{+2}Hgb ferromethemoglobin

Fe^{+3}Hgb ferrimethemoglobin

FeHV felid herpesvirus

FEIBA factor eight bypassing activity

FEKG fetal electrocardiogram

FEL familial erythrophagocytic lymphohistiocytosis

FELASA Federation of European Laboratory Animal Science Association

FELC Friend erythroleukemia cells

FeLV feline leukemia virus

FEM female; femur, femoral; finite element method [algorithm]; finite element model

fem female; femur, femoral

FEMA Federal Emergency Management Agency

FEMINA Felodipine ER and Metoprolol in the Treatment of Angina Pectoris

fem intern at inner side of the thighs [Lat. *femoribus internus*]

FEN flap endonuclease [protein]

Fen fenfluramine

FENa, FE$_{Na}$ fractional excretion of sodium

FEO familial expansile osteolysis

FE$_{O_2}$, F$_{EO_2}$ fractional concentration of oxygen in expired gas

FEOBV fluoroethoxybenzylvesamicol

FEP fluorinated ethylene-propylene; free erythrocyte protoporphyrin; front-end processing; front-end processor

FEPB functional electronic peroneal brace

FEPP free erythrocyte protoporphyrin

FER flexion, extension, rotation; fractional esterification rate; functional entity-relationship

fert fertility, fertilized

FES family environment scale; fat embolism syndrome; flame emission spectroscopy; forced expiratory spirogram; functional electrical stimulation

Fe/S iron/sulfur [protein]

FESO$_4$ ferrous sulfate

FESS functional endoscopic sinus surgery

FEST Fosinopril Efficacy/Safety Trial; Fosinopril on Exercise Tolerance [study]; Framework for European Services in Telemedicine

FeSV feline sarcoma virus

FET field-effect transistor; forced expiratory time

FETE Far Eastern tick-borne encephalitis

FETs forced expiratory time in seconds

FEUO for external use only
FEV familial exudative vitreoretinopathy; forced expiratory volume
FEV1, FEV₁ forced expiratory volume in one second
FEV₁% ratio of FEV_1 to FVC
fev fever
FEVB frequency ectopic ventricular beat
FEVR familial exudative vitreoretinopathy
FF degree of fineness of abrasive particles; fat-free; father factor; fecal frequency; fertility factor; field of Forel; filtration fraction; fine fiber; fine focus; finger flexion; finger-to-finger; fixation fluid; flat feet; flip-flop; fluorescent focus; follicular fluid; force fluids; forearm factor; forearm flow; forward flexion; foster father; free fraction; fresh frozen; fundus firm
F2F face-to-face
F-F femoro-femoral
ff⁺ fertility inhibition positive
ff⁻ fertility inhibition negative
FFA Fellow of the Faculty of Anaesthetists; free fatty acid
FFAP free fatty acid phase
FFARCS Fellow of the Faculty of Anaesthetists of the Royal College of Surgeons
FFB fat-free body; flexible fiberoptic bronchoscopy
FFC fixed flexion contracture; fluorescence flow cytometry; free from chlorine
FFCM Fellow of the Faculty of Community Medicine
FFD Fellow in the Faculty of Dentistry; finger-to-floor distance; focus-film distance; free-form deformations
FFDCA Federal Food, Drug, and Cosmetic Act
FFDD focal facial dermal dysplasia
FFDM full field digital mammography
FFDSRCS Fellow of the Faculty of Dental Surgery of the Royal College of Surgeons
FFDW fat-free dry weight
FFE fast field echo; fecal fat excretion
FFF degree of fineness of abrasive particles; field-flow fractionation; flicker fusion frequency
FFG free fat graft
FFGA Fonseca and Flaming algorithm
FFHC federally funded health center
FFHom Fellow of the Faculty of Homeopathy

FFI family function index; fatal familial insomnia; free from infection; fundamental frequency indicator
FFIT fluorescent focus inhibition test
FFL flexible fiberoptic laryngoscopy
FFM fat-free mass; friction force microscopy; fundus flavimaculatus
FFMDXA fat-free mass dual energy x-ray absorptiometry
FFMHYD fat-free mass hydrodensitometry
FFOM Fellow of the Faculty of Occupational Medicine
FFP freedom from progression; fresh frozen plasma
FFQ food frequency questionnaire
FFR Fellow of the Faculty of Radiologists
FFROM full and free range of motion
FFS failure-free survival; fat-free solids; fee for service; femoro-facial syndrome
FFT fast Fourier transform; finite Fourier transform; flicker fusion test or threshold
FFU femur-fibula-ulna [syndrome]; focal forming unit
FFV feline foamy virus; fruit fly virus
FFW fat-free weight
FFWC fractional free water clearance
FFWW fat-free wet weight
FG fasciculus gracilis; fast-glycolytic [fiber]; Feeley-Gorman [agar]; fibrinogen; Flemish giant [rabbit]
fg femtogram; flammable gas detector
FGA fibrinogen alpha
FGB fibrinogen beta
FGC fibrinogen gel chromatography
FGD fatal granulomatous disease
FgDP fibrinogen degradation products
FGDS fibrogastroduodenoscopy
FGDY faciogenital dysplasia
FGF father's grandfather; fibroblast growth factor; fresh gas flow
FGF1 fibroblast growth factor 1 [acidic]
FGF2 fibroblast growth factor 2 [basic]
FGFA fibroblast growth factor, acidic
FGFB fibroblast growth factor, basic
FGFR fibroblast growth factor receptor
FGG fibrinogen gamma; focal global glomerulosclerosis; fowl gamma-globulin
FGGM finite generalized gaussian mixture
FGH formylglutathione hydrolase
FGL fasting gastrin level; fasting glucose level

FGM father's grandmother; female genital mutilation

FGN fibrinogen; focal glomerulonephritis; fractional gaussian noise

FGP fundic gland polyp

FGR familial glucocorticoid resistance; finite time growth

FGS fibrogastroscopy; focal glomerular sclerosis; formal genesis syndrome

FGT fluorescent gonorrhea test

FH facial hemihyperplasia; familial hypercholesterolemia; familial hypertension; family history; fasting hyperbilirubinemia; favorable histology; femoral hernia; femoral hypoplasia; femur head; fetal head; fetal heart; fibromuscular hyperplasia; field hospital; flat hyperplasia; follicular hyperplasia; Frankfort horizontal [plane]; fumarate hydratase

FH$^+$ family history positive

FH$^-$ family history negative

FH$_4$ tetrahydrofolic acid

fh fostered by hand [experimental animal]

FHA familial hypoplastic anemia; Fellow of the Institute of Hospital Administrators; filamentous hemagglutinin

FHADES Farm Hazard and Demographic Enumeration Survey

FHB flexor hallucis brevis

FH/BC frontal horn/bicaudate [ratio]

FHC familial hypercholesterolemia; familial hypertrophic cardiomyopathy; family health center; Ficoll-Hypaque centrifugation; Fuchs heterochromic cyclitis

FHD familial histiocytic dermatoarthritis; family history of diabetes; femoral head diameter

FHF fetal heart frequency; fulminant hepatic failure

fHg free hemoglobin

FHH familial hypocalciuric hypercalcemia; fawn-hooded hypertensive [rat]; fetal heart heard

FHI Fuchs' heterochromic iridocyclitis

FHIP family health insurance plan

FHIS Farm Health Interview Survey

FHIT fragile histidine triad [gene]

FHL flexor hallucis longus; Food Hygiene Laboratory [UK]; functional health literacy; functional hearing loss

FHM familial hemiplegic migraine; fathead minnow [cells]

FHN family history negative

FHNH fetal heart not heard

FHP family history positive; functional health pattern

FHPMHP family history of physical and mental health problems

FHPSAT Functional Health Pattern Screening Assessment Tool

FHR familial hypophosphatemic rickets; fetal heart rate

fH-R factor H receptor

FHRDC family history research diagnostic criteria

FHRNST fetal heart rate nonstress test

FHRS Familial Hypercholesterolemia Regression Study

FHS Family Heart Study; fetal heart sound; fetal hydantoin syndrome; Floating Harbor syndrome; Framingham Heart Study

FH-S soluble fumarate hydratase

FHSA Family Health Service Authority [UK]

FHSD family history of sudden death

FHT fast Hartley transform; fetal heart; fetal heart tone

FHTG familial hypertriglyceridemia

FH-UFS femoral hypoplasia-unusual facies syndrome

FHV falcon herpesvirus; flock house virus

FHVP free hepatic vein pressure

FHx family history

FI fasciculus intrafascicularis; fever caused by infection; fibrinogen; fixed interval; flame ionization; follicular involution; food intolerance; forced inspiration; frontoiliac; full scan with interpolation

FIA fistula in ano; fluorescent immunoassay; focal immunoassay; Freund incomplete adjuvant

FIAC 2'-fluoro-5-iodo-aracytosine

FIB Fellow of the Institute of Biology; fibrin; fibrinogen; fibrositis; fibula

fib fiber; fibrillation; fibrin; fibrinogen; fibula

FIC finite-sample information criterion; Fogarty International Center; fractional inhibitory concentration

FICA Federal Insurance Contributions Act; fluoroimmunocytoadherence

FicCV *Ficus carica* virus

FICD Fellow of the Institute of Canadian Dentists; Fellow of the International College of Dentists

FiCO₂, FI_CO₂ fractional concentration of carbon dioxide in inspired gas

FICS Fellow of the International College of Surgeons

FICSIT Frailty and Injuries: Cooperative Studies of Intervention Techniques

FICU fetal intensive care unit

FID flame ionization detector; free induction decay; fungal immunodiffusion

FIDD fetal iodine deficiency disorder

FIELD Fenofibrate Intervention and Event Lowering in Diabetes [trial]

FIF feedback inhibition factor; fibroblast interferon; forced inspiratory flow; formaldehyde-induced fluorescence

FIF₅₀ forced inspiratory flow at 50% of forced vital capacity

FIFO first in, first out

FIFR fasting intestinal flow rate

FIFRA Federal Insecticide, Fungicide, and Rodenticide Act

FIG Flosequinan Investigator Group

FIGD familial idiopathic gonadotropin deficiency

FIGE field inversion gel electrophoresis

FIGLEAF Fine Grained Lexical Analysis Facility

FIGLU, FIGlu formiminoglutamate, formiminoglutamic acid

FIGLU-uria formiminoglutaminaciduria

FIGO International Federation of Gynecology and Obstetrics [Fédération Internationale de Gynécologie et d'Obstetrique]

FIH familial isolated hypoparathyroidism; fat-induced hyperglycemia

fil filament; filial

filt filter, filtration

FIM familial infantile myasthenia; field ion microscopy; fimbria; fluorescence imaged microdeformation; functional independence measure

FIMG familial infantile myasthenia gravis

FIMLT Fellow of the Institute of Medical Laboratory Technology

FIN fine intestinal needle

FINCC familial idiopathic nonarteriosclerotic cerebral calcification

FIND finding [UMLS]

FINESS First International New Intravascular Rigid-Flex Endovascular Stent Study

FINMONICA Finnish Monitoring Trends and Determinants in Cardiovascular Diseases

FINRISK Finland Cardiovascular Risk Study

FINV Fin V 707 virus

FI_O₂, forced inspiratory oxygen; fractional concentration of oxygen in inspired gas

FIO₂, FiO₂ fractional concentration of oxygen in inspired gas

FIP feline infectious peritonitis

FIPA familial intestinal polyatresia [syndrome]

FIPS Federal information processing standards; Frankfurt Isoptin Progression Study

FIPV feline infectious peritonitis virus

FIQ full-scale intelligence quotient

FIR far infrared; finite impulse response; fold increase in resistance; fractional intramural retention

FIRDA frontal, intermittent rhythmic delta activity

FIRM formal inference-based recursive modeling

FIRST Flolan International Randomized Survival Trial

FIS fatigue interview schedule; forced inspiratory spirogram; free induction signal

fis fission

FISAC Federal Information Services and Application Council

FISH Finnish Isradipine Study in Hypertension; fluorescence in situ hybridization

FISP fast imaging with steady state precision

FISS Fraxiparine in Stroke Study

fist fistula

FIT fluorescein isothiocyanate; Fracture Intervention Trial; fusion inferred threshold

FITC fluorescein isothiocyanate

FIUO for internal use only

FIV feline immunodeficiency virus; forced inspiratory volume

FIV₁ forced inspiratory volume in one second

FIVC forced inspiratory vital capacity

FIVE familial isolated vitamin E [deficiency]

FIV-O feline immunodeficiency virus (Oma)

FIV-P feline immunodeficiency virus (Petaluma)

FIXAg factor IX antigen

FJN familial juvenile nephrophthisis

FJRM full joint range of movement

FJS finger joint size

FK feline kidney

FK506 tacrolimus [drug]

FKBP FK506 [macrolide] binding protein

FK-NN fuzzy K-nearest neighbor [algorithm]

FKT Fukunaga-Koontz transform

FL false lumen; fatty liver; feline leukemia; femur length; fibers of Luschka; fibroblast-like; filtration leukapheresis; focal length; follicular lymphoma; Friend leukemia; frontal lobe; full liquid [diet]; functional length; fuzzy logic

FL-2 feline lung [cells]

Fl fluid; fluorescence

fL femtoliter

fl filtered load; flexion, flexible; flow; fluid; fluorescent; flutter; foot lambert

FLA fluorescent-labeled antibody; left frontoanterior [fetal position]

FLAC, FL/AC femur length/abdominal circumference [ratio]

flac flaccidity, flaccid

FLAIR fluid attenuated inversion recovery

FLAIR-FLASH fluid-attenuated inversion recovery-fast low angle shot

FLAK flow artifact killer

FLAP 5-lipoxygenase activating protein

FLARE Fluvastatin Angioplasty Restenosis [trial]

FLASH fast low angle shot

FLAV Flanders virus

FLC family life cycle; fatty liver cell; fetal liver cell; Fourier linear combiner; Friend leukemia cell

FICV flame chlorosis virus

FLD fibrotic lung disease; field hospital; Fisher's linear discriminate [pattern classification]

fld fluid

fl dr fluid dram

FLDV flounder lymphocystis disease

FLE fiducial localization error

FLEQUIN Flecainide Compared to Oral Quinidine [study]

FLEV Flexal virus

FLEX Federation Licensing Examination

flex flexor, flexion

FLEXOR Focused Lesion Expansion Optimizes Result [trial]

FLG filaggrin

FLIC functional living index-cancer

FLICC Federal Library and Information Center Committee

FLK funny looking kid

FLKS fatty liver and kidney syndrome

FLM fasciculus longitudinalis medialis; fraction of labeled mitosis

FLO Fourier linear combiner

floc flocculation

Flops floating point operations per second

fl oz fluid ounce

FLP fixed linear paralleling [computer-assisted surgery]; functional limitations profile; left frontoposterior [fetal position]

FLR fluorescent-labeled reference; funny looking rash

FLS fatty liver syndrome; Fellow of the Linnean Society; fibrous long-spacing [collagen]; filmless system; fixed least squares [algorithm]; flow-limiting segment

FLSP fluorescein-labeled serum protein

FLT left frontotransverse [fetal position]

FLU flumazenil; flunitrazepam; 5-fluorouracil; fluphenazine; flutamide

flu influenza

FLUAV Influenza A virus

FLUBV Influenza B virus

FLUCV Influenza C virus

FLUENT Fluvastatin Long-Term Extension Trial

fluor fluorescence; fluorescent; fluorometry; fluoroscopy

fluoro fluoroscope, fluoroscopy

FLV feline leukemia virus; Friend leukemia virus; fuzzy linguistic value

FM face mask; facilities management; family medicine; fat mass; feedback mechanism; fetal movement; fibrin monomer; fibromuscular; fibromyalgia; Fielding-Magliato [classification]; filtered mass; flavin mononucleotide; flowmeter; foramen magnum; forensic medicine; foster mother; frequency modulation; functional movement

FM2 flunitrazepam

Fm fermium

fM full mutation

f-M free metanephrine

fm femtometer; femtomole

FMA fluid movement; fluorescent microscopy; Frankfort mandibular plane angle; free of microcalcifications; full relaxation matrix analysis; functional motor activity

FMAP feeding mean arterial pressure

FMAT fetal movement acceleration test

f$_{max}$ maximum frequency

FMC family medicine center; field medical card; flight medicine clinic; focal macular choroidopathy; foundation for medical care

FMCG fetal magnetocardiography

FMD facility medical director; family medical doctor; fibromuscular dysplasia; foot and mouth disease; frontometaphyseal dysplasia

FMDI frequency modulation detection interference

FMDV foot and mouth disease virus

FME full mouth extraction

FMEA failure modes and effects analysis

Fmed median frequency

FMEG fetal magnetoencephalography

FMEL Friend murine erythroleukemia

FMEN familial multiple endocrine neoplasia

F-met, fMet formyl methionine

FMF familial Mediterranean fever; fetal movement felt; flow microfluorometry; forced midexpiratory flow

FMFD V familial multiple coagulation factor deficiency V

FMFM full mutation/full methylation

FMG five-mesh gauze; foreign medical graduate

FMGEMS Foreign Medical Graduate Examination in Medical Sciences

FMH family medical history; fat-mobilizing hormone; fetomaternal hemorrhage; fibromuscular hyperplasia; first metatarsal head

FMI fat mass index; Foods and Moods Inventory

FMIBMA fiber movement induced biological movement artifacts

FML flail mitral leaflet; fluorometholone

FMLA Family and Medical Leave Act

FMLP N-formyl-methionyl-leucyl-phenyl-alanine; formylpeptide

f-MLP N-formyl-methionyl-leucyl-phenyl-alanine

FMN first malignant neoplasm; flavin mononucleotide; frontomaxillonasal [suture]

FMNH, FMNH$_2$ reduced form of flavin mononucleotide

FMO flavin monooxygenase; Fleet Medical Officer; Flight Medical Officer

fmol femtomole

FMP faculty mentorship program; first menstrual period; fructose monophosphate

FMPIR fast multiplanar inversion recovery [imaging]

FMPM full mutation/partial methylation

FMPP familial male precocious puberty

FMPSPGR fast multiplanar spoiled gradient-recalled imaging [imaging]

FMR fragile site mental retardation [syndrome]; Friend-Moloney-Rauscher [antigen]

fMRA functional magnetic resonance angiography

F MRI fluorine magnetic resonance imaging

fMRI functional magnetic resonance imaging

FMRP fragile site mental retardation [syndrome] protein

FMS fat-mobilizing substance; fatty meal sonogram; Fellow of the Medical Society; fibromyalgia syndrome; Finnish Multicenter Study; Fragmin Multicenter Study; full mouth series

FMT Fragmin Multicenter Trial; frequency modulation detection threshold

FMTC familial medullary thyroid cancer

FMU first morning urine

F-MuLV Friend murine leukemia virus

FMX full mouth x-ray

FMZ flumazenil

FN false negative; fecal nitrogen; fibronectin; FitzHugh-Nagumo [model]; fluoride number

F-N finger to nose

fn function

FNA fine-needle aspiration

FNAB fine-needle aspiration biopsy

FNAC fine-needle aspiration cytology

fNaDC flounder sodium dicarboxylate [symporter]

FNB fine needle biopsy; food and nutrition board

FNBMD femoral neck bone mineral density

FnBPA fibronectin-binding protein A

FnBPB fibronectin-binding protein B

FNC fatty nutritional cirrhosis

FNCJ fine needle catheter jejunostomy

FND febrile neutrophilic dermatosis; frontonasal dysplasia; functional neck dissection

f-NE free norepinephrine

Fneg false negative

FNF false-negative fraction; femoral neck fracture

FNFMG foreign national foreign medical school graduate

FNH focal nodular hyperplasia

FNHR febrile nonhemolytic reaction

FNHTR febrile nonhemolytic transfusion reaction

FNIC Food and Nutrition Information Center [National Agricultural Library]

FNL fibronectin-like

f-NM free normetanephrine

FNN false nearest neighbor [pulse wave monitoring]

FNP family nurse practitioner

FNR false-negative rate; fibronectin receptor

FNRA fibronectin receptor alpha

FNRB fibronectin receptor beta

FNRBL fibronectin receptor beta-like

FNS frontier nursing service; functional neuromuscular stimulation

FNT false neurochemical transmitter; farnesyltransferase

FNTA farnesyltransferase alpha

FNTB farnesyltransferase beta

FNTC fine-needle transhepatic cholangiography

FNZ flunarizine

FO fiberoptic; fish oil; foot arthrosis; foramen ovale; forced oscillation; fronto-occipital

Fo fomentation, fomenting

FOA Federation of Orthodontic Associations

FOAR facio-oculo-acoustico-renal [syndrome]

FOAVF failure of all vital forces

FOB fecal occult blood; feet out of bed; fiberoptic bronchoscopy; foot of bed; functional observational battery

FOBT fecal occult blood test

FOC fronto-occipital circumference

FOCAL formula calculation

FOD figure of demerit [radiotherapy]; focus-to-object distance; free of disease

F-ODN fluorescein-labeled oligodeoxyribonucleotide

FOG fast oxidative glycolytic [fiber]

FOL folate

FOLR folate receptor

FOM figure-of-merit

FOMi 5-fluorouracil, vincristine, and mitomycin C

F-OMP fluorescein-labeled oligonucleoside methylphosphonate

FOOB fell out of bed

FOOD Feed or Ordinary Diet [trial]

FOOSH fell onto [his or her] outstretched hand

FOP fibrodysplasia ossificans progressiva; forensic pathology

FOPR full outpatient rate

F-OPT fluorescein-labeled oligonucleoside phosphorothioate

For foramen; forensic

for foreign; formula

FORECAST Fractional Flow Reserve or Relative Fractional Velocity Reserve Evaluation of Coronary Artery Stenosis vs Thallium

FORIMG foreign national international medical school graduate

form formula

FORT Fish Oil Restenosis Trial

FORTRAN formula translation

FORV Forecariah virus

FOS fast orthogonal search; fiberoptic sigmoidoscopy; fixation-off sensitivity; fractional osteoid surface; Framingham Offspring Study

FOSIT Fosamax International Trial

Fos-R foscarnet-resistant

Fos-R HIV foscarnet-resistant human immunodeficiency virus

FOSS Framingham Offspring-Spouse Study

FOUV Foula virus

FOV field of view

FOX ferrous xylenol orange

FP false positive; familial porencephaly; family physician; family planning; family practice; family practitioner; Fanconi pancytopenia; fast pathway [heart electrical activity]; femoropopliteal; fetoprotein; fibrinolytic potential; fibrinopeptide; fibrous proliferation; field pronouncement; filling pressure; filter paper; finite particle; fixation protein; flank pain; flash point; flavin phosphate; flavoprotein; flexor profundus; flow probe; fluid percussion; fluid pressure; fluorescence polarization; fluorescent probe; fluticazone propionate; food poisoning; food processing; forearm pronated; freezing point; frontoparietal; frontopolar; frozen plasma; full period; fusion peptide; fusion point

F-P fronto-popliteal

F:P fluorescence:protein [ratio]

F1P, F-1-P fructose-1-phosphate

F6P, F-6-P fructose-6-phosphate

Fp fibrinopeptide; frontal polar electrode placement in electroencephalography

fp flexor pollicis; foot-pound; forearm pronated; freezing point

FPA Family Planning Association; Federal Privacy Act; fibrinopeptide A or alpha; filter paper activity; fluorophenylalanine; foot progression angle

FpA fibrinopeptide A or alpha

FPB femoral popliteal bypass; fibrinopeptide B or beta; flexor pollicis brevis

FpB fibrinopeptide B or beta

FPBA fluorescence photobleaching analysis

FPBC false-positive blood culture

FPC familial polyposis coli; family planning clinic; fish protein concentrate

FPCA family practice comfort assessment

FpCA 1-fluoromethyl-2-*p*-chlorophenylethylamine

FPD feto-pelvic disproportion; flame photometric detector; flat panel detector

FPDM fibrocalculous pancreatic diabetes mellitus

FPE fatal pulmonary embolism; field placement error; final prediction error

F-18-PET fluoride ion-positron emission tomography

FPF false positive fraction; fibroblast pneumocyte factor

FPG fasting plasma glucose; fluorescence plus Giemsa; focal proliferative glomerulonephritis

FPGA field programmable gate array; field programmable generic array

FPGS folylpolyglutamate synthetase

FPH₂ reduced form of flavin phosphate

FPHE formaldehyde-treated pyruvaldehyde-stabilized human erythrocytes

FPHT fosphenytoin

FPI femoral pulsatility index; flat panel imager; fluid percussion injury; formula protein intolerance; Freiburg Personality Identification Questionnaire

FPIA fluorescence polarization immunoassay

FPK fructose phosphokinase

FPL familial partial lipodystrophy; fasting plasma lipids; flexor pollicis longus

FPLC fast protein liquid chromatography

FPLV feline panleukemia virus

FPM filter paper microscopic [test]; fine particle mass; full passive movements

fpm feet per minute

FPN ferric chloride, perchloric acid, and nitric acid [solution]; fuzzy Petri net

FPO faciopalatoosseous [syndrome]; Federation of Prosthodontic Organizations; freezing point osmometer

FPP faculty practice plan; free portal pressure

FPPH familial primary pulmonary hypertension

FPR false-positive rate; finger peripheral resistance; fluorescence photobleaching recovery; *N*-formylpeptide receptor; fractional proximal resorption

FPRA first pass radionuclide angiogram

FPRH *N*-formylpeptide receptor homolog

FPS farnesylpyrophosphate synthetase; Fellow of the Pathological Society; Fellow of the Pharmaceutical Society; fetal PCB (polychlorinated biphenyl) syndrome; footpad swelling; frames per second

fps feet per second; frames per second

FPSA fractional positive surface area

FPSL farnesylpyrophosphate synthetase-like

FPSTS false-positive serologic test for syphilis

FPT farnesyl protein transferase

FPTase farnesyl-protein transferase

FPV Facey's Paddock virus; feline parvovirus; feline pseudoleukemia virus; feline pseudoleukopenia virus; fowl plague virus; fowlpox virus; Fraser point virus

FPVB femoral popliteal vein bypass

FQHC federally qualified health center

FQPA Food Quality Protection Act

fQSR filtered QSR [ECG]

FR faculty rater; failure rate; fasciculus retroflexus; febrile reaction; feedback regulation; film-screen radiograph; Fischer-Race [notation]; fixed ratio; flocculation reaction; flow rate; fluid restriction; fluid resuscitation; fluid retention; framework region [immunoglobulin]; free radical; frequency of respiration; frequent relapses

F2R [blood coagulation] factor II receptor

F&R force and rhythm [pulse]

Fr fracture; francium; franklin [unit charge]; French; frequency or frequent

Fr1 first fraction

f$_R$ respiratory frequency

FRA fibrinogen-related antigen; fluorescent rabies antibody

fra fragile [site]

FRAC Food Research and Action Center

frac fracture

fract fracture

FrAdV frog adenovirus

F( )R:Ag factor ( ) related antigen

FRAME Fund for the Replacement of Animals in Medical Experiments

FRAMI Fragmin in Acute Myocardial Infarction [study]

FRAP fluorescence recovery after photobleaching

FRAT free radical assay technique

FRAX fragile [chromosome] X

fra(X) chromosome X fragility; fragile X chromosome, fragile X syndrome

FRAXA fragile X syndrome A

FRAXE fragile X syndrome E

FRAXIDIS Fraxiparine in Post-Hospital Discharge [study]

FRAXIS Fraxiparine in Ischemic Syndromes [study]

FRAX-MR fragile X-mental retardation [syndrome]

FRAXODI Fraxiparine Once Daily Injection [study]

Fr BB fracture of both bones

FRC Federal Radiation Council; frozen red cells; functional reserve capacity; functional residual capacity

F( )R:C factor ( ) related cofactor activity

FRCD Fellow of the Royal College of Dentists; fixed ratio combination drug

FRCGP Fellow of the Royal College of General Practitioners

FRCOG Fellow of the Royal College of Obstetricians and Gynaecologists

FRCP Fellow of the Royal College of Physicians

FRCPA Fellow of the Royal College of Pathologists of Australia

FRCPath Fellow of the Royal College of Pathologists

FRCP(C) Fellow of the Royal College of Physicians of Canada

FRCPE Fellow of the Royal College of Physicians of Edinburgh

FRCPI Fellow of the Royal College of Physicians of Ireland

FRCPsych Fellow of the Royal College of Psychiatrists

FRCS Fellow of the Royal College of Surgeons

FRCS(C) Fellow of the Royal College of Surgeons of Canada

FRCSEd Fellow of the Royal College of Surgeons of Edinburgh

FRCSEng Fellow of the Royal College of Surgeons of England

FRCSI Fellow of the Royal College of Surgeons of Ireland

FRCVS Fellow of the Royal College of Veterinary Surgeons

FRD fumarate dehydrogenase

frd fumarate dehydrogenase [gene]

FRDA Friedreich ataxia

FRD A fumarate dehydrogenase A

FRDA-Acad Acadian Friedreich ataxia

FRD B fumarate dehydrogenase B

FRD C fumarate dehydrogenase C

FRD D fumarate dehydrogenase D

FRE Fischer rat embryo; flow-related enhancement

FREFLEX force reflecting exoskeleton

FREIR Federal Research on Biological and Health Effects of Ionizing Radiation

frem fremitus

freq frequency

FRES Fellow of the Royal Entomological Society

FRESCO Florence Randomized Elective Stenting in Acute Coronary Occlusion [study]

FRESH food re-education for elementary school health [program]

FRET fluorescence resonance energy transfer

FRF Fertility Research Foundation; follicle-stimulating hormone-releasing factor

FRFC functional renal failure of cirrhosis

FRH follicle-stimulating hormone-releasing hormone

FRh fetal rhesus monkey [kidney cell]

FRhK fetal rhesus monkey kidney [cell]

FRHS fast-repeating high sequence

FRIC Fragmin in Unstable Coronary Artery Disease [trial]

frict friction

FRIPHH Fellow of the Royal Institute of Public Health and Hygiene

FRISC Fragmin During Instability in Coronary Artery Disease [trial]

FRISCII Fragmin and/or Revascularization during Instability in Coronary Artery Disease [trial]

FRIV frijoles virus

FRJM full range joint movement

FRMedSoc Fellow of the Royal Medical Society

FrMLV Friend murine leukemia virus

FRMS Fellow of the Royal Microscopical Society

FrMV Frangipani mosaic virus

FRNN fuzzy rough nearest neighbor [algorithm]

FRNS Fryns syndrome

FRO floor reaction orthosis

fROAT flounder renal organic anion transporter

FROC free receiver operating characteristic

FROG French Rotablator Group [study]

FROM full range of movements

FROST French Optimal Stenting Trial

FRP follicle-stimulating hormone releasing protein; functional refractory period

FRS Fellow of the Royal Society; ferredoxin-reducing substance; first rank symptom; fragment separator; furosemide

FRSH Fellow of the Royal Society of Health

FRT Family Relations Test; full recovery time

Fru fructose

FRV full-length retroviral [sequence]; functional residual volume

Frx fracture

FS factor of safety; Fanconi syndrome; feasibility study; febrile seizures; Felty syndrome; fetoscopy; fibrin sealant; fibromyalgia syndrome; fibrosarcoma; field stimulation; file server; fine structure; Fisher syndrome; flexible sigmoidoscope; fluorescence spectrometry; food service; forearm supination; fractional shortening; fracture site; fragile site; frequency-shifted [imaging]; Friesinger score; frozen section; full scale [IQ]; full sensitivity; full soft [diet]; full strength; functional shortening; function study; functional system; human foreskin [cells]; simple fracture

%FS percent fractional shortening

F/S female, spayed [animal]; frozen section

FSA fast simulated annealing; flexible spending account

FSB fetal scalp blood

FSBA fluorosulfonylbenzoyladenosine

FSBP finger systolic blood pressure

FSBT Fowler single breath test

FSC finite sample criterion; Food Standards Committee; forward scatter

FSCCL follicular small cleaved cell lymphoma

FSCR flexible surface coil-type resonator

FSD focus-skin distance

FSE fast spin echo; feline spongiform encephalopathy; filtered smoke exposure

FSE-IR fast spin echo-inversion recovery [imaging]

FSEV *Figulus subleavis* entomopoxvirus

FSF fibrin stabilizing factor; front surface fluorescence

FSG fasting serum glucose; focal segmental sclerosis

FSGHS focal segmental glomerular hyalinosis and sclerosis

FSGN focal sclerosing glomerulonephritis

FSGS focal segmental glomerulosclerosis

FSH fascioscapulohumeral; focal and segmental hyalinosis; follicle-stimulating hormone

FSHB follicle-stimulating hormone, beta chain

FSHD facioscapulohumeral muscular dystrophy

FSH/LR-RH follicle-stimulating hormone and luteinizing hormone releasing hormone

FSHR follicle-stimulating hormone receptor

FSH-RF follicle-stimulating hormone-releasing factor

FSH-RH follicle-stimulating hormone-releasing hormone

FSHSMA facioscapulohumeral spinal muscular atrophy

FSI foam stability index; Food Sanitation Institute; functional status index

FSIQ full-scale intelligence quotient

FSL fasting serum level

FSM finite state machine

FSMB Federation of State Medical Boards

FSMC forward support medical company

FSN functional stimulation, neuromuscular

FSOP free-standing surgical outpatient facility

FSP familial spastic paraplegia; femoral hole sagittal positioning; fibrinogen split products; fibrin split products; fine suspended particles

F-SP special form [Lat. *forma specialis*]

FSPB finite-size pencil beam [radiation]

FSPGR fast spoiled gradient-recalled acquisition in steady state [MRI]

FSQ Functional Status Questionnaire

FSR Fellow of the Society of Radiographers; film screen radiography; force sensing resistor; force sensing retractor; forward stepping regression; fragmented sarcoplasmic reticulum; full scale range; fusiform skin revision

FSRS functional status rating system

FSS focal segmental sclerosis; Freeman-Sheldon syndrome; French steel sound; functional system scale; fuzzy shell segmentation [algorithm]

FST foam stability test

FSU family service unit; functional spine unit; functional subunit

FSUM focused segmented ultrasound machine

FSV feline fibrosarcoma virus; Fort Sherman virus; forward stroke volume

FSW female sex worker; field service worker

FT Fallot tetralogy; false transmitter; family therapy; farnesyl transferase; fast twitch; fatigue trial; femorotibial; fibrous tissue; fingertip; follow through; force target; Fourier transform; free testosterone; free thyroxine; full term; function test

FT$_3$ free triiodothyronine

FT$_4$ free thyroxine

Ft ferritin

fT free testosterone

ft foot, feet

FTA femorotibial angle; fibrin tissue adhesive; fluorescent titer antibody; fluorescent treponemal antibody

FTA-ABS, FTA-Abs fluorescent treponemal antibody, absorbed [test]

FTAG, F-TAG fast-binding target-attaching globulin

FTAS familial testicular agenesis syndrome

FTase farnesyl transferase

FTAT fluorescent treponemal antibody test

FTB front-to-back [visualization]

FTBD fit to be detained; full-term born dead

FTBE focal tick-borne encephalitis

FTBI fractionated total body irradiation

FTBS Family Therapist Behavioral Scale

FTC Federal Trade Commission; Fibrinolysis Trialists Collaboration; fibulotalocalcaneal [ligament]; follicular thyroid carcinoma; frequency threshold curve; frequency tuning curve

ftc foot candle

FTD femoral total density; frontotemporal dementia

FTDS familial testicular dysgenesis syndrome

FTE full-time equivalent

FTEE full-time employee equivalent

FTF finger to finger

FTFT fast time frequency transform

FTG full-thickness graft

FTH ferritin heavy chain; fracture threshold

FTI farnesyl transferase inhibitor; free thyroxine index

FT$_3$I free triiodothyronine index

FT$_4$I free thyroxine index

FTIR Fourier transform infrared; functional terminal innervation ratio

FTKA failed to keep appointment

FTL ferritin light chain
ftL foot lambert
FTLB full-term live birth
ft lb foot pound
FTLV feline T-lymphotropic lentivirus
FTM fluid thioglycolate medium; fractional test meal
FTMS Fourier transform mass spectrometry
FTN finger to nose
FTNB full-term newborn
FTND full-term normal delivery
FTO fructose-terminated oligosaccharide
FTP file transfer protocol [sending and receiving files from remote computers on the Internet]
FTQ Fagerström Tolerance Questionnaire
FTR fractional tubular reabsorption
FTS family tracking system; feminizing testis syndrome; fetal tobacco syndrome; fissured tongue syndrome; flexor tenosynovitis; thymulin [Fr. *facteur thymique sérique*]
FTSG full thickness skin graft
FTT failure to thrive; fat tolerance test; Fibrinolytic Therapy Trialist [collaboration]
FTU fluorescence thiourea
FTVD full term vaginal delivery
FU fecal urobilinogen; fetal urobilinogen; fluorouracil; flux unit [ion]; follow-up; fractional urinalysis; fundus
Fu Finsen unit
F/U follow-up, fundus of umbilicus
F&U flanks and upper quadrants
5-FU 5-fluorouracil
FUB functional uterine bleeding
FUC fucosidase
Fuc fucose
FUCA fucosidase alpha
FUCA1 alpha-L-fucosidase gene
FUDR, FUdR fluorodeoxyuridine
FUF functional unification formalism
FUFA free volatile fatty acid
FUKAV Fukuoka virus
FULL fully formed anatomical structure [UMLS]
FUM 5-fluorouracil and methotrexate; fumarate; fumigation
FUMIR 5-fluorouracil, mitomycin C, radiation
FUMP fluorouridine monophosphate
FUN follow-up note

FUNC functional concept [UMLS]
funct function, functional
FUO fever of unknown origin
FUOV follow-up office visit
FUR 5-fluorouracil and radiation; fluorouracil riboside; fluorouridine; follow-up report; furin membrane-associated receptor
FUS feline urologic syndrome; first-use syndrome; focused ultrasound surgery; fusion
FuSV Fujinami sarcoma virus
FUT fibrinogen uptake test; fucosyl transferase
FUTP fluoridine triphosphate
FV femoral vein; fetal vaccinia; fever virus; fibroma virus; filiform virus; flow velocity; fluid volume; foamy virus; Fomede virus; Friend virus; Frog virus
Fv variable region antibody fragment
F(v) velocity distribution function
FVA Friend virus anemia
FVB Friend virus B-type
FVC false vocal cord; femoral vein cannulation; forced vital capacity
FVCC First Virtual Congress of Cardiology
FVE forced volume expiration
fVEP flash-evoked visual potential
FVI flow velocity interval
FVL factor V Leiden mutation; femoral vein ligation; flow volume loop; force, velocity, length
FVOP finger venous opening pressure
FVP Friend virus polycythemia
FVPF Family Violence Prevention Fund
FVR feline viral rhinotracheitis; forearm vascular resistance
FVS fetal valproate syndrome; Fig virus S
FVT follicular-variant-translocation
f/V$_T$ frequency-to-tidal volume ratio
FW Felix-Weil [reaction]; Folin-Wu [reaction]; fragment wound
Fw F wave
fw fresh water
FWA Family Welfare Association
FWB full weight bearing
FWHM full width at half maximum [resolution or measurement]
FWPCA Federal Water Pollution Control Administration
FWPV fowlpox virus

FWR Felix-Weil reaction; Folin-Wu reaction

FWTM full width tenth maximum

FX factor X; fluoroscopy; fornix; fracture; frozen section

Fx fracture

fx fracture; friction

FXa factor Xa

FXD fexofenadine

Fx-dis fracture-dislocation

FXN function

FXS fragile X syndrome

fx/V$_T$ frequency/tidal volume [ratio]

FY fiscal year; full year

FYI for your information

FYMS fourth-year medical student

FZ focal zone; furazolidone

Fz frontal midline placement of electrodes in electroencephalography

FZS Fellow of the Zoological Society

G

G acceleration [force]; conductance; free energy; gallop; ganglion; gap; gas; gastrin; gauge; gauss; genome, genomic; geometric efficiency; giga; gingiva, gingival; glabella; globular; globulin; glucose; glycine; glycogen; goat; gold inlay; gonidial; good; goose; grade [TNM (tumor-node-metastasis) classification: **GX** grade cannot be assessed, **G1** well differentiated tumor, **G2** moderately differentiated tumor, **G3** poorly differentiated tumor, **G4** undifferentiated tumor]; Grafenberg spot; gram; gravida; gravitation constant; Greek; green; guanidine; guanine; guanosine; gynecology; unit of force of acceleration

G- giga- [10^9]

G$_0$ quiescent phase of cells leaving the mitotic cycle

1G first generation

G1 well differentiated tumor [TNM (tumor-node-metastasis) classification]

G$_1$ presynthetic gap [phase of cells prior to DNA synthesis]

GI primigravida

2G second generation

G2 moderately differentiated tumor [TNM (tumor-node-metastasis) classification]

G$_2$ postsynthetic gap [phase of cells following DNA synthesis]

GII secundigravida

G3 poorly differentiated tumor [TNM (tumor-node-metastasis) classification]

GIII tertigravida

G4 undifferentiated tumor [TNM (tumor-node-metastasis) classification]

G° standard free energy

g force [pull of gravity]; gap; gauge; gender; grain; gram; gravity; group; ratio of magnetic moment of a particle to the Bohr magneton; standard acceleration due to gravity, 9.80665 m/s^2

g relative centrifugal force

γ see *gamma*

GA Gamblers Anonymous; gastric analysis; gastric antrum; general anesthesia; general angiography; general appearance; genetic algorithm; gentisic acid; germ-cell antigen; gestational age; gibberellic acid; gingivoaxial; glucoamylase; glucose; glucose/acetone; glucuronic acid; Golgi apparatus; gramicidin A; granulocyte adherence; granuloma annulare; guessed average; gut-associated; gyrate atrophy

GA1 genetic algorithm 1 [based on algebraic rules]

GA2 genetic algorithm 2 [fuzzy logic based on mutation strategy]

G/A globulin/albumin [ratio]

Ga gallium; granulocyte agglutination

Gα G protein subunit alpha complex

ga gauge

GAA gossypol acetic acid

GAAS Goldberg Anorectic Attitude Scale

GABA, gaba gamma-aminobutyric acid

GABA$_A$ gamma-aminobutyric acid ionotropic receptor family A

GABA$_B$ gamma-aminobutyric acid ionotropic receptor family B

GABA$_C$ gamma-aminobutyric acid ionotropic receptor family C

GABAT, GABA-T gamma-aminobutyric acid transaminase

GABHS group A beta-hemolytic streptococcus

GABI German Angioplasty Bypass Intervention [trial]; German Angioplasty Bypass Surgery Investigation

GABOA gamma-amino-beta-hydroxybutyric acid

GABRA gamma-aminobutyric acid alpha receptor

GAC general ambulatory care

GACELISA immunoglobulin G [IgG] capture enzyme-linked immunosorbent assay [ELISA]

GACT government activity [UMLS]

GAD generalized anxiety disorder; glutamic acid decarboxylase

GADFLI general absorbed [radiation] dose and fluence investigation

GADH gastric alcohol dehydrogenase

GADS gonococcal arthritis/dermatitis syndrome

GAdV goat [caprine] adenovirus

GAEIB Group of Advisors on the Ethical Implications of Biotechnology [European Economic Community]

GAERS genetic absence epilepsy rats from Strasbourg

GAF global assessment of functioning [scale]

GAFeSV Gardner-Arnstein feline sarcoma virus

GAFG goal attainment follow-up guide

GAG glycosaminoglycan; group-specific antigen

GAH glyceraldehyde

GAHS galactorrhea-amenorrhea hyperprolactinemia syndrome

GaHV gallid herpesvirus

GAIN Glycine Antagonist GV150526 in Acute Stroke [trial]

GaIN Georgia Interactive Network for Medical Information

GAIP human G_α interacting protein

GAIPAS General Audit Inpatient Psychiatric Assessment Scale

GAIT-ER-AID Gait Explanation and Reasoning Aid [computer gait analysis system]

GAL galactose; galactosyl; glucuronic acid lactone

Gal galactose

gal galactose; gallon

GALBP galactose-binding protein

GALC, GalC galactocerebroside

GALE galactose epimerase

GALK galactokinase

GalN galactosamine

GalNAc *N*-acetylgalactosamine

GALNS galactosamine-4-sulfatase

Gal-1-P galactose-1-phosphate

GalR galanin receptor

GALT galactose-1-*p*-uridyltransferase; gut-associated lymphoid tissue

GALV gibbon ape leukemia virus

Galv, galv galvanic

Gα G protein subunit alpha complex

GAM geographical analysis machine

GAME immunoglobulins G, A, M, and E

GAMIS German-Austrian Myocardial Infarction Study

GAMM generalized abstract medical model

γ Greek letter *gamma*; a carbon separated from the carboxyl group by two other carbon atoms; a constituent of the gamma protein plasma fraction; heavy chain of immunogammaglobulin; a monomer in fetal hemoglobin; photon

*γ*G immunoglobulin G

GAMP German-Austrian Multicenter Project

GAMS German-Austrian Multicenter Study

GAMV Gamboa virus

GAN giant axon neuropathy

G and D growth and development

gang, gangl ganglion, ganglionic

GANS granulomatous angiitis of the nervous system

GAO general accounting office

GAP glottal area patency; D-glyceraldehyde-3-phosphate; growth associated protein; guanosine triphosphatase-activating protein

GAPD, GAPDH glyceraldehyde-3-phosphate dehydrogenase

GAPDP glyceraldehyde-3-phosphate dehydrogenase pseudogene

GAPO growth retardation, alopecia, pseudo-anodontia, and optic atrophy [syndrome]

GAPST global average peri-stimulus time

GarCLV garlic common latent virus

GarLV garlic latent virus

GarMbFV garlic mite-borne filamentous virus

GarMbLV garlic mite-borne latent virus

GARS German-Austrian Reinfarction Study; glycine amide phosphoribosyl synthetase

GART genotype antiretroviral resistance test

GARV Garba virus

GAS galactorrhea-amenorrhea syndrome; gastric acid secretion; gastrin; gastroenterology; general adaptation syndrome; generalized arteriosclerosis; global anxiety score; global assessment scale; goal attainment scale; group A *Streptococcus*; growth arrest-specific [gene]

GASA growth-adjusted sonographic age

GASCIS German-Austrian Space-occupying Cerebellar Infarction Study

GASP Group Against Smoking Pollution [study]

gastroc gastrocnemius [muscle]

GAT gamma aminobutyric acid transporter; gelatin agglutination test; geriatric assessment team; Gerontological Apperception Test; group adjustment therapy

GATB Global Alliance for TB Drug Development

GATR group attribute [UMLS]

GAUS German Activator Urokinase Study

GAVI Global Alliance for Vaccines and Immunization

GAWTS genomic amplification with transcript sequencing

GAXS German and Austrian Xamoterol Study

GB gallbladder; gigabyte; glial bundle; goof balls; Guillain-Barré [syndrome]

Gb gigabit; gilbert

gB glycoprotein B

GBA ganglionic blocking agent; gingivobuccoaxial

GBAP glucocerebrosidase pseudogene

GBD gallbladder disease; gender behavior disorder; glass blower's disease; Global Burden of Disease [study]; granulomatous bowel disease

Gβ G protein subunit beta complex

GBF/DIME Geographic Base File Dual Independent Map Encoding [Bureau of Census file]

GBG glycine-rich beta-glycoprotein; gonadal steroid-binding globulin

GBH gamma-benzene hexachloride; graphite benzalkonium-heparin

GBHA glyoxal-bis-(2-hydroxyanil)

GBI globulin-binding insulin

GBIA Guthrie bacterial inhibition assay

GBL glomerular basal lamina

GBM glioblastoma multiforme; glomerular basement membrane

GBP gabapentin; galactose-binding protein; gastric bypass; gated blood pool

GBpd gigabits per day

Gbps gigabits per second

Gbq gigabequerel

GBR guided bone regeneration

GBS gallbladder series; gastric bypass surgery; general biopsychosocial screening; glycerine-buffered saline [solution]; group B *Streptococcus*; Guillain-Barré syndrome

GBSS Gey's balanced saline solution; Guillain-Barré-Strohl syndrome

GC ganglion cell; gas chromatography; general circulation; general closure; general condition; generalizability coefficient; generalized coherence; genetic counseling; geriatric care; germinal center; giant cell; glucocerebrosidase; glucocorticoid; goblet cell; Golgi cell; gonococcus; gonorrhea; granular casts; granulomatous colitis;

granulosa cell; group-specific component; guanine cytosine; guanylate (or guanylyl) cyclase

Gc galactocerebroside; gigacycle; gonococcus; group-specific component

gC glycoprotein C

GCA gastric cancer area; giant cell arteritis

g-cal gram calorie

GCAP germ-cell alkaline phosphatase

GCAT Guideline Compliance Assessment Tool

GCB gonococcal base

GC-B guanylate cyclase B

gCBF global cerebral blood flow

GCBM glomerular capillary basement membrane

GCD graft coronary disease

GCDFP gross cystic disease fluid protein

GCF growth-rate-controlling factor

GCFT gonococcal/gonorrhea complement fixation test

GCFV ginger chlorotic fleck virus

GCG galactosyl ceramide beta-galactosidase; Genetics Computer Group; glucagon

GCGR glucagon receptor; glucocorticoid receptor

GCH granular clinical history

GCI General Cognitive Index; glottal closure instant

GCIIS glucose controlled insulin infusion system

GCK glomerulocystic kidney; glucokinase

GCL giant-cell lesion; globoid cell leukodystrophy

GCLO gastric *Campylobacter*-like organism

GCM Gorlin-Chaudhry-Moss [syndrome]

g-cm gram-centimeter

gCMRO₂ global cerebral oxygen uptake

GC-MS gas chromatography-mass spectrometry

GC/MS gas chromatography/mass spectrometry

GCN geometric constraint network; giant cerebral neuron

GCNA Genetic Confidentiality and Non-discrimination Act

GCNF glial cell-derived neurotrophic factor

g-coef generalizability coefficient

GCOP glucocorticoid-induced osteoporosis

GCP geriatric cancer population; German Cardiovascular Prevention [study]; good clinical practices; granulocyte chemotactic protein

GCPS Greig cephalopolysyndactyly syndrome

GCR glucocorticoid receptor; Group Conformity Rating

GCRC General Clinical Research Center [of NIH]

GCRG giant-cell reparative granuloma

GCRS gynecological chylous reflux syndrome

GCS general clinical services; Gianotti-Crosti syndrome; Glasgow Coma Scale; global coordinate system [computer-assisted surgery]; glucocorticosteroid; glutamylcysteine synthetase; glycine cleavage system

GCSA Gross cell surface antigen

GCSE generalized convulsive status epilepticus

G-CSF granulocyte colony-stimulating factor

GCSFR granulocyte colony-stimulating factor receptor

GCSP glycine cleavage system protein

GCT general care and treatment; germ-cell tumor; giant cell thyroiditis; giant cell tumor

GC(T)A giant cell (temporal) arteritis

GC-TEA gas chromatography thermal energy analyzer

GCTTS giant cell tumor of tendon sheath

GCU gonococcal urethritis

GCV ganciclovir; great cardiac vein

GCVF great cardiac vein flow

GCV-TP ganciclovir triphosphate

GCW glomerular capillary wall

GCWM General Conference on Weights and Measures

GCY gastroscopy

GD gadolinium; gastroduodenal; Gaucher disease; general diagnostics; general dispensary; gestational day; Gianotti disease; gonadal dysgenesis; Graves disease; growth and development; growth delay

Gd gadolinium

gD glycoprotein D

gD2 glycoprotein D2

G&D growth and development

GDA gastroduodenal artery; general daily activity; germine diacetate; Graves disease autoantigen

GDAC Generic Drugs Advisory Committee [FDA]

GDB gas density balance; Genome Database; guide dogs for the blind

GDC General Dental Council; giant dopamine-containing cell; Guglielmi detachable coil [x-ray imaging]

Gd-CDTA gadolinium-cyclohexane-diamine-tetraacetic acid

GDCMS German Dilated Cardiomyopathy Study

Gd-DOTA gadolinium-tetra-azacyclo-dodecatetraacetic acid

Gd-DTPA gadolinium-diethylene-triamine-pentaacetic acid

GDE Genetic Data Environment

Gd-EDTA gadolinium diethylene-triamine-pentaacetic acid

GDEP general dielectrophoretic [force]

GDF gel diffusion precipitin; growth differentiation factor

GDH glucose dehydrogenase; glutamate dehydrogenase; glycerophosphate dehydrogenase; glycol dehydrogenase; gonadotropin hormone; growth and differentiation hormone

GDI common gateway interface; guanidine nucleotide dissociation inhibitor

GDID genetically determined immunodeficiency disease

g/dL grams per deciliter

GDM gestational diabetes mellitus

GDMO General Duties Medical Officer

GdMP gadolinium mesoporphyrin

GDMS glow discharge mass spectrometry

gDNA genomic deoxyribonucleic acid

GDNF glial cell line derived neutrophilic factor

GDP gel diffusion precipitin; gross domestic product; guanosine diphosphate

GDS General Dental Service [UK]; geriatric depression scale; Global Deterioration Scale; Gordon Diagnostic System [for attention disorders]; gradual dosage schedule; guanosine diphosphate dissociation stimulator

GDT geometrically deformable template

GDU gastroduodenal ulcer

GDV garlic dwarf virus

GDW glass-distilled water

GDXY XY gonadal dysgenesis

GE gastric emptying; gastroemotional; gastroenteritis; gastroenterology; gastroenterostomy; gastroesophageal; gastrointestinal endoscopy; gel electrophoresis; generalized epilepsy; generator of excitation; genetic enhancement; genome equivalent; gentamicin; glandular epithelium; grade of evidence; gradient echo; guanidoethyl

G-E gradient-echo [imaging]

G/E granulocyte/erythroid [ratio]

Ge germanium

gE glycoprotein E

GEA gastric electrical activity; gastroepiploid artery

GEART Gemfibrozil Atherosclerosis Regression Trial

GEB gum elastic bougie

GEC galactose elimination capacity; glomerular epithelial cell

GECC Government Employees' Clinic Centre

GEE generalized estimating equation

GEF gastroesophageal fundoplication; glossoepiglottic fold; gonadotropin enhancing factor; guanosine nucleotide exchange factor

Ge^{-G} Gerbich negative

GEH glycerol ester hydrolase

GEHR Good European Health Record

GEJ gastroesophageal junction

gel gelatin

GELIA German Experience with Low-Intensity Anticoagulation

GEM guidelines element model

GEMISCH Generalized Medical Information System for Community Health

GEM-Q guidelines element model-quality

GE-MRI gradient echo magnetic resonance imaging

GEMS gel electrophoresis mass spectrometry; generic error-modeling system

GEMS/Food [WHO] Global Environment Monitoring System-Food Contamination Monitoring and Assessment Programme

GEMSS glaucoma-lens ectopia-microspherophakia-stiffness-shortness syndrome

GEMT German Eminase Multicenter Trial

GEN gender; generation

Gen genetic, genetics; genus

gen general; genital

GeneCIS Genetic Clinical Information System [UK]

GENESIS General Ethnography and Needs Evaluations; Genes in Stroke [study]

genet genetic, genetics

GENE-TOX Genetic Toxicology [database]

genit genitalia, genital

GENNET Genetic Network

GENOA Genetics of Atherosclerosis [study]

GENOVA generalized analysis of variance

GENPS genital neoplasm-papilloma syndrome

GenRF gene reference into function

GENT gentamicin

GEO Gene Expression Omnibus [data repository]; genetically enhanced organism

GEP gastroenteropancreatic; gustatory evoked potential

GEPG gastroesophageal pressure gradient

GEPIC granulocyte elastase alpha-1 proteinase inhibitor complex

GER gas exchange region; gastroesophageal reflux; geriatrics; granular endoplasmic reticulum

Ger geriatric(s); German

GERD gastroesophageal reflux disease

geriat geriatrics, geriatric

GeriROS geriatric review of systems

GERL Golgi-associated endoplasmic reticulum lysosome

GEROD Generator of Body Data [computer program]

Geront gerontology, gerontologist, gerontologic

GERRI geriatric evaluation by relative rating instrument

GERV Germiston virus

GES gastroesophageal sphincter; glucose-electrolyte solution

GEST, gest gestation, gestational

GET gastric emptying time; general endotracheal [anesthesia]; graded treadmill exercise test

GETV Getah virus

GEU geriatric evaluation unit

Gev giga electron volt

GEWS Gianturco expandable wire stent

GEX gas exchange

G$_{exg}$ exogenous glucose

GF gastric fistula; gastric fluid; germ-free; glass factor; glomerular filtration; gluten-free; grandfather; growth factor; growth failure

Gf gastric fluid

gf gram-force

GFA genetic function approximation [algorithm]; glial fibrillary acidic [protein]

GF-AAS graphite furnace atomic absorption spectroscopy

GFAP glial fibrillary acidic protein

GFAT glutamine:fructose-6-phosphate amidotransferase

GFCI ground-fault circuit-interrupter

GFD gingival fibromatosis-progressive deafness [syndrome]; gluten-free diet

GFFS glycogen and fat-free solid

GFH glucose-free Hanks [solution]

GFI glucagon-free insulin; goodness-of-fit index; ground-fault interrupter

GfIV *Glypta fumiferanae* ichnovirus

GFL giant follicular lymphoma

Gflops gigaflops [billions of floating point operations per second]

GFP gamma-fetoprotein; gel-filtered platelet; glomerular filtered phosphate; green fluorescent protein

GFR glomerular filtration rate

GFRP growth factor response protein

GFS global focal sclerosis; guafenesin

GFV Gabek Forest virus

GG gamma globulin; genioglossus; glycylglycine

gG glycoprotein G

gg gynogenetic

GGA general gonadotropic activity

Gγ G protein subunit gamma complex

GGC gamma-glutamyl carboxylase

GGCS, g-GCS gamma-glutamyl cysteine synthetase

GGE generalized glandular enlargement; gradient gel electrophoresis

GGED Graphical Gene-Expression Database

GGFC gamma-globulin-free calf [serum]

GGG glycine-rich gamma-glycoprotein

GGH glycine-glycine-histidine

GGM glucose-galactose malabsorption

GGMRF generalized gaussian Markov random field

GGO ground glass opacification

GG or S glands, goiter, or stiffness [of neck]

GGPNA gamma-glutamyl-*p*-nitroanilide

GGR global genomic repair

GGT gamma-glutamyl transferase; gamma-glutamyl transpeptidase; geranyl-geranyltransferase

GGTB glycoprotein 4-beta-galactosyl transferase

GGTP gamma-glutamyl transpeptidase

GGV *Gaeumannomyces graminis* virus; Gan Gan virus; generalized gross validation

GgV *Gaeumannomyces graminis* virus

GGVB gelatin, glucose, and veronal buffer

GGYV Gadgets Gully virus

GH general health; general hospital; genetic hemochromatosis; genetic hypertension; genetically hypertensive [rat]; geniohyoid; growth hormone

GHA generalized harmonic analysis; glucoheptanoic acid; Group Health Association

GHAA Group Health Association of America

GHAP Global Health Care Application Project

GHAT German Hip Arthroplasty Trial

GHB gamma hydroxybutyrate

GHb glycated hemoglobin

GHBA gamma-hydroxybutyric acid

GHBMO general hazardous materials behavior model

GHBP growth hormone binding protein

GHC group health cooperative

GHCH giant hepatic cavernous hemangioma

GHD growth hormone deficiency

GHDD Ghosal hematodiaphyseal dysplasia

GHDNet Global Health Disaster Network

GHEI Global Health Equity Initiative

GHEV *Goeldichironomus holoprasinus* entomopoxvirus

GHF growth hormone factor

GHL growth hormone-like

GHMM Generalized Hidden Markov Model [DNA sequences]

GHNet Global Health Network

GHP growth hormone promotor [locus]; group health plan

GHPM general health policy model

GHPQ General Health Perception Questionnaire

GHQ General Health Questionnaire

GHR granulomatous hypersensitivity reaction; growth hormone receptor

GHRA geriatric health risk appraisal [survey]

GHRF growth hormone-releasing factor

GHRFR growth hormone-releasing releasing factor

GH-RH growth hormone-releasing hormone

GHRHR growth hormone-releasing hormone receptor

GHRI general health rating index

GH-RIF growth hormone-release inhibiting factor

GH-RIH growth hormone-release inhibiting hormone

GHRP growth hormone releasing peptide

GHT generalized Hough transform

GHV goose hepatitis virus; growth hormone variant

GHz gigahertz

GI galvanic isolation; gastrointestinal; gelatin infusion [medium]; giant interneuron; gingival index; globin insulin; glomerular index; glucose intolerance; granuloma inguinale; growth inhibition

GI$_{50}$ concentration required to inhibit cell growth by 50%

G$_i$ inhibitory guanyl-nucleotide-binding protein

gi gill

GIA gastrointestinal anastomosis

GIB gastrointestinal bleeding

GIBF gastrointestinal bacterial flora

GIBS generalized iterative Bayesian simulation

GICA gastrointestinal cancer

GID gender identity disorder

GIF gastric intrinsic factor; gonadotropin-inhibiting factor; graphic interchange format [imaging]; growth hormone–inhibiting factor

GIFB growth hormone inhibitory factor, brain

GIFIC graphical interface for intensive care

GIFT gamete intrafallopian transfer; granulocyte immunofluorescence test

GIGO garbage in, garbage out

GIH gastrointestinal hemorrhage; growth-inhibiting hormone

GIHINA Genetic Information Health Insurance Nondiscrimination Act

GII gastrointestinal infection

GIK Glucose-Insulin-Kalium [pilot trial]; glucose-insulin-potassium [solution]

GIM general internal medicine; gonadotropin-inhibiting material

GIMC general internal medicine clinic

GIN Grosse Isle Anthrax Project [Canada]

GINA Global Initiative for Asthma

Ging, ging gingiva, gingival

g-ion gram-ion

GIP gastric inhibitory polypeptide; giant cell interstitial pneumonia; glucose-dependent insulinotropic peptide; gonorrheal invasive peritonitis

GIPR gastric inhibitory polypeptide receptor

GIPSI Gradual Inflation at Optimum Pressure vs Stent Implantation [study]

GIR global improvement rating; Grosse Isle Rinderpest Project [Canada]

GIS gas in stomach; gastrointestinal series; geographic information system; guaranteed income supplement

GISSI Grupo Italiano per lo Studio della Streptochinasi nell'Infarto Miocardico

GIST gastrointestinal stromal tumor

GIT gastrointestinal tract

GITS gastrointestinal therapeutic system

GITSG Gastrointestinal Tumor Study Group

GITT gastrointestinal transit time; glucose insulin tolerance test

GIV Great Island virus

GJ gap junction; gastric juice; gastrojejunostomy

gJ glycoprotein J

GJA-S gastric juice aspiration syndrome

GK galactokinase; glomerulocystic kidney; glycerol kinase

GKD glycerol kinase deficiency

GKI glucose potassium insulin

GKRS gamma knife radiosurgery

GL gland; glomerular layer; glomerulus; glycolipid; glycosphingolipid; glycyrrhizin; graphics library; greatest length; gustatory lacrimation

4GL fourth generation [computer] language

GL-4 glycophospholipid

Gl glabella

gL glycoprotein L
gl gill; gland, glandular
g/l grams per liter
GLA galactosidase A; gamma-linolenic acid; gingivolinguoaxial
glac glacial
GLAD gold-labeled antigen detection
gland glandular
GLAP D-glyceraldehyde-3-phosphate
GLAT galactose + activator
GLB galactosidase beta
GLC gas-liquid chromatography
Glc glucose
glc glaucoma
GlcA gluconic acid
GLCB beta-glucuronidase
GLCLC glutamylcysteine synthase
GLC-MS gas-liquid chromatography-mass spectrometry
GlcN glucosamine
GlcNAc N-acetylglucosamine
GlcUA D-glucuronic acid
GLD globoid-cell leukodystrophy; glutamate dehydrogenase
GLDH glutamic dehydrogenase
GLH germinal layer hemorrhage; giant lymph node hyperplasia; gray level histogram
GLI glicentin; glioblastoma; glucagon-like immunoreactivity; guideline interchange format
GLIF guideline interchange format
GLIIRA green light induced infrared absorption
GLIM generalized linear interactive model
GLM general linear model
GLN glutamine
Gln glucagon; glutamine
gln glutamine
GLNH giant lymph node hyperplasia
GLNN galanin
GlnRS glutaminyl transfer ribonucleic acid synthase
GLO glyoxylase
GLO1 glyoxylase 1
glob globular; globulin
G-LOC G-induced loss of consciousness
GLOM glenoid labrum ovoid mass
GLP glucagon-like peptide; glucose-L-phosphate; glycolipoprotein; good laboratory practice; group living program
GLPC gas liquid phase chromatography
GLPR glucagon-like peptide receptor

GLR generalized likelihood ratio; graphic level recorder
GLRA glycine receptor alpha
GLRB glycine receptor beta
GLS generalized least square [estimator]; generalized lymphadenopathy syndrome
GLTN glomerulotubulonephritis
GLTT glucose-lactate tolerance test
GLU glucose; glucuronidase; glutamate; glutamic acid
GLU-5 five-hour glucose tolerance test
Glu glucuronidase; glutamic acid; glutamine
Glu2 glucose transporter 2
glu glucose; glutamic acid
Glu-A glutathione-agarose
GLUC glucosidase
gluc glucose
GLUD glutamate dehydrogenase
GLUDP glutamate dehydrogenase pseudogene
GLUL glutamate (ammonia) ligase
GluproRS glupropyl transfer ribonucleic acid synthase
GLUR, GluR glutamate receptor
GLUS granulomatous lesion of unknown significance
GLUT glucose transporter
GLV *Giardia lamblia* virus; gibbon ape leukemia virus; Gross leukemia virus
GLVR gibbon ape leukemia virus receptor
Glx glucose; glutamic acid
GLY, Gly, gly glycine
glyc glyceride
GlyCAM glycosylation-dependent cell adhesion molecule
GM gastric mucosa; gastrocnemius [muscle]; Geiger-Müller [counter]; general medicine; genetic manipulation; geometric mean; giant melanosome; glyceryl methacrylate; gram; grand mal [epilepsy]; grandmother; grand multiparity; granulocyte-macrophage; graph-based model; Grateful Med [NLM database]; gray matter; growth medium
G-M Geiger-Müller [counter]
G/M granulocyte/macrophage
GM⁺ gram-positive
GM⁻ gram-negative
Gm an allotype marker on the heavy chains of immunoglobins
gM glycoprotein M
gm gram

g-m gram-meter
GMA glyceral methacrylate
GMB gastric mucosal barrier; granulo-membranous body
GMBF gastric mucosa blood flow
GMC general medical clinic; general medical council; giant migratory contraction; grivet monkey cell
gm cal gram calorie
gm/cc grams per cubic centimeter
GMCD grand mal convulsive disorder
GM-CFC granulocyte-macrophage colony forming cell
GM-CFU granulocyte-macrophage colony forming unit
GM-CSA granulocyte-macrophage colony-stimulating activity
GM-CSF, (GM)-CSF granulocyte-macrophage colony-stimulating factor
GMD general message description; geometric mean diameter; glycopeptide moiety modified derivative
GME graduate medical education
GMENAC Graduate Medical Education National Advisory Committee
G-MEPP giant miniature end-plate potential
GMF gastric magnetic field; glial maturation factor
GMH germinal matrix hemorrhage
GMHA glycidyl methacrylate modified hyaluronic acid
GMK green monkey kidney [cells]
GMKV Gomoka virus
GML gut mucosa lymphocyte
g/ml grams per milliliter
gm/l grams per liter
gm-m gram-meter
GMN gradient moment nulling; moment reduction gradient
GMO genetically modified organism
g-mol gram-molecule
GMoV glycine mottle virus
GMP genetically modified product; glucose monophosphate; good manufacturing practice; granule membrane protein; guanosine monophosphate
3′,5′-GMP guanosine 3′,5′-cyclic phosphate
GMPR guanine monophosphate reductase
GMPS guanosine 5′-monophosphate synthetase

GMR gallops, murmurs, rubs; gradient moment reduction; gradient motion rephasing
GMRH germinal matrix related hemorrhage
GMRI gated magnetic resonance imaging
GMS General Medical Service; geriatric mental state; Gilbert-Meulengracht syndrome; glyceryl monostearate; Gomori methenamine silver [stain]; goniodysgenesis-mental retardation-short stature [syndrome]
GM&S general medicine and surgery
GMSC General Medical Services Committee
GMSP Galen Model for Surgical Procedures
GMT geometric mean titer; gingival margin trimmer; Göteborg Metoprolol Trial
GMV glycine mosaic virus; golden mosaic virus; gram molecular volume; green mottle virus
GMW gram molecular weight
GN gaze nystagmus; glomerulonephritis; glucose nitrogen [ratio]; gnotobiote; graduate nurse; gram-negative; guanine nucleotide
G/N glucose/nitrogen ratio
Gn gnathion; gonadotropin
GNA general nursing assistance
GNAT guanine nucleotide-binding protein, alpha-transducing
GNAZ guanosine nucleotide-binding alpha Z polypeptide
GNB ganglioneuroblastoma; gram-negative bacillus; guanine nucleotide-binding [protein]
GNBM gram-negative bacillary meningitis
GNBT guanine nucleotide-binding protein, beta transducing
GNC general nursing care; General Nursing Council; geriatric nurse clinician
GND gram-negative diplococci
GNDF giant cell-derived neurotropic factor
GNDFR giant cell-derived neurotropic factor-responsive
GNG gluconeogenesis
GNID gram-negative intracellular diplococci
GNN genetic neural network

GNP geriatric nurse practitioner; gerontologic nurse practitioner

GNR gram-negative rods

GnRF gonadotropin-releasing factor

GnRH gonadotropin-releasing hormone

GnRHR gonadotropin-releasing hormone receptor

GNRP guanine-nucleotide releasing protein

GNS German Nutrition Study

G/NS glucose in normal saline [solution]

GNSWA Genetic Nurses and Social Worker's Association

GNTP Graduate Nurse Transition Program

GNUDI gerontological nursing U-diagnose instrument

GO gastro-[o]esophageal; geroderma osteodysplastica; glutamic oxylacetic [acid]; gonorrhea; glucose oxidase

G&O gas and oxygen

Go gonion

GOA generalized osteoarthritis

GoAdV goose adenovirus

GOAT Galveston Orientation and Amnesia Test

GOBAB gamma-hydroxy-beta-aminobutyric acid

GOBI Growth and Development Charting the Road to Health, Oral Rehydration Therapy, Breast Feeding, Immunization [WHO program]

GOC granulose cell oocyte

GOE gas, oxygen, and ether

GOG Gynecologic Oncology Group

GOH geroderma osteodysplastica hereditaria

GOLD Global Initiative on Obstructive Lung Disease

GOMBO growth retardation-ocular abnormalities-microcephaly-brachycephaly-oligophrenia [syndrome]

Gω gigaohm [one billion ohms]

GON gonococcal ophthalmia neonatorum; greater occipital nerve

GOND glaucomatous optic nerve damage

GOQ glucose oxidation quotient

GOR general operating room

GOS Glasgow outcome score; gum optical shield

GOSIP Government Open Systems Intercommunications Profile

GOT aspartate aminotransferase; glucose oxidase test; glutamate oxaloacetate transaminase; goal of treatment

GOTM glutamic-oxaloacetic transaminase, mitochondrial

GOTS geriatric outpatient telephone screening

GOx glucose oxidase

GP gangliocytic paraganglioma; gastroplasty; general paralysis, general paresis; general practice, general practitioner; genetic prediabetes; genetic programming; geometric progression; globus pallidus; glucose phosphate; glutamic pyruvic [acid]; glutathione peroxidase; glycerophosphate; glycopeptide; glycophorin; glycoprotein; Goodpasture syndrome; gram-positive; grass pollen; guinea pig; gutta percha

G-P Grassbeger-Procaccia [algorithm]

G/P gravida/para

G-1-P glucose-1-phosphate

GP1 genetic programming 1 [with logical rules]

GPI glycoprotein I

GP2 genetic programming 2 [with algebraic rules]

G3P, G-3-P glyceraldehyde-3-phosphate; glycerol-3-phosphate

G6P, G-6-P glucose-6-phosphate

Gp glycoprotein

G$_p$ guanine nucleotide-binding protein

gp gene product; glycoprotein; group

GPA Global Program on AIDS; glycophorin A; Goodpasture antigen; grade point average; Group Practice Association; guinea pig albumin

GpA glycophorin A

GPAIS guinea pig anti-insulin serum

G6Pase, G-6-Pase glucose-6-phosphatase

GPASS General Practice Administration System for Scotland

GPB glossopharyngeal breathing; glycophorin B

GPC gastric parietal cell; gel permeation chromatography; giant papillary conjunctivitis; glycerolphosphorylcholine; glycophorin C; granular progenitor cell; guinea pig complement

GPCA gastrin-producing cell antibody

GPCI geographic practice cost index

GPCOV guinea pig type C oncovirus

GPCR G protein–coupled receptor

GPD glucose-6-phosphate dehydrogenase; glycerol-phosphate dehydrogenase

G3PD glucose-3-phosphate dehydrogenase

G6PD, G-6-PD glucose-6-phosphate dehydrogenase

G-6-PDA glucose-6-phosphate dehydrogenase enzyme variant A

G6PDH, G-6-PDH glucose-6-phosphate dehydrogenase reduced

G6PDL glucose-6-phosphate dehydrogenase-like

GPE globus pallidus externus; granulocyte colony-stimulating factor promoter element; guinea pig embryo

GPEBP granulocyte colony-stimulating factor promoter element binding protein

GPEP General Professional Education of the Physician

GP/ES gait pathology expert system [automatic data preprocessing]

GPET graphic plan evaluation tool

GPF glomerular plasma flow; greater palatine foramen; granulocytosis-promoting factor

GPGG guinea pig gamma-globulin

GPh Graduate in Pharmacy

GPHN giant pigmented hairy nevus

GPHIN Global Public Health Intelligence Network

GP-HPLC gel permeation high-performance liquid chromatography

GPHV guinea pig herpesvirus

GPI general paralysis of the insane; globus pallidus internus; glucose phosphate isomerase; glycosylphosphatidylinositol; guinea pig ileum

GP-IB general purpose-interface bus [CT scanner-radiotherapy machine interface]

GPIbα glycoprotein Ib alpha

GPIbβ glycoprotein Ib beta

GPII General Practice Immunisation Incentives [Australia]

GPIMH guinea pig intestinal mucosal homogenate

GPIPID guinea pig intraperitoneal infectious dose

GPK guinea pig kidney [antigen]

GPKA guinea pig kidney absorption [test]

GPLV guinea pig leukemia virus

Gply gingivoplasty

GPM general preventive medicine; giant pigmented melanosome

GPm medial globus pallidus

GPMAL gravida, para, multiple births, abortions, and live births

GPN glossopharyngeal nerve; graduate practical nurse

GPNA Genetic Privacy Nondiscrimination Act

GPOA primary open angle glaucoma

GPP generalist physician program; gross primary production

GPPQ General Purpose Psychiatric Questionnaire

GPPT Göteborg Primary Prevention Trial

GPRBC guinea pig red blood cell

GPS global positioning system; Goodpasture syndrome; gray platelet syndrome; guinea pig serum

GPSYCH geriatric psychiatry

GPT General Population Trial; glutamate-pyruvate transaminase; glutamic-pyruvic transaminase

GpTh group therapy

GPU guinea pig unit

GPUT galactose phosphate uridyl transferase

GPV Global Programme for Vaccines and Immunization [WHO]; goose parvovirus

GPVI glycoprotein VI

GPWW group practice without wall

GPX, GPx glutathione peroxidase

GQAP general question-asking program

GQAQ guidelines quality assessment questionnaire

GQL GALEN Representation and Integration Language [GRAIL] query language

GR gamma rays; gastric resection; general relief; general research; generalized rash; glucocorticoid receptor; glutathione reductase; good recovery; graded response; gravid; gravity resistance; growth rate

GR II Gianturco Roubin Second Generation Coronary Stent Trial

gr grade; graft; grain; gram; gravity; gray; gross

gr⁺ gram-positive

gr⁻ gram-negative

GRA gated radionuclide angiography; glucocorticoid-remedial aldosteronism; gonadotropin-releasing agent

GRABS group A beta-hemolytic streptococcal pharyngitis

GRACE Gianturco Roubin Stent in Acute Closure Evaluation

grad gradient; gradually; graduate

GRAE generally regarded as effective

GRAIL Gene Recognition and Analysis Internet Link

GRAMI Gianturco Roubin Second Generation Coronary Stent in Acute Coronary Infarction

gran granule, granulated

GRAND Glaxo Receptor Antagonist Against Nottingham Deep Vein Thrombosis Study

GRANDDAD growth delay-aged facies-normal development-deficiency of subcutaneous fat [syndrome]

GRAPE Glycoprotein Receptor Antagonist Potency Evaluation [study]

GRAS generally recognized as safe

GRASP Glaxo Restenosis and Symptoms Project

GRASS gradient recalled acquisition in a steady state

GRASSIC Grampian Asthma Study of Integrated Care

grav gravid

grav I pregnancy one, primigravida

grav II pregnancy two, secundagravida

GRB growth factor receptor-binding protein

GRC growth factor-regulated [ion] channel

GRD gastroesophageal reflux disease; gender role definition

grd ground

GRE global relative entropy; glucocorticoid response element; gradient-recalled echo; gradient-refocused echo; Graduate Record Examination

GREAT Genome Recognition and Exon Assembly Tool; Grampian Region Early Antistreplase Trial

GRECC Geriatric Research and Education Clinical Center

GRECO German Recanalization of Coronary Occlusion [trial]; German Recombinant Plasminogen Activator [study]

GREP get regular expression and print

GRF gastrin-releasing factor; gelatin-resorcinol-formalin; genetically related macrophage factor; Gibbs random field; glutamyl transpeptidase [GTP] releasing factor; gonadotropin-releasing factor; ground reaction force; growth hormone-releasing factor

GRG glucocorticoid receptor gene; glycine-rich glycoprotein; guidelines review group

GRH growth hormone-releasing hormone

GRHR gonadotropic-releasing hormone receptor

GrHV gruid herpesvirus

GRIA glutamate receptor, ionotropic, ampa

GRID gay-related immunodeficiency [syndrome]

GRIF growth hormone release-inhibiting factor

GRIFFIN Graphics Investigation of Familial Information

GRIK glutamate receptor, ionotropic, kainate

GRINA glutamate receptor, ionotropic, N-methyl-D-aspartate A

GRINB glutamate receptor, ionotropic, N-methyl-D-aspartate B

GRIPS Göttingen Risk, Incidence and Prevalence Study

GRL glass reflection light

GRMP granulocyte membrane protein

GRN granules; granulin

GrN gram-negative

Grn green

gRNA genomic ribonucleic acid; guide ribonucleic acid

GRO growth-related [protein]

GROB growth-related protein beta

GROD granular osmophilic deposit

GROG growth-related protein gamma

GROU group [UMLS]

GRP gastrin-releasing peptide; glucose-regulated protein

GrP gram-positive

Gr₁P₀AB₁ $Gr_1P_0AB_1$ one pregnancy, no births, one abortion

GRPR gastrin-releasing peptide receptor

GRPS glucose-Ringer-phosphate solution

GRS Golabi-Rosen syndrome

GRV ground reaction vector

GRW giant ragweed [test]

gr wt gross weight

GS gallstone; Gardner syndrome; gas spectrometry; gastric shield; gastrocnemius; general surgery; gestational score;

Gilbert syndrome; Gitelman syndrome; glomerular sclerosis; glucagon secretion; glucosamine; glucosamine sulfate; glutamine synthetase; glycogen synthase; goat serum; Goldenhar syndrome; Goodpasture syndrome; graft survival; granulocytic sarcoma; grip strength; Griselli syndrome; group section; group-specific

G/S glucose and saline

G6S glucosamine-6-sulfatase

G$_s$ stimulatory G protein

gs group specific

g/s gallons per second

GSA generalized simulated annealing; general somatic afferent; Gerontological Society of America; group-specific antigen; Gross virus antigen; guanidinosuccinic acid

Gsa G protein stimulatory alpha subunit

GSBG gonadal steroid-binding globulin

G-SBS guanosine substrate-binding strand

GSC gas-solid chromatography; germline stem cell; gravity settling culture

GSCN giant serotonin-containing neuron

GSD genetically significant dose; Gerstmann-Sträussler disease; glutathione synthetase deficiency; glycogen storage disease

GSD-0 glycogen storage disease-zero

GSE general somatic efferent; gluten-sensitive enteropathy

GSEV *Geotrupes sylvaticus* entomopoxvirus

GSF galactosemic fibroblast; generalized structure function; genital skin fibroblast

GSFR granulocyte colony-stimulating factor receptor

GSH glomerulus-stimulating hormone; golden Syrian hamster; reduced glutathione; L-alpha-glutamyl-L-cysteinylglycine

GSH-Px glutathione peroxidase

GSHV ground squirrel hepatitis B virus

GSI global severity index

GSIV Great Saltee Island virus

GSM generic semantic [data] modeling; global system for mobile communication [telemedicine]; group sequential method

GS-MS gas spectrography-mass spectrophotometry

GSN gelsonin; giant serotonin-containing neuron

GSoA Gerontological Society of America

GSP galvanic skin potential

GSPECT, gSPECT gated single photon emission computed tomography

GspIV *Glypta* sp. ichnovirus

GSR galvanic skin response; generalized Shwartzman reaction; glutathione reductase

GSS gamete-shedding substance; General Social Survey; genome survey sequence; Gerstmann-Sträussler-Scheinker [disease]; glutathione synthetase

GSSD Gerstmann-Sträussler-Scheinker disease

GSSG oxidized glutathione

GSSG-R glutathione reductase

GSSI general solvent-solute interaction

GSSR generalized Sanarelli-Shwartzman reaction

GST glutathione-*S*-transferase; gold salt therapy; gold sodium thiomalate; graphic stress telethermometry; group striction

GSTA glutathione-*S*-transferase, α

GST1L glutathione-*S*-transferase-1-like

GSTM glutathione-*S*-transferase, μ

GSTP glutathione-*S*-transferase π

GSTT glutathione-*S*-transferase θ

GSV gestational sac volume; greater saphenous vein

GSVD general singular value decomposition

GSVT greater saphenous vein thrombophlebitis

GSW gunshot wound

GSWA gunshot wound, abdominal

GSWH gunshot wound to head

GSYY Grimsey virus

GT gait training; galactosyl transferase; gastrostomy; generation time; genetic therapy; gingiva treatment; Glanzmann thrombasthenia; glucose therapy; glucose tolerance; glucose transport; glucuronyl transferase; glutamyl transpeptidase; glycityrosine; granulation tissue; great toe; greater trochanter; group tensions; group therapy

G&T gowns and towels

GT1-GT10 glycogen storage disease, types 1 to 10

gt drop [Lat. *gutta*]

g/t granulation time; granulation tissue

GTA gene transfer agent; Glanzmann thrombasthenia; glycerol teichoic acid

GTB gastrointestinal tract bleeding

GTCS generalized tonic-clonic seizures

GTD gestational trophoblastic disease

GTDS Giesen Tumor Documentation System

GTEM gigahertz transverse electromagnetic [cell]

GTF general transcription factor; glucose tolerance factor; glucosyl-transferase

GTH gonadotropic hormone

GTHR generalized thyroid hormone resistance

GTI grid tiler

GTM generalized tendomyopathy

GTN gestational trophoblastic neoplasia; glomerulotubulonephritis; glyceryl trinitrate

GTO Golgi tendon organ

GTP glutamyl transpeptidase; guanosine triphosphate

GTPase guanosine triphosphatase

gt-PET ground-truth positron emission tomography

GTPV goatpox virus

GTR galvanic tetanus ratio; granulocyte turnover rate; guided tissue regeneration

GTS Gilles de la Tourette syndrome; glucose transport system

GTT gelatin-tellurite-taurocholate [agar]; glucose tolerance test

GTV gross tumor volume

GTX *Goniopora* toxin; gonyautoxin

GTX$_2$ gonyautoxin II

GTX$_3$ gonyautoxin III

GU gastric ulcer; genitourinary; glucose uptake; glycogenic unit; gonococcal urethritis; gravitational ulcer; guanethidine

GUA group of units of analysis

Gua guanine

GUARANTEE Global Unstable Angina Registry and Treatment Evaluation

GUCA guanylate cyclase activator

GUD genitourinary dysplasia

GUI graphic user interface

GUIDE Guidance by Ultrasound Imaging for Decision Endpoints [trial]

GUIDE II Guidance by Ultrasound for Interventional Decision Endpoints II [trial]

GUK guanylate kinase

GULHEMP general physique, upper extremity, lower extremity, hearing, eyesight, mentality, and personality [workplace evaluation scale]

GUM genitourinary medicine

GUNM Georgetown University Nursing Model

Guo guanosine

GURV Gurupi virus

GUS genitourinary sphincter; genitourinary system

GUSTO Globus Ubiquitous Supercomputing Testbed Organization

GUSTO-I Global Utilization of Streptokinase and Tissue Plasminogen Activator for Occluded Coronary Arteries [trial]

GUSTO-IIa Global Use of Strategies to Open Occluded Arteries [trial]

GUSTO-IIb Global Use of Strategies to Open Occluded Arteries in Acute Coronary Syndromes [trial]

GUSTO-III Global Use of Strategies to Open Occluded Coronary Arteries [trial]

GUSTO-IV Global Use of Streptokinase and Tissue Plasminogen Activator for Occluded Arteries [trial]

GV gastric volume; gas ventilation; generalized vaccinia; gentian violet; germinal vesicle; granulosis virus; griseoviridin; Gross virus

GVA general visceral afferent [nerve]

GVB gelatin-Veronal buffer

GVBD germinal vesicle breakdown

GVE general visceral efferent [nerve]

GVF good visual fields; gradient vector flow

GVG gamma-vinyl-gamma-aminobutyric acid

GVH, GvH graft-versus-host

GVHD, GvHD graft-versus-host disease

GVHR, GvHR graft-versus-host reaction

GVL graft versus leukemia

G vs HD graft versus host disease

GVTY gingivectomy

GW germ warfare; gigawatt; glycerin in water; gradual withdrawal; group work; guidewire

G/W glucose in water

GWAFD Genée-Wiedemann acrofacial dysostosis

GWB general well-being [schedule]

GWDT gray-weighted distance transformation [imaging]

GWE glycerol and water enema

GWG generalized Wegener granulomatosis

GWN gaussian white noise

GWTG Get with the Guidelines [American Heart Association]

GWUHP George Washington University Health Plan

GX glycinexylidide; histopathologic grade of tumor cannot be assessed [TNM (tumor-node-metastasis) classification]

GXD Gene-Expression Database

GXT graded exercise test

Gy gray

GY-1 graduate year one

GYN, Gyn, gyn gynecologic, gynecologist, gynecology

GypV gypsy virus

GZ Guilford-Zimmerman [test]

H

H bacterial antigen in serologic classification of bacteria [Ger. *Hauch*, breath]; deflection in the His bundle in electrogram [spike]; dose equivalent; draft [Lat. *haustus*]; electrically induced spinal reflex; enthalpy; fucosal transferase-producing gene; heart; heavy [strand]; height; hemagglutination; hemisphere; hemolysis; *Hemophilus*; henry; heparin; heroin; high; hippocampus; histidine; *Histoplasma*; histoplasmosis; Holzknecht unit; homosexual; horizontal; hormone; horse; hospital; Hounsfield unit; hour; human; hydrogen; hydrolysis; hygiene; hyoscine; hypermetropia; hyperopia; hypodermic; hypothalamus; magnetic field strength; magnetization; mustard gas; oersted; the region of a sarcomere containing only myosin filaments [band; Ger. *heller*, lighter]

H$_0$ null hypothesis

H1/2 half-value layer

H1 first [heart] sound; halistatin; protium

^{1}H, H^1 protium

H$_1$ alternate hypothesis [statistics]

H2 deuterium; second [heart] sound

^{2}H, H^2 deuterium

H3, ^{3}H, H^3 tritium

4H hypothalamic hamartoblastoma-hyperphalangeal hypoendocrine-hypoplastic anus [syndrome]

H$^+$ hydrogen ion

[H$^+$] hydrogen ion concentration

h hand-rearing [of experimental animals]; heat transfer coefficient; hecto; height; henry; hour [Lat. *hora*]; human; hundred; hypodermic; negatively staining region of a chromosome; Planck constant; secondary constriction; specific enthalpy

h- hecto- [10^2]

HA H antigen; Hakim-Adams [syndrome]; halothane anesthesia; Hartley [guinea pig]; headache; health affairs; health alliance; hearing aid; height age; hemadsorption; hemagglutinating antibody; hemagglutination; hemagglutinin; hemolytic anemia; hemophiliac with adenopathy; hepatic adenoma; hepatic artery; hepatitis A; hepatitis-associated; heteroduplex analysis; heterophil antibody; Heyden antibiotic; high anxiety; hippocampal asymmetry; hippuric acid; histamine; histocompatibility antigen; Horton arteritis; hospital administration; hospital admission; hospital apprentice; Hounsfield unit; human albumin; hyaluronic acid; hydroxyapatite; hydroxylamine; hyperalimentation; hyperandrogenism; hypersensitivity alveolitis; hypothalamic amenorrhea

H/A head to abdomen; headache

1HA hydroxyapatite; hydroxylamine

HA2 hemadsorption virus 2

Ha absolution hypermetropia; hafnium; hamster; Hartmann number

ha hectare

HAA hearing aid amplifier; hemolytic anemia antigen; hepatitis-associated antigen; hepatitis-associated aplastic anemia; hospital activity analysis

HA Ag hepatitis A antigen

HAART highly active antiretroviral therapy

HAAS Honolulu-Asia Aging Study

hAAT human α_1-antitrypsin

HAB harmful algal bloom; histoacryl blue

HABA 2(4′-hydroxyazobenzene) benzoic acid

HABF hepatic artery blood flow

HA-BP high affinity binding protein

HACCP hazard analysis and critical control point system [food safety]

HACE high-altitude cerebral edema

HACEK *Haemophilus, Actinobacillus, Cardiobacterium, Eikenella, Kingella*

HACER hypothalamic area controlling emotional response

HAChT high affinity choline transport

HACR hereditary adenomatosis of the colon and rectum

HACS Hazard-Assessment Computer System; hyperactive child syndrome

hACSP human adenylate cyclase-stimulating protein

HACT health care activity [UMLS]

HAD health care alternatives development; hemadsorption; HIV-associated dementia; hospital administration, hospital administrator; hospital anxiety and depression [scale]; human immunodeficiency virus-associated dementia

HAd hemadsorption; hospital administrator

HADD hydroxyapatite deposition disease

HADH hydroxyacyl CoA dehydrogenase

HAd-I hemadsorption-inhibition

HADS hospital anxiety and depression scale

HAdV 1–51 human adenoviruses 1 to 51

HAdV-A, B, C, D, E, F human adenoviruses A, B, C, D, E, and F

HAE health appraisal examination; hearing aid evaluation; hepatic artery embolism; hereditary angioneurotic edema

Hae *Haemophilus influenzae aegyptius*

HAEC Hirschsprung-associated enterocolitis; human aortic endothelial cell

HAF hepatocellular altered focus; hyperalimentation fluid

HaF Hageman factor

HAFP human alpha-fetoprotein

HAG heat-aggregated globulin

HAGG hyperimmune antivariola gammaglobulin

HAGH hydroxyacyl-glutathione hydrolase

HAGL humeral avulsion of glenohumeral ligament

HAH halogenated aromatic compound

HAHS Harvard Alumni Health Study

HAHTG horse antihuman thymus globulin

HAI hemagglutination inhibition; hepatic arterial infusion; hospital-acquired infection

H&A Ins health and accident insurance

HAIR-AN hyperandrogenism, insulin resistance, and acanthosis nigricans [syndrome]

HaK hamster kidney

HAL hand-assisted laparoscopy; Heart Attacks in London [study]; hepatic artery ligation; hybrid artificial liver; hypoplastic acute leukemia

hal halogen; halothane

HALC high affinity-low capacity

HALF high amplitude low frequency; Homocysteine, Atherosclerosis, Lipid and Familial Hypercholesterolemia [study]

HALFD hypertonic albumin-containing fluid demand

halluc hallucinations

HALO Halotestin

HALP hyperalphalipoproteinemia

HALT Hypertension and Lipid Trial

HALT MI Hu23F2G Anti-Adhesion to Limit Cytotoxic Injury Following Acute Myocardial Infarction [study]

HALV human acquired immunodeficiency syndrome lymphotropic virus

HaLV hamster leukemia virus

HAM hearing aid microphone; helical axis in motion; hemolymph anticoagulation medium; human albumin microsphere; human alveolar macrophage; human T-cell lymphotropic virus associated myelopathy; hypoparathyroidism, Addison disease, and mucocutaneous candidiasis [syndrome]

HAM-1, 2 histocompatibility antigen modifier types 1 and 2

HAm human amnion

HAMA Hamilton anxiety [scale]; human anti-murine antibody

HA-MA methacrylated hyaluronic acid

HAMD Hamilton depression [scale]

HAMDCT Hospital Authority Master Disease Code Table [Hong Kong]

HAMIT Heparin in Acute Myocardial Infarction Trial

HaMSV, Ha-MSV Harvey murine sarcoma virus

HAN heroin-associated nephropathy; hyperplastic alveolar nodule

HANA hemagglutinin neuraminidase

H and E hematoxylin and eosin [stain]

HANDI Hemophilia and AIDS/HIV Network for the Dissemination of Information

Handicp handicapped

HANE hereditary angioneurotic edema; Hydrochlorothiazide, Atenolol, Nitrendipine, Enalapril [study]

HANES Health and Nutrition Examination Survey

hANF human atrial natriuretic factor

h ANP human atrial natriuretic peptide

HANSA Healthcare Advanced Networked System Architecture

HAODM hypoplasia anguli oris depressor muscle

HAP Handicapped Aid Program; Hazardous Air Pollutants [List]; hazardous air pollution; health alliance plan; hepatic arterial phase; heredopathia atactica polyneuritiformis; high-altitude peristalsis; histamine acid phosphate; hospital-acquired pneumonia; hospital admissions program; humoral antibody production; hydrolyzed animal protein; hydroxyapatite

HAp hydroxyapatite

HAPA hemagglutinating anti-penicillin antibody

HAPC high-amplitude peristaltic contraction; hospital-acquired penetration contact

HAPE high-altitude pulmonary edema

HAPI Heparin as an Alternative to Promote Patency in Acute Myocardial Infarction [study]

HAPORT Heart Attack Patient Outcome Research Team [study]

HAPPHY Heart Attack Primary Prevention in Hypertension

HAPS hepatic arterial perfusion scintigraphy

HAPSA Home Assessment Program for Successful Aging

HaPV hamster polyomavirus

HAPVC hemi-anomalous pulmonary venous connection

HAPVD hemi-anomalous pulmonary venous drainage

HAPVR hemi-anomalous pulmonary venous return

HaPyV hamster polyomavirus

HAQ health assessment questionnaire

HAR head airway region; high-altitude retinopathy

HARD hydrocephalus-agyria-retinal dysplasia [syndrome]

HARD +/− E hydrocephalus-agyria-retinal dysplasia plus or minus encephalocele [syndrome]

HAREM heparin assay rapid easy method

HARH high-altitude retinal hemorrhage

HARM harmonics from the injected signal; heparin assay rapid method

HAROLD Hypertension and Ambulatory Recording in the Old

HARP Harvard Atherosclerosis Reversibility Project; homeless and at-risk population; hospital admission risk profile

HARS histidyl-ribonucleic acid [RNA] synthetase; human AIDS [acquired immunodeficiency syndrome] reporting system

HART Heparin-Aspirin Reperfusion Trial; hyperfractionated accelerated radiation therapy; Hypertension Audit of Risk Factor Therapy [study]

HART II Heparin and Reperfusion Therapies [study]

HARTS Hoechst Adverse Reaction Terminology System

HAS Hamilton Anxiety Scale; health advisory service; health-assessment system; Helsinki Ageing Study; Hemostatic System Activation Substudy; highest asymptomatic [dose]; Hirulog Angioplasty Study; hospital administrative service; hospital advisory service; human albumin solution; hydrocephalus due to stenosis of the aqueduct of Sylvius; hyperalimentation solution; hypertensive arteriosclerotic

HASCVD hypertensive arteriosclerotic cardiovascular disease

HASHD hypertensive arteriosclerotic heart disease

HASI Hirulog Angioplasty Study Investigators

HASM human airway smooth muscle

HASMC human aortic smooth muscle cell

HASP Hospital Admissions and Surveillance Program

HASS highest anxiety subscale score

HASTE half-Fourier acquisition single shot turbospin echo

HAstV 1-8 human astroviruses 1 to 8

HAT Halsted Aphasia Test; head, arm, trunk; heparin-associated thrombocytopenia; heterophil antibody titer; histone acetyltransferase; home asthma telemonitoring; hospital arrival time; human African trypanosomiasis; hypoxanthine, aminopterin, and thymidine; hypoxanthine, azaserine, and thymidine

3-HAT 3-hydroxyanthranilic acid

HATG horse antihuman thymocyte globulin

HATH Heterosexual Attitudes Toward Homosexuality [scale]

HATT heparin-associated thrombocytopenia and thrombosis

HATTS hemagglutination treponemal test for syphilis

HaTx hanatoxin

HAU hemagglutinating unit

HAV hemadsorption virus; hepatitis A virus

HAVOC Hematoma and Vascular Outcome Complications [study]

HAVS hand-arm vibration syndrome

HAWIC Hamburg-Wechsler Intelligence Test for Children

HAZ height-for-age Z-score

HAZMAT hazardous material
HAZOP hazard and operability
HAZR hazardous substance [UMLS]
HAZUS Hazard US [loss estimation methodology]
HAZWOPER hazardous waste operations and emergency response
HB health board; heart block; heel to buttock; held back; hemoglobin; hepatitis B; His bundle; hold breakfast; housebound; hybridoma bank; hyoid body
Hb hemoglobin
HBA bundle of His electrogram; heated blood agar [test]
HbA hemoglobin A, adult hemoglobin
HBA₁ glycosylated hemoglobin
HBAb hepatitis B antibody
HBABA hydroxybenzeneazobenzoic acid
HbA1c, HbA₁c glycosylated hemoglobin
HBAg hepatitis B antigen
HB₅AG hepatitis B surface virus
HBB hemoglobin beta-chain; hospital blood bank; hydroxybenzyl benzimidazole
HbBC hemoglobin binding capacity
HBBW hold breakfast blood work
HBC hereditary breast cancer
HBC, HBc, HB_c hepatitis B core [antigen]
HbC hemoglobin C
HBCAB, HBcAb hepatitis B core antibody
HBCAG, HBcAg, HB_cAg hepatitis B core antigen
HBCG heat-aggregated Calmette-Guérin bacillus
HbCO carboxyhemoglobin
Hb CS hemoglobin Constant Spring
HBCT helical biphasic contrast-enhanced computed tomography
HbCV *Haemophilus influenzae* conjugate vaccine
HBD has been drinking; homozygous-by-descent; hydroxybutyric dehydrogenase; hypophosphatemic bone disease
HbD hemoglobin D
HBDH hydroxybutyrate dehydrogenase
hBDNF human brain derived neurotrophic factor
HBDT human basophil degranulation test
HBE His bundle electrogram
HbE hemoglobin E
HB_e hepatitis B early antigen
HBeAb/Ag hepatitis B e antibody/antigen

HBEAG, HB_eAg, HBeAg hepatitis B early antigen
HBEC human brain endothelial cell
HB-EGF heparin-binding epidermal growth factor
HBF hand blood flow; hemispheric blood flow; hemoglobinuric bilious fever; hepatic blood flow; hypothalamic blood flow
HbF fetal hemoglobin, hemoglobin F
Hbg hemoglobin
HBGF heparin-binding growth factor
HBGM home blood glucose monitoring
HBGR hemoglobin-gamma regulator
HbH hemoglobin H
HBHC hospital-based home care
HBHCT hospital-based home care team
Hb-Hp hemoglobin-haptoglobin [complex]
HBI hemibody irradiation; high serum-bound iron
HBIG, HBIg hepatitis B immunoglobulin
HBL hepatoblastoma
HBLA human B-cell lymphocyte antigen
H₂ blockers histamine blockers
HBLV human B-cell lymphotropic virus
HBM health belief model; hypertonic buffered medium
HbM hemoglobin Milwaukee
HBMEC human brain microvascular endothelial cell
HbMet methemoglobin
HBMP Human Brain Map Project
hBNP human brain natriuretic peptide
HBO hyperbaric oxygen, hyperbaric oxygenation
HbO oxyhemoglobin
HbO₂ oxyhemoglobin
HBOC hereditary breast-ovarian cancer
HBOT hyperbaric oxygen therapy
HBP heartbeat period; hepatic binding protein; high blood pressure; hospital-based practice
HbP primitive hemoglobin
HBPV HB virus
HBr hydrobromic acid
HbR reduced hemoglobin
HBS hepatitis B surface [antigen]; hyperkinetic behavior syndrome
HB_s hepatitis B surface [antigen]
HbS hemoglobin S, sickle-cell hemoglobin
HBsAb hepatitis B surface antibody

HBsAb/Ag hepatitis B surface antibody/ antigen

HBSAG, HBsAg, HB$_s$AG, HB$_s$Ag hepatitis B surface antigen

HBsAg/adr hepatitis B surface antigen manifesting group-specific determinant *a* and subtype-specific determinants *d* and *r*

HBSC hematopoietic blood stem cell

HBSS Hank's balanced salt solution

HbSS hemoglobin SS

HBT brevetoxin; human brain thromboplastin; human breast tumor

HBT-B brevetoxin B

Hb$_{tot}$ total hemoglobin

HBV hepatitis B vaccine; hepatitis B virus; high biological value

HBV-MN membranous nephropathy associated with hepatitis B virus

HBVS hepatitis B virus integration site

HBW Healthbeat Wales [study]; high birth weight

HbZ hemoglobin Z, hemoglobin Zürich

HC hair cell; hairy cell; Hajdu-Cheney [disease]; handicapped; head circumference; head compression; health care; health checkup; healthy control; heart catheterization; heart cycle; heat conservation; heavy chain; hematochromatosis; hemicholinium; hemoglobin concentration; hemorrhagic colitis; heparin cofactor; hepatic catalase; hepatitis C; hepatocellular; hepatocellular cancer; hereditary coproporphyria; hexachloroethane; Hickman catheter; high-calorie [diet]; hippocampus; histamine challenge; histochemistry; home care; homocystinuria; Hospital Corps; house call; Huntington chorea; hyaline casts; hybrid capture [assay]; hydraulic concussion; hydrocarbon; hydrocortisone; hydroxycorticoid; hyoid cornu; hypercholesterolemia; hypertrophic cardiomyopathy

H&C hot and cold

4HC 4-hydroperoxy-cyclophosphamide

Hc hexachloroethane; *Histoplasma capsulatum*; hybrid capture [assay]; hydrocolloid

HCA healthcare associate; heart cell aggregate; hepatocellular adenoma; hierarchical clustering analysis; home care aide; Hospital Corporation of America; hybrid capture assay; hydrocortisone acetate; hypothermic circulatory arrest

HCa high calcium [diet]

HC/AC head circumference/abdominal circumference ratio

hCaCC human calcium-sensitive chloride channel

HCAEC human coronary artery endothelial cell

HCAP handicapped

HCATT hyperbaric care air transport team

HCA/W home care aide or worker

HCB hexachlorobenzene

HCC health call center [telemedicine]; healthcare related common component; hepatitis contagiosa canis; hepatocellular carcinoma; history of chief complaint; hospital computer center; hydroxycholecalciferol

25-HCC 25-hydroxycholecalciferol

HCCA healthcare commuting area; 4-hydroxycinnamic acid

HCCAA hereditary cysteine C amyloid angiopathy

HCCH hexachlorocyclohexane

HCCS hereditary cancer consulting service

HCD health care delivery; heavy-chain disease; high-calorie diet; high-carbohydrate diet; homologous canine distemper; human Chagas disease

HCE healthcare establishment; healthcare expertise; hypoglossal carotid entrapment

HC-EAS hybrid capture expansion analysis system

HCF [fetal] head-to-cervix force; healthy control female; heparin cofactor; hereditary capillary fragility; highest common factor; hypocaloric carbohydrate feeding

HCFA Health Care Financing Administration [pronounced "Hickfa"]

hCFSH human chorionic follicle-stimulating hormone

HCG, HcG, hCG human chorionic gonadotropin

HCH Health Care for the Homeless; hexachlorocyclohexane; hemochromatosis; hygroscopic condenser humidifier

HCHB hemichorea-hemiballismus

HCHP Harvard Community Health Plan

HCHWA hereditary cerebral hemorrhage with amyloidosis

HCHWA-D hereditary cerebral hemorrhage with amyloidosis-Dutch type

HCI Health Commons Institute; human collagenase inhibitor; human-computer interface

HcImp hydrocolloid impression
HCIN high-grade cervical intraepithelial neoplasia
HCIS Health Care Information System
HCK hematopoietic cell kinase
HCL hairy-cell leukemia; human cultured lymphoblasts
HCl hydrogen chloride
HCLF high carbohydrate, low fiber [diet]
HCLU health care libraries unit
HCM health care management; hospital communication module; hypertrophic cardiomyopathy
HCMM hereditary cutaneous malignant melanoma
HCMV human cytomegalovirus
HCN health communication network; hereditary chronic nephritis
HCO health care organization
HCO$_3^-$ bicarbonate
HCOP health center opportunity program
HCoV human coronavirus
HCP handicapped; health care provider; hematopoietic cell phosphatase; hepatocatalase peroxidase; hereditary coproporphyria; hexachlorophene; high cell passage; home care platform; hydrophobic class pair; hyperplasia with chronic pancreatitis
H&CP hospital and community psychiatry
HCPCS Healthcare Common Procedure Coding System
HCPH hematopoietic cell phosphatase
HCPOTP health care professionals other than physicians
HCPP health care prepayment plan
HCQI health care quality improvement (pronounced Hicky)
HCQIA Health Care Quality Improvement Act
HCR heme-controlled repressor; host-cell reactivation; hysterical conversion reaction
HCRE Homeopathic Council for Research and Education
hCRH human corticotropin-releasing hormone
Hcrit hematocrit
H-CRT high-resolution cathode ray tube
HCS Hajdu-Cheney syndrome; Hazard Communication Standard; health care support; hemocystic spot; high confidence

[information] system; hourglass contraction of the stomach; human chorionic somatotropin; human cord serum
17-HCS 17-hydroxycorticosteroid
hCS human chorionic somatomammotropin
HCSD Health Care Studies Division
hCSM human chorionic somatomammotropin
HCSS hypersensitive carotid sinus syndrome
HCSUS human immunodeficiency virus [HIV] Cost and Services Utilization Study
HCT health check test; helical computed tomography; hematocrit; historic control trial; homocytotrophic; human calcitonin; hydrochlorothiazide; hydrophobic class torsion; hydroxycortisone
Hct hematocrit
hCT human calcitonin; human chorionic thyrotropin
HCTA health care technology assessment; helical compound tomographic angiography
HCTC Health Care Technology Center
HCTD hepatic computed tomography density
HCTS high cholesterol and tocopherol supplement
HCTU home cervical traction unit
HCTZ hydrochlorothiazide
HCU healthcare unit; homocystinuria; hyperplasia cystica uteri
HCUP Healthcare Cost and Utilization Project [database]
HCUPnet Healthcare Cost and Utilization Project Network
HCV hepatitis C virus; hog cholera virus
HCVD hypertensive cardiovascular disease
HCVE human cardiac valve endothelium
HCVS human coronavirus sensitivity
HCW health care worker
Hcy homocysteine
HD distilled mustard [war gas]; Haab-Dimmer [syndrome]; Hajna-Damon [broth]; Hansen disease; hard disk; hearing distance; heart disease; helix destabilizing [protein]; hemidesmosome; hemidiaphragm; hemodialysis; hemolytic disease; hemolyzing dose; hemorrhagic dengue; herniated disk; high density; high dose; hip disarticulation; Hirschsprung disease;

histopathologic damage; Hodgkin disease; homeodomain; hormone-dependent; house dust; human diploid [cells]; Huntington disease; hydatid disease; hydrodensitometry; hydroxydopamine

H&D Hunter and Driffield [curve]

HD$_{50}$ 50% hemolyzing dose of complement

HDA heteroduplex analysis; Huntington Disease Association; hydroxydopamine

HDAC histone deacetylase

HDAd helper-dependent adenovirus

HD-AF hemidesmosome-anchoring filament

HDAg hepatitis delta antigen

HDARAC high-dose cytarabine

HDBH hydroxybutyric dehydrogenase

HDC hand drive control; Health Care Financing Administration [HCFA] Data Center; high-dose chemotherapy; histidine decarboxylase; hospital dialysis center; human diploid cell; hypodermoclysis

HDCS human diploid cell strain

HDCT high-dose chemotherapy

HDCV human diploid cell rabies vaccine

HDD hard disk device; high-dosage depth; Higher Dental Diploma

HDDRISC Heart Disease and Diabetes Risk Indicators in a Screened Cohort [study]

HDES Heidelberg Diet and Exercise Study

HDF hemodiafiltration; host defense factor; human diploid fibroblast

HDFP Hypertension Detection and Follow-up Program

3H-DFP tritiated diisopropyl-fluorophosphonate

HDG high-dose group

HDH heart disease history

Hdh huntingtin; Huntington disease homolog

3H-DHE tritiated dihydroergocryptine

HDI Hamilton depression inventory; hemorrhagic disease of infants; hexamethylene diisocyanate; high definition imaging; hospital discharge index

HDIC hepatodiaphragmatic interposition of colon

HDIR high isodose range [radiosurgery]

HDIVIG high-dose intravenous immunoglobulin

HDL hardware description language; high-density lipoprotein

HDLBP high-density lipoprotein binding protein

HDL-C high-density lipoprotein-cholesterol complex

HDL-c high-density lipoprotein-cell surface

HDLP high-density lipoprotein

HDLS hereditary diffuse leukoencephalopathy with spheroids

HDLW distance from which a watch ticking is heard by left ear

HDM house dust mite

HDML health checkup data makeup language

HDMP high-dose methylprednisolone

HDMTX high-dose methotrexate

HDMTX-CF high-dose methotrexate citrovorum factor

HDMTX-LV high-dose methotrexate leucovorin

HDN health data network; hemolytic disease of the newborn

hDNA heteroduplex deoxyribonucleic acid [DNA]; hybrid deoxyribonucleic acid

HDP heart disease program [computerized diagnosis]; hexose diphosphate; high-density polyethylene; hydrogen diphosphonate; hydroxydimethylpyrimidine

HDPAA heparin-dependent platelet-associated antibody

HDPE high-density polyethylene

HDR high dose radiation; high dose rate [brachytherapy]

HDRBC head-damaged red blood cells

HDRF Heart Disease Research Foundation

HDRS Hamilton Depression Rating Scale

HDRV human diploid rabies vaccine

HDRW distance from which a watch ticking is heard by right ear

HDS Hamilton Depression Scale; Health Data Services; health delivery system; Healthcare Data Systems; herniated disk syndrome; Hospital Discharge Survey; Hypertension in Diabetes Study

HDSCR health deviation self-care requisites

HDU hemodialysis unit; high dependency unit

HDV hemorrhagic disease virus; hepatitis D virus, hepatitis delta virus

HDZ hydralazine

HE half-scan with extrapolation; hard exudate; hektoen enteric [agar]; hemagglutinating encephalomyelitis; hematoxylineosin [stain]; hemoglobin electrophoresis; hepatic encephalopathy; hereditary elliptocytosis; high exposure; hollow enzyme; human enteric; hydroxyethyl [cellulose]; hyperextension; hypertensive encephalopathy; hypogonadotropic eunuchoidism

H&E hematoxylin and eosin [stain]; hemorrhage and exudate; heredity and environment

H/E hematoxylin-eosin [staining]

He heart

HEA hexone-extracted acetone; human erythrocyte antigen

HEADDFIRST Hemicraniectomy and Durotomy from Massive Hemispheric Infarctions: A Proposed Multicenter, Prospective Randomized Study

HEADLAMP Health and Environment Analysis for Decision-Making: Linkage and Monitoring Project

HEAL health education assistance loan; Hospital and Emergency Ambulance Link [Singapore]

HealSB Health Standards Board

HEALTH ABC Dynamics of Health, Aging and Body Composition [study]

HealthSTAR Health Services, Technology, Administration, and Research [NLM database]

HEAP heparin and early patency

HEART Healing and Early Afterload Reducing Therapy [study]; Health Education and Research Trial; Hyperlipidemia, Epidemiology, Atherosclerosis Risk-Factor Trial; Hypertension and Ambulatory Recording Venetia Study

HEAT human erythrocyte agglutination test

HEB hemato-encephalic barrier

HEBSWEB Health Education Board for Scotland's Website

HEC hamster embryo cell; Health Education Council; human endothelial cell; hydroxyergocalciferol; hydroxyethyl cellulose

HECC high-end computing and computation

HECCWG High End Computing and Computation Working Group

HED hereditary ectodermal dysplasia; hydrotropic electron-donor; hydroxyephedrine; hypohidrotic ectodermal dysplasia; unit skin dose [of x-rays, Ger. *Haut-Einheits-Dosis*]

HEDH hypohidrotic ectodermal dysplasia-hypothyroidism [syndrome]

HEDIS health employer data and information set

HEENT head, ears, eyes, nose, and throat

HEEP health effects of environmental pollutants

HEF hamster embryo fibroblast; human embryo fibroblast

HeFT heart failure trial

HEG hemorrhagic erosive gastritis; hexaethylene glycol

HEHR highest equivalent heart rate

HEI Health Effects Institute; high-energy intermediate; highly exposed individual; homogeneous enzyme immunoassay; human embryonic intestine [cells]

HEI-AR Health Effects Institute-Asbestos Research

HEIR health effects of ionizing radiation; high-energy ionizing radiation

HEIS high-energy ion scattering

HEK human embryo kinase; human embryonic kidney

HEL hen egg white lysozyme; human embryonic lung; human erythroleukemia

HeLa Helen Lake [human cervical carcinoma cells]

Heliox helium and oxygen

HELF human embryo lung fibroblast

HELLIS Health, Literature, Library and Information Services

HELLP hemolysis, elevated liver enzymes, and low platelet count [syndrome]

HELP Hawaii early learning profile; Health Education Library Program; Health Emergency Loan Program; Health Evaluation and Learning Program; Health Evaluation Through Logical Processing; Heart European Leaders Panel [study]; heat escape lessening posture; heparin-induced extracorporeal low-density lipoprotein precipitation [treatment]; Heroin Emergency Life Project; Hospital Equipment Loan Project; Hospitalized Elderly Longitudinal Project

HELP NSAID *Helicobacter* Eradication for Lesion Prevention with Nonsteroidal Anti-inflammatory Drugs [study]

HELPS Hypertension, Exercise and Lifestyle Programs for Seniors [study]

HELVETICA Hirudin in European Restenosis Prevention Trial vs Heparin Treatment in Percutaneous Transluminal Coronary Angioplasty

HEM hematology, hematologist; hematuric; hemophilia; hemorrhage; hemorrhoids; high-electrolyte meal

HEMA health data manager application; Health Education Media Association; 2-hydroxyethyl methacrylate

hemat hematology, hematologist

HEMB hemophilia B

hemi hemiparalysis, hemiparesis; hemiplegia

HEMO, hemo hemodialysis

HEMOA Hemophilia A Mutation Database

HEMOSTAT Hemostasis with ProstarXL vs Angioseal After Coronary Intervention Trial

HEMPAS hereditary erythrocytic multinuclearity with positive acidified serum

HEMRI hereditary multifocal relapsing inflammation

HEMS hospital engineering management system

HEN home enteral nutrition

hENaC human epithelial sodium channel

HeNe helium neon [laser]

HEP hemolysis end point; hepatic; hepatoerythropoietic porphyria; high egg passage [virus]; high-energy phosphate; human epithelial cell; Hypertension in Elderly Persons [trial]

HEp-1 human cervical carcinoma cells

HEp-2 human laryngeal tumor cells

Hep hepatic; hepatitis

hEP human endorphin

HEPA high-efficiency particulate air [filter]

HEP A, HepA hepatitis A

HEP B, HepB hepatitis B

HEPBsAg hepatitis B surface antigen

HEP C hepatitis C

HEP D hepatitis D

HEPES *N*-2-hydroxyethylpiperazine-*N*-2-ethanesulfonic [acid]

HEPM human embryonic palatal mesenchymal [cell]

HEPOD hereditary expansile polyostotic dysplasia

HEPT 1-[(2-hydroxyethoxy)methyl]-6-(phenylthio)thymine

HER hemorrhagic encephalopathy of rats; hernia; human epidermal growth factor receptor

Her-2 human epidermal growth factor receptor-2 [breast cancer]

hered heredity, hereditary

HERN Human T-cell Leukemia Virus European Research Network

hern hernia, herniated

HERO Hirulog Early Reperfusion/Occlusion [study]

HEROICS How Effective Are Revascularization Options in Cardiogenic Shock? [trial]

HERS Health Evaluation and Referral Service; Heart and Estrogen-Progestin Replacement Study; hemorrhagic fever with renal syndrome; Human Immunodeficiency Virus [HIV] Research Study; Hysterectomy Educational Resources and Services [Foundation]

HERT hospital emergency response team

HES health examination survey; hematoxylin-eosin stain; human embryonic skin; human embryonic spleen; hydroxyethyl starch; hypereosinophilic syndrome; hyperprostaglandin E syndrome

HeSCA Health Sciences Communications Association

HESI Health and Environmental Sciences Institute

HET Health Education Telecommunications; helium equilibration time

Het heterophil

het heterozygous

HETA health evaluation and technical assistance

HETE hydroxy-eicosatetraenoic [acid]

HETP height equivalent to a theoretical plate; hexaethyltetraphosphate

HEV health and environment; hemagglutinating encephalomyelitis virus; hemorrhagic enteritis virus; hepatitis E virus; hepato-encephalomyelitis virus; high endothelial venule; high endothelial vessel; human enterovirus

HeV hepatitis virus

HEV-A, B, C, D human enteroviruses A, B, C and D
HEW [Department of] Health, Education, and Welfare
HEX hexaminidase; hexosaminidase
Hex hexamethylmelamine
HEXA Hexosaminidase A Locus Database
HEX A, hex A hexosaminidase A
HEX B, hex B hexosaminidase B
HEX C, hex C hexosaminidase C
HF Hageman factor; half-Fourier; haplotype frequency; hard filled [capsule]; hay fever; head forward; head of fetus; heart failure; helper factor; hemofiltration; hemorrhagic factor; hemorrhagic fever; Hertz frequency; high fat [diet]; high flow; high frequency; hippocampal formation; human factor; human fibroblast; humidifier fever; hydrogen fluoride; hyperflexion
Hf hafnium; hippocampal formation
hF half-Fourier
hf half; high frequency
HFA Health for All [WHO]; high-functioning autism
HFAK hollow-fiber artificial kidney
HFB human fetal brain
HFBA heptafluorobutyric acid
HFC hard filled capsule; high-frequency component; high-frequency current; histamine-forming capacity; hydrofluorocarbon
HFD hemorrhagic fever of deer; high-fiber diet; high-flux dialysis; high forceps delivery; high-frequency Doppler; hospital field director; human factors design
HFDA high film density area
HFDK human fetal diploid kidney
HFDL human fetal diploid lung
HFE hemochromatosis
HFe hemochromatosis
HFEC human foreskin epithelial cell
HFECG high frequency electrocardiography
HFF human foreskin fibroblast
HFG hand-foot-genital [syndrome]
HFGC human fetal glial cell
HFH hemifacial hyperplasia
HFHV high frequency, high volume
HFI hereditary fructose intolerance; high-Fourier imaging; high-frequency information; human fibroblast interferon
HFIF human fibroblast interferon

HFIFPPV high frequency interrupted flow positive pressure ventilation
HFIS high-frequency insertion system [electrosurgery]
HFJV high-frequency jet ventilation
HFK human foreskin keratinocyte
HFL human fetal lung
HFM hand, foot and mouth [disease]; hemifacial microsomia
HFMA Healthcare Financial Management Association
HFO high-frequency oscillator; high-frequency oscillatory [ventilation]
HFO-A high-frequency oscillatory [ventilation]-active [expiratory phase]
HFOV high-frequency oscillatory ventilation
HFP hexafluoropropylene; high-frequency pulsation; hypofibrinogenic plasma
HFPPV high-frequency positive pressure ventilation
HFPV high-frequency percussive ventilation
HFR high-frequency recombination
Hfr heart frequency; high frequency
HFRND high frequency and responsibility nursing diagnosis
HFRS hemorrhagic fever with renal syndrome
HFS hemifacial spasm; Hospital Financial Support
hfs hyperfine structure
hFSH, HFSH human follicle-stimulating hormone
HFSP Hanukah factor serine protease
HFST hearing for speech test
HFT high-frequency transduction; high-frequency transfer
Hft high-frequency transfer
HFTT high-frequency induced thermotherapy
HFU hand-foot-uterus [syndrome]
HFV high-frequency ventilation; human foamy virus
HG hand grip; herpes gestationis; Heschl's gyrus; high glucose; human gonadotropin; human growth; hypoglycemia
hg hectogram; hemoglobin
HGA homogentisic acid
HGAC high gain adaptive control
hGalR human galanin receptor
Hgb hemoglobin
HGD high grade dysplasia

HGDB Human Genome Database
Hge hemorrhage
HGF hematopoietic growth factor; hepatocyte growth factor; human gingival fibroblast; hyperglycemic-glucogenolytic factor
Hg-F fetal hemoglobin
HGFL hepatocyte growth factor–like [protein]
HGF-R hepatocyte growth factor receptor
HGF/SF hepatocyte growth factor/scatter factor
HGG herpetic geniculate ganglionitis; human gammaglobulin; hypogammaglobulinemia
HGH, HgH, hGH human growth hormone
HGHRF human growth hormone releasing factor
HGI Human Gene Index
HGL heregulin
HGM hog gastric mucosa; human gene mapping; human glucose monitoring
HGMCR human genetic mutant cell repository
HGMD, HGMDB Human Gene Mutation Database
HGMP Human Genome Mapping Project
HGMPRC Human Genome Mapping Project Resource Centre [UK]
HGO hepatic glucose output; human glucose output
HGP hepatic glucose production; Human Genome Project; hyperglobulinemic purpura
HGPRT hypoxanthine guanine phosphoribosyl transferase
HGPS hereditary giant platelet syndrome; Hutchinson-Gilford progeria syndrome
HGPT hypoxanthine-guanosine phosphoribosyl transferase
hGR human glucocorticoid receptor
hGRH human growth hormone–releasing hormone
HGS hand grip strength
HGTS Human Gene Therapy Subcommittee
HGV hepatitis G virus
HH halothane hepatitis; handheld; hard-of-hearing; healthy hemophiliac; healthy human; Henderson-Hasselbalch equation; hiatal hernia; Hodgkin-Huxley [model]; holistic health; home help; hydralazine acid-labile hydrazone; hydroxyhexamide; hypergastrinemic hyperchlorhydria; hyperhidrosis; hypogonadotropic hypogonadism; hyporeninemic hypoaldosteronism
H&H hematocrit and hemoglobin
Hh hedgehog
HHA health hazard appraisal; hereditary hemolytic anemia; home health agency; home health aid; hypothalamo-hypophyseo-adrenal [system]
HHANES Hispanic Health and Nutrition Examination Survey
HHAV human hepatitis A virus
HHb hypohemoglobinemia; un-ionized hemoglobin
HHC home health care; household contact; hypocalciuric hypercalcemia
HHCC home health care classification
HHCS high-altitude hypertrophic cardiomyopathy syndrome
HHD high heparin dose; home hemodialysis [telemedicine]; hypertensive heart disease
HHE health hazard evaluation; hemiconvulsion-hemiplegia-epilepsy [syndrome]; hypotonic hyporesponsive episode
HHG hypertrophic hypersecretory gastropathy; hypogonadotropic hypogonadism
HHH hyperornithinemia, hyperammonemia, homocitrillinuria [syndrome]
HHHH hereditary hemihypotrophy-hemiparesis-hemiathetosis [syndrome]
HHHO hypotonia, hypomentia, hypogonadism, obesity [syndrome]
HHI hereditary hearing impairment
HHIE Hearing Handicap Inventory for the Elderly
HHIE-S Hearing Handicap Inventory for the Elderly-Screening Version
HHIS [function of] hospital in home information system
HHM high humidity mask; Hodgkin-Huxley equation for muscles; humoral hypercalcemia of malignancy
H + Hm compound hypermetropic astigmatism
HHMI Howard Hughes Medical Institutes
HHMMTV human homologue of mouse mammary tumor virus
HHN handheld nebulizer
HHNC hyperosmolar nonketotic diabetic coma

HHNK hyperglycemic hyperosmoler non-ketotic [coma]

HHNS hyperosmolar hyperglycemic non-ketotic syndrome

HHP Honolulu Heart Program

HHR hydralazine, hydrochlorothiazide, and reserpine

HHRG home health resource group

HHRH hereditary hypophosphatemic rickets with hypercalciuria; hypothalamic hypophysiotropic releasing hormone

HHS [Department of] Health and Human Services; Hearing Handicap Scale; Helsinki Heart Study; hereditary hemolytic syndrome; Honolulu Heart Study; human hypopituitary serum; hyperglycemic hyperosmolar syndrome; hyperkinetic heart syndrome

HHSSA Home Health Services and Staffing Association

HHT head halter traction; hereditary hemorrhagic telangiectasia; heterotopic heart transplantation; homoharringtonine; hydroxyheptadecatrienoic acid

HHV human herpesvirus

HHV 1 to 8 human herpesviruses 1 to 8

HI half-scan with interpolation; hazard index; head injury; health informatics; health insurance; hearing impaired; heart infusion; hemagglutination inhibition; hepatobiliary imaging; high impulsiveness; histidine; hormone-independent; hormone insensitivity; hospital insurance; humoral immunity; hydroxyindole; hyperglycemic index; hypomelanosis of Ito; hypothermic ischemia

H-I hemagglutination-inhibition

Hi histamine; histidine

HIA Hearing Industries Association; heat infusion agar; hemagglutination inhibition antibody or assay

HIAA Health Insurance Association of America

5-HIAA 5-hydroxyindoleacetic acid

HIB heart infusion broth; hemolytic immune body; *Haemophilus influenzae* type B [vaccine]

Hib *Haemophilus influenzae* type B [vaccine]

HIBAC Health Insurance Benefits Advisory Council

HIBC health industry bar code

HIBCC Health Industry Business Communications Council

HIC handling-induced convulsions; health insurance claim; Heart Information Center; hydrophobic-interaction chromatography

HICA hydroxyisocaproic acid

HIC-CPR high-impulse compression cardiopulmonary resuscitation

HICH hypertensive intracranial hemorrhage

HiCn cyanmethemoglobin

HICPAC Hospital Infection Control Practices Advisory Committee [CDC]

HI-CPR high-impulse cardiopulmonary resuscitation

HID headache, insomnia, depression [syndrome]; herniated intervertebral disk; human infectious dose; hyperkinetic impulse disorder; hypertension in diabetes

HIDA Health Industry Distributors Association; hepato-iminodiacetic acid (lidofenin) [nuclear medicine scan]

HIDAC high density avalanche chamber

HIDDEL health information disclosure, description, and evaluation language

HIE human intestinal epithelium; hyperimmunoglobulin E; hypoxic-ischemic encephalopathy

HIES hyper-immunoglobulin E [IgE] syndrome

HIF higher integrative functions; hypoxia-inducible factor

HIFBS heat-inactivated fetal bovine serum

HIFC hog instrinsic factor concentrate

HIFCS heat-inactivated fetal calf serum

HiFOS High-Frequency Oscillation Study

HIFU high-intensity focused ultrasound

HIG, hIG human immunoglobulin

HIg hyperimmunoglobulin

HIH hypertensive intracerebral hemorrhage

HIHA high impulsiveness, high anxiety

HiHb hemiglobin (methemoglobin)

HII Health Industries Institute; health information infrastructure; Health Insurance Institute; hemagglutination inhibitor immunoassay

HIL health information locator

HILA high impulsiveness, low anxiety

HILDA human interleukin in DA [cells]

HIM health information management; hepatitis-infectious mononucleosis; hexosephosphate isomerase; hyperimmunoglobulin M

HIMA Health Industry Manufacturers Association

HIMAC heavy ion medical accelerator in Chiba [radiotherapy]

HIMC hepatic intramitochondrial crystalloid

HIMO Healthcare Information Management Officer [Japan]

HIMP high-dose intravenous methylprednisolone

HIMS healthcare information management system

HIMSS Healthcare Information Management and Support System; Healthcare Information Management Systems Society

HIMT hemagglutination inhibition morphine test

HIN health information network; Hemophilia in the Netherlands [study]

HI:NC health information: nursing component

HINF health information science

HINT healthcare information networks and technologies; hierarchical interpolation; Holland Interuniversity Nifedipine/Metoprolol Trial

Hint Hinton [test]

HIO health insuring organization; hypoiodism

HIOMT hydroxyindole-*O*-methyl transferase

HIOS high index of suspicion

HIP health illness profile; health insurance plan or program; help for incontinent people; heparan sulfate/heparin interacting protein; homograft incus prosthesis; hospital insurance program; hydrostatic indifference point

HIPA heparin-induced platelet activation

HIPAA Health Insurance Portability and Accountability Act

HIPC Health Information Policy Council; health insurance purchasing collective; health insurance purchasing cooperative

HIPDM *N*-trimethyl-*n*-(2-hydroxyl-3-methyl-5-iodobenzyl)-1,3-propendiamine

HIPE Hospital Inpatient Enquiry

HiPIP high potential iron protein

HIPO hemihypertrophy, intestinal web, preauricular skin tag, and congenital corneal opacity [syndrome]; Hospital Indicator for Physicians Orders

HIPOS Hypertension in Pregnancy: Offspring Study

HiPPI high-performance parallel interface

HiPRF high pulse repetition frequency

HIPS health information processing system; Heparin Delivery with Infusasleeve Catheter Prior to Stent Implantation [study]; Heparin Infusion Prior to Stenting [study]

HIR head injury routine; healthcare information repository; homogeneity isodose range [radiosurgery]

HIRL₁ homogeneity isodose range limited to the inferior [radiosurgery]

HIRMIT High-Risk Myocardial Ischemia Trial

HIRS healthcare-specific incident reporting scheme

HIS health information system; Health Interview Survey; Hemodilution in Stroke [study]; histatin; histidine; Hormones in Stroke [study]; hospital information system; Hungarian Isradipine Study; hyperimmune serum

His, his histidine

HISA healthcare information system architecture

HISAAP Hunter Illawarra Study of Airways and Air Pollution

HISB Health Insurance Standards Board

HISCC Healthcare Information Standards Coordinating Committee

HISKEW Health Information Skeletonized Eligibility Write-off [Medicare]

HISP Health Information System Programme [South Africa]

HIS-PACS hospital information system-picture archiving and communication system

HISPP Healthcare Informatics Standards Planning Panel

HISSG Healthcare Information System Sharing Group; Hospital Information Systems Sharing Group

HIST hospital in-service training

hist histamine; history

HISTLINE History of Medicine Online [NLM database]

Histo histoplasmin skin test

histol histological, histologist, histology

HIT health integration team; hemagglutination inhibition test; heparin-induced thrombocytopenia; High-Density Lipoprotein Cholesterol Intervention Trial; Hirudin for the Improvement of Thrombolysis [study]; histamine inhalation test; hypertrophic infiltrative tendinitis

HITB, HiTB *Haemophilus influenzae* type B

HITF Health Insurance Trust Fund

HITS high intensity transient signal

HIT-SK Hirudin for the Improvement of Thrombolysis with Streptokinase

HITT heparin-induced thrombocytopenia and thrombosis

HITTS heparin-induced thrombosis-thrombocytopenia syndrome

HIU hyperplasia interstitialis uteri

HIV human immunodeficiency virus

HIV1 human immunodeficiency virus type 1

HIV-1.ANT70 human immunodeficiency virus 1 ANT70

HIV 1.ARV2/SF2 human immunodeficiency virus 1 ARV2/SF2

HIV 1.93BR020 human immunodeficiency virus 1 93BR020

HIV 1.BRU(LAI) human immunodeficiency virus 1 BRU(LAI)

HIV-1.90CR056 human immunodeficiency virus 1 90CR056

HIV-1.ELI human immunodeficiency virus 1 ELI

HIV-1.ETH2220 human immunodeficiency virus 1 ETH2220

HIV-1.HXB2 human immunodeficiency virus 1 HXB2

HIV-1MN human immunodeficiency virus 1 MN

HIV-1.NDK human immunodeficiency virus 1 NDK

HIV-1.RF human immunodeficiency virus 1 RF

HIV-1.U455 human immunodeficiency virus 1 U455

HIV-2 human immunodeficiency virus type 2

HIV-2.BEN human immunodeficiency virus 2 BEN

HIV-2.D205 human immunodeficiency virus 2 D205

HIV-2.EHOA human immunodeficiency virus 2 EHOA

HIV-2.ISY human immunodeficiency virus 2 ISY

HIV-2.ROD human immunodeficiency virus 2 ROD

HIV-2.ST human immunodeficiency virus 2 ST

HIV-2.UC1 human immunodeficiency virus 2UC1

HIV Ag human immunodeficiency virus antigen

HIV/AIDS human immunodeficiency virus/acquired immunodeficiency syndrome

HIVAN human immunodeficiency virus–associated nephropathy

HIV-G human immunodeficiency virus–associated gingivitis

HIVRAD HIV Vaccine Research and Design

HIVRT human immunodeficiency virus [HIV] reverse transcriptase

HIZ high intensity zone

HJ Henderson-Jones [disease]; Highlands J [virus]; Howell-Jolly [bodies]

HJB high jugular bulb

HJR hepatojugular reflex

HJV Highlands J virus

HK hand to knee; heat-killed; heel-to-knee; hexokinase; human kidney

H-K hand to knee

hK2 human glandular kallikrein 2

HKAFO hip-knee-ankle-foot orthosis

HKAO hip-knee-ankle orthosis

HKB hybrid knowledge base

HKC human kidney cell

HKLM heat-killed *Listeria monocytogenes*

HKS hyperkinesis syndrome

HL hairline; hairpin loop; hairy leukoplakia; half life; hallux limitus; health level; hearing level; hearing loss; heparin lock; hepatic lipase; histiocytic lymphoma; histocompatibility locus; Hodgkin lymphoma; human leukocyte; hydrolethalus [syndrome]; hyperlipidemia; hypermetropia, latent; hypertrichosis lanuginosa

H&L heart and lung [machine]

H/L hydrophil/lipophil [ratio]

Hl hypermetropia, latent

hl hectoliter

HL7 health level 7

HLA histocompatibility leukocyte antigen; histocompatibility locus antigen; homologous leukocyte antibody; horizontal long axis [imaging]; human leukocyte antigen; human lymphocyte antigen

HL-A human leukocyte antigen

HLAA human leukocyte antigen A

HLAB human leukocyte antigen B

HLAC human leukocyte antigen C

HLAD human leukocyte antigen D

HLA-DP human leukocyte antigen, DP subregion

HLA-DQ human leukocyte antigen, DQ subregion

HLA-DR human leukocyte antigen, DR subregion

HLA-LD human lymphocyte antigen-lymphocyte defined

HLA-SD human lymphocyte antigen-serologically defined

HLB hydrophilic-lipophilic balance; hypotonic lysis buffer

HLBI human lymphoblastoid interferon

HLC heat loss center

HLCL human lymphoblastoid cell line

HLD hepatolenticular degeneration; herniated lumbar disk; Hippel-Lindau disease; hypersensitivity lung disease

HLDH heat-stable lactic dehydrogenase

HLDM high-level data model

HLEG hydrolysate lactalbumin Earle glucose

HLF heat-labile factor; hepatic leukemia factor; high-level fluoroscopy

HLH helix-loop-helix; hemophagocytic lymphohistiocytosis

hLH human luteinizing hormone

HLHS hypoplastic left heart syndrome

HLI human leukocyte interferon

H-L-K heart, liver, and kidneys

HLL hypoplastic left lung

HLLAPI high-level language application programming interface

HLM heart-lung machine

HLN hilar lymph node; hyperplastic liver nodules

HLP hepatic lipoperoxidation; hind leg paralysis; holoprosencephaly; hyperkeratosis lenticularis perstans; hyperlipoproteinemia

HLQ high-level question

HLR heart-lung resuscitation; heart-to-lung ratio; high-level resistance

HLS Health Learning System; high-level segmentation [module]; Hippel-Lindau syndrome

HLT heart-lung transplantation; high-L-leucine transport; human lipotropin; human lymphocyte transformation

HLTx heart-lung transplant

HLV hamster leukemia virus; herpes-like virus; hypoplastic left ventricle

HLVS hypoplastic left ventricle syndrome

HM hand movements; health maintenance; heart murmur; hemifacial microsomia; hemodynamic monitoring; hemosiderin-laden macrophages [siderophages]; Holter monitoring; home management; homosexual male; hospital management; human milk; hydatidiform mole; hyperbaric medicine; hyperimmune mouse

Hm manifest hypermetropia

hm hectometer

HMA health care management alternatives; heteroduplex mobility assay; human monocyte antigen; hydroxymethionine analog

HMAB human monocyte antigen B

HMAC Health Manpower Advisory Council

HMAS hyperimmune mouse ascites

HMB homatropine methobromide; human milk bank; hydroxymethylbilane

HMBA hexamethylene bisacetamide

7-HMBA 7-hydroxymethyl-7-methylbenz[α]anthracene

HMBANA Human Milk Bank Association of North America

HMBS hydroxymethylbilane synthetase

HMC hand-mirror cell; health maintenance cooperative; heroin, morphine, and cocaine; hospital management committee; human mesotheial cell; hypertelorism-microtia-clefting [syndrome]

HMCA hydroxymethyl-cyclophenyl adenine

HMCCMP human mammary carcinoma cell membrane proteinase

HMD head-mounted display [computer graphics]; hyaline membrane disease

HMDC health maintenance and diagnostic center

HMDP hydroxymethylenediphosphonate

HME Health Media Education; heat and moisture exchanger; heat, massage, and exercise; hemimegalencephaly

HMEC human mammary epithelial cell

HMEF heat and moisture exchanger filter

HMF hydroxymethylfurfural

HMFG human milk fat globulin

HMG high-mobility group; human menopausal gonadotropin; 3-hydroxy-3-methylglutaryl

hMG human menopausal gonadotropin

HMG CoA 3-hydroxy-3-methylglutaryl coenzyme A

HMH health level [HL] message handling

HMI healed myocardial infarct; health and medical informatics; human-machine interface; hypomelanosis of Ito

HMIC Health Management Information Consortium

HMIG hazardous materials identification guide

HMIS hazardous materials identification system; hazardous materials information system; hospital management information system

HMK high molecular weight kininogen

HML human milk lysosome

HMM heavy meromyosin; hexamethylmelamine; hidden Markov model

HMMA 4-hydroxy-3-methoxymandelic acid

HMMER hidden Markov marker and profiles

HMMF human monocyte-derived macrophage

HMN hereditary motor neuropathy

H-MNPM [Department of] Health Education and Welfare-Medicus Nursing Process Methodology

HMO health maintenance organization; heart minute output

HMOX heme oxygenase

HMP hexose monophosphate pathway; hot moist packs

HMPA hexamethylphosphoramide

HMPAO, HM-PAO hexamethyl-propyleneamine oxime

HMPG hydroxymethoxyphenylglycol

HMPS hexose monophosphate shunt

HMPT hexamethylphosphorotriamide

HMQC heteronuclear multiple-quantum correlation

HMR health maintenance record; health maintenance recommendations; health management resources; histiocytic medullary reticulosis

HMRI Hospital Medical Records Institute [Canada]

H-mRNA H-chain messenger ribonucleic acid

HMRT hazardous materials response team

HMRTE human milk reverse transcriptase enzyme

HMRU hazardous materials response unit

HMS hexose monophosphate shunt; Household Multipurpose Survey; hypermobility syndrome

HMSA health manpower shortage area; hydroxymethanesulfonate

HMSAS hypertrophic muscular subaortic stenosis

hMSH human Mut S homologue

HMSN hereditary motor and sensory neuropathy

HMSS Hospital Management Systems Society

HMT hematocrit; histamine-N-methyltransferase; hospital management team

HMTA hexamethylenetetramine

HMU hydroxymethyl-uracil

5-HMU 5-hydroxymethyl uridine

HMVEC human dermal microvascular endothelial cell

HMW high-molecular-weight

HMW-BCGF high-molecular-weight B cell growth factor

HMWC high-molecular-weight component

HMWGP high-molecular-weight glycoprotein

HMWK high-molecular-weight kininogen

HMX heat, massage, and exercise

HN head and neck; head nurse; hemagglutinin neuraminidase; hematemesis neonatorum; hemorrhage of newborn; hereditary nephritis; high necrosis; hilar node; histamine-containing neuron; home nursing; human nutrition; hypertrophic neuropathy

H&N head and neck

HNA healthcare network architecture; heparin neutralizing activity

HNAD hyperosmolar nonacidotic diabetes

HNB human neuroblastoma

HNBD has not been drinking

HNC hypernephroma cell; hyperosmolar nonketotic coma; hypothalamoneurohypophyseal complex

HNF hepatocyte nuclear factor

HNF1A hepatocyte nuclear factor-1-alpha

HNKC hyperosmolar nonketotic coma

HNKDS hyperosmolar nonketotic diabetic state

HNL histiocytic necrotizing lymphadenitis

HNMT histamine *N*-methyltransferase

HNN hierarchical neural network

HNP hereditary nephritic protein; herniated nucleus pulposus; human neurophysin

HNPCC hereditary nonpolyposis colorectal cancer; Hereditary Non-Polyposis Colorectal Cancer [Database]; human nonpolyposis colorectal cancer

HNPP hereditary neuropathy with liability to pressure palsies

HNR harmonic-to-noise ratio

hnRNA heterogeneous nuclear ribonucleic acid

hnRNP, HNRP heterogeneous nuclear ribonucleoprotein

HNRPG heterogeneous nuclear ribonucleoprotein peptide G

HNS head and neck surgery; home nursing supervisor

HNSCC head and neck squamous cell carcinoma

HNSHA hereditary nonspherocytic hemolytic anemia

HNTD highest nontoxic dose

HNV has not voided; health network venture

HO hand orthosis; heterotopic ossification; high oxygen; hip orthosis; history of; Holt-Oram [syndrome]; house officer; hyperbaric oxygen

H/O, h/o history of

Ho horse; [Cook-Medley] hostility scale

HOA hip osteoarthritis; hypertrophic osteoarthropathy

HoaRhLG horse anti-rhesus lymphocyte globulin

HoaTTG horse anti-tetanus toxoid globulin

HOB head of bed

HOC human ovarian cancer; hydroxycorticoid; hypertrophic obstructive cardiomyopathy

HOCA high osmolar contrast agent

HOCAP Hypertrophic Obstructive Cardiomyopathy Ablation Pacing [study]

HOCM high-osmolar contrast medium; hypertrophic obstructive cardiomyopathy

HOD hyperbaric oxygen drenching

HOF hepatic outflow

HofF height of fundus

HOGA hyperornithinemia with gyrate atrophy

HOH hard of hearing

HOI hospital onset of infection

HoIg horse immunoglobulin

HOKPP hypokalemic periodic paralysis

HOLON health object library online

HOM high osmolar medium

HOME Home Observations for Measurement of the Environment

Homeop homeopathy

HOMER-D home rehabilitation-dialysis

HOMO highest occupied molecular orbital; homosexual

homo homosexual

HOMSTRAD Homologous Structure Alignment Database [proteins]

HON Health on the Net [Foundation]

HONC hyperosmolar nonketotic coma

HONK hyperosmolar nonketosis

HoNOS Health of the Nation Outcome Scale

HOOD hereditary onycho-osteodysplasia

HOODS hereditary onycho-osteodysplasia syndrome

HOOE heredopathia ophthalmo-oto-encephalica

HOOP Health Online Outreach Project

HOP high oxygen pressure; holoprosencephaly-polydactyly [syndrome]

HOPE Health Outcomes Prevention Evaluation; Healthcare Options Plan Entitlement; health-oriented physical education; holistic orthogonal parameter estimation; Hospital Outcomes Project for the Elderly; Hypertensive Old People in Edinburgh [study]

HOPG highly oriented pyrolytic graphite

HOPI history of present illness

HOPP hepatic occluded portal pressure

HOPWA housing opportunities for people with AIDS

hor horizontal

HORG health care organization [UMLS]

HOS health opinion survey; high-order spectrum; Holt-Oram syndrome; human osteosarcoma; hypoosmotic swelling [test]

HoS horse serum

HOSE Hierarchically Ordered Spherical Description of Environment

Hosp, hosp hospital

HOST healthcare open systems and trials; hybrid open system technology; hypo-osmotic shock treatment

HOT health-oriented telecommunication; Hormones Opposed by Tamoxifen [trial]; human old tuberculin; hyperbaric oxygen therapy; Hypertension Optimal Treatment [study]

HOT MI Hyperbaric Oxygen and Thrombolysis in Myocardial Infarction [study]

HOTS hypercalcemia–osteolysis–T-cell syndrome

HOVERGEN Homologous Vertebrate Genes [database]

HOX, Hox homeobox [protein]

Ho:YAG holmium:yttrium-aluminum-garnet [laser]

HP halogen phosphorus; handicapped person; haptoglobin; hard palate; Harvard pump; health profession(al); health profile; health promotion; heat production; heel to patella; *Helicobacter pylori*; hemiparkinsonism; hemipelvectomy; hemiplegia; hemoperfusion; *Hemophilus pleuropneumoniae*; heparin; hepatic porphyria; high permeability; high potency; high power; high pressure; high protein; highly purified; horizontal plane; horsepower; hospital participation; hot pack; house physician; human pituitary; hydrophilic petrolatum; hydrostatic pressure; hydroxypyruvate; hyperparathyroidism; hypersensitivity pneumonitis; hypophoria

H&P history and physical examination

Hp haptoglobin; hematoporphyrin; hemiplegia

HPA Health Care Practice Act; Health Policy Agenda for the American People; health promotion advocates; *Helix pomatia* agglutinin; hemagglutinating penicillin antibody; *Histoplasma capsulatum* polysaccharide antigen; human platelet alloantigen; human platelet antigen; humeroscapular periarthritis; hybridization protection assay; hypertrophic pulmonary arthropathy; hypophyseal-adrenal axis; hypothalamo-pituitary-adrenocortical [system]; hypothalamopituitary axis

HPAA hydroperoxyarachidonic acid; hydroxyphenylacetic acid; hypothalamo-pituitary-adrenal axis

HPAC high-performance affinity chromatography; hypothalamo-pituitary-adrenocortical

HPAE high performance anion exchange [chromatography]

HPAEC high performance anion exchange chromatography

HPAEC-PAD high performance anion exchange chromatography with pulsed amperometric detection

HPAFT hereditary persistence of alfa-feto-protein

H-PAGE horizontal polyacrylamide gel

HPAH hydralazine pyruvic acid hydrazone

HPASE high-performance application for science and engineering

HPB hepatobiliary

HPBC hyperpolarizing bipolar cell

HPBF hepatotrophic portal blood factor

HPBL human peripheral blood leukocyte

HPC health professional card; hemangiopericytoma; high-performance computing; hippocampal pyramidal cell; history of present complaint; holoprosencephaly; hydroxypropylcellulose

HPCA human progenitor cell antigen

HPCC high-performance computing and communications

HPCE high performance capillary electrophoresis

HPCHA high red-cell phosphatidylcholine hemolytic anemia

HPD hearing protective device; hereditary progressive dystonia; high-protein diet; home peritoneal dialysis

HPDR hypophosphatemic D-resistant rickets

HPE hepatic portoenterostomy; high-permeability edema; history and physical examination; holoprosencephaly; hydrostatic permeability edema

HPETE hydroxyperoxy-eicosatetranoic [acid]

HPeV human parechovirus

HPF heparin-precipitable fraction; hepatic plasma flow; high-pass filter; high-performance FORTRAN; high-power field [microscope]; hypocaloric protein feeding

hpf high-power field [microscope]

HPFH hereditary persistence of fetal hemoglobin

hPFSH, HPFSH human pituitary follicle-stimulating hormone

HPG high purity germanium

hPG, HPG human pituitary gonadotropin

HpGe hyperpure germanium

HPGL Hewlett Packard graphic language

HPH *Helix pomatia* hemocyanin; hygromycin B phosphotransferase

Hp-HB haptoglobulin-hemoglobulin complex

HPI hepatic perfusion index; high pathogenicity island; history of present illness

HPIEC high performance ion-exchange chromatography

HPIV 1, 2, 3, 4 human parainfluenza viruses 1, 2, 3, 4

HPL human parotid lysozyme; human peripheral lymphocyte; human placental lactogen

hPL human placental lactogen; human platelet lactogen

HPLA hydroxyphenyl lactic acid

HPLAC high-pressure liquid-affinity chromatography

HPLC high-performance liquid chromatography; high-power liquid chromatography; high-pressure liquid chromatography

HPLC-MS high performance liquid chromatography–mass spectrometry

HPLE hereditary polymorphic light eruption

HPLH hypoplastic left heart

HPM high-performance membrane

HPMC human peripheral mononuclear cell; hydroxypropylmethylcellulose

hPMS human postmeiotic segregation

HPN Health Provider Network; hepsin; home parenteral nutrition; hypertension

hpn hypertension

HPNAT high-performance networking application team

HPNS high pressure neurological syndrome

HPNSP high performance network service provider

HPO high-pressure oxygen; hydroperoxide; hydrophilic ointment; hypertrophic pulmonary osteoarthropathy

HPOA hypertrophic pulmonary osteoarthropathy

HPP hereditary pyropoikilocytosis; history of presenting problems

HPP, hPP human pancreatic polypeptide; hydroxyphenylpyruvate; hydroxypyrozolopyrimidine

HPPA hydroxyphenylpyruvic acid

HPPC health plan purchasing cooperative

HPP-CFC high proliferative potential colony-forming cell

HPPD hours per patient day; hydroxyphenylpyruvate dioxygenase

hppd hours per patient day

HPPH 5-(4-hydroxyphenyl)-5-phenylhydantoin

HPPK 6-hydroxymethyl-7,8-dihydropterin pyrophosphokinase

HPPO high partial pressure of oxygen; hydroxyphenyl pyruvate oxidase

HPQ Health Perceptions Questionnaire

HPR haptoglobin-related gene; health practices research

HPr human prolactin

hPRL human prolactin

HPRP human platelet-rich plasma

HPRT hypoxanthine phosphoribosyltransferase

HpRz hairpin ribozyme

HPS Hantavirus pulmonary syndrome; [Simvastatin] Heart Protection Study; Helsinki Policemen Study; hematoxylin, phloxin, and saffron; Hermansky-Pudlak syndrome; high-protein supplement; His-Purkinje system; Hopkins Precursors Study; human platelet suspension; hypertrophic pyloric stenosis; hypothalamic pubertal syndrome

HPSA health professional shortage area

HPSL health professions student loan

HPSS high-performance storage system

HPT histamine provocation test; human placental thyrotropin; hyperparathyroidism; Hypertension Prevention Trial; hypothalamo-pituitary-thyroid [system]

1°HPT primary hyperparathyroidism

2°HPT secondary hyperparathyroidism

HPTH hyperparathyroid hormone

HPTIN human pancreatic trypsin inhibitor

HPTLC high-performance thin-layer chromatography

HPU heater probe unit

HPV *Hemophilus pertussis* vaccine; hepatic portal vein; human papillomavirus;

human parvovirus; hypoxic pulmonary vasoconstriction

HPVD hypertensive pulmonary vascular disease

HPV-DE high-passage virus-duck embryo

HPV-DK high-passage virus-dog kidney

HPVG hepatic portal venous gas

HPVM high-performance virtual machine

HPW hypergammaglobulinemic purpura of Waldenström

HP/W health promotion/wellness [program]

HPX high peroxidase [content]; hypophysectomized

Hpx hemopexin

HPZ high pressure zone

[3H] QNB (−)-[3H]quinuclidinyl benzilate

HQSAR hologram quantitative structure-activity relationship

HR hairpin ribozyme; hallux rigidus; handwriting recognition [algorithm]; hazard ratio; heart rate; hematopoietic reconstitution; hematopoietic resistance; hemorrhagic retinopathy; hepatorenal; higher rate; high resolution; high risk; histamine receptor; histamine release; hormonal response; hospital record; hospital report; hospitalization rate; human resources; hydroxyethylrutoiside; hyperimmune reaction; hypersensitive response; hypertensive rat; hypophosphatemic rickets; hypoxic reaction

H&R hysterectomy and radiation

hr hairless [mouse]; homologous repeat; host-range [mutant]; hour

HRA health record analyst; health risk appraisal; heart rate audiometry; heart-reactive antibody; hereditary renal adysplasia; high right atrium; histamine release activity; Human Resources Administration

HRAE high right atrium electrogram

HRBC horse red blood cell

HRC health reference center; hereditary renal cancer; high-resolution chromatography; horse red cell; human rights committee

h/rCRF human recombinant corticotropin-releasing factor

HRCT, HR-CT high-resolution computed tomography

HRE hepatic reticuloendothelial [cell]; high-resolution electrocardiography; hormone receptor enzyme; hormone response element

HR-EEG high resolution electroencephalography

HREH high-renin essential hypertension

HREM high-resolution electron microscopy

HRF health-related facility; heart rate fluctuations; histamine-releasing factor; homologous restriction factor [erythrocyte surface protein]; human readable format

HRG histidine-rich glycoprotein

HRGP histidine-rich glycoprotein

HRH2 histamine receptor H2

HR-HPV high risk human papillomavirus [infection]

HrHRF human recombinant histamine-releasing factor

HRI high resolution imaging

HRIG, HRIg human rabies immunoglobulin

HRL head rotation to the left

HRLA human reovirus-like agent

HRM health risk management; Heidelberg Retracing Model

HRmax maximal heart rate

HRMS health records management system; high resolution multisweep [imaging]

hRNA heterogeneous ribonucleic acid

HRNB Halstead-Reitan Neuropsychological Battery

hROAT human renal organic anion transporter

HRP high-risk patient; high-risk pregnancy; histidine-rich protein; horseradish peroxidase

HRPC hormone-resistant prostatic cancer

HRPD Hamburg Rating Scale for Psychiatric Disorders

hr-PET high-resolution positron emission tomography

HRPT hyperparathyroidism

HRQOL health-related quality of life

HRR Hardy-Rand-Rittler [color vision test]; head rotation to the right; heart rate range

HRRI heart rate retardation index

HRS Hamilton Rating Scale; Hamman-Rich syndrome; Haw River syndrome; health and rehabilitative services; Health and Retirement Study; hepatorenal syndrome; high rate of stimulation; hormone receptor site; humeroradial synostosis

HRSA Health Resources and Services Administration

HRSD Hamilton Rating Scale for Depression; Hirschsprung disease

HRSP high-resolution storage phosphor

HRSUB submaximal heart rate

HRT heart rate; Heidelberg retinal tomography; hormone replacement therapy; Hormone Replacement Trial

HRTE human reverse transcriptase enzyme

HRTEM high-resolution transmission electron microscopy

HRV heart rate variability; human reovirus; human rhinovirus; human rotavirus

HRV-A, B human rhinoviruses A and B

HS Haber syndrome; half-scan; half strength [JCAHO unapproved abbreviation]; Hallopeau-Siemens [syndrome]; hamstring; hand surgery; harmonic scalpel; Hartmann solution; head sling; health services; health statistics; healthy subject; heart sounds; heat-stable; heavy smoker; Hegglin syndrome; heme synthetase; hemorrhagic septicemia; hemorrhagic shock; Henoch-Schönlein [purpura]; heparan sulfate; hereditary spherocytosis; herpes simplex; hidradenitis suppurativa; hippocampal system; home surgeon; homologous serum; horizontally selective; Horner syndrome; horse surgeon; hospital ship; hospital staff; hospital stay; hours of sleep; house surgeon; human serum; Hurler syndrome; hybrid sign; hypereosinophilic syndrome; hypersensitive site; hypersensitivity; hypertonic saline; hypothalamic syndrome

H/S helper-suppressor [ratio]; hysterosalpingography

H&S hemorrhage and shock; hysterectomy and sterilization

hs history; hospitalization

HSA Hazardous Substances Act; Health Services Administration; Health Services Australia; health systems agency; hereditary sideroblastic anemia; horse serum albumin; human serum albumin; hypersomnia-sleep apnea

HSAG *N*-2-hydroxyethylpiperazine-*N*-2-ethanesulfonate-saline-albumin-gelatin

HSAM highly selective affinity modification

HSAN hereditary sensory and autonomic neuropathy

HSAP heat-stable alkaline phosphatase

HSAS hydrocephalus due to stenosis of aqueduct of Sylvius; hypertrophic subaortic stenosis

HSC Hand-Schüller-Christian [syndrome]; Health and Safety Commission; health sciences center; health screening center; hematopoietic stem cell; human skin collagenase

HSCD Hand-Schüller-Christian disease

HSCL Hopkins Symptom Check List

HS-CoA reduced coenzyme A

HSCR Hirschsprung disease

HSCS health state classification system; Hypertension-Stroke Cooperative Study

HSCSG Hypertension-Stroke Cooperative Study Group [trial]

HSCT hematopoietic stem cell transplantation

HSD Hallervorden-Spatz disease; high speed data; highly sulfated domain; honestly significant difference; hydroxysteroid dehydrogenase; hypertonic saline and dextran

H(SD) Holtzman Sprague-Dawley [rat]

HSDB Hazardous Substances Database [NLM]

HSDD hypoactive sexual desire disorder

HSDO health services delivery organization

HSE health, safety, and environment; heat stress element; hemorrhagic shock and encephalopathy; herpes simplex encephalitis; human serum esterase

hSEAP human secreted alkaline phosphatase

HSEES Hazardous Substances Emergency Events Surveillance [system]

HSEP heart synchronized evoked potential

HSES hemorrhagic shock-encephalopathy syndrome

HSF heat shock factor; hepatocyte stimulatory factor; histamine sensitizing factor; hypothalamic secretory factor

HSG Health Service Guideline [UK]; herpes simplex genitalis; human salivary gland; hysterosalpingogram, hysterosalpingography

hSGF human skeletal growth factor

HSGP human sialoglycoprotein

HSH Health Smart Home [database]; hypomagnesemia with secondary hypocalcemia

HSHC hydrocortisone hemisuccinate

HSI health service indicator; health supervision index; heat stress index; hue saturation intensity [imaging]; human seminal plasma inhibitor

HSIL high-grade squamous intraepithelial lesion

HSIL/CA high-grade squamous intraepithelial lesion/cancer

HSIS Health Services Information System

HSK herpes simplex keratitis

HSL hormone-sensitive lipase

HSLC high-speed liquid chromatography

HSM health system model; heparin surface-modified [intra-ocular lens]; hepatosplenomegaly; hierarchical storage management; holosystolic murmur

HSMHA Health Services and Mental Health Administration

HSN hereditary sensory neuropathy; hospital satellite network

HSO health service organization

hSOD human superoxide dismutase

HSP Health Systems Plan; healthcare security policy; heat shock protein; Hemorrhagic Stroke Project; hemostatic screening profile; Henoch-Schönlein purpura; high scoring segment pair [molecular genetics database searching algorithm]; hereditary spastic paraparesis; Hospital Service Plan; human serum prealbumin; human serum protein

hsp heat shock protein [gene]

HS PACS high-speed picture archive and communication system

HSPG, HS-PG heparan sulfate-proteoglycan

HSPM hippocampal synaptic plasma membrane

HSPN Henoch-Schönlein purpura nephritis

HSP$_p$ heat shock protein promoter

HSQ health status questionnaire; home screening questionnaire

HSQB Health Standards and Quality Bureau

HSQC heteronuclear single-quantum correlation

HSR Harleco synthetic resin; health services research; heated serum reagin;

homogeneously staining region; hypersensitivity reaction

HSRC Health Services Research Center; Human Subjects Review Committee

HSRCCT high spatial resolution cine computed tomography

HSRD hypertension secondary to renal disease

HSR&D health services research and development

HS-RDEB recessively inherited dystrophic epidermolysis bullosa of Hallopeau and Siemens

HSRI Health Systems Research Institute

HSRPROJ Health Services Research Project in Progress [NLM database]

HSRS Health-Sickness Rating Scale

HSRV human spuma retrovirus

HSS Hallermann-Streiff syndrome; Hallervorden-Spatz syndrome; health services support; Henoch-Schönlein syndrome; high-speed supernatant; hyperstimulation syndrome; hypertrophic subaortic stenosis

HSSCC hereditary site-specific colon cancer

HSSD hospital sterile supply department

HSSU hospital sterile supply unit

HST health sciences and technology

HSTAR health services and technology assessment research

HSTAT Health Science/Technology Assessment Text [NLM database]

HSTF heat shock transcription factor; heat stress transferring factor; human serum thymus factor

HSTM health state transition matrix

HSUS Health Services Utilization Study

HSV herpes simplex virus; high selective vagotomy; hop stunt viroid; hyperviscosity syndrome

HSV-1 herpes simplex virus type 1

HSV-2 herpes simplex virus type 2

HSVd hop stunt viroid

HSVE herpes simplex virus encephalitis

HSVT high speed valve tester

HSVTK, HSVtk herpes simplex virus [HSV] thymidine kinase

HSyn heme synthase

HT Hashimoto thyroiditis; head trauma; hearing test; hearing threshold; heart; heart transplantation, heart transplant; hemagglutination titer; hereditary tyrosinemia; hierarchical term [UMLS]; high-frequency transduction; high temperature; high tension; high threshold; histologic technician; home treatment; hospital treatment; Hough transform; Hubbard tank; human thrombin; hydrocortisone test; hydrotherapy; hydroxytryptamine; hypermetropia, total; hypertension; hypertensive; hypertext; hyperthyroidism; hypertransfusion; hypodermic tablet; hypothalamus; hypothyroidism

H&T hospitalization and treatment
³HT tritiated thymidine
5-HT 5-hydroxytryptamine [serotonin]
Ht height of heart; heterozygote; hyperopia, total; hypothalamus
H, dose equivalent to individual tissues
hT human telomerase
ht heart; heart tones; height; high tension
HTA health technology assessment; heterophil transplantation antigen; human thymocyte antigen; hydroxytryptamine; hypophysiotropic area
HTACS human thyroid adenyl-cyclase stimulator
ht aer heated aerosol
HT(ASCP) Histologic Technician certified by the American Society of Clinical Pathologists
HTB house tube feeding; human tumor bank
HTC hepatoma cell; hepatoma tissue culture; home telecare; homozygous typing cell
Htc hematocrit
HTCMS home telecare management system
HTCVD hypertensive cardiovascular disease
HTD human therapeutic dose
HTDW heterosexual development of women
HTF heterothyrotropic factor; house tube feeding; HpaII tiny fragment
HTG hypertriglyceridemia
HTGL hepatic triglyceride lipase
HTGS high-throughput genomic sequence
HTH helix-turn-helix; high-test hypochlorite; homeostatic thymus hormone; hypothalamus
Hth hypothermic
HTHD hypertensive heart disease
HTIG human tetanus immune globulin
HTK heel to knee

HTL hamster tumor line; hearing threshold level; histotechnologist; human T-cell leukemia; human thymic leukemia
HTLA high-titer, low avidity [antibody]; human T-lymphocyte antigen
HTL(ASCP) Histotechnologist certified by the American Society of Clinical Pathologists
HTLF human T-cell leukemia virus enhancer factor
HTLV human T-lymphotropic virus
HTLV 1, 2 human T-lymphotropic viruses 1 and 2
HTLV-III human T-cell lymphotrophic virus type III
HTLV-MA cell membrane antigen associated with human T-lymphotropic virus
HTLVR human T-lymphotropic virus receptor
HTML hypertext markup language
HTMT hybrid technology multi-threaded technology
HTN Hantaan [-like virus]; histatin; hypertension; hypertensive nephropathy
HTO high tibial osteotomy; high turnover osteoporosis; hospital transfer order
HTOF healthy tissue overdose factor [radiotherapy]
HTOR 5-hydroxytryptamine oxygenase regulator
HTP House-Tree-Person [test]; hydroxytryptophan; hypothromboplastinemia
5-HTP 5-hydroxy-L-tryptophan
HtPA hexahydrophthalic anhydride
HTPN home total parenteral nutrition
HTR hemolytic transfusion reaction; histidine transport regulator; 5-hydroxytryptamine receptor
hTR human thyroid receptor
HTRAK health maintenance tracking system
hTRb human thyroid receptor beta
HTRCCT high temporal resolution cine computed tomography
HTS Hamilton Twin Study; head traumatic syndrome; HeLa tumor suppression; high-throughput screening; high-titer screening; Home Telecare System [Australia]; human thyroid-stimulating hormone, human thyroid stimulator; hypertonic saline [solution]
hTS human thymidylate synthase

HTSAB human thyroid-stimulating antibody

HTSC home telecare service center

hTSC human thiazide-sensitive sodium-chloride cotransporter

HTSH, hTSH human thyroid-stimulating hormone

HTST high temperature, short time

HTT 5-hydroxytryptamine transformer

HTTP hypertext transfer protocol

HTTPD hypertext transfer protocol daemon

HTTPS secure hypertext transfer protocol; support hypertext transfer protocol

HTV herpes-type virus

HTVD hypertensive vascular disease

HTX heterotaxy, X-linked; histrionicotoxin

HTx heart transplantation

HU heat unit; hemagglutinating unit; hemolytic unit; Hounsfield unit; human urine, human urinary; hydroxyurea; hyperemia unit

Hu human

HUAA home uterine activity assessment

HUB HELIOS unification bus

HUBNET Hospital and University of Buffalo Library Resource Network

HUC human uroepithelial cell; hypouricemia

HuCS human-centered system

HuEPO human erythropoietin

HU-FSH human urinary follicle-stimulating hormone

HUGO Human Genome Organization

HUGV Hughes virus

HUI headache unit index; Health Utilities Index

HUIFM human leukocyte interferon milieu

HuIFN human interferon

HUK human urinary kallikrein

HUM Hilbert uniqueness method

Hum humerus

HUMAN hyper utilities mechatronic assistant [microscopic neurosurgical manipulator]

HUMANE human-oriented universal medical assessment system under network environment

HUP Hospital Utilization Project

HUR hydroxyurea

HURA health in underserved rural areas

HURT hospital utilization review team

HUS heel ultrasonography; hemolytic uremic syndrome; hyaluronidase unit for semen

HuSA human serum albumin

HuSMC human smooth muscle cell

HUT head-up tilt

hut histidine utilization [gene]

HUTHAS human thymus antiserum

HuTV human torovirus

HUV human umbilical vein

HUVEC human umbilical vein endothelial cell

HV hallux valgus; Hantaan virus; has voided; heart volume; hepatic vein; hepatitis virus; herpesvirus; high voltage; high volume; histologically verified; His ventricle; hospital visit; hyperventilation; hypervolemia; hypovirus

H&V hemigastrectomy and vagotomy

H$_v$ heat of evaporation

hv hypervariable region

HVA hallux valgus angle; homovanillic acid

HVAC heating, ventilating, and air conditioning

HVC Health Visitor's Certificate

HVCT helical volume scan computed tomography

HVD Hantavirus [HV] disease; hypertensive vascular disease

HVDRR hypocalcemic vitamin D–resistant rickets

HVE hepatic venous effluence; high-voltage electrophoresis

HVEM herpesvirus [HV] entry mediator

HVG host versus graft [disease]

HVGS high-voltage galvanic stimulation

HVJ hemagglutinating virus of Japan

HVL, hvl half-value layer

HVLP high volume, low pressure

HVM high-velocity missile

HVPC high-voltage pulsed current

HVPE high-voltage paper electrophoresis

HVPG hepatic venous pressure gradient

HVPGS high voltage pulsed galvanic stimulation

HVR hepatic vascular resistance; hypervariable region; hypoxic ventilation response

HVS herpesvirus of Saimiri; herpesvirus sensitivity; high vaginal swab; high-voltage spike-and-wave [discharge]; high-voltage stimulation; high-volume screening; hyperventilation syndrome; hyperviscosity syndrome

HVSD hydrogen-detected ventricular septal defect

HVT half-value thickness; herpesvirus of turkeys

HVTEM high-voltage transmission electron microscopy

HVUS hypocomplementemic vasculitis urticaria syndrome

HVWP hepatic vein wedge pressure

HW half-width; healing well; heart weight; hypertriglyceridemic waist

HWB hot water bottle

HWBW heart weight to body weight [ratio]

HWC Health and Welfare, Canada

HWCD Hans-Weber-Christian disease

HWD heartworm disease

HWE Hardy-Weinberg equilibrium [population genetics]; healthy worker effect; hot water extract

HWML health and welfare makeup language

HWP hepatic wedge pressure; hot wet pack

HWS hot water-soluble

HX histiocytosis X; hydrogen exchange; hypophysectomized; hypoxanthine

Hx hallux; Hemopexin; history; hypoxanthine

hx hospitalization

HXB hexabrachion

HXIS hard x-ray imaging spectrometry

HXM hexamethylmelamine

HXR hypoxanthine riboside

Hy hypermetropia; hyperopia; hypophysis; hypothenar; hysteria

HYC hycanthone methylsulfonate

Hy-C Hydralazine vs Captopril [trial]

HYCAT Hytrin Community Assessment Trial

HYCONES Hybrid Connectionist Expert System

HYCX hydrocephalus due to congenital stenosis of aqueduct of Sylvius

HYD hydralazine; hydration, hydrated; hydrocortisone; hydrodensitometry; hydroxyurea

hydr hydraulic

hydro hydrotherapy

HYE healthy years equivalent

hyg hygiene, hygienic, hygienist

HYL, Hyl hydroxylysine

HYNON Hypertension Non-Drug treatment [cooperative study]

HYP hydroxyproline; hypnosis

Hyp hydroxyproline; hyperresonance; hypertrophy; hypothalamus

hyp hypophysis, hypophysectomy

HyperGEN Hypertension Genetic Epidemiology Network

hyper-IgE hyperimmunoglobulinemia E

hypn hypertension

hypno hypnosis

Hypo hypodermic, hypodermic injection

hypox hypophysectomized

HYPP hyperkalemic periodic paralysis

HYPPOS Hypertensive Population Survey

HYPREN Hypertension under Prazosin and Enalapril [study]

HypRF hypothalamic releasing factor

Hypro hydroxyproline

hys, hyst hysterectomy; hysteria, hysterical

HYSTENOX Enoxaparin Following Hysterectomy [study]

HyTk hybromycin-thymidine kinase

HYVET Hypertension in the Very Elderly Trial

HZ herpes zoster

Hz hertz

HZFesV Hardy-Zuckerman feline sarcoma virus

Hz/G hertz/gauss

HZO herpes zoster ophthalmicus

HZV herpes zoster virus

I

I carcinoma of the vaginal wall [International Federation of Gynecologists and Obstetricians (FIGO) classification]; electric current; endometrial carcinoma in situ confined to the corpus uteri [International Federation of Gynecologists and Obstetricians (FIGO) classification]; immediate; implantation; impression; inactive; incisor [permanent]; increase; independent; index; indicated; indirect; induction; inertia; inhalation; inhibited [pacemaker]; inhibition, inhibitor; inosine; insoluble; inspiration, inspired; insulin; intake; intensity; intermediate; intermittent; internal; internal medicine; intervention; intestine; involvement of a single lymph node [Ann Arbor staging system for Hodgkin disease]; iodine; ionic current; ionic strength; iris; ischemia; isochromosome; isoleucine; isotope; isotropic; nuclear spin quantum number; region of a sarcomere that contains only actin filaments

I2 intervention implementation [AIDS prevention]

I-131 iodine-131

i electric current; incisor [deciduous]; insoluble; isochromosome; optically inactive

ι see *iota*

IA ibotenic acid; image analysis; immediately available; immune adherence; immunoadsorbent; immunobiologic activity; impedance angle; indolaminergic accumulation; indole acetic acid; indolic acid; indulin agar; infantile autism; infected area; inferior angle; information assurance; inhibitory antigen; inpatient admission; intelligent agent [decision support model]; internal auditory; intra-alveolar; intra-amniotic; intra-aortic; intra-arterial; intra-articular; intra-atrial; intra-auricular; intracellular anchor [segment]; intrinsic activity; irradiation area; isopropyl alcohol

I&A identification and authentication; irrigation and aspiration

Ia endometrial carcinoma in situ, length of uterine cavity less than 8 cm [International Federation of Gynecologists and Obstetricians (FIGO) classification]; immune response gene-associated antigen

IAA imidazoleacetic acid; indoleacetic acid; infectious agent, arthritis; insulin autoantibody; International Antituberculosis Association; interruption of the aortic arch; iodoacetic acid

IAAA inflammatory abdominal aortic aneurysm

IAAR imidazoleacetic acid ribonucleotide

IAB Industrial Accident Board; intra-abdominal; intra-aortic balloon

IABA intra-aortic balloon assistance

IABC, IABCP intra-aortic balloon counterpulsation

IABM idiopathic aplastic bone marrow

IABP intra-aortic balloon pump

IABS International Association for Biological Standards

IAC image analysis cytometry; immunoaffinity chromatography; ineffective airway clearance; internal auditory canal; interposed abdominal compression; intra-arterial catheter; intra-arterial chemotherapy

IAC CPR interposed abdominal compression cardiopulmonary resuscitation

IACD implantable automatic cardioverter-defibrillator; intra-arterial conduction defect

IACI idiopathic arterial calcification of infancy

IACOV Iaco virus

IACP intra-aortic counterpulsation

IACS International Academy of Cosmetic Surgery

IACUC institutional animal care and utilization committee

IACV International Association of Cancer Victims and Friends

IAD inactivating dose; instructional advance directive; internal absorbed dose; internal age distribution; intraset distance

IADH inappropriate antidiuretic hormone

IADHS inappropriate antidiuretic hormone syndrome

IADL instrumental or intermediate activities of daily living

IADR International Association for Dental Research

IAds immunoadsorption

IADSA, IA-DSA intra-arterial digital subtraction angiography

IAEA International Atomic Energy Agency

IAET International Association for Enterostomal Therapy

IAF idiopathic alveolar fibrosis; 5-iodoacetamidofluorescein

IAFC International Association of Fire Chiefs

IAFF International Association of Fire Fighters

IAFI infantile amaurotic familial idiocy

IAG International Association of Gerontology; International Academy of Gnathology

IAGP International Association of Geographic Pathology

IAGUS International Association of Genito-Urinary Surgeons

IAH idiopathic adrenal hyperplasia; implantable artificial heart

IAHA idiopathic autoimmune hemolytic anemia; immune adherence hemagglutination

IAHD idiopathic acquired hemolytic disorder

IAHS infection-associated hemophagocytic syndrome; International Association of Hospital Security

IAI integral access interface [telemedicine]; intra-abdominal infection; intra-abdominal injury

IAIMS Integrated Academic Information Management System; Integrated Advanced Information Management System

IAIS insulin autoimmune syndrome

IAM immune adhesion molecule; Institute of Aviation Medicine; internal auditory meatus

i am intra-amniotic

IAMA Infection in Atherosclerosis and Use of Macrolide Antibiotics [study]

IAMM International Association of Medical Museums

IAMS International Association of Microbiological Societies

IAN idiopathic aseptic necrosis; indole acetonitrile

iANP immunoreactive atrial natriuretic peptide

IAO immediately after onset; intermittent aortic occlusion; International Association of Orthodontists

IA OCA oculocutaneous albinism type IA

IAOM International Association of Oral Myology

IAP idiopathic acute pancreatitis; immunosuppressive acidic protein; incident action plan; inosinic acid pyrophosphorylase; Institute of Animal Physiology; integrin-associated protein; intermittent acute porphyria; International Academy of Pathology; International Academy of Proctology; International Atherosclerosis Project; intra-abdominal pressure; intra-arterial pressure; intracellular action potential; intracisternal A-type particle; islet-activating protein

IAPB International Association for Prevention of Blindness

IAPG interatrial pressure gradient

IAPM International Academy of Preventive Medicine

IAPP International Association for Preventive Pediatrics; islet amyloid polypeptide

IAPSRS International Association of Psychosocial Rehabilitation Services

IAPV intermittent abdominal pressure ventilation

IAQ indoor air quality

IAR immediate asthma reaction; inhibitory anal reflex; iodine-azide reaction

IARC International Agency for Research on Cancer

IARF ischemic acute renal failure

IARG International Anticoagulant Review Group [study]

IARS image archival and retrieval system

IARSA idiopathic acquired refractory sideroblastic anemia

IAS immunosuppressive acidic substance; infant apnea syndrome; insulin autoimmune syndrome; interatrial septum; interatrial shunting; internal anal sphincter; International Acquired Immune Deficiency Syndrome Society; intra-amniotic saline

IASA interatrial septal aneurysm

IASD interatrial septal defect; inter-auricular septal defect

IASH isolated asymmetric septal hypertrophy

IASHS Institute for Advanced Study in Human Sexuality

IASL International Association for Study of the Liver

IASLC International Association for the Study of Lung Cancer

IASP International Association for Study of Pain

IASSH Italian Acute Stroke Study with Hemodilution

IAT instillation abortion time; intrinsic accuracy test; invasive activity test; iodine azide test

IATI, IaTI inter-alpha-trypsin inhibitor

IATIL inter-alpha-trypsin inhibitor, light chain

IAV intermittent assisted ventilation; intra-arterial vasopressin

IAVB incomplete atrioventricular block

IAVI International AIDS Vaccine Initiative

IAVM intramedullary arteriovenous malformation

IB idiopathic blepharospasm; immune body; inclusion body; index of body build; infectious bronchitis; instantaneous boundary; Institute of Biology; interface bus; ipratropium bromide

Ib endometrial carcinoma in situ, length of uterine cavity more than 8 cm [International Federation of Gynecologists and Obstetricians (FIGO) classification]

I$_b$ background sodium current [heart electrical activity]

ib in the same place [Lat. *ibidem*]

IBAT intravascular bronchoalveolar tumor

IBAV Ibaraki virus

IBB intestinal brush border

IBBB intra-blood-brain barrier

IBBBB incomplete bilateral bundle branch block

IBC inflammatory breast cancer; inflammatory breast carcinoma; Institutional Biosafety Committee; iodine-binding capacity; iron-binding capacity; isobutyl cyanoacrylate

IBCA isobutyl-2-cyanoacrylate

IBC-R Injury Behavior Checklist-Revised

IBD identical-by-descent; inflammatory bowel disease; integrated balloon display; irritable bowel disease

IBDlist Inflammatory Bowel Disease List [database]

IBDQ Inflammatory Bowel Disease Questionnaire

IBDV infectious bursal disease virus

IBE immunoreactive beta-endomorphin; International Bureau for Epilepsy

IBED Inter-African Bureau for Epizootic Diseases

IBEN individual behavior [UMLS]

IBF immature brown fat; immunoglobulin-binding factor; Insall-Burstein-Freeman [total knee instrumentation]; intestinal blood flow

IBG insoluble bone gelatin

IBI intermittent bladder irrigation; ischemic brain infarction

ibid in the same place [Lat. *ibidem*]

IBIDS ichthyosis-brittle hair-impaired intelligence-decreased fertility-short stature [syndrome]; International Bibliographic Information on Dietary Supplements [NIH database]

IBIS Invasive Bacterial Infection Surveillance [study]

IBK infectious bovine keratoconjunctivitis

IBM inclusion body myositis; intact bridge mastoidectomy

IBMP International Board of Medicine and Psychology

IBMTR International Bone Marrow Transplantation Registry

IBMX 3-isobutyl-1-methylxanthine

IBNR incurred but not reported

IBO information-bearing object

IB OCA oculocutaneous albinism type IB

IBP insulin-like growth factor binding protein; International Biological Program; intra-aortic balloon pumping; iron-binding protein

IBPMS indirect blood pressure measuring system

IBQ Illness Behavior Questionnaire

IBR infectious bovine rhinotracheitis

IBRO International Brain Research Organization

IBRV infectious bovine rhinotracheitis virus

IBS identical-by-state; imidazole buffered saline; immunoblastic sarcoma; integrated backscatter; Iowa Breakfast Study; irritable bowel syndrome; isobaric solution

IBSA iodinated bovine serum albumin

IBSN infantile bilateral striated necrosis

IBSP integrin-binding sialoprotein

IBSS International Bibliography of the Social Sciences

IBT ink blot test

IBTR ipsilateral breast tumor recurrence

IbTX iberiotoxin

IBU ibuprofen; international benzoate unit

i-Bu isobutyl

IBV infectious bronchitis vaccine; infectious bronchitis virus; Ivorian bacilliform virus

IBW ideal body weight

IC icteric, icterus; immune complex; immunoconjugate; immunocytochemistry; immunocytotoxicity; impedance cardiogram; imprinting center; indirect calorimetry; individual counseling; infection control; inferior colliculus; information and communication; informed consent; inner canthal [distance]; inorganic carbon; inspiratory capacity; inspiratory center; institutional care; integrated circuit; integrated concentration; intensive care; intercostal; intermediate care; intermittent catheterization; intermittent claudication; internal capsule; internal carotid; internal conjugate; interstitial cell; intracapsular; intracardiac; intracarotid; intracavitary; intracellular; intracerebral; intracisternal; intracranial; intracutaneous; intraoperative cholangiography; irritable colon; islet cells; isovolumic contraction

IC 1/2/3 intermediate care 1/2/3

IC$_{50}$ inhibitory concentration of 50%

ICA immunocytochemical analysis; independent component analysis; internal carotid artery; intracranial aneurysm; islet cell antibody

ICAA International Council on Alcohol and Addictions; Invalid Children's Aid Association

ICAAC Interscience Conference on Antimicrobial Agents and Chemotherapy

ICAb islet cell antibody

IC-AFM intermittent-contact mode atomic force microscopy

ICAI intelligent computer-aided instruction

ICAM improved chemical agent monitor; induced endothelial cell adhesion molecule; integrated computer-aided manufacturing

ICAM-1, -2, -3 intracellular adhesion molecule 1, 2, 3

ICAMI International Committee Against Mental Illness

ICAO internal carotid artery occlusion

ICARIS Intervention Cardiology Risk Stratification [study]

ICARUS Islet Cell Antibody Register User Study

ICASO International Committee of Acquired Immunodeficiency Syndrome Service Organisations

ICAT International Comprehensive Anatomical Terminology

ICBDMS International Clearinghouse for Birth Defects Monitoring Systems

ICBF inner cortical blood flow

ICBG idiopathic calcification of basal ganglia

ICBM International Consortium for Brain Mapping

ICBP intracellular binding protein

ICBPG improved chemical and biological protective glove

ICBR increased chromosomal breakage rate

ICC immunocompetent cells; immunocytochemistry; Indian childhood cirrhosis; infection control committee; intensive coronary care; interchromosomal crossing over; interclass correlation coefficient; intercluster constraint; internal conversion coefficient; International Certification Commission; interventional cardiac center; intraclass correlation coefficient; intracranial cavity; invasive cervical cancer; Italian [Committee for TNM] Cancer Classification

ICCE intracapsular cataract extraction

iCCK immunoreactive cholecystokinin

ICCM idiopathic congestive cardiomyopathy

ICCR International Committee for Contraceptive Research

ICCS International Classification of Clinical Services

ICCU intensive coronary care unit; intermediate coronary care unit

ICD I-cell disease; immune complex disease; impedance cardiogram; implantable cardioverter-defibrillator; impulse-control disorder; induced circular dichroism; initial cardioverter-defibrillator; Institute for Crippled and Disabled; intercanthal distance; International Center for the Disabled; International Classification of Diseases, Injuries, and Causes of Death;

International Statistical Classification of Diseases and Health-related Problems; intracardiac defibrillator; intracervical device; intrauterine contraceptive device; ischemic coronary disease; isocitrate dehydrogenase; isolated conduction defect

ICD-10 International Statistical Classification of Diseases and Health-related Problems, 10th Revision

ICDA International Classification of Diseases, Adapted

ICD/BPA International Classification of Diseases as adapted by the British Paediatric Association

ICDC implantable cardioverter-defibrillator catheter

ICD-9-CM International Classification of Diseases, 9th Revision-Clinical Modification

ICDH isocitrate dehydrogenase

ICD-O International Classification of Diseases-Oncology

ICDRC International Contact Dermatitis Research Center

ICDREC International Computer Database for Radiation Accident Case Histories

ICDS Integrated Child Development Scheme; International Cardiac Doppler Society

ICE ice, compression, elevation; ichthyosis-cheek-eyebrow [syndrome]; immunochemical evaluation; integrated clinical encounter; integration, codification and evaluation; interleukin converting enzyme; intracardiac echocardiography; iridocorneal endothelial [syndrome]

ICECA International Committee for Electronic Communication on Acquired Immunodeficiency Syndrome

ICECG intracardiac electrocardiography

ICED Index of Co-existent Diseases

ICEEG intracranial electroencephalography

ICER inducible cyclic adenosine monophosphate [cAMP] early repressor

ICES information collection and evaluation system

ICET induced current electrical impedance tomography

ICEUS intracaval endovascular ultrasound

ICF immunodeficiency-centromeric; instability-facial anomalies [syndrome];

indirect centrifugal flotation; intensive care facility; intercellular fluorescence; interciliary fluid; intermediate-care facility; International Cardiology Foundation; intracellular fluid; intravascular coagulation and fibrinolysis

ICFA incomplete Freund adjuvant; induced complement-fixing antigen

ICFF important clinical field finding

ICF(M)A International Cystic Fibrosis (Mucoviscidosis) Association

ICF-MR intermediate-care facility for the mentally retarded

ICF/MR intensive care facilities for mental retardation

ICG impedance cardiogram; impedance cardiography; indocyanine green; isotope cisternography

ICGC indocyanine-green clearance

ICGN immune-complex glomerulonephritis

ICH idiopathic cortical hyperostosis; immunocompromised host; infectious canine hepatitis; Institute of Child Health [UK]; International Conference on Harmonisation [of technical requirements for registration of pharmaceuticals for human use]; intracerebral hematoma; intracranial hemorrhage; intracranial hypertension

ICHD Inter-Society Commission for Heart Disease Resources

ICHPPC International Classification of Health Problems in Primary Care

IcHV Ictalurid herpesvirus

ICI intracardiac infection

ICi intracisternal

ICIC International Classification of Primary Care

ICIDH International Classification of Impairments, Disabilities, and Handicaps

ICIN Intracoronary Streptokinase Trial of the Interuniversity Cardiology Institute of the Netherlands

ICIS imaging center information system

iCJD iatrogenic Creutzfeldt-Jakob disease

ICL idiopathic CD4 T-cell lymphocytopenia; implantable contact lens; intracranial lesion; iris-clip lens; isocitrate lyase

I$_{cl}$ chloride ionic current [heart electrical activity]

ICLA International Committee on Laboratory Animals

ICLAS International Council for Laboratory Animal Science

ICLH Imperial College, London Hospital

ICM inner cell mass; integrated conditional model; intelligent cardiovascular monitor; intercostal margin; International Confederation of Midwives; intersecting core model; intracellular multiplication; intracytoplasmic membrane; introduction to clinical medicine; ion conductance modulator; isolated cardiovascular malformation

icm intracellular multiplication

ICMA immunochemiluminometric assay

ICMI Inventory of Childhood Memories and Imaginings

ICML International Congress on Medical Librarianship

ICMP Internet control message protocol

ICMSF International Commission on Microbiological Specifications for Foods

ICN intensive care nursery; International Council of Nurses

ICNa intracellular concentration of sodium

ICNB International Committee on Nomenclature of Bacteria

ICNC intracerebral nuclear cell

ICNIRP International Commission on Nonionizing Radiation Protection

ICNND Interdepartmental Committee on Nutrition in National Defense

ICNP International Classification of Nursing Practice

ICNV International Committee on Nomenclature of Viruses

ICO idiopathic cyclic oedema; impedance cardiac output; infection control officer

ICOHCS Ishi Town Preschool Children Oral Health Care Study [Japan]

ICOMS input, constraints, output, and mechanisms

ICOPER International Cooperative Pulmonary Embolism Registry

ICP incident command post; incubation period; indwelling catheter program; infantile cerebral palsy; infection-control practitioner; infectious cell protein; inflammatory cloacogenic polyp; insecticidal crystal protein; integrated care pathway or planning; interactive closest point [algorithm]; interdisciplinary care plan; intermittent catheterization protocol; intracranial pressure; intracytoplasmic; intrahepatic cholestasis of pregnancy; iterative closest point [algorithm]

ICPA International Commission for the Prevention of Alcoholism

ICPB International Collection of Phytopathogenic Bacteria

ICPC International Classification of Primary Care

ICPC-PLUS International Classification of Primary Care with extension and electronic version

ICPEMC International Commission for Protection against Environmental Mutagens and Carcinogens

ICPI Intersociety Committee on Pathology Information

ICP-MS inductively coupled plasma mass spectrometer; inductively coupled plasma mass spectrometry

ICPR International Commission on Stage Grouping and Presentation of Results [cancer]

ICR [distance between] iliac crests; Institute for Cancer Research; intermittent catheter routine; International Congress of Radiology; international consensus report; intracardiac catheter recording; intracavitary radium; intracorneal ring; intracranial reinforcement; ion cyclotron resonance

ICRAC calcium release-activated calcium current

ICRC infant care review committee; International Committee of the Red Cross; Islet Cell Resource Center

ICRD Index of Codes for Research Drugs

ICRE International Commission on Radiological Education

ICRETT International Cancer Research Technology Transfer

ICREW International Cancer Research Workshop

ICRF Imperial Cancer Research Fund [UK]

I-CRF immunoreactive corticotropin-releasing factor

ICRF-159 razoxane

ICRP International Commission on Radiological Protection; International Committee on Radiation Protection

ICRS Index Chemicus Registry System

ICRT intracoronary radiation therapy

ICRU International Commission on Radiation Units and Measurements

ICS ileocecal sphincter; image criteria score; immotile cilia syndrome; immunocytochemical staining; impulse-conducting system; incident command system; information and communication system; inhaled corticosteroids; integrated case study; intensive care, surgical; intercellular space; intercostal space; intercuspidation splint; International College of Surgeons; International Cytokine Society; intracellular segment; intracranial stimulation; Iohexol Cooperative Study; irritable colon syndrome

I&CS information and communication system

ICSA islet cell surface antibody

ICSB International Committee on Systematic Bacteriology

ICSC idiopathic central serous choroidopathy

ICS$_f$ final intercuspidation splint

ICSG International Cooperative Study Group

ICSH International Committee for Standardization in Hematology; interstitial cell-stimulating hormone

ICS-HSH Information and Communication System-Health Smart Home

ICSI Institute for Clinical Systems Integration; intracytoplasmic sperm injection

ICSK intracoronary streptokinase

ICSO intermittent coronary sinus occlusion

ICSP Interagency Council on Statistical Policy; International Council of Societies of Pathology

ICSS intracranial self-stimulation

I/CSS informed consent support system

ICSTI International Council for Scientific and Technical Information

ICSU International Council of Scientific Unions

ICT icteric, icterus; indirect Coombs test; induction chemotherapy; inflammation of connective tissue; information and communications technology; insulin coma therapy; intensive conventional therapy; intermittent cervical traction; interstitial cell tumor; intracardiac thrombus; intracranial tumor; isovolumic contraction time

Ict icterus

iCT immunoreactive calcitonin

ICTDR International Centers for Tropical Disease Research

ICTMM International Congress on Tropical Medicine and Malaria

ICTS idiopathic carpal tunnel syndrome

ICTV International Committee for the Taxonomy of Viruses

ICTVdB International Committee on Taxonomy of Viruses Database

ICTX intermittent cervical traction

ICU infant care unit; immunologic contact urticaria; intensive care unit; intermediate care unit

ICUS intracoronary ultrasound

ICV internal cerebral vein; intracellular volume; intracerebroventricular

icv intracerebroventricular

ICVA intracranial vertebral artery

ICVS International Cardiovascular Society

ICW intensive care ward; intermediate care ward; intracellular water

ICWS integrated clinical workstation

ICx immune complex; inter-cartridge exchange

ID identification; identifier; idiotype; iditol dehydrogenase; immunodeficiency; immunodiffusion; immunoglobulin deficiency; inappropriate disability; incapacitating dose; inclusion disease; index of discrimination; individual dose; infant death; infectious disease; infective dose; inhibitory dose; initial diagnosis; initial dose; initial dyskinesia; injected dose; inside diameter; interdigitating; interhemispheric disconnection; internal diameter; interstitial disease; intradermal; intraduodenal

ID$_{50}$ median incapacitating dose; median infective dose

I-D intensity-duration

I&D incision and drainage

Id infradentale; interdentale

id the same [Lat. *idem*]

IDA idamycin; iduronidase; image display and analysis; iminodiacetic acid; insulin-degrading activity; intelligent data analysis; iron deficiency anemia

IDAMAP intelligent data analysis in medicine and pharmacology

IDAV immunodeficiency-associated virus

IDB image data baser

IDBS infantile diffuse brain sclerosis

IDC idiopathic dilated cardiomyopathy; infiltrating ductal carcinoma; interdigitating cell

iDC immature dendritic cell

IDCI intradiplochromatid interchange

IDCOP idealized design of clinical office practice

IDCS Idiopathic Dilated Cardiomyopathy Study

IDCT inverse discrete cosine transform

IDD idealized dose distribution [radiotherapy]; insulin-dependent diabetes; intraluminal duodenal diverticulum; Inventory to Diagnose Depression

IDDF investigational drug data form

IDDM insulin-dependent diabetes mellitus

IDDM-MED insulin-dependent diabetes mellitus-multiple epiphyseal dysplasia [syndrome]

IDDP immediate drug development project

IDDT immune double diffusion test

IDE insulin-degrading enzyme; integrated development environment; intelligent drive electronics; investigational device exemption

IDEA Individuals with Disabilities Education Act; Internet Database of Evidence-based Abstracts and Articles

IDEF Integrated [Computer-Aided Manufacturing] Definition

i-DENT Internet Dental Epidemiology System Produced by Tokushima University [Japan]

IDF inverse document frequency

IDFT inverse discrete Fourier transform

IDG intermediate dose group

IDH intraductal hyperplasia; isocitrate dehydrogenase

IDHS Indian Diet Heart Study

IDI immunologically detectable insulin; induction-delivery interval; inter-dentale inferius

I-5DI type I 5′deiodinase

IDIC Internal Dose Information Center

idic isodicentric

IDIS International Drug Information Service; intraoperative digital substraction angiography

IDISA intraoperative digital substraction angiography

IDK internal derangement of knee

IDL Index to Dental Literature; interface definition language; intermediate density lipoprotein; intermediate differentiation of lymphocytic lymphoma; isodose line [radiotherapy]

IDL-C, IDL-c intermediate density lipoprotein-cholesterol complex

IDLH immediate danger to life and health

IDM idiopathic disease of myocardium; immune defense mechanism; indirect method; infant of diabetic mother; intermediate-dose methotrexate; inverse different moment

ID-MS isotope dilution-mass spectrometry

IDN integrated delivery network

iDNA intercalary deoxyribonucleic acid

IDP imidodiphosphonate; immunodiffusion procedure; inflammatory demyelinating neuropathy; initial dose period; inosine diphosphate

IDPH idiopathic pulmonary hemosiderosis

IDPN iminodipropionitrile; inflammatory demyelinating polyneuropathy

IDQ Individualized Dementia Questionnaire

IDR intradermal reaction; item discrimination ratio

IDS iduronate sulfatase; immune deficiency state; infectious diseases service; inhibitor of DNA synthesis; integrated delivery system; International Documentation System; intraduodenal stimulation; Inventory for Depressive Symptomatology; investigational drug service

IdS interdentale superius

IDSA Infectious Diseases Society of America; intraoperative digital subtraction angiography

IDSAN International Drug Safety Advisory Network

IDS-CRC International Documentation System-Colorectal Cancer

IDSRN Integrated Delivery System Research Network

IDS-SR Inventory for Depressive Symptomatology-Systems Review

IDT immune diffusion test; instillation delivery time; interdisciplinary team; intradermal typhoid [vaccine]

IDU idoxuridine; injecting drug use; injection or intravenous drug user; iododeoxyuridine
IDUA iduronidase
IdUA iduronic acid
IDUR idoxuridine
IdUrd idoxuridine
IDUS injecting drug users
IDV intermittent demand ventilation
IDVC indwelling venous catheter
IDW initial deflection width [respiratory sounds]
IDWT inverse discrete wavelet transform
IDX 4′-iodo-4′-deoxyoxorubicin
Idx cross-reactive idiotype
IE imaging equipment; immediate early [genes]; immunizing unit [Ger. *Immunitäts Einheit*]; immunoelectrophoresis; infective endocarditis; information economics; information engineering; inner ear; intake energy; internal elastica; intraepithelial
ie that is [Lat. *id est*]
I/E inspiratory/expiratory [ratio]; internal/external
I$_E$ involvement of a single extrahepatic organ or site [Ann Arbor staging system for Hodgkin disease]
I:E inspiratory/expiratory [ratio]
IEA immediate early antigen; immunoelectroadsorption; immunoelectrophoretic analysis; infectious equine anemia; inferior epigastric artery; International Epidemiological Association; intravascular erythrocyte aggregation
IEBC International Entomopathogenic Bacillus Center
IEC information, education, communication; injection electrode catheter; inpatient exercise center; International Electrotechnical Commission; intestinal epithelial cell; intraepithelial carcinoma; ion-exchange chromatography
IECa intraepithelial carcinoma
IECG intracardiac electrocardiography
IED inherited epidermal dysplasia; intermittent explosive disorder
IEE inner enamel epithelium
IEEE Institute of Electrical and Electronics Engineers
IEEG intracranial electroencephalography
IEF International Eye Foundation; isoelectric focusing
IEG immediate early gene

IEGM intracardiac electrogram
I-EHR integrated electronic health record
IEI isoelectric interval
IEL internal elastic lamina; intraepithelial lymphocyte
IEM immuno-electron microscopy; inborn error of metabolism
IEMA immunoenzymatic assay
IEMCT individualized epidural morphine conversion tool
IEMG integrated electromyogram; integrated electromyography
IEOP immunoelectro-osmophoresis
IEP immunoelectrophoresis; individualized education program; isoelectric point
IERIV Ieri virus
IES impact of events scale; inferior esophageal sphincter
IESS Intergroup Ewing Sarcoma Study
IET intrauterine exchange transfusion
IETF Internet Engineering Task Force
IETT immediate exercise treadmill testing
IF idiopathic fibroplasia; idiopathic flushing; immersion foot; immunofluorescence; impact factor; indirect fluorescence; infrared; inhibiting factor; initiation factor; instantaneous flow; instantaneous frequency [ECG]; integrate and fire [neuron]; intensifying factor; interbody fusion; interferon; interior facet; intermediate filament; intermediate frequency; internal fixation; interstitial fluid; interventional fluoroscopy; intrinsic factor; involved field [radiotherapy]
IF1, IF2, IF3 interferon 1, 2, 3
I$_f$ hyperpolarization-activated current [heart electrical activity]
IFA idiopathic fibrosing alveolitis; immunofluorescence assay; immunofluorescent antibody; incomplete Freund's adjuvant; indirect fluorescent antibody; indirect fluorescent assay; International Fertility Association; International Filariasis Association
IFAA International Federation of Associations of Anatomists
IFABP intestinal fatty acid binding protein
IFAP ichthyosis follicularis-atrichia-photophobia [syndrome]
IFAT indirect fluorescent antibody test
IFBC International Food Biotechnology Council

IFC intermittent flow centrifugation; intrinsic factor concentrate

IFCC International Federation of Clinical Chemistry

IFCR International Foundation for Cancer Research

IFCS inactivated fetal calf serum

IFDS isolated follicle-stimulating hormone deficiency syndrome

IFE immunofixation electrophoresis; interfollicular epidermis

IFEV Ife virus

IFF inner fracture face

IFFH International Foundation for Family Health

IFG inferior frontal gyrus; interferon gamma

IFGO International Federation of Gynecology and Obstetrics

IFGS interstitial fluid and ground substance

IFGT irradiation and fusion gene transfer

IFHGS International Federation of Human Genetics Societies

IFHNOS International Federation of Head and Neck Oncologic Societies

IFHP International Federation of Health Professionals

IFHPMSM International Federation for Hygiene, Preventive Medicine, and Social Medicine

IFI immune interferon; intensified followup indicator [pacemaker]

IFIP International Federation for Information Processing

IFL immunofluorescence

IFLrA recombinant human leukocyte interferon A

IFM internal fetal monitor; isoleucine, phenylalanine, and methionine

IFMBE International Federation for Medical and Biological Engineering

IFME International Federation for Medical Electronics

IFMP International Federation for Medical Psychotherapy

IFMSA International Federation of Medical Student Associations

IFMSS International Federation of Multiple Sclerosis Societies

IFN interferon

IFNA interferon alpha

IFN α, β, γ interferon alpha, beta, and gamma

If nec if necessary

IFNG interferon gamma

IFNGT interferon gamma transducer

IFOS International Federation of ORL Societies

IFP inflammatory fibroid polyp; insulin, compound F [hydrocortisone], prolactin; interactive filtered projection [radiotherapy]; intermediate filament protein; intimal fibrous proliferation; intrapatellar fat pad

IFPM International Federation of Physical Medicine

IFR infrared; inspiratory flow rate

IFRA indirect fluorescent rabies antibody [test]

IFRP International Fertility Research Program

IFRT involved field radiotherapy

IFS interstitial fluid space

IFSE International Federation of Science Editors

IFSM information system; International Federation of Sports Medicine

IFSP individualized family service plan

IFSSH International Federation of Societies for Surgery of the Hand; International Forum for Social Sciences in Health

IFT immunofluorescence test; inverse Fourier transform

IFU interferon unit

IFV interstitial fluid volume; intracellular fluid volume

IG immature granule; immunoglobulin; insulin and glucose; intergenic; interstitial glucose; intragastric; irritable gut

Ig immunoglobulin

IGA infantile genetic agranulocytosis

IgA immunoglobulin A

IgA1, IgA2 subclasses of immunoglobulin A

IgAGN immunoglobulin A glomerulonephritis

IgAN immunoglobulin A nephropathy

IGC immature germ cell; intragastric cannula

IG-CAM immunoglobulin of cell adhesion molecule

IGCP intraglomerular capillary pressure

IGD idiopathic growth hormone deficiency; Integrated Genome Database;

interglobal distance; isolated gonadotropin deficiency

IgD immunoglobulin D

IgD1, IgD2 subclasses of immunoglobulin D

IGDM infant of mother with gestational diabetes mellitus

IGE idiopathic generalized epilepsy; impaired gas exchange

IgE immunoglobulin E

IgE1 subclass of immunoglobulin E

IGF insulin-like growth factor

IGF-I insulin-like growth factor-I

IGFBP insulin-like growth factor binding protein

IGF-I-BP insulin-like growth factor I binding protein

IGFBP-3 IGF-binding protein 3

IGFET insulated gate field effect transistor

IGF-I-KIRA insulin-like growth factor I kinase receptor activation

IGFL integral green fluorescence

IGFR insulin-like growth factor receptor

IGF1R insulin-like growth factor receptor type 1

IgG immunoglobulin G

IgG1, IgG2, IgG3, IgG4 subclasses of immunoglobulin G

IgG-SC immunoglobulin G secreting cells

IGH immunoreactive growth hormone

IgH immunoglobulin heavy chain

IgHC immunoglobulin heavy chain constant region

IGHD immunoglobin delta heavy chain; isolated growth hormone deficiency

IGHE immunoglobulin epsilon heavy chain

IGHV immunoglobulin heavy chain variable region

IGI intelligent graphic interface

IGIF interferon-γ-inducing factor

IGIV immune globulin intravenous

IGKDEL immunoglobulin kappa deleting element

IGL immunoglobulin lambda; immunoglobulin light chain

IGLJ immunoglobulin lambda light chain J

IGLL immunoglobulin lambda-like

IGLLC inferior glenohumeral ligament labral complex

iGluR ionotropic glutamate receptor

IGM Internet Grateful Med

IgM immunoglobulin M

IgM1 subclass of immunoglobulin M

IgMN immunoglobulin M nephropathy

IGNS image-guided neurosurgery

IGO1 immunoglobulin kappa orphan 1

IGOS Image Guided Orthopaedic Surgery [project]

IGP intestinal glycoprotein

IGR immediate generalized reaction; integrated gastrin response

iGrid international grid

IGS image-guided surgery; inappropriate gonadotropin secretion; internal guide sequence

Igs immunoglobulins

IgSC immunoglobulin-secreting cell

IGSF immunoglobulin superfamily

IGSS immuno-gold silver staining

IGT impaired glucose tolerance

IGTT intravenous glucose tolerance test

IGUV Iguape virus

IGV intrathoracic gas volume

IH idiopathic hirsutism; idiopathic hypercalciuria; immediate hypersensitivity; incompletely healed; indirect hemagglutination; industrial hygiene; infantile hydrocephalus; infectious hepatitis; inguinal hernia; inhibiting hormone; in hospital; inner half; inpatient hospital; intermittent heparinization; intimal hyperplasia; intracranial hematoma; iron hematoxylin

IHA idiopathic hyperaldosteronism; indirect hemagglutination; indirect hemagglutination antibody; intrahepatic atresia

IHAC Industrial Health and Advisory Committee

IHAPS interactive health appraisal system

IHBT incompatible hemolytic blood transfusion

IHC idiopathic hemochromatosis; idiopathic hypercalciuria; immunohistochemical [staining assay]; immunohistochemistry; inner hair cell; interactive health communication system; Internet Healthcare Coalition; intrahepatic cholestasis

IHCA individual health care account; isocapnic hyperventilation with cold air

IHCM ichthyosis hystrix, Curth-Macklin [type]

IHCP Institute of Hospital and Community Psychiatry

IHD in-center hemodialysis; intermittent hemodialysis; ischemic heart disease

IHDI ischemic heart disease index

IHDP Infant Health and Development Program

IHDPORT Ischemic Heart Disease Patient Outcomes Research Team

IHD SDP Ischemic Heart Disease Shared Decision-Making Program

IHES idiopathic hypereosinophilic syndrome

IHF Industrial Health Foundation; integration host factor; interhemispheric fissure; International Hospital Foundation

IHGD isolateral human growth deficiency

IHH idiopathic hypogonadotropic hypogonadism; idiopathic hypothalamic hypogonadism; infectious human hepatitis

IHHS idiopathic hyperkinetic heart syndrome

IHI Institute for Healthcare Improvement

IHIS integrated hospital information system

IHL International Homeopathic League

IHM in-hospital malnutrition

IHN integrated health care network

IHO idiopathic hypertrophic osteo-arthropathy

IHOU in-hospital observation unit

IHP idiopathic hypoparathyroidism; idiopathic hypopituitarism; individualized health plan; inositol hexaphosphate; interhospitalization period; inverted hand position

IHPC intrahepatic cholestasis

IHPH intrahepatic portal hypertension

IHPP Intergovernmental Health Project Policy

IHQL index of health-related quality of life

IHR International Health Regulations; intrahepatic resistance; intrinsic heart rate

IHRA isocapnic hyperventilation with room air

IHRB Industrial Health Research Board

IHS idiopathic hypereosinophilic syndrome; inactivated horse serum; Indian Health Service; innovative health care system; integrated health system; International Headache Society; International Health Society; intracranial hypotension syndrome

IHSA iodinated human serum albumin

IHSC immunoreactive human skin collagenase

IHSS idiopathic hypertrophic subaortic stenosis

IHT insulin hypoglycemia test; intravenous histamine test; ipsilateral head turning

I5HT intraplatelet serotonin

IHW International Histocompatibility Workshop

II carcinoma of the subvaginal tissue without involving the pelvic wall [International Federation of Gynecologists and Obstetricians (FIGO) classification]; endometrial carcinoma involving the corpus and cervix but no other tissues [International Federation of Gynecologists and Obstetricians (FIGO) classification]; icterus index; image intensification or intensifier; involvement of two or more lymph nodes on the same side of the diaphragm [Ann Arbor staging system for Hodgkin disease]

I&I illness and injuries

Ii incision inferius

IIA internal iliac artery

IIC ineffective individual coping

IICP increased intracranial pressure

IID independent identically distributed [nucleotides]; insulin-independent diabetes

IIDM insulin-independent diabetes mellitus

IIE idiopathic ineffective erythropoiesis

II$_E$ localized involvement of an extrahepatic organ or site [Ann Arbor staging system for Hodgkin disease]

IIEF International Index of Erectile Function

i-IEL intestinal intraepithelial lymphocyte

IIF immune interferon; indirect immunofluorescence; intracellular ice formation; isolated intraperitoneal fluid

IIFT intraoperative intraarterial fibrinolytic therapy

IIG imagineering interest group; interactive image-guided [surgery]

IIGR ipsilateral instinctive grasp reaction

IIH idiopathic infantile hypercalcemia

IIHD Israeli Ischemic Heart Disease [study]

III endometrial carcinoma extending outside the uterus but not outside the true pelvis [International Federation of Gynecologists and Obstetricians (FIGO) classification]; involvement of two or more lymph node regions on both sides of the diaphragm [Ann Arbor staging system for Hodgkin disease]; vaginal carcinoma extending to pelvic wall [International Federation of Gynecologists and Obstetricians (FIGO) classification]

III$_E$ localized involvement of an extrahepatic organ or site [Ann Arbor staging system for Hodgkin disease]

III-para tertipara

III$_S$ localized involvement of the spleen [Ann Arbor staging system for Hodgkin disease]

III$_{SE}$ localized involvement of an extrahepatic organ and spleen [Ann Arbor staging system for Hodgkin disease]

IIME Institute of International Medical Education

IIMS Interest in Internal Medicine Scale

IIOP Internet inter object request broker protocol

IIP idiopathic interstitial pneumonia; idiopathic intestinal pseudo-obstruction; increased intracranial pressure

II-para secundipara

I-123 IPPA I-123 Iodo-Phenylpentadecanoic Acid [Viability Multicenter Study]

IIR infinite impulse response; Internet information retrieval

IIS intensive immunosuppression; International Institute of Stress; Internet information server; [Microsoft] Internet Information Service

IIT induction of immune tolerance; ineffective iron turnover; intensive insulin therapy; interactive image tool

IITF Information Infrastructure Task Force

IIUK Intraoperative Intra-Arterial Urokinase [study]

IIVS Institute for In-Vitro Sciences

IJ ileojejunal; internal jugular; intrajejunal; intrajugular

IJCAI International Joint Conference on Artificial Intelligence

IJD inflammatory joint disease

IJP inhibitory junction potential; internal jugular pressure

IJV internal jugular vein

IK immobilized knee; immune body [Ger. *Immunekörper*]; *Infusoria* killing [unit]; interstitial keratitis

I-K immunoconglutinin

I$_K$ potassium current [heart electrophysiology]

I$_k$ delayed rectifier current [heart electrophysiology]

I$_{K(AC, Adoi)}$ acetylcholine and adeno-sensitive potassium current [heart electrophysiology]

I$_{K-Ach}$ acetylcholine-induced potassium current [heart electrophysiology]

I$_{KAdo}$ outward inwardly rectifying potassium current [heart electrophysiology]

I$_{K(ATP)}$, I$_{K-ATP}$ ATP-sensitive potassium current [heart electrical activity]

IKE Internet key exchange protocol; ion kinetic energy

I$_{KI}$ inward rectifier current [heart electrophysiology]

I$_{Kp}$ plateau potassium current [heart electrophysiology]

I$_{Kr}$ rectified potassium current [heart electrophysiology]

IKU *Infusoria* killing unit

IL ileum; iliolumbar; immature lung; incisolingual; independent laboratory; inguinal ligament; inspiratory load; instant library; intensity load; interleukin; internal loop; intestinal lymphocyte; intracellular loop; intralumbar; intraocular lens

IL-1 to 15 interleukin 1 to 15

ILA insulin-like activity; International Leprosy Association

ILa incisolabial

ILAE International League Against Epilepsy

ILAR Institute of Laboratory Animal Research

ILB infant, low birth [weight]; initial lung burden

ILBBB incomplete left bundle branch block

ILBW infant, low birth weight

ILC ichthyosis linearis circumflex; incipient lethal concentration; interstitial laser coagulation

ILD interstitial lung disease; intraoperative localization device; ischemic leg disease; ischemic limb disease; isolated lactase deficiency

ILDBP interleukin-dependent deoxyribonucleic acid-binding protein

ILE information-laden event; isoleucine

ILe, Ile isoleucine

ILED infrared light emission diode

IIeRS isoleucyl ribonucleic acid synthetase
ILEV Ilesha virus
ILGA International Lesbian and Gay Association
ILGF insulin-like growth factor
ILH immunoreactive luteinizing hormone
ILHV Ilheus virus
ILIS intelligent laboratory information system
ILL interlibrary loan; intermediate lymphocytic lymphoma
ILLE inverted [position] with lower limbs extended
ILM insulin-like material; internal limiting membrane
ILMA, I-LMA intubating laryngeal mask airway
ILMS Israel Longitudinal Mortality Study
ILNR intralobar nephrogenic rest
ILo iodine lotion
ILP inadequate luteal phase; insufficiency of luteal phase; insulin-loaded polymer; interstitial laser photocoagulation; interstitial lymphocytic pneumonia; isolated limb perfusion
ILR interleukin receptor; irreversible loss rate
IL-1R to 15R interleukin 1 to 15 receptors
ILRA interleukin receptor alpha
IL1-RA interleukin-1 receptor antagonist
ILRB interleukin receptor beta
ILRCFS Iowa Lipid Research Clinics Family Study
ILS idiopathic leucine sensitivity; idiopathic lymphadenopathy syndrome; increase in life span; infrared liver scanner; integrated library system; intermittent light stimulation; intralobal sequestration
ILSA Italian Longitudinal Study on Aging
ILSI International Life Sciences Institute
ILSS integrated life support system; intraluminal somatostatin
ILT iliotibial tract
ILTV infectious laryngotracheitis virus
ILUS intraluminal ultrasound
ILV independent lung ventilation; instantaneous lung volume [recording]
ILVEN inflamed linear verrucous epidermal nevus
ILY intermedilysin
IM idiopathic myelofibrosis; immunosuppressive method; implementation monitoring; Index Medicus; indomethacin;

industrial medicine; infection medium; infectious mononucleosis; information management; inner membrane; innocent murmur; inspiratory muscles; intensity modulated; intermediate; intermediate megaloblast; intermediate metabolizer; internal malleolus; internal mammary [artery]; internal margin [imaging]; internal medicine; internal monitor; intramedullary; intrametatarsal; intramuscular; invasive mole; isolated microcalcification
I-M incudomalleolar
2IM 2-ipomeanol
Im imidazole
im intramuscular
IMA immunometric assay; Industrial Medical Association; inferior mesenteric artery; installation medical authority; Interchurch Medical Assistance; intermetatarsal angle; internal mammary artery; internal maxillary artery; Irish Medical Association
IMAA iodinated macroaggregated albumin
IMAB internal mammary artery bypass
IMAC image management archiving and communications; immobilized metal affinity capture; information management, archiving, and communication; Intervention in Myocarditis and Acute Cardiomyopathy [study]
IMACS image archiving and communication system; image management and communication system
IMAGE integrated molecular analysis of gene expression; International Metoprolol/Nifedipine Angina Exercise Trial; International Multicenter Angina Exercise [study]; International Multicenter Aprotinin Graft Patency Experience [trial]
IMAGES Intravenous Magnesium Efficacy in Stroke [trial]
IMAI internal mammary artery implant
IMAP Internet mail access protocol
I_{max} maximum [drug-induced] inhibition
IMB intensity-modulated beam [radiotherapy]; intermenstrual bleeding
IMBC indirect maximum breathing capacity
IMBI Institute of Medical and Biological Illustrators
IMC indigent medical care; information-memory-concentration [test]; intelligent

monitoring and control; interdigestive migrating contractions; internal mammary chain; internal medicine clinic; internal model control; International Medical Corps; intestinal mast cell

IMCD inner medullary collecting duct

IMCI Integrated Management of Childhood Illness [PAHO]

IMCT Information-Memory-Concentration Test; International Multicentre Trial

IMCU intermediate medical care unit

IMD immunodeficiency; immunologically mediated disease; information management department; institution for mentally disabled

ImD$_{50}$ median immunizing dose

IMDC intramedullary metatarsal decompression

IMDD idiopathic midline destructive disease

IMDDI individual molecular dataset diversity index

IMDG International Maritime Dangerous Goods [code]

IMDM Iscove's modified Dulbecco's medium

IMDP imidocarb diproprionate

IME independent medical examination; indirect medical education

IMEG innovations in medical education grant

IMEL International Medical Electronic Link [telemedicine]

IMEM improved minimum essential medium

IMEP Investigation in Menopausal Women of the Effect of Estradiol and Progesterone on Cardiovascular Risk Factors

IMET isometric endurance test

IMEX image segmentation [radiotherapy]

IMF idiopathic myelofibrosis; immunofluorescence; inframammary fold; installation medical facility; intermaxillary fixation; intermediate filament; intramaxillary fixation

IMG inferior mesenteric ganglion; internal medicine group [practice]; international medical graduate

IMGG intramuscular gammaglobulin

IMGT International Immuno-Genetics Database

IMH idiopathic myocardial hypertrophy; indirect microhemagglutination [test]

IMHP 1-iodomercuri-2-hydroxypropane

IMHT indirect microhemagglutination test

IMI immunologically measurable insulin; impending myocardial infarction; Imperial Mycological Institute [UK]; inferior myocardial infarction; intermeal interval; internal motility index; intramuscular injection

Imi imipramine

IMIA International Medical Informatics Association

IMIA-NI International Medical Informatics Association-Nursing Informatics

IMIA-NI/SIG International Medical Informatics Association-Nursing Informatics, Special Internet Group

IMIC International Medical Information Center

IMIMC interdigestive migrating myoelectric complex

IMIS Integrative Molecular Information System [database]

IML intermediolateral

IMLA intramural left anterior [artery]

IMLAD intramural left anterior descending [artery]

IMLNS idiopathic minimal lesion nephrotic syndrome

ImLy immune lysis

IMM immunization [database]; inhibitor-containing minimal medium; inner mitochondrial membrane; internal medial malleolus

immat immaturity, immature

IMMC interdigestive migrating motor complex

IMO idiopathic multicentric osteolysis

imoa instantaneous maximum over the array [transformation]

immobil immobilization, immobilize

immun immune, immunity, immunization

IMN internal mammary node

IMP idiopathic myeloid proliferation; impression; incomplete male pseudohermaphroditism; individual Medicaid practitioner; inosine 5'-monophosphate; intramembranous particle; intramuscular compartment pressure; *N*-isopropyl-*p*-iodoamphetamine

Imp impression

imp impacted, impaction

IMPA incisal mandibular plane angle

IMPAC Information for Management, Planning, Analysis and Coordination

IMPACT Immunisation Monitoring Programme Active [Canada]; Initiatives to Mobilize for the Prevention and Control of Tobacco Use; Integrilin to Minimize Platelet Aggregation and Prevent Coronary Thrombosis [trial]; Interdisciplinary Maternal Perinatal Australasian Clinical Trials; International Mexiletine and Placebo Antiarrhythmia Coronary Trial

IMPACT-II Integrilin to Minimize Platelet Aggregation and Coronary Thrombosis [trial]

IMPACT-AMI Integrilin to Minimize Platelet Aggregation and Prevent Coronary Thrombosis-Acute Myocardial Infarction [trial]

IMPACT-Stent Integrilin to Minimize Platelet Aggregation and Coronary Thrombosis in Stenting [trial]

IMPATH interactive microcomputer patient assessment tool for health

IMPC International Myopia Prevention Center

IMPD inosine-5'-monophosphate dehydrogenase

IMPDH inosine-5'-monophosphate dehydrogenase

IMPDHL inosine-5'-monophosphate dehydrogenase-like

IMPG interphotoreceptor matrix proteoglycan

IMPR integrated microscopy resource

IMPRESS Intramural Low Molecular Weight Heparin for Prevention of Restenosis Study

IMPROVED Influence of Introduction of Mycophenolate Mofetil and Reduction of Cyclosporine on Renal Dysfunction After Cardiac Transplantation [study]

IMPS Inpatient Multidimensional Psychiatric Scale; intact months of patient survival

Impx impacted

IMR individual medical record; infant mortality rate; infant mortality risk; Institute for Medical Research; institution for mentally retarded; integrated microscopy resource; intelligent medical record

IMRI intraoperative magnetic resonance imaging

IMRT intensity modulated radiotherapy

IMS image management system; immunomagnetic separation; incurred in military service; Indian Medical Service; industrial methylated spirit; information management system; integrated medical services; international metric system; Internet map server; ion mobility spectrometry

IMS/DL1 information management system/data language one

IMSI international mobile subscriber identity [telemedicine]

iMSP ideal midsagittal plane

IMSS in-flight medical support system

IMT indomethacin; induced muscular tension; inspiratory muscle training; intimal mean thickness

IM&T information management and technology

IMU Index of Medical Underservice

IMV inferior mesenteric vein; informative morphogenetic variant; intelligent magic view [imaging]; intermittent mandatory ventilation; intermittent mechanical ventilation; intracellular mature virion; isophosphamide, methotrexate, and vincristine

IMViC, imvic indole, methyl red, Voges-Proskauer, citrate [test]

IMVP idiopathic mitral valve prolapse

IMVS Institute of Medical and Veterinary Science

IN icterus neonatorum; impetigo neonatorum; incidence; incompatibility number; infundibular nucleus; insulin; integrase; interneuron; interstitial nephritis; intranasal; irritation of nociceptors

In index; indium; inion; insulin; inulin

in inch

in² square inch

in³ cubic inch

INA infectious nucleic acid; inferior nasal artery; instrumentation amplifier; International Neurological Association

I$_{Na}$ sodium current [heart electrical activity]

INAA instrumental neutron activation analysis

INABIS First Internet World Congress for Biomedical Sciences

INAD infantile neuroaxonal dystrophy

INAH isonicotinic acid hydrazide

INB internuclear bridging; ischemic necrosis of bone

inbr inbreeding
INC inside needle catheter; internodular cortex
inc incision; inclusion; incompatibility; incontinent; increase, increased; increment; incurred
INCB International Narcotics Control Board
IncB inclusion body
INCD infantile nuclear cerebral degeneration
IN-CHF Italian Network Congestive Heart Failure
INCL infantile neuronal ceroid lipofuscinosis
incl inclusion or include
INCLEN International Clinical Epidemiology Network
incr increase, increased; increment
incur incurable
IND indomethacin; industrial medicine; investigational new drug
ind indirect; induction
INDANA Individual Data Analysis of Antihypertensive Intervention Trials
indic indication, indicated
indig indigestion
indiv individual
INDO indoleamine-2,3-dioxygenase; indomethacin
INDOR internuclear double resonance
indust industrial
INE infantile necrotizing encephalomyelopathy
INEPT insensitive nuclei enhanced by polarization transfer
INET image network
INF infant, infantile; infection, infective, infected; inferior; infirmary; infundibulum; infusion; interferon
Inf influenza
inf infant, infantile; inferior
INF APC infero-apical
infect infection, infected, infective
INFH ischemic necrosis of femur head
Inflamm inflammation, inflammatory
inf mono infectious mononucleosis
InfoMAP information management and assessment process
INFORMM Information Network for Online Retrieval and Medical Management
INFSEC information security

INFV Inner Farne virus
ING isotope nephrogram
ing inguinal
InGP indolglycerophosphate
INH Indian hedgehog homolog; inhalation; inhibitor; isoniazid; isonicotinic acid hydrazide
INHA inhibin alpha
inhal inhalation
INHB inhibin beta
INHBA inhibitin beta A
INHBB inhibitin beta B
INHBC inhibitin beta C
inhib inhibition, inhibiting
INH-PT isonicotinic acid hydrazide preventive therapy
INI intranuclear inclusion
INIRC International Non-Ionizing Radiation Committee
inj injection; injury, injured, injurious
INJECT International Joint Efficacy Comparison of Thrombolytics [trial]; International Joint Evaluation of Coronary Thrombolysis [trial]
inject injection
INJR injury or poisoning [UMLS]
INK injury not known
INKV Inkoo virus
INL International Nursing Library
INLINIS Ireland-Netherlands Lisinopril-Nifedipine Study
INLSD ichthyosis and neutral lipid storage disease
i-NMDS international nursing minimum data set
INN International Nonproprietary Names; intestinal noise
innerv innervation, innervated
innom innominate
INNOVO Inhaled Nitric Oxide Compared to Ventilatory Support Without Inhaled Nitric Oxide [trial; for neonates with severe respiratory failure]
INO inosine; internuclear ophthalmoplegia
Ino inosine
INOC isonicotinoyloxycarbonyl
inoc inoculation, inoculated
inorg inorganic
iNOS inducible macrophage-type nitric oxide synthase
Inox inosine, oxidized
INP idiopathic neutropenia

INPAV intermittent negative-pressure assisted ventilation

INPC isopropyl *N*-phenyl carbamate

INPEA isopropyl nitrophenylethanolamine

INPH iproniazid phosphate

INPHO Integrated Network for Public Health Officials

INPP1 inositol polyphosphate 1-phosphatase

INPV intermittent negative-pressure ventilation

INQ interior nasal quadrant

InQ inquiry mode questionnaire

InQ(R) inquiry mode questionnaire, reliability assessment

INR international normalized ratio [prothrombin time]

INREM internal roentgen-equivalent, man

INRIA Institut National de la Recherche Informatique et Automatique [National Institute for Research in Computers and Automation (France)]

INROAD In-Stent Restenosis Optimal Angioplasty Device [trial]

INS idiopathic nephrotic syndrome; implantable neurostimulator; information networking system; insulin; insurance

Ins insulin; insurance, insured

ins insertion; insulin; insurance, insured

INSECT intensity normalized stereotaxic environment for classification of tissues

insem insemination

INSIGHT International Nifedipine Study Intervention as a Goal in Hypertension Treatment

insol insoluble

INSP, Insp inspiration

INSPIRE increasing participation in cardiac rehabilitation; Intravascular Ultrasound Study Predictor of Restenosis [trial]

INSR insulin receptor

INSRR insulin receptor-related receptor

INSS international neuroblastoma staging system

Inst institute

instab instability

instill instillation

insuf insufflation

insuff insufficient, insufficiency; insufflation

INT interference; intermediate; intermittent; intern, internship; internal; interval; intestinal; intima; *p*-iodonitrotetrazolium

Int international; intestinal

int internal

INTACT International Nifedipine Trial on Antiatherosclerotic Therapy

INTEG integument

INTEL-SAT international communication satellite

INTERCEPT Incomplete Infarction Trial of European Research Collaborators Evaluating Prognosis Post-Thrombolysis

INTERHEALTH Integrated Programme for Community Health and Noncommunicable Diseases

INTERMAP International Study of Macronutrients and Blood Pressure

intern internal

Internat international

INTERSALT International Study of Salt and Blood Pressure

INTERSEPT International Sepsis Trial

intes intestine

Intest intestine, intestinal

Int/Ext internal/external

INTH intrathecal

INTIMA Infusion of Tissue Plasminogen-Activator in Myocardial Infarction at the Acute Phase [study]

in-TIME Intravenous Lanoteplase for Treating Infarcting Myocardium Early [trial]

Intmd intermediate

Int Med internal medicine

INTOX, Intox intoxication

INTR intermittent

INTRO-AMI Integrilin and Reduced Dose of Thrombolysis in Acute Myocardial Infarction

Int Rot internal rotation

INTRP Inventory of Negative Thoughts in Response to Pain

INTRUC Introducing Catheter [study]

Int trx intermittent traction

intub intubation

INV inferior nasal vein; Inini virus

Inv, inv inversion; involuntary

INVEST International Verapamil SR/Trandolapril [study]

invest investigation

Inv/Ev inversion/eversion

inv ins inverted insertion

INVM isolated noncompaction of left ventricular myocardium

invol involuntary

involv involvement, involved

inv(p + q −) pericentric inversion

inv(p − q +) pericentric inversion

IO incisal opening; inferior oblique; inferior olive; internal os; interorbital; intestinal obstruction; intraocular; intraoperative; intra-osseous

IO₂ inspired oxygen

I&O in and out; intake and output

I/O input/output; intake/output

Io ionium; onset of inspiration

IOA inner optic anlage; International Osteopathic Association

IOC International Organizing Committee on Medical Librarianship; intern on call; intraoperative cholangiography

IOCG intraoperative cholangiogram

IOCM isosmolar contrast medium

IOD information object model; injured on duty; integrated optical density; interorbital distance

IOE intraoperative echocardiography

IOECS intraoperative electrocortical stimulation

IOERT intraoperative electron beam radiation therapy

IOFB intraocular foreign body

IOH idiopathic orthostatic hypotension

IOHDR intraoperative high dose rate

IOL induction of labor; intraocular lens

IOM inferior orbitomental [line]; infraorbital margin; Institute of Medicine [National Research Council]; Institute of Occupational Medicine [UK]; interosseous membrane; intraoperative monitoring

IOML infraorbitomeatal line

IOMP International Organization for Medical Physics

ION ischemic optic neuropathy

IONDT Ischemic Optic Neuropathy Decompression Trial

IOP improving organizational performance; intraocular pressure

IOPR intra-operative patient representation

IOR index of refraction; index of response; interoperable object reference

IORT intraoperative radiotherapy

IOS infant observation scale; International Organization for Standardization; intraoperative sonography

IOS RF intact outlet strut resonance frequency

IOT intraocular tension; intraocular transfer; ipsilateral optic tectum

IOTA information overload testing aid

ɩ Greek letter *iota*

IOTF International Obesity Task Force [WHO]

IOU intensive care observation unit; international opacity unit

IOUS intraoperative ultrasound [examination]

IOV inside-out vesicle

IOVA intraocular vision aid

IP icterus praecox; imaging plate; immune precipitate; immunoblastic plasma; immunoperoxidase technique; inactivated pepsin; incisoproximal; incisopulpal; incontinentia pigmenti; incubation period; induced potential; induction period; infection prevention; inflation point; infundibular process; infusion pump; inhibition period; inorganic phosphate; inosine phosphorylase; inositol phosphate; inpatient; instantaneous pressure; intermediate purity; International Pharmacopoeia; Internet protocol; interpeduncular; interphalangeal; interpupillary; intestinal pseudoobstruction; intramuscular pressure; intraperitoneal; intrapulmonary; inverse planning [radiotherapy]; inverted papilloma; ionization potential; ischemic preconditioning; isoelectric point; isoproterenol; L'Institut Pasteur

IP1 incontinentia pigmenti 1

IP₁ inositol-1-phosphate

IP2 incontinentia pigmenti 2

IP₃ inositol triphosphate

IP₄ inositol 1,3,4,5-tetraphosphate

Ip peak of inspiratory effort

I_p ionic current pump

ip intraperitoneal

i/p inpatient

IPA idiopathic pulmonary arteriosclerosis; immunoperoxidase assay; incontinentia pigmenti achromians; independent physician or practice association; independent practice organization; individual practice association; infantile papular acrodermatitis; International Pediatric Association;

International Pharmaceutical Association; International Psychoanalytical Association; International Psychogeriatric Association; intrapleural analgesia; isopropyl alcohol

I_pa pulse average intensity

IPAA International Psychoanalytical Association

IPAC Information Policy Advisory Committee

IPAG The Influenza and Pneumonia Action Group

IPAP inspiratory positive airway pressure

I-para primipara

IPAT Institute of Personality and Ability Testing; Iowa Pressure Articulation Test

IPB injury-prone behavior; integrated problem-based curriculum

IPBH intraparenchymal brain hemorrhage

IPC intermittent pneumatic compression; International Poliomyelitis Congress; interpeduncular cistern; interpersonal process of care; ion pair chromatography; isopropyl carbamate; isopropyl chlorophenyl

IPCD infantile polycystic disease

IPCP interdisciplinary patient care plan

IPCS International Program on Chemical Safety; intrauterine progesterone contraception system

IPD idiopathic Parkinson disease; idiopathic protracted diarrhea; immediate pigment darkening; impedance plethysmography; increase in pupillary diameter; incurable problem drinker; inflammatory pelvic disease; intermittent peritoneal dialysis; intermittent pigment darkening; International Pharmacopeal Database; interocular phase difference; interpupillary distance; Inventory of Psychosocial Development

IPE infectious porcine encephalomyelitis; interstitial pulmonary emphysema

IPEH intravascular papillary endothelial hyperplasia

IPF idiopathic pulmonary fibrosis; infection-potentiating factor; insulin promoter factor; interstitial pulmonary fibrosis

IPFM integral pulse frequency modulation

IPFM/SDC integral pulse frequency modulation/Smith delay compensator

IPG impedance plethysmography; inspiration-phase gas

iPGE immunoreactive prostaglandin E

IPH idiopathic portal hypertension; idiopathic pulmonary hemosiderosis; idiopathic pulmonary hypertension; inflammatory papillary hyperplasia; International Partnership for Health; interphalangeal; intraparenchymal hemorrhage; intraperitoneal hemorrhage

IΦE International Partnership in Health Information Education

IPHR inverted polypoid hamartoma of the rectum

IPI interpotential interval; interpulse interval

IPIA immunoperoxidase infectivity assay

IPITA International Pancreas and Islet Transplant Association

IPJ interphalangeal joint

IPK intractable plantar keratosis

IPKD infantile polycystic kidney disease

IPL inner plexiform layer; intrapleural

IPM impulses per minute; inches per minute; interphotoreceptor matrix

IPMI information processing in medical imaging

IPMS inhibited power motive syndrome

IPMT intraductal papillary mucinous tumor

IPN infantile polyarteritis nodosa; infectious pancreatic necrosis [of trout]; interductal papillary neoplasm; intern progress note; interpeduncular nucleus; interstitial pneumonitis

IPNA isopropyl noradrenalin

IPNV infectious pancreatic necrosis virus

IPO improved pregnancy outcome

IPOF immediate postoperative fitting

IPOP immediate postoperative prosthesis

IPP independent practice plan; individual patient profile; inflatable penile prosthesis; inorganic pyrophosphate; inspiratory plateau pressure; intermittent positive pressure; intracisternal A particle-promoted polypeptide; intrahepatic partial pressure; intrapericardial pressure

Ipp interpulse potential

IPPA inspection, palpation, percussion, and auscultation; iodophenylpentadecanoic acid

IPPB intermittent positive-pressure breathing

IPPB-I intermittent positive-pressure breathing-inspiration

IPPHS International Primary Pulmonary Hypertension Study

IPPI interruption of pregnancy for psychiatric indication

IPPO intermittent positive-pressure inflation with oxygen

IPPPSH International Prospective Primary Prevention Study in Hypertension

IPPR integrated pancreatic polypeptide response; intermittent positive-pressure respiration

IPPV intermittent positive-pressure ventilation

IPPYV Ippy virus

IPQ intimacy potential quotient

IPR imidozaline preferring receptor; immediate phase reaction; independent professional review; Institute of Process Control and Robotics [Germany]; insulin production rate; interval patency rate; intraparenchymal resistance; ipratropium; iproniazid

IP₃R IP_3R inositol 1,4,5-triphosphate receptor

i-Pr isopropyl

IPRD intellectual product [UMLS]

IPRL isolated perfused rat liver or lung

iProClass integrated protein classification

IPRT interpersonal reaction test

IPS idiopathic pain syndrome; idiopathic postprandial syndrome; immersive projection system; inches per second; infundibular pulmonary stenosis; initial prognostic score; intensive care unit point system; intermittent photic stimulation; interpractice system; intrapartum stillbirth; intraperitoneal shock; ischiopubic synchondrosis

ips inches per second

IPSB index of proximity to stability boundary

IPSC inhibitory postsynaptic current

IPSC-E Inventory of Psychic and Somatic Complaints in the Elderly

IPsec Internet protocol security

IPSF immediate postsurgical fitting

IPSID immunoproliferative small intestine disease

IPSP inhibitory postsynaptic potential

IPT immunoperoxidase technique; immunoprecipitation; information processing theory; interpersonal psychotherapy; isoniazid preventive therapy; isoproterenol

IPTG isopropyl-β-thiogalactopyranoside; isopropyl thiogalactose

iPTH immunoassay for parathyroid hormone; immunoreactive parathyroid hormone

IPTT Initiative for Pharmaceutical Technology Transfer

IPTX intermittent pelvic traction

IpTX imperatoxin

IpTxa imperatoxin A

IpTxi imperatoxin I

IPU inpatient unit

IPV inactivated poliomyelitis vaccine or virus; infectious pustular vaginitis; infectious pustular vulvovaginitis; interpersonal violence; intimate partner violence; intrapulmonary vein

IPW interphalangeal width

IPZ insulin protamine zinc

IQ inhibitory quotient; institute of quality; intelligence quotient

IQAS internal quality assurance system

IQB individual quick blanch

IQCODE information questionnaire on cognitive decline in the elderly

IQOLA International Quality of Life Assessment [project]

IQR interquartile range

IQ&S iron, quinine, and strychnine

IQW interactive query workstation

IR drop of voltage across a resistor produced by a current; ileal resection; immune response; immunization rate; immunoreactive; immunoreagent; in room; index of response; impedance rheography; individual reaction; inferior rectus [muscle]; inflow resistance; information retrieval; infrared; infrarenal; inside radius; insoluble residue; inspiratory reserve; inspiratory resistance; insulin resistance; intermediate representation; internal resistance; internal rotation; interventional radiology; intrarectal; intrarenal; inversion recovery; inverted repeat; irritant reaction; ischemia-reperfusion; isovolumic relaxation

I-R Ito-Reenstierna [reaction]

I/R ischemia/reperfusion

Ir immune response [gene]; iridium

ir immunoreactive; intrarectal; intrarenal

IRA ileorectal anastomosis; immunoradioassay; immunoregulatory alpha-globulin; inactive renin activity; individual regression analysis; infarct-related artery; inwardly rectifying [current]

IR-ACTH immunoreactive adrenocorticotropic hormone

IRAD International Registry of Aortic Dissection

IrANP, ir-ANP immunoreactive atrial natriuretic peptide

IR-APAP immediate-release acetaminophen

IRAR Immunization Registry Annual Report

IRAS Insulin Resistance Atherosclerosis Study

IR-AVP immunoreactive arginine-vasopressin

IRB immunoreactive bead; institutional review board

IRBBB incomplete right bundle branch block

IRBC immature or infected red blood cell

ir-BNP immunoreactive brain natriuretic peptide

IRBP intestinal retinol-binding protein

IRC inspiratory reserve capacity; instantaneous resonance curve; International Red Cross; International Research Communications System

IRCA intravascular red cell aggregation

IRCC International Red Cross Committee

IRCU intensive respiratory care unit

IRD infantile Refsum disease; isorhythmic dissociation

IrDA infrared data association

IRDP insulin-related DNA polymorphism

IRDS idiopathic respiratory distress syndrome; infant respiratory distress syndrome

IRE intelligent rules element; internal rotation in extension; iron regulatory element; iron-responsive element; isolated rabbit eye

IREBP iron-responsive element binding protein

IRED infrared emission detection; infrared light-emitting diode

IRES internal ribosome entry site; ischemia residua

IRF idiopathic retroperitoneal fibrosis; impulse response function; installation response force; interferon regulatory factor; internal rotation in flexion

IRFL integral red fluorescence

IRFPA infrared focal plan array

IRG immunoreactive gastrin; immunoreactive glucagon

IRGH immunoreactive growth hormone

IRGl immunoreactive glucagon

IRH Institute for Research in Hypnosis; Institute of Religion and Health; intrarenal hemorrhage

IRHCS immunoradioassayable human chorionic somatomammotropin

IRhGH immunoreactive human growth hormone

IRhPL immunoreactive human placental lactogen

IRI immunoreactive insulin; [near]-infrared interreactance; insulin resistance index

IRIA indirect radioimmunoassay

IRIg insulin-reactive immunoglobulin

IRIS Integrated Risk Information System [NLM database]; interleukin regulation of immune system; International Research Information Service; Isostents for Reperfusion Intervention Study

IRIV immuno-potentiating reconstituted influenza virosome; Irituia virus

IRK inwardly rectifying potassium [channel]

IRLED, IR-LED infrared light emitting diode

IRM information resource management; innate releasing mechanism; insect resistance management; Institute of Rehabilitation Medicine

IRMA immunoradiometric assay; intraretinal microvascular abnormalities

iRNA immune ribonucleic acid; informational ribonucleic acid

ir-NP immunoreactive natriuretic peptide

IROS intelligent robots and systems; ipsilateral routing of signal

IROX iridium oxide

IRP immunoreactive plasma; immunoreactive proinsulin; incus replacement prosthesis; insulin-releasing polypeptide; interstitial radiation pneumonitis; intraocular retinal prosthesis

IRPA International Radiation Protection Association

IRPA/INIRC International Radiation Protection Association's International Non-Ionizing Radiation Committee

IRPTC International Registry of Potentially Toxic Chemicals

IRR insulin receptor-related receptor; intrarenal reflux

Irr irradiation; irritation

IRRD Institute for Research in Rheumatic Diseases

irreg irregularity, irregular

irrig irrigation, irrigate

IRS immunoreactive secretion; incident reporting scheme; infrared sensor; infrared spectrophotometry; insulin receptor species; insulin receptor substrate; insulin-related substrate; Intergroup Rhabdomyosarcoma Study; internal resolution site; International Rhinologic Society; Invasive Reperfusion Study; ionizing radiation sensitivity

IRS-1 insulin receptor substrate 1

IRS-2 insulin receptor substrate 2

IRSA idiopathic refractory sideroblastic anemia; iodinated rat serum albumin

IRSE inversion recovery spin-echo

IRT immunoreactive trypsin; interresponse time; interstitial radiotherapy; item response theory

IRTIS Integrated Radiation Therapy Information System

IRTO immunoreactive trypsin output

IRTU integrating regulatory transcription unit

IRU industrial rehabilitation unit; interferon reference unit

IRV inferior radicular vein; inspiratory reserve volume; intelligent radiology workstation; inverse ratio ventilation; Italian ringspot virus

IrVd Iresine viroid

IRW intelligent radiology workstation

IRX Information Retrieval Experimental Workbench

IS ileal segment; iliosacral; immediate sensitivity; immune serum; immunostaining; immunosuppression; impingement syndrome; incentive spirometer; index of sexuality; infant size; infantile spasms; information services; information system; infundibular septum; insertion sequence; in situ; insulin secretion; interaction site; intercellular space; intercostal space;

interictal spike; international standards; interstitial space; interventricular system; intracardial shunt; intraspinal; intrasplenic; intrastriatal; intraventricular septum; invalided from service; inversion sequence; ischemic score; isoproterenol

I-S incudostapedial

Is incision superius

is in situ; island; islet; isolated

ISA ileosigmoid anastomosis; industry standard architecture [computer interconnection]; Information Science Abstracts; Instrument Society of America; intracarotid sodium amytal; intraoperative suture adjustment; intrinsic simulating activity; intrinsic stimulation activity; intrinsic sympathomimetic activity; iodinated serum albumin; irregular spiking activity

I$_{sa}$ spatial average intensity [pulse]

ISAAA International Service for the Acquisition of Agri-Biotech Applications

ISAAC International Study of Asthma and Allergies in Childhood

ISADH inappropriate secretion of antidiuretic hormone

ISAGA immunosorbent agglutination assay

ISAKEMP Internet Security Association and Key Management Protocol

ISAM indexed sequential access manager; Intravenous Streptokinase in Acute Myocardial Infarction [trial]

I$_{sapa}$ spatial average pulse average

ISAPI Internet server application program interface

ISAPS International Society of Aesthetic Plastic Surgery

ISAR Intracoronary Stenting and Antithrombotic Regimen [trial]

I$_{sata}$ spatial average, temporal average intensity [pulse]

ISB incentive spirometry breathing

ISBI International Society for Burn Injuries

ISBN international standard book number

ISBP International Society for Biochemical Pharmacology

ISBT International Society for Blood Transfusion

ISC immunoglobulin-secreting cells; innerstrand crosslink; information system center; insoluble collagen; International Society of Cardiology; International

Society of Chemotherapy; intensive supportive care; intershift coordination; interstitial cell; irreversibly sickled cell

IS&C image save and carry

Isc short circuit current

ISCAB Israeli Coronary Artery Bypass [study]

ISCAS International Society for Computer-Aided Surgery

ISCB International Society of Computational Biology

ISCD International Society of Clinical Densitometry

ISCF interstitial cell fluid

ISCL integrated secure communication layer

ISCLT International Society for Clinical Laboratory Technology

ISCM International Society of Cybernetic Medicine

ISCN International System for Human Cytogenetic Nomenclature

ISCO immunostimulating complex [vaccine]; Information System for Clinical Oncology [UK]

ISCOAT Italian Study on Complications of Oral Anticoagulant Therapy

ISCOM immune stimulatory complexes in matrix

ISCP infection surveillance and control program; International Society of Comparative Pathology

ISCVS International Society for Cardiovascular Surgery

ISCW immunosuppression of streptococcal wall [antigen]

ISD immunosuppressive drug; implant support device; Information Services Division; inhibited sexual desire; intermediate sulfate domain; interset distance; interstimulus distance; interventricular septal defect; isosorbide dinitrate

ISDB information source database

ISDN integrated services digital network; isosorbide dinitrate

iSDR inducible stable DNA replication

ISE inhibited sexual excitement; intelligent synthesis environment; International Society of Endocrinology; International Society of Endoscopy; inversion spin-echo pulse sequence; ion-selective electrode

ISEFT ion-sensitive field effect transistor

ISEK International Society of Electromyographic Kinesiology

ISEM immunosorbent electron microscopy

ISF interstitial fluid

ISFC International Society and Federation of Cardiology

ISFV interstitial fluid volume; Isfahan virus

ISG Ibopamine Study Group [trial]; immune serum globulin

ISGE International Society of Gastroenterology

ISH icteric serum hepatitis; in situ hybridization; internal self helper; International Society of Hematology; International Society of Hypertension; isolated septal hypertrophy; isolated systolic hypertension

ISHAM International Society for Human and Animal Mycology

ISHT International Society for Heart Transplantation [registry]

ISHTAR Implementing Secure Healthcare Telematics Application

ISI infarct size index; information science innovations; initial slope index; injection scan interval; injury severity index; Institute for Scientific Information; insulin sensitivity index; International Sensitivity Index; International Standardized Index; interstimulus interval

ISIH interspike interval histogram

ISIS image selected in vivo spectroscopy; imaging science and information system; Information Society Initiative for Standardization; information system-imaging system; integrated survey information system; intelligent selection and imaging studies; interactive system for image selection; International Infarct Survival [Trial]; International Study of Infarct Survival

ISIS-2 Second International Infarct Survival [Trial]

ISIT interactive simulation and identification tool

ISKDC International Study of Kidney Diseases in Childhood

ISKV Issyl-Kul virus

ISL inner scapular line; instrumental spatial linkage; interspinous ligament; isoleucine

ISLAND Infant Size Limitation: Acute *N*-Acetylcysteine Defense [trial]

ISLAV Isla Vista virus

ISM industrial-scientific-medical [telemedicine, wireless transmission]; Information Source Map [UMLS]; International Society of Microbiologists; intersegmental muscle

ISMB Intelligent System for Molecular Biology

ISMED International Society on Metabolic Eye Disorders

ISMH International Society of Medical Hydrology

ISMHC International Society of Medical Hydrology and Climatology

ISMHO International Society of Mental Health Online

ISMN isosorbide mononitrate

ISMO International Society of Mental Health Online [telemedicine]

ISN integrated service network; International Society of Nephrology; International Society of Neurochemistry

ISO incident safety officer; International Organization for Standardization; isoprenaline

iso isoproterenol; isotropic

ISOBM International Society of Oncodevelopmental Biology and Medicine

isol isolation, isolated

isom isometric

ISO-OSI International Organization for Standardization-Open Systems Interconnect

ISP distance between iliac spines; international standardized profile; Internet service provider; interspace; interstitial pressure; intraspinal; isoproterenol

I$_{sp}$ spatial peak intensity [pulse]

ISPCR in situ polymerase chain reaction

ISPI integrated services protocol instrument

ISPO International Society for Prosthetics and Orthotics

ISPOCD International Study of Postoperative Cognitive Dysfunction

ISPOT International Study of Perioperative Transfusion

I$_{sppa}$ spatial peak, pulse average intensity

I$_{spta}$ spatial peak, temporal average intensity [pulse]

ISPS International Society of Pediatric Surgery

ISPT interspecies ovum penetration test

isq unchanged [Lat. *in status quo*]

ISR image service representative; information storage and retrieval; Institute for Sex Research; Institute of Surgical Research; insulin secretion rate; intelligent stroke registry

ISRE interferon-stimulated response element

ISRI Information Science Research Institute

ISRM International Society of Reproductive Medicine

ISS idiopathic short stature; infantile sialic acid storage [disease]; inferior sagittal sinus; injury severity scale; injury severity score; instructional support services; International Society of Surgery; invasive surgical staging; ion-scattering spectroscopy; ion surface scattering; isotonic saline solution

ISSCBW Inter-Service Sub-Committee on Biological Warfare [UK]

ISSD infantile sialic acid storage disease

ISSHP International Society for the Study of Hypertension in Pregnancy

ISSI interspinous surgical staging; interview schedule for social interaction; Israeli Study of Surgical Infections

ISSIR International Society of Sexual and Impotence Research

ISSN international standard serial number

ISSX International Society for the Study of Xenobiotics

IST inappropriate sinus tachycardia; insulin sensitivity test; insulin shock therapy; International Society on Toxicology; International Stroke Trial; Internet Security Team; isometric systolic tension

IS&T Society for Imaging Science and Technology

ISTAHC International Society of Technology Assessment in Healthcare

ISTC [Department of] Industry, Science and Technology of Canada

ISTD International Society of Tropical Dermatology

ISTU isometric strength testing unit

ISU International Society of Urology

I-sub inhibitor substance

ISUP International Society of Urological Pathology

ISV integrated simulation and verification

ISVP infectious subviral particle; intermediate subviral particle

ISW interstitial water

ISWI incisional surgical wound infection

ISY intrasynovial

IT iliotibial; immunological test; immunotherapy; immunotoxin; implantation test; individual therapy; inferior turbinate; information technology; inhalation test; inhalation therapy; injection time; insulin therapy; intensive therapy; intentional tremor; intermittent traction; internal telomere; interstitial tissue; intradermal test; intratesticular; intrathecal; intrathoracic; intratracheal; intratracheal tube; intratuberous; intratumoral; ischial tuberosity; isolation transformer; isomeric transition

I/T information technology; intensity/time

I&T intolerance and toxicity

IT² Internet technology for the twenty-first century

I-T interrupter technique

ITA inferior temporal artery; information transmission analysis; internal thoracic artery; International Tuberculosis Association

I$_{ta}$ temporal average intensity [pulse]

ITAM immunoreceptor tyrosine activation motif

ITAV Itaituba virus

ITB iliotibial band

ITC imidazolyl-thioguanine chemotherapy; inferior temporal cortex; Interagency Testing Committee; information and communication technology; in the canal [hearing aid]; intrathecal chemotherapy; isothermal titration calorimetry; isothiocyanate

ITc International Table calorie

ITCM information technology for crises management teams

ITCP idiopathic thrombocytopenic purpura

ITCVD ischemic thrombotic cerebrovascular disease

ITD idiopathic torsion dystonia; intensely transfused dialysis; iodothyronine deiodinase

ITE information technology equipment; insufficient therapeutic effect; in the ear [hearing aid]; in-training examination; intrapulmonary interstitial emphysema

ITEA intermittent thoracic epidural anesthesia

ITEM information and communication technology for medicine

ITET isotonic endurance test

ITF Interagency Tack Force [Department of Health and Human Services]; interferon

ITFS iliotibial tract friction syndrome; incomplete testicular feminization syndrome

ITG integrin

ITGA integrin alpha

ITGB integrin beta

ITH interstitial hyperthermia

ITh, ith intrathecal

IThP intrathyroidal parathyroid

ITI inter-alpha-trypsin inhibitor; International Trachoma Initiative; intertrial interval

ITIH2 inter-alpha-trypsin inhibitor, heavy chain 2

ITIL inter-alpha-trypsin inhibitor, light chain

ITIM immunoreceptor tyrosine-based inhibition motif

ITIV Itimirim virus

ITL information technology laboratory

ITLC instant thin-layer chromatography

ITM improved Thayer-Martin [medium]; intermediate transient memory; intrathecal methotrexate; Israel turkey meningoencephalitis

ITMTX intrathecal methotrexate

ITO indium tin oxide

I$_{(to)}$ transient outward current [heart electrical activity]

ITOU intensive therapy observation unit

ITP idiopathic thrombocytopenic purpura; immune thrombocytopenia; immunogenic thrombocytopenic purpura; increased torque production; individualized treatment plan; inosine triphosphate; inositol 1,4,5-triphosphate; islet-cell tumor of the pancreas; isotachophoresis

I$_{tp}$ temporal peak intensity [pulse]

ITPA Illinois Test of Psycholinguistic Abilities; inosine triphosphatase

ITPASMT International Tissue Plasminogen Activator/Streptokinase Mortality Trial

ITPK inositol 1,4,5-triphosphate-3-kinase

ITPKA inositol 1,4,5-triphosphate-3-kinase A

ITPKB inositol 1,4,5-triphosphate-3-kinase B

ITPR inositol 1,4,5-triphosphate receptor

ITPV intratracheal pulmonary ventilation; Itaporanga virus

ITQ inferior temporal quadrant

ITQV Itaqui virus

ITR intraocular tension recorder; intratracheal; inverted terminal repeat; isotretinoin

ITRI Inhalation Toxicology Research Institute

ITS infective toxic shock; insulin-transferrin-selenium; intelligent [computer-assisted] tutoring system; International Twin Study; Israeli Thrombolytic Survey

ITSHD isolated thyroid-stimulating hormone deficiency

ITT insulin tolerance test; intent to treat; internal tibial torsion

IT&T information technology and telematics

ITU intensive therapy unit; International Telecommunication Union; international toxic unit

ITUV Itupiranga virus

ITV inferior temporal vein

IU immunizing unit; infection unit; integral uniformity; international unit [JCAHO unapproved abbreviation]; intrauterine; in utero; 5-iodouracil

iu infectious unit

IUA intrauterine adhesions

IUAT International Union Against Tuberculosis

IUB International Union of Biochemistry

IUBS International Union of Biological Sciences

IUC idiopathic ulcerative colitis; intrauterine catheter; inward unidirectional current

IUCD intrauterine contraceptive device

IUD intrauterine death; intrauterine device

IUDR, IUdR iodeoxyuridine

IUF isolated ultrafiltration

IUFB intrauterine foreign body

IUG infusion urogram; intrauterine gas; intrauterine growth

IUGR intrauterine growth rate; intrauterine growth retardation

IUI intrauterine insemination

IUIS International Union of Immunological Societies

IU/L international units per liter

IUM internal urethral meatus; intrauterine [fetus] malnourished; intrauterine membrane

IU/min international units per minute

IUP intrauterine pregnancy; intrauterine pressure

IUPAC International Union of Pure and Applied Chemistry

IUPAP International Union of Pure and Applied Physics

IUPAT intrauterine pregnancy at term

IUPD intrauterine pregnancy delivered

IUPESM International Union for Physical and Engineering Sciences in Medicine

IUPHAR International Union of Pharmacology

IUPS International Union of Physiological Sciences

IUPTB intrauterine pregnancy, term birth

IURES International Union of Reticuloendothelial Societies

IUT intrauterine transfusion

IUVDT International Union against Venereal Diseases and the Treponematoses

IV endometrial carcinoma extending outside the true pelvis or involving the bladder and rectum [International Federation of Gynecologists and Obstetricians (FIGO) classification]; ichnovirus; ichthyosis vulgaris; immunodeficiency virus; initial visit; interventricular; intervertebral; intravaginal; intravascular; intravenous; intraventricular; intravertebral; invasive; in vivo; in vitro; involvement of one or more extralymphatic organs [Ann Arbor staging system for Hodgkin disease]; iodine value; iridescent virus; iridovirus; isometric virus; symbol for class 4 controlled substances

iv intravascular; intravenous

IVA interpretative value analysis; intraoperative vascular angiography; isovaleric acid

IVa endometrial carcinoma spreading to adjacent organs [International Federation of Gynecologists and Obstetricians (FIGO) classification]; vaginal carcinoma with metastases to adjacent organs [International Federations of Gynecologists and Obstetricians (FIGO) classification]

IVACG International Vitamin A Consultative Group

IVAP in-vivo adhesive platelet

IVAS intracorporeal ventricular assist system

IVB intraventricular block

IVb endometrial carcinoma spreading to distant organs [International Federation of Gynecologists and Obstetricians (FIGO) classification]; vaginal carcinoma with metastases to distant organs [International Federation of Gynecologists and Obstetricians (FIGO) classification]

IVBAT intravascular bronchioalveolar tumor

IVBC intravascular blood coagulation

IVC inferior vena cava; inspiratory vital capacity; integrated vector control; intravascular coagulation; intravenous cholangiogram, intravenous cholangiography; intraventricular catheter

IVCC intravascular consumption coagulopathy

IVCD intraventricular conduction defect

IVCH intravenous cholangiography

IVC-LA inferior vena cava and left atrium

IVCP inferior vena cava pressure

IVCR inferior vena cava reconstruction

IVCT inferior vena cava thrombosis; intravenously enhanced computed tomography

IVCV inferior venacavography; Ivy vein clearing virus

IVD interactive videodisk; intervertebral disc; in vitro diagnostic device

IVDA/IVDU intravenous drug abuse/abuser—intravenous drug use/user

IVDSA intravenous digital subtraction angiography

IVET in vivo expression technology

IVF interventricular foramen; intervertebral foramen; intravascular fluid; intravenous fluid; in vitro fertilization

IVFA intravenous fluorescein angiography

IVF-ET in vitro fertilization-embryo transfer

IVGG intravenous gammaglobulin

IVGTT intravenous glucose tolerance test

IVH intravenous hyperalimentation; intraventricular hemorrhage; in vitro hyperploidy

IVI intravenous infusion

IVIG, IVIg, ivIG intravenous immunoglobulin

IVISTAT Intravenous Immunoglobulin or Sulfamethaxazole/Trimethoprim as Additional Therapy for Systemic Vasculitis [study]

IVJC intervertebral joint complex

IVL intravascular lymphomatosis; involucrin

I-VLBW intubated very low birthweight

IVM intravascular mass; in vitro maturation

IVMG intravenous magnesium sulfate

IVMP intravenous methylprednisolone

IVN intravenous nutrition

IVNA in vivo neutron activation [analysis]

IVNAA in vivo neutron activation analysis

IVNR interventional neuroradiology

IVOTTS Irvine viable organ-tissue transport system

IVOX intravascular oxygenator

IVP intravenous push; intravenous pyelogram, intravenous pyelography; intraventricular pressure

IVPB intravenous piggyback

IVPF isovolume pressure flow curve

IVPSB International Veterinary Pathology Slide Bank

IVR idioventricular rhythm; interactive voice response; intravaginal ring; isolated volume responder

IVRA intravenous regional anesthesia

IVRT isovolumic relaxation time

IVS inappropriate vasopressin secretion; intervening sequence; interventricular septum; intervillous space

IVSA International Veterinary Students Association

IVSCT in vitro skin corrosivity test

IVSD interventricular septal defect; intraventricular septum in diastole

IVST intraventricular septal thickness

IVT index of vertical transmission; interventional video tomography; interventricular trigone; intrasound vibration test; intravenous transfusion; intraventricular; in vitro tetraploidy; isovolumetric time

IVTT in vitro transcription and translation

IVTTT intravenous tolbutamide tolerance test

IVU intravenous urography

IVUS intravascular ultrasound

IVUS/QCA Intravascular Ultrasound Quantitative Coronary Angiography [study]

IVV influenza virus vaccine; intravenous vasopressin

IVW image-viewing workstation

IW inner wall; inpatient ward; input word

IWB indeterminate Western blot [test]; index of well being

IWGMT International Working Group on Mycobacterial Taxonomy

IWHS Iowa Women's Health Study

IWI inferior wall infarction; interwave interval

IWL insensible water loss; inter-wave latency

IWMI inferior wall myocardial infarct

IWPS info-window presentation system

IWRP Individualized Written Rehabilitation Program

IWS Index of Work Satisfaction

IXDB X Chromosome Integrated Database

IZ infarction zone

J

J dynamic movement of inertia; electric current density; flux density; joint; joule; journal; juvenile; juxtapulmonary-capillary receptor; magnetic polarization; a polypeptide chain in polymeric immunoglobulins; a reference point following the QRS complex, at the beginning of the ST segment, in electrocardiography; sound intensity
J flux [density]
j jaundice [rat]
JA jet area; judgment analysis; juvenile atrophy; juxta-articular
JAAS Java Authentication and Authorization Service
JACADS Johnston Atoll chemical agent destruction system
JACV Jacareacanga virus
JAE juvenile absence epilepsy
JAHIS Japanese Association of Healthcare Information System
JAI Java Advanced Imaging; juvenile amaurotic idiocy
JAK Janus kinase
JAK-STAT Janus kinase-signal transducers and activators of transcription
JAM junction-associated membrane
JAMG juvenile autoimmune myasthenia gravis
JAMIA Journal of the American Medical Informatics Association
JaMSPUK Japanese Multicenter Study for Pro-Urokinase
JAMV Jamanxi virus
JAN Japanese accepted name
JANET Joint Academic Network [UK]
JAPV Japanaut virus
JARIV Jari virus
JAS Jenkins Activity Survey; juvenile ankylosing spondylitis
JASTRO Japanese Society for Therapeutic Radiology and Oncology
jaund jaundice
JAV Johnston Atoll virus
JB jugular bulb
JBE Japanese B encephalitis
JBS Johanson-Blizzard syndrome

JC Jakob-Creutzfeldt; joint contracture
J/C joules per coulomb
jc juice
JCA juvenile chronic arthritis
JCAE Joint Committee on Atomic Energy
JCAH Joint Commission on Accreditation of Hospitals
JCAHO Joint Commission on Accreditation of Healthcare Organizations
JCAI Joint Council of Allergy and Immunology
JCC Joint Committee on Contraception
JCD Jakob-Creutzfeldt disease
JcDNV *Junonia coenia* densovirus
JCE Java Cryptography Extension
JCF juvenile calcaneal fracture
JCM Japanese Collection of Microorganisms
JCML juvenile chronic myelogenous leukemia
JCN Jefferson Cancer Network
JCP juvenile chronic polyarthritis
JCPyV JC polyomavirus
JCQ job contentment questionnaire
JCRB Japanese Collection of Research Bioresources
jct junction
JCV Jakob-Creutzfeldt virus; Jamestown Canyon virus
JD jejunal diverticulitis; juvenile delinquent; juvenile diabetes
JDBC Java Database Connectivity
JDF Juvenile Diabetes Foundation
JDM juvenile diabetes mellitus
JDMS juvenile dermatomyositis
JDV Juan Diaz virus
JE Japanese encephalitis; junctional escape
JEB junctional epidermolysis bullosa
JECFA Joint Expert Committee on Food Additives [FAO/WHO]
JEE Japanese equine encephalitis
J2EE Java 2 Platform Enterprise Edition
Jej, jej jejunum
JEMBEC agar plates for transporting cultures of gonococci
JER junctional escape rhythm
JES junkies ex-users substitutes
JET Joint Engineering Team; junctional ectopic tachycardia
JEV Japanese encephalitis virus

JF joint fluid; jugular foramen; junctional fold

JFET junction field effect transistor

JFS jugular foramen syndrome

JG, jg juxtaglomerular

JGA juxtaglomerular apparatus

JGC juxtaglomerular cell

JGCT juvenile granulosa cell tumor; juxtaglomerular cell tumor

JGI jejunogastric intussusception; juxtaglomerular granulation index

JGP juvenile general paresis

JH juvenile hormone

J$_H$ heat transfer factor

JHA juvenile hormone analog

JHITA Joint Healthcare Information Technology Association

JHMO Junior Hospital Medical Officer

JHPS Johns Hopkins Precursors Study

JHR Jarisch-Herxheimer reaction

JI jejunoileal; jejunoileitis; jejunoileostomy

JIB jejunoileal bypass

JIC joint information center

JIH joint interval histogram

JIMI Japanese Intervention Trial in Myocardial Infarction

JIPID Japan International Protein Information Center

JIS Japanese industrial standard; juvenile idiopathic scoliosis

JISK Joint Information Systems Committee [UK]

JIT just-in-time [real time database]

JJ jaw jerk; jejunojejunostomy

J/K joule per kelvin

J/kg joules per kilogram

JL jet length

J-LN Jervell and Lange-Nielsen [syndrome]

JLO judgment of line orientation

JLP juvenile laryngeal papilloma

JLRCPS Jerusalem Lipid Research Clinic Prevalence Study

JMD juvenile macular degeneration

JME juvenile myoclonic epilepsy; juvenile myoclonus epilepsy

JMHTS Japanese Society of Multiphasic Health Testing and Service

J-MIX Japanese medical record information exchange

JMS Juberg-Marsidi syndrome; junior medical student

JN Jamaican neuropathy

Jn junction

JNA Jena Nomina Anatomica

JNC Joint National Committee

JNC-V Fifth Report of the Joint National Committee on Detection, Evaluation and Treatment of High Blood Pressure

JNC-VI Sixth Report of the Joint National Committee on Detection, Evaluation and Treatment of High Blood Pressure

JND just noticeable difference

JNK Jun N-terminal kinase

JNP Jadassohn nevus phakomatosis

JNPA juvenile nasopharyngeal angiofibroma

JNPV juncopox virus

jnt joint

JOAG juvenile open-angle glaucoma

JOAV Joa virus

JOC joint operations center

JOD juvenile-onset diabetes

JODM juvenile-onset diabetes mellitus

JOIV Joinjakaka virus

JOR jaw opening response

JOS jaw osteosarcoma

jour journal

JP Jackson-Pratt [drain]; Japanese Pharmacopeia; joining peptide; juvenile periodontitis

JPA juvenile pilocytic astrocytoma

JPB junctional premature beat

JPC junctional premature contraction

JPD juvenile plantar dermatosis

JPEG Joint Photographic Experts Group

JPI Jackson Personality Inventory

JPS Japanese Pancreatic Society; joint position sense

JPSTH joint peristimulus histogram

JR Jolly reaction; junctional rhythm

JRA juvenile rheumatoid arthritis

JRC-CVT Joint Review Committee on Education in Cardiovascular Technology

JRC DMS Joint Review Committee on Diagnostic Medical Sonography

JRC/EMT Joint Review Committee for Emergency Medical Technicians

JROM joint range of motion

JRT junctional recovery time

JS jejunal segment; Job syndrome; junctional slowing

J/s joules per second

JSAIR Japanese Society of Angiography and Interventional Radiology

JSATO₂ jugular vein oxygen saturation

JSDN Japan Standardized Disease Names

JSLIST joint service lightweight integrated suit technology

JSP Java server pages

JSRT Japanese Society of Radiologic Technology

JSRV jaagsiekte sheep retrovirus

JSSE Java Secure Socket Extension

JSV Jerry-Slough virus

JT jejunostomy tube; junctional tachycardia

J/T joules per tesla

jt joint

JTPS juvenile tropical pancreatitis syndrome

Ju jugale

JUA Joint Underwriting Association

jug jugular

JUGV Jugra virus

junct junction

JUNV Junin virus

JURV Jurona virus

JUTV Jutiapa virus

juv juvenile

juxt near [Lat. *juxta*]

JV jugular vein; Junin virus

JVC jugular venous catheter

JVD jugular venous distention

JVM Java Virtual Machine

JVP jugular vein pulse; jugular venous pressure; jugular venous pulsations

JVPT jugular venous pulse tracing

JWG Joint Working Group [American National Standards Institute, for common data model]

JWS Jackson-Weiss syndrome

Jx junction

JXG juvenile xanthogranuloma

K

K absolute zero; a burst of diphasic slow waves in response to stimuli during sleep [in electroencephalography]; capsular antigen [Ger. *Kapsel*, capsule]; carrying capacity; cathode; coefficient; constant; constant improvement factor [in imaging]; electron capture; electrostatic capacity; equilibrium constant; ionization constant; kallikrein inhibiting unit; kanamycin; Kell factor; kelvin; kerma; kidney; Kilham [virus]; killer [cell]; kilo-; kilodalton; kinetic energy; *Klebsiella*; knee; lysine; modulus of compression; the number 1024 in computer core memory; potassium [Lat. *kalium*]; vitamin K

K_1 phylloquinone

K_1, K_2 empirical Rohrer constants

K4 fourth Korotkoff sound

K5 fifth Korotkoff sound

17-K 17-ketosteroid

°K degree on the Kelvin scale

k Boltzmann constant; constant; kilo; kilohm

κ see *kappa*

KA alkaline phosphatase; kainic acid; keratoacanthoma; keto acid; ketoacidosis; King-Armstrong [unit]; knowledge acquisition; knowledge aggregate

K/A ketogenic/antiketogenic ratio

K_A association constant

Ka cathode

K_a absorption rate constant; acid ionization constant; affinity constant; association constant

kA kiloampere

ka cathode

KAAD kerosene, alcohol, acetic acid, and dioxane

KAAS Keele assessment of auditory style

KABC Kaufman Assessment Battery for Children

KADV Kadam virus

KAF conglutinogen-activating factor; killer-assisting factor; kinase activating factor

KAFO knee-ankle-foot orthosis

KAIV Kaikalur virus

KAL Kallmann [syndrome]

KAL1 Kallmann gene

KALP Kallmann pseudogene

KAMI Koch Acute Myocardial Infarction [study]

KAMIT Kentucky Acute Myocardial Infarction Trial

KAMV Kamese virus

kan kanamycin

KanR, kan^r kanamycin resistance

KANV Kannamangalam virus

KAO knee-ankle orthosis

KAP knowledge, attitudes, and practice

κ Greek letter *kappa*; magnetic susceptibility

kappa a light chain of human immunoglobulins [chain]

KAPS Kuopio Atherosclerosis Prevention Study

KARV Karimabad virus

KAS Katz Adjustment Scales; Kennedy-Alter-Sung [syndrome]

KASV Kasba virus; Kasokero virus

KAT kanamycin acetyltransferase; knowledge acquisition tool; Kuopio Angioplasty Gene Transfer Trial

kat katal

kat/l katals per liter

K_{ATP} adenosine triphosphate [ATP] potassium channel

KAU King-Armstrong unit

KaV Kawino virus

KB human oral epidermoid carcinoma cells; Kashin-Bek [disease]; ketone body; kilobase; kilobyte; Kleihauer-Betke [test]; knee brace; knowledge [data] base

K-B Kleihauer-Betke [test]; Kuo-Bean [sodium channel model]

Kb kilobit

K_b base ionization constant; binding constant

kb kilobase; kilobyte

KBD knowledge base dictionary

KBG syndrome of multiple abnormalities designated with the original patient's initials

KBI knowledge-based information

KBM knowledge base manager

kbp kilobase pair

Kbps kilobits per second

kBq kilobecquerel

KBS Klüver-Bucy syndrome; knowledge-based system

KBTA knowledge-based temporal abstraction

KBV Kachemak Bay virus

KC cathodal closing; keratoconus; keratoconjunctivitis; knee-to-chest; Kupffer cell

kC kilocoulomb

kc kilocycle

K Cal, Kcal, kcal kilocalorie

KCC cathodal closing contraction; Kulchitzky cell carcinoma

KCCT kaolin-cephalin clotting time

KCD kinostatic change detector

K cell killer cell

KCF key clinical finding

KCG kinetocardiogram

kCi kilocurie

KCO transfer coefficient

KCP knowledge, concern, and first aid practices

kcps kilocycles per second

KCS Kenny-Caffey syndrome; keratoconjunctivitis sicca

kc/s kilocycles per second

KCSS Keio Cooperative Stroke Study

KCT, KCTe cathodal closing tetanus

KCV Kern Canyon virus

KD cathodal duration; Kawasaki disease; Kennedy disease; killed; Krabbe disease

K$_D$ dissociation constant

K$_d$ degradation constant; dissociation constant; distribution coefficient; partition coefficient

kd, kDa kilodalton

KDA known drug allergies

KDAPPIMT Kawasaki Disease Aneurysm Prevention Protocol and Italian Multicenter Trial

KDB knowledge database

KDC kidney disease treatment center

KDD knowledge discovery in databases

KDD-R knowledge discovery in databases using rough sets

KDI knowledge and distributed intelligence

kdn kidney

KDNA kinetoblast deoxyribonucleic acid

KDO ketodeoxyoctonate

KDS Kaufman Developmental Scale; King-Denborough syndrome; knowledge data system; Kocher-Debré-Semelaigne [syndrome]; Kupfer-Detre system

KDT cathodal duration tetanus

KDV Kadipiro virus

kdyn kilodyne

KE Kendall compound E; kethoxal; kinetic energy; Krining estimator

K$_e$ exchangeable body potassium

KED Kendrick extrication device

KEDV Kedougou virus

Kel elimination constant

K$_{em}$ elimination rate constant

KEMRI Kenyan Medical Research Institute

KEMV Kemerovo virus

KENV Kenai virus

Kera keratitis

KERMA kinetic energy released per unit mass

KERV Kentucky equine respiratory virus

KETV Ketapang virus

KEUV Keuraliba virus

keV kiloelectron volt

KEYV Keystone virus

KF Kenner-fecal medium; kidney function; Klippel-Feil [syndrome]; knowledge finder

KF, K-F Kayser-Fleischer [rings]

K$_f$ Klenow fragment

kf flocculation rate in antigen-antibody reaction; kilogram force

KFAB kidney-fixing antibody

KFAO knee-foot-ankle orthosis

KFC Ketanserin for Carcinoid [trial]; Ketanserin on Fibroblast Culture [study]

K$_{fc}$ filtration coefficient

KFD Kyasanur forest disease

KFDV Kyasanur Forest disease virus

KFR Kayser-Fleischer ring

KFS Klippel-Feil syndrome

KFSD keratosis follicularis spinulosa decalvans

KG ketoglutarate; knowledge graph

kG kilogauss

kg kilogram

KG-1 Koeffler Golde-1 [cell line]

kg-cal kilocalorie

kg/cm^2 kilogram per square centimeter

KGD ketoglutarate dehydrogenase

KGF keratocyte growth factor

kgf kilogram-force

KGFR keratocyte growth factor receptor

kg/L kilograms per liter

KGM keratinocyte growth medium

kg-m kilogram-meter

kg/m kilograms per meter

kg-m/s² kilogram-meter per second squared
Kgn kininogen
kgps kilograms per second
KGS ketogenic steroid
17-KGS 17-ketogenic steroid
KH K-homologous; K-homology [domain]; Krebs-Henseleit [buffer]
K24H potassium, urinary 24-hour
KHAV Khabarovsk virus; Kharagysh virus; Khasan virus
KHB Krebs-Henseleit buffer
KHb potassium hemoglobinate
KHC kinetic hemolysis curve
KHD kinky hair disease
KHF Korean hemorrhagic fever
KHM keratoderma hereditaria mutilans
KHN Knoop hardness number
KHP King's Honorary Physician
KHS King's Honorary Surgeon; kinky hair syndrome; Krebs-Henseleit solution
kHz kilohertz
KI karyopyknotic index; Krönig's isthmus
KIA Kligler iron agar
KIC ketoisocaproate; keto isocaproic acid
KICB killed intracellular bacteria
KID keratitis, ichthyosis, and deafness [syndrome]; kinase insert domain
KIDI knowledge of infant development inventory
KIF knowledge information format; knowledge interchange format
KIHD Kuopio Ischemic Heart Disease Risk Factor Study
kilo kilogram
KIMSA Kirsten murine sarcoma
KIMSV, KiMSV Kirsten murine sarcoma virus
KIMV Kimberley virus
KIN keratinocytic intraepidermal neoplasia
KIND Kyushu University Hospital Information Network Database
KINDS Kinmen Neurologic Disorders Survey
KINV Kindia virus
KIP key intermediary protein
KiP kilopascal
KIPS key indicators, probes, and scoring method [for evaluating compliance with requirements for accreditation]
KIR killer immunoglobulin receptor
Kir inward rectified potassium [channel]

KIRA kinase receptor activation
KISS keep it simple and safe; keep it simple, stupid; key integrative social system; Kobe Idiopathic Cardiomyopathy Survival Study; saturated solution of potassium iodide
KIST Korea Institute of Science and Technology
KISV Kismayo virus
KIT Kahn Intelligence Test
KIU kallikrein inactivation unit
KIVA keto isovaleric acid
KJ, kj knee jerk
kJ kilojoule
KK knee kick
kkat kilokatal
KKS kallikrein-kinin system
KKV Kaeng Khoi virus
KL Karhunen-Loéve [transform]; kidney lobe; Kit ligand; Klebs-Loeffler [bacillus]; Kleine-Levin [syndrome]
kl kiloliter
KLAV Klamath virus
KLC Karhunen-Loéve coefficient
Klebs *Klebsiella*
KLH keyhole limpet hemocyanin
KLK kallikrein
KLKR kallikrein
KLM killed *Mycobacterium*
KLS kidneys, liver, and spleen; Kreuzbein lipomatous syndrome
KLT Karhunen-Loéve transform
KLV Kalanchoe latent virus
KM kanamycin; knowledge management; Knowledge Map [UMLS]
K_m Michaelis-Menten constant
km kilometer
km² square kilometer
k_m metabolic constant
KMC K-means clustering analysis
kMc kilomegacycle
K-MCM potassium-containing minimum capacitation medium
kMc/s kilomegacycles per second
KMEF keratin, myosin, epidermin, and fibrin
kmps kilometers per second
KMPV Kammavanpettai virus
Km^R kanamycin residue
KMS kabuki make-up syndrome; knowledge management system; kwashiorkor-marasmus syndrome
K-MSV Kirsten murine sarcoma virus

KMV killed measles virus vaccine
KN knowledge networking
Kn kanamycin; knee; Knudsen number
kN kilonewton
kn knee
K nail Küntscher nail
KNG kininogen
KNN K-nearest neighbor; Kohonen neural network
k-NN K-nearest neighbor
KnoME knowledge management environment
KNRK Kirsten sarcoma virus in normal rat kidney
KNS kinesin
KNSL kinesin-like
KO keep on; keep open; killed organism; knee orthosis; knock out
kΩ kilohm
KOC cathodal opening contraction
KO-DMEM Knockout Dulbecco Modified Eagle Medium
k$_{off}$ off-rate constant
KOH potassium hydroxide
KOKV Kokobera virus
KOLV Kolongo virus
KOOLV Koolpinyah virus
KOOV Koongol virus
KOPS thousand of operations per second
KOTV Kotonkan virus
KOUV Koutango virus
KOWV Kowanyama virus
KP Kaufmann-Peterson [base]; keratitic precipitate; keratitis punctata; kidney protein; killed parenteral [vaccine]; *Klebsiella pneumoniae*
K$_p$ partition coefficient
kPa kilopascal
kPas/l kilopascal seconds per liter
KPB ketophenylbutazone; potassium phosphate buffer
KPC keratoconus posticus circumscriptus
KPE Kelman pharmacoemulsification
KPI kallikrein-protease inhibitor; karyopyknotic index
kpm kilopodometer
KPR key pulse rate
KPS Karnofsky Performance Status
KPT kidney punch test
KPTI Kunitz pancreatic trypsin inhibitor
KPTT kaolin partial thromboplastin time

KPV kangaroo poxvirus; key process variable; killed parenteral vaccine; killed polio vaccine
KPWIN KnowledgePro for Windows
KPyV Kilham polyomavirus
KQC key quality characteristics
KQML knowledge query and manipulation language
KR key-ridge; knowledge representation; Kopper-Reppart [medium]
Kr krypton
kR kiloroentgen
KRB Krebs-Ringer buffer
KRBG Krebs-Ringer bicarbonate buffer with glucose
KRBS Krebs-Ringer bicarbonate solution
KRDU Knowledge Resources Development Unit [UK]
KRIS Kaunas-Rotterdam Intervention Study
KRIV Kairi virus
KRP Kolmer test with Reiter protein [antigen]; Krebs-Ringer phosphate
KRR knowledge representation and reasoning
KRRS kinetic resonance Raman spectroscopy
KRS knowledge representation syntax
KRT keratin
KRV Kilham rat virus
KS Kabuki [make-up] syndrome; Kallmann syndrome; Kaposi sarcoma; Kartagener syndrome; Kawasaki syndrome; keratan sulfate; ketosteroid; Klinefelter syndrome; Korsakoff syndrome; Kozhevnikov syndrome; Kveim-Siltzbach [test]
K-S Kearns-Sayre [syndrome]
17-KS 17-ketosteroid
ks kilosecond
KSC cathodal closing contraction
KSHV Kaposi sarcoma-associated herpesvirus
KSIV Karshi virus
KS/OI Kaposi sarcoma with opportunistic infection
KSOM Kohonen's self-organizing map
KSOV Kaisodi virus
K$_{sp}$ solubility product
KSP Karolinska Scales of Personality; kidney-specific protein
17-KSR 17-ketosteroid reductase

KSS Kearns-Sayre syndrome; Kearns-Sayre-Shy [syndrome]; knowledge source server [UMLS]
KSSO knowledge support system zero
KST cathodal closing tetanus; kallistatin
KSV Kao Shuan virus
KT kidney transplant, kidney transplantation
K$_t$ turnover rate constant
KTA kidney transplant alone
KTI kallikrein-trypsin inhibitor
KTM Kops Tissot Monro [mask]
KTRV Keterah virus
KTS Klippel-Trenaunay syndrome
KTSA Kahn test of symbol arrangement
KTSV Kalanchoe top-spotting virus
KTU knowledge transfer and utilization
KTW, KTWS Klippel-Trenaunay-Weber [syndrome]
KTX kaliotoxin
KTx kidney transplant
KU kallikrein unit; Karmen unit
Ku kurchatovium; Peltz factor
K$_u$ urinary rate coefficient
KUB kidneys and upper bladder; [x-ray examination of the] kidneys, ureters, and bladder
KUf ultrafiltration coefficient
KUMIS Kumamoto University Myocardial Infarction Study
KUN Kunjin [virus]
KUNV Kunjin virus
KUS kidney, ureter, spleen
KV kanamycin and vancomycin; kidney vacuolating virus; killed vaccine
K$_v$ voltage-gated potassium [channel]
kV, kv kilovolt

kVA kilovolt-ampere
kvar kilovar
KVBA kanamycin-vancomycin blood agar
kVcp, kvcp kilovolt constant potential
KVE Kaposi varicelliform eruption
KVLBA kanamycin-vancomycin laked blood agar
KVM Kilobyte Virtual Machine
KVO keep vein open
kVp, kvp kilovolt peak
KW Keith-Wagener [ophthalmoscopic finding]; Kimmelstiel-Wilson [syndrome]; Kugelberg-Welander [syndrome]
Kw weighted kappa
K$_w$ dissociation constant of water
kW, kw kilowatt
KWAV Kwatta virus
KWB Keith-Wagener-Barker [hypertension classification]
KWD Kimmelstiel-Wilson disease
KWE Kumar-Welti-Ernst [method]
kWh, kW-hr, kw-hr kilowatt-hour
KWIC key word in context
K wire Kirschner wire
KWK Kids Who Know [Johns Hopkins]
KWord 32-bit word
KWS Kimmelstiel-Wilson syndrome; Kugelberg-Welander syndrome
K-XRF K x-ray fluorescence
KYCS Kiryat Yovel Community Study
KYN kynurenic acid
KYN-OH kynurenine-3-hydrooxylase
KYSMI Kyoto Shiga Myocardial Infarction [study]
KZ ketoconazole

L

L angular momentum; Avogadro constant; boundary [Lat. *limes*]; coefficient of induction; diffusion length; inductance; *Lactobacillus*; lambda; lambert; latent heat; latex; Latin; leader sequence; left; *Legionella*; *Leishmania*; length; lente insulin; lethal; leucine; levo-; lewisite; lidocaine; ligament; light; light sense; lingual; *Listeria*; liter; liver; low; lower; lumbar; luminance; lymph; lymphocyte; outer membrane layer of cell wall of gram-negative bacteria [layer]; pound [Lat. *libra*]; radiance; self-inductance; syphilis [Lat. *lues*]; threshold [Lat. *limen*]

L0 no evidence of lymph node metastases [TNM (tumor node-metastasis) classification]

L$_0$ limes zero [limes nul, the largest amount of toxin which will not produce a toxic reaction]

L$_+$ limes tod [the smallest amount of toxin which will produce a toxic reaction]

L1 acute lymphoblastic leukemia with lymphoblasts, scanty cytoplasm and inconspicuous nucleoli [FAB (Franco-American-British) classification]; lymph node metastases assessed [TNM (tumor-node-metastasis) classification]

L1, L2, L3, L4, L5 first, second, third, fourth, and fifth lumbar vertebrae

LI, LII, LIII first, second, third stage of syphilis

L2 acute lymphoblastic leukemia with large pleomorphic blasts, abundant cytoplasm, and prominent nucleoli [FAB (Franco-American-British) classification]

L$_2$ area [length square]

L3 acute lymphoblastic leukemia having blast with basophilic vacuolated cytoplasm [FAB (Franco-American-British) classification]

L$_3$ volume [length cube]

L/3 lower third

l azimuthal quantum number; left; length; lethal; levorotatory; liter; long; longitudinal; specific latent heat

Λ see *lambda*

λ see *lambda*

LA lactic acid; lactic acidemia; large amount; laser angioplasty; late abortion; late antigen; latex agglutination; left angle; left arm; left atrium; left auricle; leucine aminopeptidase; leukemia antigen; leukoagglutination; leuprolide acetate; levator ani; Lightwood-Albright [syndrome]; linear addition; linguo-axial; linoleic acid; lobuloalveolar; local anesthesia; local anesthetic; long-acting [drug]; long arm; long axis; low anxiety; Ludwig angina; lupus anticoagulant; lymphocyte antibody

L&A light and accommodation; living and active

L/A liver/aorta

LA50 total body surface area of burn that will kill 50% of patients (lethal area)

La labial; lambda; lambert; lanthanum

LAA left atrial appendage; left atrial area; left auricular appendage; leukemia-associated antigen; leukocyte ascorbic acid

LAAM L-alpha acetyl methadol; levo-alpha-acetylmethadol

LAAO L-amino acid oxidase

LA/Ao left atrial/aortic [ratio]

LAB, lab laboratory

LABA long-acting beta agonist

LabBase laboratory database

LABBB left anterior bundle branch block

LABC locally advancing breast cancer

LABE labetalol

LABP laboratory procedure [UMLS]

LA-BP low affinity binding protein

LABV left atrial ball valve

LabVISE Laboratory Reporting Scheme in Virology and Serology [Australia]

LAC La Crosse [virus]; lactase; lansoprazole, amoxicillin, clarithromycin; large area coverage; left atrial circumflex [artery]; left atrial contraction; linear attenuation coefficient; linguoaxiocervical; long-arm cast; low-amplitude contraction; lung adenocarcinoma cells; lupus anticoagulant

LaC labiocervical

Lac laceration; lactation

LACD left apex cardiogram, calibrated displacement

LACI lacidipine; lipoprotein-associated coagulation inhibitor

LACN local area communications network

LacR lactose repressor

Lacr lacrimal
LACS long chain acyl-coenzyme A synthetase
Lact lactate, lactating, lactation; lactic
Lact hyd lactalbumin hydrolysate
LACV La Crosse virus
LAD lactic acid dehydrogenase; left anterior descending [coronary artery]; left atrial defect; left axis deviation; leukocyte adhesion deficiency; ligament augmentation device; linoleic acid depression; lipoamide dehydrogenase; lymphocyte-activating determinant
LADA laboratory animal dander allergy; latent autoimmune diabetes in the adult, latent autoimmune diabetes of adults; left acromio-dorso-anterior [position]; left anterior descending artery
LADB left [coronary] descending branch
LADCA left anterior descending coronary artery
LADD lacrimo-auriculo-dento-digital [syndrome]; left anterior descending diagonal [coronary artery]
LADH lactic acid dehydrogenase; liver alcohol dehydrogenase
LAD-MIN left axis deviation, minimal
LADP left acromio-dorso-posterior [position]; left anterior descending arterial pressure
LADS Lors American Data System
LAE left atrial enlargement
LAEDV left atrial volume in end diastole
LAEI left atrial emptying index
LAESV left atrial volume in end systole
LAF laminar air flow; Latin American female; left anterior fascicle; leukocyte-activating factor; lymphocyte-activating factor
LAFB left anterior fascicular block
LAFR laminar air flow room
LAFU laminar air flow unit
LAG labiogingival; leukocyte antigen group; linguo-axiogingival; lymphangiogram; lymphocyte activation gene
LaG labiogingival
LAH lactalbumin hydrolysate; left anterior hemiblock; left atrial hypertrophy; Licentiate of Apothecaries Hall; lithium, aluminum, hydroxide
LAHB left anterior hemiblock
LAHC low affinity-high capacity
LAHF low amplitude high frequency

LAHT laser-assisted hair transplantation
LAHV leukocyte-associated herpesvirus
LAI latex particle agglutination inhibition; leukocyte adherence inhibition
Lal labioincisal
LAID left anterior internal diameter
LAIF leukocyte adherence inhibition factor
LAIT latex agglutination inhibition test
LAK lymphokine-activated killer [cells]
LAL left axillary line; limulus amebocyte lysate; low air loss; lysosomal acid lipase
LaL labiolingual
LALB low air-loss bed
LALI lymphocyte antibody-lymphocytolytic interaction
LALL lymphomatous acute lymphoblastic leukemia
LALR lexically assign, logically refine [computer strategy]
LALV Lucerne Australian latent virus
LAM laminectomy; laminin; lamivudine; late ambulatory monitoring; Latin American male; left anterior measurement; left atrial myxoma; linear associative memory; lipoarabinomannan; lymphangioleiomyomatosis; lymphocyte adhesion molecule
Lam laminectomy
LAMA laminin A
LAMB laminin B; lentigines, atrial myxoma, mucocutaneous myxomas, blue nevi [syndrome]
L-AmB liposomal AmBisome [amphotericin]
Λ Greek capital letter *lambda*
λ Greek lowercase letter *lambda*; craniometric point; decay constant; an immunoglobulin light chain; mean free path; microliter; thermal conductivity; wavelength
LAMBR laminin B receptor
LAMC laminin C
LAMMA laser microprobe mass analyzer
LAMP limbic system-associated membrane protein; lysosome-associated membrane protein
LAN local area network; long-acting neuroleptic [agent]
LANC long-arm navicular cast
LANE lidocaine, atropine, naloxone, epinephrine [drugs that may be administered via endotracheal tube]
LANV Laguna Negra virus; left atrial neovascularization

LAO left anterior oblique; left atrial overload; Licentiate of the Art of Obstetrics

LAP laboratory accreditation program; laparoscopy; laparotomy; latency-active promoter; latency-associated protein; left arterial pressure; left atrial pressure; leucine aminopeptidase; leukemia-associated phenotype; leukemia-associated phosphoprotein; leukocyte alkaline phosphatase; liver-enriched transcriptional activator protein; low atmospheric pressure; lyophilized anterior pituitary

Lap laparoscopy; laparotomy

Lap & dye laparoscopy and injection of dye

LAPIS Late Potentials in Myocardial Infarction Study

LAPSE long-term ambulatory physiologic surveillance

LAPSS Los Angeles Prehospital Stroke Screen

LAPW left atrial posterior wall

LAR laryngology; late asthmatic response; late reaction; left arm recumbent; legally authorized representative; leukocyte antigen-related; low anterior resection

Lar larynx; left arm reclining

LARA Low-Dose Aspirin Trial on Restenosis after Angioplasty

LARab laryngeal abductor

LARad laryngeal adductor

LARC leukocyte automatic recognition computer

LARD lacrimoauriculoradiodental [syndrome]

ʟ-Arg L-arginine

LARIS laser atomization resonance ionization spectroscopy

LARS laparoscopic antireflux surgery; laser angioplasty in the treatment of restenosis developing within coronary stents; leucyl-tRNA synthetase

Laryngol laryngology

LAS laboratory automation system; lateral amyotrophic lateral sclerosis; laxative abuse syndrome; left anterior-superior; leucine acetylsalicylate; linear alkylsulfonate; local adaptation syndrome; long arm splint; lower abdominal surgery; lymphadenopathy syndrome; lymphangioscintigraphy

LASA linear-analogue self assessment; lipid-associated phenotype

LASAF low quantities of acetylsalicylic acid in atrial fibrillation

LASA-P linear-analogue self-assessment-Pristman

LASAR Local Alcohol and Stent Against Restenosis [trial]

LASA-S linear-analogue self-assessment-Selby

LASE laser-assisted spinal endoscopy

LASER light amplification by stimulated emission of radiation

LASH left anterior superior hemiblock

LA SI linearly additive spatially invariant [image]

LASIK laser-assisted in situ keratomileusis

L-ASP L-asparaginase

LASS labile aggregation stimulating substance

LAST Left Anterior Small Thoracotomy [study]

LASTAC laser transluminal angioplasty catheter

LASTLHY Latin American Study of Lacidipine in Hypertension

LASV Lassa virus

LAT lactic acidosis threshold; latency-associated transcript; lateral; lateral atrial tunnel; latex agglutination test; latissimus dorsi [muscle]; left anterior trigone; left atrial thrombus; less acute mode of transportation; limbal autograft transplantation; L-type amino acid transporter; lysolecithin acyltransferase

Lat Latin

Lat latent; lateral

Lat bend lateral bending

LATC lateral talocalcaneal

LATCH literature attached to charts

LATE Late Assessment of Thrombolytic Efficacy [trial]

L · atm liter atmosphere

LATP left atrial transmural pressure

LATPT left atrial transesophageal pacing test

LATS long-acting thyroid stimulator

LATS-P long-acting thyroid stimulator-protector

LATu lobulo-alveolar tumor

LAUP laser-assisted uvulopalatoplasty

LAV liquid-assisted ventilation; lymphadenopathy-associated virus

Lav lavoratory

LAVA laser angioplasty vs. angioplasty; Leiden Artificial Valves and Anticoagulation [study]

LAVH laparoscopy-assisted vaginal hysterectomy

LAW left atrial wall

LAX, LAx long axis

Lax laxative; laxity

LAX-DSS long axis-discrete subaortic stenosis

Lax oc laxative of choice

LB lamellar body; large bowel; left breast; left bronchus; left bundle; left buttock; leiomyoblastoma; lipid body; live birth; liver biopsy; loose body; low back [pain]; lung biopsy; Luria-Bertani [medium]

L&B left and below

Lb *Leishmania brasiliensis*; pound [Lat. *libra*]; pound force

LBA laser balloon angioplasty; left basal artery

LBB left bundle branch; low back bending

LBBB left bundle branch block

LBBsB left bundle branch system block

LBC lidocaine blood concentration; liquid-based cytology; lymphadenosis benigna cutis

LBCD left border of cardiac dullness

LBCF Laboratory Branch complement fixation [test]

LBD lamellar body density; large bile duct; left border of dullness; Lewy body dementia; ligand-binding domain; lower back disorder; lumbar body density

LBF *Lactobacillus bulgaricus* factor; limb blood flow; liver blood flow

Lbf pound force

Lbf-ft pound force foot

LBH length, breadth, height

LBI low back injury; low serum-bound iron

Lb/in² pounds per square inch

LBL labeled lymphoblast; lymphoblastic lymphoma

LbL layer-by-layer

LBM last bowel movement; lean body mass; loose bowel movement; lung basement membrane

L-BMAA L-beta-*N*-methylamino-L-alanine

LBMT lansoprazole, bismuth, metronidazole, tetracycline

LBNP lower body negative pressure

LBO large bowel obstruction

LBP lipopolysaccharide-binding protein; local binary pattern; low back pain; low blood pressure; lumbar back pain

LBPF long bone or pelvic fracture

LBPP lower body positive pressure

LBPQ Low Back Pain Questionnaire

LBRF louse-borne relapsing fever

LBS low back syndrome; Lübeck Blood [Pressure] Study; lumbar back strain; Lutheran Brotherhood Study; lysine-binding site

LBSA lipid-bound sialic acid

LBT low back tenderness or trouble

LBTI lima bean trypsin inhibitor

Lb tr pound troy

LBV Lagos bat virus; left brachial vein; lung blood volume

LB-V left bundle-ventricle

LBW lean body weight; low birth weight

LBWI low-birth-weight infant

LBWR lung-body weight ratio

LC Laënnec cirrhosis; Langerhans cell; laparoscopic cholecystectomy; large chromophobe; late clamped; lateral canthotomy; lateral cortex; lecithin cholesterol acyltransferase; left circumflex [coronary artery]; lethal concentration; Library of Congress; life care; light chain; linguocervical; lipid cytosomes; liquid chromatography; liquid crystal; liver cirrhosis; living children; location component; locus ceruleus; long chain; low calorie; low contrast; lower calyceal; lung cancer; lung cell; lymphocyte count

LC₀ maximum sublethal concentration

LC₅₀ median lethal concentration

LCA Leber congenital amaurosis; left carotid artery; left circumflex artery; left coronary artery; leukocyte common antigen; lithocholic acid; liver cell adenoma; lymphocyte chemotactic activity

LCa low calcium [diet]

LCAH lipoid congenital adrenal hyperplasia

LCAL large-cell anaplastic lymphoma

LCAM liver cell adhesion molecule

L1CAM L1CAM Mutation Database

LCAO linear combination of atomic orbitals

L-CAPS Low-Density Lipoprotein Coronary Atherosclerosis Prospective Study

LCAR late cutaneous anaphylactic reaction

LCAS Lipoprotein and Coronary Atherosclerosis Study

LCAT lecithin cholesterol acyltransferase

LCATA lecithin cholesterol acetyltransferase alpha

LCB Laboratory of Cancer Biology; Leber congenital blindness; left costal border; lymphomatosis cutis benigna

LCBF local cerebral blood flow

LCBI laboratory-confirmed bloodstream infection

LCC lactose coliform count; left circumflex coronary (artery); left common carotid; left coronary cusp; life cycle cost [analysis]; lipid-containing cell; liver cell carcinoma; L-type calcium channel

LCCA late cortical cerebellar atrophy; leukoclastic angiitis

LCCME Liaison Committee on Continuing Medical Education

LCCS lower cervical cesarean section

LCCSCT large-cell calcifying Sertoli cell tumor

LCD lattice corneal dystrophy; liquid crystal diode; liquid crystal display; coal tar solution [liquor carbonis detergens]; localized collagen dystrophy; low-calcium diet

LC-DCP low contact dynamic compression plate

LCDD light chain deposition disease

LCDV lymphocystis disease virus

LCE leg cycle ergometry

LCED liquid chromatography with electrochemical detection

LCF least common factor; left circumflex [coronary artery]; lymphocyte culture fluid

LCFA, L-cFA long-chain fatty acid

LCFU leukocyte colony-forming unit

LCG Langerhans cell granule; Langerhans cell granulomatosis

LCGL large-cell granulocytic leukemia

LCGME Liaison Committee on Graduate Medical Education

LCGR lutropin-choriogonadotropin receptor

LCGU local cerebral glucose utilization

LCH Langerhans cell histiocytosis

LCh Licentiate in Surgery

L-CHAD long-chain 3-hydroxyacyl coenzyme A dehydrogenase

LCI length complexity index

LCIN low-grade cervical intraepithelial neoplasia

LCIS lobular carcinoma in situ

LCL lateral collateral ligament; left coronary leaflet; Levinthal-Coles-Lillie [body]; lower confidence limit; lower control limit; lymphoblastoid cell line; lymphocytic lymphosarcoma; lymphoid cell line

LCLC large-cell lung carcinoma

LCLo lowest lethal concentration

LCM laser-capture microdissection; latent cardiomyopathy; left costal margin; leukocyte-conditioned medium; lowest common multiple; lymphatic choriomeningitis; lymphocytic choriomeningitis

LCME Liaison Committee on Medical Education

LCMG long-chain monoglyceride

L/cm H₂O liters per centimeter of water

LC-MS liquid chromatography-mass spectrometry

LC/MS liquid chromatography/mass spectrometry

LCMV lymphocytic choriomeningitis virus

LCN lateral cervical nucleus; left caudate nucleus; line correlated noise; lipocalin

LCNB large core needle biopsy

LCO left coronary ostium; low cardiac output

LCOS low cardiac output syndrome

LCP Legg-Calvé-Perthes [syndrome]; long-chain polysaturated [fatty acid]; lymphocyte cytosol polypeptide

LCPD Legg-Calvé-Perthes disease

LCPS Licentiate of the College of Physicians and Surgeons

LCQ Learning Climate Questionnaire

LCR late cutaneous reaction; lifetime clinical record; ligase chain reaction; locus control region [genomic sequencing]; long control region

Lcr low calcium response

LCRB locus control region beta

LCRI limit cycle reciprocal interaction

LCRUS Leigh Clinical Research Unit Study

LCrv retroventral lateral cortex

LCS cerebrospinal fluid [Lat. *liquor cerebrospinalis*]; laboratory of computer science; laparoscopic coagulating shear; left coronary sinus; Leydig cell stimulation; lichen chronicus simplex; life care service;

Life Closure Scale; longest common substring; low constant suction; low continuous suction; lymphocyte culture supernatants

LCSB Liaison Committee for Specialty Boards

LCSC local community service centre [Canada]

LCSD left cardiac sympathetic denervation

LCSG Lung Cancer Study Group

LCSS lethal congenital contracture syndrome

LcSSc limited cutaneous systemic sclerosis

LCST low critical solution temperature

LCSW licensed clinical social worker

LCT laser dynamic compliance measurement technique; liquid crystal thermography; liver cell tumor; long-chain triglyceride; lymphocytotoxicity; lymphocytotoxin

LCt$_{50}$ median lethal vapor or aerosol concentration

LCTA lymphocytotoxic antibody

LCU laparoscopic contact ultrasonography; life change unit

LCuV leaf curl virus

LCV Lake Clarendon virus; lecithovitellin; leukocytoclastic vasculitis; lymphocytic choriomeningitis virus

LCWI left cardiac work index

LCX left circumflex [coronary artery]

LCXB left [coronary] circumflex branch

LD label dictionary; labor and delivery; laboratory data; labyrinthine defect; lactate dehydrogenase; Lafora disease; L-dopa (levodopa); laser Doppler; learning disability; learning disorder; left deltoid; Legionnaires' disease; lethal dose; levodopa; light differentiation; limited disease; linear dichroism; linear discriminate; linguodistal; linkage disequilibrium; lipodystrophy; liver disease; living donor; loading dose; Lombard-Dowell [agar]; longitudinal diameter; low density; low dose; Lyme disease; lymphocyte-defined; lymphocyte depletion

L-D Leishman-Donovan [body]

L/D light/darkness [ratio]

L&D labor and delivery

LD$_1$ isoenzyme of lactate dehydrogenase found in the heart, erythrocytes, and kidneys

LD$_2$ isoenzyme of lactate dehydrogenase found in the lungs

LD$_3$ isoenzyme of lactate dehydrogenase found in the lungs

LD$_4$ isoenzyme of lactate dehydrogenase found in the liver

LD$_5$ isoenzyme of lactate dehydrogenase found in the liver and muscles

LD$_{50}$ median lethal dose

LD$_{50/30}$ a dose that is lethal for 50% of test subjects within 30 days

LD$_{100}$ lethal dose in all exposed subjects

Ld *Leishmania donovani*

LDA laser Doppler anemometry; left dorso-anterior [fetal position]; linear discriminant analysis; low density area; lymphocyte-dependent antibody

LDAC low-dose cytosine arabinoside

LDAR latex direct agglutination reaction

LDB lamb dysentery bacillus; Legionnaires' disease bacillus; Location Database [genetics]

LDC lactose digestion capacity; limited assistance dialysis center; lymphoid dendritic cell; lysine decarboxylase

L-dC L-deoxycytidine

LDCC lectin-dependent cellular cytotoxicity

LDCF lymphocyte-derived chemotactic factor

LDCI low-dose continuous infusion

LDCMC Lady Davis Carmel Medical Center

LdCPV *Lymantria dispar* cypovirus

LDCT late distal cortical tubule

LDD late dedifferentiation; light-dark discrimination; liquefy, digest, and discharge

LDDB London Dysmorphology Database

LDDE low-dose dobutamine echo

LDER lateral-view dual-energy radiography

LD-EYA Lombard-Dowell egg yolk agar

LDF laser Doppler flowmetry; laser Doppler flux, laser Doppler fluxometry; limit dilution factor

LDFA linear discrimination functional analysis

LDG lactic dehydrogenase; limit grid displacement; lingual developmental groove

L-dG L-deoxyguanosine

LDH lactate dehydrogenase; low-dose heparin

LDHA lactic dehydrogenase A

LDHB lactic dehydrogenase-B

LDHC lactic dehydrogenase-C

LDHSPS Low Dose Heparin Stroke Prevention Study

LD im lethal intramuscular dose

LD ip lethal intraperitoneal dose

LDL loudness discomfort level; low-density lipoprotein

LDLA low-density lipoprotein apheresis

LDL A low-density lipoprotein receptor class A

LDL B low-density lipoprotein receptor class B

LDL-C, LDL-c low-density lipoprotein/cholesterol complex

LDL/HDL low-density lipoproteins/high-density lipoproteins ratio

LD$_{Lo}$ lowest lethal dose

LDLP low-density lipoprotein

LDLR, LDL-R low-density lipoprotein receptor; Low-Density Lipoprotein Receptor Mutation Database

LDM lactate dehydrogenase, muscle; limited dorsal myeloschisis

LDMF latissimus dorsi myocutaneous flap

LD-NEYA Lombard-Dowell neomycin egg yolk agar

ʟ-DOPA, ʟ-dopa [levo-3, 4-dihydroxyphenylalanine] levodopa

LDP left dorsoposterior [fetal position]; lumbodorsal pain

LDR labor, delivery, recovery; lifetime data repository; low dose rate

LDRI leukotriene D4 receptor inhibitors

LDRPS labor-delivery-recovery-postpartum suite

LDRS labor-delivery-recovery suite

LDS Licentiate in Dental Surgery; lightweight decontamination system; Lipids in Diabetes Study; locked door seclusion

LDSc Licentiate in Dental Science

LDT left dorsotransverse [fetal position]

LDUB long double upright brace

LDUH low-dose unfractionated heparin

LDV lactate dehydrogenase-elevating virus, lactic dehydrogenase virus; large dense-cored vesicle; laser Doppler velocimetry; lateral distant view; Le Dantec virus; Lordsdale virus

LE lactate extraction; law enforcement; left ear; left eye; leukocyte elastase; leukoerythrogenic; life expectancy; linkage equilibrium [population genetics]; live embryo;

Long Evans [rat]; low exposure; lower extremity; lupus erythematosus [cell]

LEA lower extremity amputation; lumbar epidural anesthesia

LEADER® Lightweight Epidemiological Advanced Detection and Emergency Response System

LEAF layman education and activation system

LEAP Lower Extremity Amputation Prevention [program]

LEAV Leanyer virus

LEBV Lebombo virus

LEC leprosy elimination campaign; leukoencephalitis; long Evans cinnamon [rat]; low energy cardioversion; lower esophageal contractility

LECP low-energy charged particle

LED light-emitting diode; lowest emitting dose; lupus erythematosus disseminatus

LEDC low-energy direct current

LEDV Lednice virus

LEE locus of enterocyte effacement

LEED low-energy electron diffraction

LEEDS low-energy electron diffraction spectroscopy

LEEP left end-expiratory pressure; loop electrosurgical excision procedure

LEER likelihood equivalent error

LEET Low-Energy Endotak Trial

LEF late expression factor; leukokinesis-enhancing factor; lupus erythematosus factor; lymphoid-enhanced binding factor; lymphoid enhancer factor

Leg legislation; legal

LEHR lifetime electronic health record

LeIF leukocyte interferon

LEIS low-energy ion scattering

LELC lymphoepithelioma-like carcinoma

LEL lower explosive limit; lowest effect level

LEM lateral eye movement; Leibovitz-Emory medium; leukocyte endogenous mediator; light electron microscope; light emission microscopy; low-electrolyte meal

LEMA least error matrix analysis

LEMO lowest empty molecular orbital

LEMS Lambert-Eaton myasthenic syndrome

Lenit lenitive

LENT late effect to normal tissues

LEOPARD lentigines, EKG abnormalities, ocular hypertelorism, pulmonary stenosis, abnormalities of genitalia, retardation of growth, and deafness [syndrome]

LEP laboratory of enteric pathogens; lethal effective phase; lipoprotein electrophoresis; low egg passage; lower esophageal pressure

Lep leptotene

LEPC local emergency planning committee

L~EPN~ effective perceived noise level

LEPR leptin receptor

Leq loudness equivalent

LER lysozomal enzyme release

LERG local electroretinogram

LERS learning from examples based on rough sets

LES Lambert-Eaton syndrome; Lawrence Experimental Station [agar]; Life Experiences Survey; lifestyle evaluation system; local excitatory state; Locke egg serum; low excitatory state; lower esophageal sphincter; lupus erythematosus, systemic

Les lesion

LESD Letterer-Siwe disease

LESP lower esophageal sphincter pressure

LESS lateral electrical spine stimulation

LESSD lupus erythematosus, specific skin disease

LESTR leukocyte-derived seven-transmembrane domain receptor

LET lidocaine, epinephrine, and tetracaine [solution]; linear energy transfer; Losartan Effectiveness and Tolerability [study]

LETD lowest effective toxic dose

LETS large external transformation-sensitive [protein]; Leiden Thrombophilia Study

LEU leucine; leucovorin; leukocyte equivalent unit

Leu, leu leucine

Leuc leukocyte

Leu-CAM leukocyte cell adhesion molecule

LeuRS leucyl ribonucleic acid synthetase

LEUT leucine transport

LEV levamisole

LEW Lewis [rat]

L/ext lower extremity

LF labile factor; lactoferrin; laryngofissure; Lassa fever; latex fixation; left foot; left forearm; lethal factor; leukotactic factor; ligamentum flavum; limit of flocculation; long frequency; low fat [diet]; low

flow; low forceps; low frequency; lymphatic filariasis

L/F Latin female

Lf limit of flocculation

Lf lactoferrin; low frequency

LFA left femoral artery; left frontal craniotomy; left fronto-anterior [fetal position]; leukocyte function associated antigen; leukotactic factor activity; logical framework analysis; low-friction arthroplasty; lymphocyte function-associated antigen

LFAB lipid-associated formation of amphotericin B

LFB luxol fast blue [stain]

LFBMA lattice function biological movement artifacts

LFC living female child; low fat and cholesterol [diet]

LFD lactose-free diet; large for date [fetus]; late fetal death; lateral facial dysplasia; least fatal dose; local field potential; low-fat diet; low-fiber diet; low forceps delivery

LFE local frequency estimation; low frequency enhancement [imaging]

LFER linear free-energy relationship

LFH left femoral hernia

LFHL low-frequency hearing loss

LFL left frontolateral; leukocyte feeder layer; lower flammable limit; lower frequency limit

LFN lactoferrin

L-[form] a defective bacterial variant that can multiply on hypertonic medium

LFP left frontoposterior [fetal position]

LFPPV low-frequency positive pressure ventilation

LFPS Licentiate of the Faculty of Physicians and Surgeons

LFR lymphoid follicular reticulosis

LFS lateral facet syndrome; latest finishing shift; Li-Fraumeni syndrome; limbic forebrain structure; liver function series

LFSE ligand field-stabilizing energy

LFT latex fixation test; latex flocculation test; left fronto-transverse [fetal position]; liver function test; low-frequency tetanus; low-frequency transduction; low-frequency transfer; lung function test

LFU lipid fluidity unit

LFV large field of view; Lassa fever virus; low-frequency ventilation

LFx linear fracture

LG lactoglobulin; lamellar granule; laryngectomy; left gluteal; Lennox-Gastaut [syndrome]; leucylglycine; linguogingival; lipoglycopeptide; liver graft; low glucose; lymphatic gland

Lg large; leg

LGA large for gestational age; left gastric artery; low grade astrocytoma

LGALS lecithin, galactoside-binding, soluble

LGB Landry-Guillain-Barré [syndrome]; lateral geniculate body

LGBS Landry-Guillain-Barré syndrome

LGD limb girdle dystrophy; limit grid displacement; low grade dysplasia

LGE Langat encephalitis

LGF lateral giant fiber

LGH lactogenic hormone

LGI large glucagon immunoreactivity; low gastrointestinal; lower gastrointestinal

LGIB low gastrointestinal bleeding

LGIC ligand gated ion channel

LGL large granular leukocyte; large granular lymphocyte; Lown-Ganong-Levine [syndrome]

LGL-NK large granular lymphocyte-natural killer

LGM left gluteus medius

3LGM three level graph-based model

LGMD limb-girdle muscular dystrophy

LGN lateral geniculate nucleus; lateral glomerulonephritis

LGP labioglossopharyngeal

LGS Langer-Giedion syndrome; Lennox-Gastaut syndrome; limb girdle syndrome

LGSIL low-grade squamous intraepithelial lesions

LGSS low-grade stromal sarcoma

LGT late generalized tuberculosis

LGTI lower genital tract infection

LGTV Langat virus

LGV large granular vesicle; lymphogranuloma venereum

LGVHD lethal graft-versus-host disease

LgX lymphogranulomatosis X

LH late healing; lateral habecular [nucleus]; lateral hypothalamic [syndrome]; lateral hypothalamus; left hand; left heart; left hemisphere; left hyperphoria; liver homogenate; loop of Henle; lower half; lues hereditaria; lung homogenate; luteinizing hormone; Lyon hypertensive [rat]

L/H lung-to-heart [ratio]

LHA lateral hypothalamic area; lay health advisor; left hepatic artery; low height for age

LHB long head of biceps [muscle]; luteinizing hormone beta chain

LHBV left heart blood volume

LHC Langerhans cell histiocytosis; left heart catheterization; left hypochondrium; light-harvesting complex; Local Health Council

LHCGR luteinizing hormone-choriogonadotropin receptor

LHD lateral head displacement [sperm]

LHe liquid helium

LHEG local healthcare executive group

LHF left heart failure

LHFA lung Hageman factor activator

LHG left hand grip; localized hemolysis in gel

LHI laboratory for healthcare informatics; lipid hydrocarbon inclusion; local health jurisdiction

LHIPS Local Heparin Infusion Pre-Stenting [trial]

LHL left hepatic lobe

LHM lysuride hydrogen maleate

LHMP Life Health Monitoring Program

LHN lateral hypothalamic nucleus

LHNCBC Lister Hill National Center for Biomedical Communication

LHON Leber hereditary optic neuropathy

LHP lifetime health plan

LHPZ low high-pressure zone

LHR leukocyte histamine release; lifetime health record; lymph node homing receptor

L-hr lumen-hour

LHRF luteinizing hormone-releasing factor

LHRH, LH-RH luteinizing hormone-releasing hormone

LHRHR luteinizing hormone-releasing hormone receptor

LHS left hand side; left heart strain; left heelstrike; Losartan Hemodynamic Study; library of health sciences; Lung Heart Study; lymphatic/hematopoietic system

LHT left hypertropia; Lifestyle Heart Trial

LHV left hepatic vein

LI labeling index; lactose intolerance; lacunar infarct; lamellar ichthyosis; Langerhans islet; large intestine; *Leptospira*

icterohaemorrhagiae; linguoincisal; link interface [telemedicine]; lithogenic index; low impulsiveness

L&I liver and iron

Li a blood group system; labrale inferius; lithium

L-I late inspiratory

LIA Laser Institute of America; left iliac artery; leukemia-associated inhibitory activity; lock-in amplifier; lymphocyte-induced angiogenesis; lysine iron agar

LIAF laser-induced arterial fluorescence; lymphocyte-induced angiogenesis factor

LIAFI late infantile amaurotic familial idiocy

Lib a pound [Lat. *libra*]

LIBC latent iron-binding capacity

LIC left internal carotid [artery]; left interventricular coronary [artery]; limiting isorrheic concentration; link interface connector [telemedicine]; local intravascular coagulation

Lic licentiate

LICA left internal carotid artery

LICM left intercostal margin

LicMed Licentiate in Medicine

LICS left intercostal space

LICU laparoscopic intracorporeal ultrasound

LID large intraluminal density; late immunoglobulin deficiency; lymphocytic infiltrative disease

LIF laser-induced fluorescence; left iliac fossa; left index finger; leukemia-inhibiting factor; leukocyte inhibitory factor; leukocytosis-inducing factor; light-induced fluorescence

LIFE lifestyle intervention, food, and exercise program; Losartan Intervention for Endpoint Reduction in Hypertension [trial]; lung imaging fluorescence endoscope

LIFO last in, first out

LIFR leukemia inhibitory factor receptor

LIFT late intervention following thrombolysis; lymphocyte immunofluorescence test

Lig ligament; ligation

LIH left inguinal hernia

LIHA low impulsiveness, high anxiety

LIHFE living with heart failure [questionnaire]

LIHPS local infusion of heparin prior to stenting

LIJ left internal jugular [vein]

LILA low impulsiveness, low anxiety

LILT low-intensity laser therapy

LIM line isolation monitor

Lim limit, limited

LIMA left internal mammary artery

LIME Leeds interactive medical education [UK]

LIMIT Laboratory for Integrated Medical Interface Technology; Leicester Intravenous Magnesium Intervention Trial

LIMIT-AMI Double Blind, Placebo-Controlled, Multicenter Angiographic Trial of RhuMAb CD 18 in Acute Myocardial Infarction

LIMITS Liquemin in Myocardial Infarction during Thrombolysis with Saruplase [trial]

LIMM lethal infantile mitochondrial myopathy

LIN linear statistical classifier

LINAC linear accelerator

LINC laboratory instrumentation computer

LINE long interspersed repetitive element

Linim, lin liniment

LINNET [medical] library information network

LIO left inferior oblique

LIP lipase; lipocortin; lithium-induced polydipsia; lower inflection point; lymphoid or lymphocytic interstitial pneumonitis

Lip lipoate

LIPA line probe assay

LIPB lipase B

LIPD lipase D

LIPID Long-Term Intervention with Pravastatin in Ischemic Disease [trial]

LipoMM lipomyelomeningocele

LIPOX lipoxygenase

LIPP laser-induced pressure pulse

LIPS Lescol Intervention Prevention Study

LIPV left inferior pulmonary vein; Lipovnik virus

LIQ low inner quadrant

Liq liquid [Lat. *liquor*]

Liq dr liquid dram

Liq oz liquid ounce

Liq pt liquid pint

Liq qt liquid quart

LIR left iliac region; left inferior rectus

LIRBM liver, iron, red bone marrow

LIS laboratory information system; lateral intercellular space; learning and intelligent system; left intercostal space; library information service; lissencephaly; lobular in situ; locked-in syndrome; low intermittent suction; low ionic strength

LISA Lescol in Severe Atherosclerosis [trial]; less invasive surgical approach; Library and Information Science Abstracts

LISF linear least square fit

LISP List Processing Language

LISREL linear structural relations

LISS less invasive stabilization system; low-ionic-strength saline

LISU library and information statistics unit

Li/SVO lithium silver vanadium oxide [defibrillator battery]

LIT Leiden Intervention Trial [with vegetarian diet for coronary atherosclerosis]; liver infusion tryptose; local immune therapy; Lopressor Intervention Trial

LITA left internal thoracic artery; Library and Information Technology Association

LITE low-intensity treadmill exercise [protocol]

LITT laser-induced interstitial thermotherapy; laser-induced thermal therapy; laser-induced thermography or thermotherapy

LIV left innominate vein; louping ill virus

Liv live, living

LIV-BP leucine, isoleucine, and valine-binding protein

LIVC left inferior vena cava

LIVE Left Ventricular Hypertrophy: Indapamide vs Enalapril [trial]

LIVEN linear inflammatory verrucous epidermal nevus

LJ Lowenstein-Jensen [medium]

LJAV Landjia virus

LJI List of Journals Indexed [in Index Medicus]

LJM limited joint mobility; Lowenstein-Jensen medium

LJNV Lanjan virus

LJV La Joya virus

LK lamellar keratoplasty; Landry-Kussmaul [syndrome]; left kidney; lichenoid keratosis; lymphokine

Lkc leukocyte

Lkcs leukocytes

LKKS liver, kidneys, spleen

LKM liver-kidney microsomal [antibody]

LKP lamellar keratoplasty

LKS Landau-Kleffner syndrome; liver, kidneys, spleen

LKSB liver, kidney, spleen, bladder

LKV laked kanamycin vancomycin [agar]

LL large lymphocyte; lateral lemniscus; left lateral; left leg; left lower; left lung; lepromatous [in Ridley-Jopling Hansen disease classification]; lepromatous leprosy; lipoprotein lipase; loudness level; lower [eye]lid; lower limb; lower lip; lower lobe; lumbar length; lymphocytic lymphoma; lymphoid leukemia; lysolecithin

LLA left lung apex; limulus lysate assay; lipid-lowering agent

LLAEP long latency auditory evoked potential

LLam lumbar laminectomy

LLAT left lateral; lysolecithin aminotransferase

L lat left lateral

LLB left lateral border; long-leg brace

LLBCD left lower border of cardiac dullness

LLC laparoscopic laser cholecystectomy; Lewis lung carcinoma; link layer controller [telemedicine]; liquid-liquid chromatography; long-leg cast; lymphocytic leukemia

LLCC long-leg cylinder cast

LLCD link layer controller detector [telemedicine]

LLC-MK1 rhesus monkey kidney cells

LLC-MK2 rhesus monkey kidney cells

LLC-MK3 *Cercopithecus* monkey kidney cells

LLC-RK1 rabbit kidney cells

LLD left lateral decubitus [muscle]; leg length discrepancy; limb length discrepancy; lipid-lowering drug; long-lasting depolarization

LLE left lower extremity

LLETZ large loop excision of the transformation zone

LLF Laki-Lorand factor; late-life forgetfulness; left lateral femoral; left lateral flexion

LLI leg length inequality; low-level interface

LLL late luminal loss; left lower [eye]lid; left liver lobe; left lower leg; left lower lobe

LLLE lower lid left eye

LLLT low-reactive level laser therapy

LLM localized leukocyte mobilization

LLMSE linear least mean square error

LLN lower limit of normal

LLNA local lymph node assay

LLO *Legionella*-like organism; listeriolysin O; lower limb orthosis

LLP late luteal phase; long-lasting potentiation

LLPV left lower pulmonary vein

LLQ left lower quadrant; low-level question

LLR large local reaction; left lateral rectus [muscle]; left lumbar region; ligation linked [polymerase chain] reaction; long intergenic region; long latency reflex

LLRE lower lid right eye

LLS lazy leukocyte syndrome; Level of Living Survey; linear least squares; long-leg splint; low-level segmentation [module]

LLSB left lower scapular border; left lower sternal border

LLSF linear least squares fit

LLSV Llano Seco virus

LLT left lateral thigh; lysolecithin

LLV lymphatic leukemia virus

LLV-F lymphatic leukemia virus, Friend associated

LLVP left lateral ventricular preexcitation

LLWC long-leg walking cast

LLX left lower extremity

LLZ left lower zone

LLZ-TB lower lung zone tuberculosis

LM labiomental; lactic acid mineral [medium]; lactose malabsorption; laminin; laryngeal mask; laryngeal melanosis; laryngeal muscle; lateral malleolus; left main [coronary artery]; left marginal [coronary artery]; left median; legal medicine; lemniscus medialis; leptomeningeal; Levenberg-Marquardt [algorithm]; Licentiate in Medicine; Licentiate in Midwifery; light microscope, light microscopy; light minimum; lincomycin; lingual margin; linguomesial; lipid mobilization; liquid membrane; *Listeria monocytogenes*; living male; localized movement; longitudinal muscle; lower motor [neuron]; lung metastases; lymphatic metastases

L/M Latin male

Lm *Listeria monocytogenes*

Lm lower midline; lumen

L/m liters per minute

LMA laryngeal mask airway; left main [coronary] artery; left mentoanterior [fetal position]; limbic midbrain area; liver cell membrane autoantibody

LMB Laurence-Moon-Biedl [syndrome]; left main bronchus; leiomyoblastoma; leukomethylene blue

LMBB Laurence-Moon-Bardet-Biedl [syndrome]

LMBS Laurence-Moon-Biedl syndrome

LMC large motile cell; lateral motor column; left main coronary [artery]; left middle cerebral [artery]; living male child; lymphocyte-mediated cytotoxicity; lymphomyeloid complex

LMCA left main coronary artery; left middle cerebral artery

LMCAD left main coronary artery disease

LMCAO left marginal coronary artery occlusion

LMCC Licentiate of the Medical Council of Canada

LMCL left midclavicular line

LMD lipid-moiety modified derivative; local medical doctor; low-molecular-weight dextran; lumbar microdiscotomy

LMDS locally multiply damaged sites

LMDX low-molecular-weight dextran

LME left mediolateral episiotomy; leukocyte migration enhancement; longitudinal mixed effects [in linear regression analysis]

LMed&Ch Licentiate in Medicine and Surgery

LMF left middle finger; lymphocyte mitogenic factor

Lm/ft² lumens per square foot

LMG lethal midline granuloma

LMH lipid-mobilizing hormone

Lmh lumen hour

LMI leukocyte migration inhibition

LMIF leukocyte migration inhibition factor

L/min liters per minute

LMK low molecular weight kininogen

LML large and medium lymphocytes; left mediolateral; left middle lobe

LMM *Lactobacillus* maintenance medium; laser microbeam microdissection; lentigo maligna melanoma; light meromyosin

Lm/m² lumens per square meter

LMMG low molecular mass G [protein]

LMMH low molecular mass heparin

LMN lower motor neuron

LMNL lower motor neuron lesion

LMO living modified organism; localized molecular orbital

LMP large multifunctional protease; last menstrual period; latent membrane potential; left mentoposterior [fetal position]; lumbar puncture

LMPS lethal multiple pterygium syndrome

LMR left medial rectus [muscle]; localized magnetic resonance; longitudinal medical record; lymphocytic meningopolyradiculitis

LMRCP Licentiate in Midwifery of the Royal College of Physicians

LMRP local medical review policy

LMS laser marker system; lateral medullary syndrome; least mean square; left main stem [coronary artery]; leiomyosarcoma; Licentiate in Medicine and Surgery

Lms lumen-second

LMS HPF least means square high pass filter

LMSSA Licentiate in Medicine and Surgery of the Society of Apothecaries

LMT left main trunk; left mentotransverse [fetal position]; leukocyte migration technique

LMV larva migrans visceralis

LMW low molecular weight

Lm/W lumens per watt

LMWD low-molecular-weight dextran

LMWH low-molecular-weight heparin

LMWP low-molecular-weight proteinuria

LMWT low molecular weight

LMZ left midzone

LN labionasal; laminin; Lesch-Nyhan [syndrome]; lipoid nephrosis; Lisch nodule; low necrosis; lung nodule; lupus nephritis; lymph node; Lyon normotensive [rat]

Ln lymph node

LN₂ liquid nitrogen

L/N letter/numerical [system]

Ln natural logarithm

LNAA large neutral amino acid

LNBx lymph node biopsy

LNC lymph node cell

LND lymph node dissection

LNDS lymph node [cancer] negative dataset

LNE lymph node enlargement

LNF laparoscopic Nissen fundoplication

LNH large number hypothesis

LNKS low natural killer syndrome

LNL lymph node lymphocyte

LNLS linear-nonlinear least squares

LNM lymph node metastasis

LNMC lymph node mononuclear cell

LNMP last normal menstrual period

LNNB Luria-Nebraska Neuropsychological Battery

LNP large neuronal polypeptide

LNPF lymph node permeability factor

LNS lateral nuclear stratum; Lesch-Nyhan syndrome

LNV last normal vertebra

LO lateral oblique; linguo-occlusal; lipoxygenase; lumbar orthosis; lysyl oxidase

5-LO 5-lipooxygenase

LOA leave of absence; Leber optic atrophy; left occipitoanterior [fetal position]

LOAEL lowest observed adverse effect level

LOC laxative of choice; level of consciousness; liquid organic compound; locus of control; loss of consciousness

LOCA low osmolarity contrast agent

Lo cal low calorie

Lo calc low calcium

LOCAT Lopid Coronary Angiography Trial

LOCF last observation carried forward

Lo CHO low carbohydrate

Lo chol low cholesterol

LOCM low molecular contrast medium

LOCS laryngoonychocutaneous syndrome

LOD line of duty; log odds ratio [score]

LOF lofexidine

LOFD low outlet forceps delivery

LOG lipoxygenase

LOG, LoG laplacian of gaussian [in imaging]

Log logarithm

LOGIC laryngeal and ocular granulations in children of Indian subcontinent [syndrome]

LOH loop of Henle; loss of heterozygosity

LOHF late-onset hepatic failure

LOI level of incompetence; level of injury; limit of impurities; loss of imprinting

LOIH left oblique inguinal hernia

LOINC Logical Observation Identifier of Names and Codes [vocabulary]

Lo k low potassium

LOKD late-onset Krabbe disease

LOKV Lokern virus

LOL left occipitolateral [fetal position]

LOM left otitis media; ligament of Marshall; limitation of motion; loss of motion

LOMC laser optical memory card

LOMIR-MCT-IL Lomir [isradipine] Multicenter Study in Israel

LOMSA left otitis media suppurativa acuta

LOMSC, LOMSCh left otitis media suppurativa chronica

Lo Na low sodium

Long longitudinal

LONIR Laboratory of Neuro-Imaging Resources

LOP leave on pass; left occipitoposterior [fetal position]

LOPAIR long path infrared [alarm]

LOPP chlorambucil, vincristine, procarbazine, prednisolone

LOPS length of patient's stay

LOQ lower outer quadrant

LOR long open reading frame; lorazepam; loricrin; loss of righting reflex

Lord lordosis, lordotic

LORETA low-resolution brain electromagnetic tomography

LORF long open reading frame

LOS length of stay; Licentiate in Obstetrical Science; lipo-oligosaccharide; low cardiac output syndrome; lower [o]esophageal sphincter

LOS(P) lower [o]esophageal sphincter (pressure)

LOT lateral olfactory tract; left occipitotransverse [fetal position]; Long-Term Outcome after Thrombolysis [study]

Lot lotion

LOV large opaque vesicle; loviride

LOWBI low-birth-weight infant

LOX liquid oxygen; lysyl oxidase

LOXL lysyl oxidase-like

LP labile peptide; labile protein; laboratory procedure; lactic peroxidase; lamina propria; laryngopharyngeal; late potential; latent period, latency period; lateralis posterior [muscle]; lateral plantar; lateral posterior; lateral pylorus; latex particle; *Legionella pneumophila*; leukocyte poor; leukocytic pyrogen; levator palati; levator palpebrae; lichen planus; ligamentum patellae; light padding; light perception; lingua plicata; linear predictive [spectral analysis]; linear programming; linguopulpal; lipoprotein; liver plasma [concentration]; longitudinal propagation; loss of privileges; low potency; low power; low pressure; low protein; lumbar puncture; lumboperitoneal; lung parenchyma; lymphocyte predominant; lymphoid plasma; lymphomatoid papulosis

L/P lactate/pyruvate [ratio]; liver plasma [concentration]; lymph/plasma [ratio]

Lp lipoprotein; sound pressure level

L$_p$ pathlength

LPA latex particle agglutination; left pulmonary artery; lipoprotein A; lysophosphatidic acid

Lp(a) lipoprotein A

LPAM L-phenylalanine mustard

LPB, Lp(b) lipoprotein B

LPBP low-profile bioprosthesis

LPC laser photocoagulation; late positive component; leukocyte-poor cell; linear predictive coding; lipocortin; longitudinal primary care [program]; lysophosphatidylcholine

LPCh latero-posterior choroidal

LPCM low-placed conus medullaris

LP/cm line pairs per centimeter

LPCT late proximal cortical tubule

LPD Lovelace Patient Database; low-protein diet; luteal phase defect; lymphoproliferative disease

LPDF lipoprotein-deficient fraction

LPDS lymph node [cancer] positive dataset

LPE lipoprotein electrophoresis; liquid phase epitaxy; lysophosphatidylethanolamine

LPF leukocytosis-promoting factor; leukopenia factor; lipopolysaccharide factor; localized plaque formation; low pass filter; low-power field; lymphocytosis-promoting factor

Lpf low-power field

LPFB left posterior fascicular block

LPFN low-pass filtered noise

LPFS low-pass filtered signal

LPG left paracolic gutter; lipophosphoglycan

LPH lactase-phlorizin hydrolase; left posterior hemiblock; lipotropic pituitary hormone

LPHA local public health agency

LPHAS limb/pelvis-hypoplasia/aplasia syndrome

LPHD lymphocyte-predominant Hodgkin disease

LPI left posterior-inferior; lysinuric protein intolerance

LPIFB left posteroinferior fascicular block

LPIH left posteroinferior hemiblock

LPK liver pyruvate kinase

LPL lethal-potentially-lethal; lichen planus-like lesion; lipoprotein lipase; local probability of lesion

LPLA lipoprotein lipase activity

LPM lateral pterygoid muscle; leverage and parallelepiped mechanism [computer-assisted surgery]; liver plasma membrane

Lpm lines per minute; liters per minute

Lp/mm line pairs per millimeter

LPN Licensed Practical Nurse

LPO lactoperoxidase; left posterior oblique; light perception only; lipid peroxidation

LPP large plaque parapsoriasis; lateral pterygoid plate

LPPH late postpartum hemorrhage

LPR lactate-pyruvate ratio; late phase reaction

Lpro longitudinal prospective [trial]

LPS lateral premotor system; levator palpebrae superioris [muscle]; linear profile scan; link power status; lipase; lipopolysaccharide; Lovastatin Pravastatin Study

Lps liters per second

LPSR lipopolysaccharide receptor

LPT Language Proficiency Test; lipotropin

LPTP Laboratory Proficiency Test Program [Canada]

LPV lapine parvovirus; left portal view; left pulmonary veins; lopinavir

LPVP left posterior ventricular preexcitation

LPW lateral pharyngeal wall

Lpw lumens per watt

LPX, Lp-X lipoprotein-X

LPyV lymphotropic polyomavirus

LQ linear quadratic; longevity quotient; lordosis quotient; lower quadrant

LQS Lexicon Query Service Specifications

LQT long QT [syndrome]

LQTS long QT syndrome

LR labeled release; laboratory references; laboratory report; labor room; lactated Ringer's [solution]; large reticulocyte; latency reaction; latency relaxation; lateral rectus [muscle]; lateral retinaculum; left hand; left-handed [person]; left rotation; level of recommendation; level of risk; light reaction; light reflex; likelihood ratio; limb reduction [defect]; limit of reaction; livedo reticularis; local recurrence; logistic regression; low renin; lymphocyte recruitment

L-R left to right

L/R left-to-right [ratio]

LR[+] positive likelihood ratio

LR[−] negative likelihood ratio

L&R left and right

Lr lawrencium; limes reacting dose [the least amount of toxin which will produce a reaction]

L$_r$ limes reacting dose [the least amount of toxin which will produce a reaction]

LRA local relevance aggregation [algorithm for insulin therapy]; low right atrium

LRC learning resource center; lipid research clinic; lower rib cage

LRC-CDPT Lipid Research Clinics Coronary Drug Project Trial

LRC-CPPT Lipid Research Clinics Coronary Primary Prevention Trial

LRCMB Laboratory of Retinal Cell and Molecular Biology

LRC-MFS Lipid Research Clinics Mortality Follow-Up Study

LRCP Licentiate of the Royal College of Physicians; low-risk chest pain

LRCS Licentiate of the Royal College of Surgeons

LRCSE Licentiate of the Royal College of Surgeons, Edinburgh

LRD living related donor

LRDT living related donor transplant

LRE lamina rara externa; leukemic reticuloendotheliosis; lymphoreticuloendothelial

LREC language resources and evaluation

LREH low renin essential hypertension

LRES long-range evaluation system

LRes limited resuscitation

Lretro longitudinal retrospective [trial]

LRF latex and resorcinol formaldehyde; liver residue factor; luteinizing hormone-releasing factor

LRG leucine-rich glycoprotein

LRH likelihood ratio for heterogeneity; luteinizing hormone-releasing hormone

LRI lamina rara interna; lower respiratory [tract] illness; lower respiratory [tract] infection; lymphocyte reactivity index

LRL lower [heart] rate limit

LRLT living-related donor transplantation

LRM left radical mastectomy; logistic regression model

LRMP last regular menstrual period

LRN Laboratory Response Network; lateral reticular nucleus

LROP lower radicular obstetrical paralysis

LRP lichen ruber planus; linear resolution pattern; lipoprotein receptor-related protein; long-range planning

LRPC Long Range Planning Committee [National Cancer Institute]

Lr-PET low resolution positron emission tomography

LRQ lower right quadrant

LRR labyrinthine righting reflex; leucine-rich repeat; light reflection rheography; local regional recurrence; lymph return rate

LRS laboratory results; lactated Ringer solution; lateral recess stenosis; lateral recess syndrome; low rate of stimulation; lumboradicular syndrome

LRSDS long range standoff detection system

LRSF lactating rat serum factor; liver regenerating serum factor

LRSS late respiratory systemic syndrome

LRT lateral reticular nucleus; living related transplant; local radiation therapy; long terminal repeat; Lovastatin Restenosis Trial; lower respiratory tract

LRTI lower respiratory tract illness; lower respiratory tract infection

LRV Lato River virus; left renal vein; *Leishmania* RNA virus

LS lateral septum; lateral suspensor; leader sequence; learning system; least; left sacrum; left septum; left side; legally separated; Leigh syndrome; leiomyosarcoma; length of stay; Leriche syndrome; Letterer-Siwe [disease]; Licentiate in Surgery; life sciences; light scanning; light scattering [technique]; light-sensitive, light sensitivity; light sensor; light sleep; Likert score; liminal sensation; linear scanning; linear scleroderma; lipid synthesis; liver and spleen; long sleep; longitudinal section; longitudinal study; Lowe syndrome; low-sodium [diet]; lower strength; lumbar spine; lumbosacral; lung surfactant; lymphosarcoma

L-S Letterer-Siwe [disease]; lipid-saccharide

L:S lecithin:sphingomyelin [ratio]

L/S lactase/sucrase [ratio]; lecithin/ sphingomyelin [ratio]; lipid/saccharide [ratio]; longitudinal section; lumbosacral

L&S liver and spleen

LSA left sacro-anterior [fetal position]; left subclavian artery; leukocyte-specific activity; lichen sclerosus et atrophicus; lymphosarcoma

LS&A lichen sclerosus et atrophicus

LSAH Longitudinal Study of Astronaut Health

LSANA leukocyte-specific antinuclear antibody

LSA/RCS lymphosarcoma-reticulum cell sarcoma

LSB least significant bit; left sternal border; left scapular border; long spike burst; lower sternal border; lumbar sympathetic block

LSBE low-segment Barrett's esophagus

LS-BMD lumbar spine bone mineral density

LSC last sexual contact; late systolic click; least significant change; left side colon cancer; left subclavian; lichen simplex chronicus; liquid scintillation counting; liquid-solid chromatography; locus subcoeruleus

LSc local scleroderma

LScA left scapulo-anterior [fetal position]

LSCL lymphosarcoma cell leukemia

LSCM laser scanning confocal microscopy

LScP left scapulo-posterior [fetal position]

LSCS lower segment cesarean section

LSCT lung cancer screening test

LSCVP left subclavian central venous pressure

LSD laryngeal sound discrimination; least significant difference; least significant digit; low-sodium diet; lysergic acid diethylamide

LSD-25 lysergic acid diethylamide

LSDIS large scale distributed information system

LSE least squares error; left sternal edge

LSect longitudinal section

LSEP left somatosensory evoked potential; lumbosacral somatosensory evoked potential

LSER linear solvation energy relationship

LSF linear spread function; low saturated fat; lymphocyte-stimulating factor

LSFB least squares forward backward

LSG labial salivary gland; losigamone

LSGP leukocyte sialoglycoprotein

LSH lutein-stimulating hormone; lympho-cyte-stimulating hormone

LSHTM London School of Hygiene and Tropical Medicine

LSI large-scale integration; latent semantic indexing; life satisfaction index; List of Serials Indexed [NLM]; lumbar spine index

LSIL low-grade intraepithelial lesion

LSK liver, spleen, kidneys

LSKM liver-spleen-kidney-megaly

LSL left sacrolateral [fetal position]; left short leg; lymphosarcoma [cell] leukemia

LSM laser scanning microscopy; late sys-tolic murmur; least square mean; least square matching [algorithm]; lymphocyte separation medium; lysergic acid morpho-lide

LSN large scale networking; left substan-tia nigra

LSNWG Large Scale Networking Work-ing Group

LSO lateral superior olive; left salpingo-oophorectomy; left superior oblique; lum-bosacral orthosis

LSP left sacroposterior [fetal position]; linguistic string project; liver-specific pro-tein; lymphocyte-specific protein

LSp life span

LS PACS low-speed picture archive and communication system

L-Spar asparaginase (Elspar)

LSP-MLP linguistic string project-medical language processor

LSPV left superior pulmonary vein

LSR lanthanide shift reagent; lecithin/sphingomyelin ratio; left superior rectus [muscle]; liver/spleen ratio

LSRA low septal right atrium

LSRO Life Sciences Research Office

LSS latest starting shift; Life Span Study; life support station; liver-spleen scan; lumbar spinal stenosis; lumbosacral spine

LSSA lipid-soluble secondary antioxidant

LS-SEDUHS Longitudinal Study on Socio-Economic Differences in Utilization of Health Services

LS-SEHD Longitudinal Study on Socio-Economic Health Differences

LSSP-PCR low-stringency single specific primer polymerase chain reaction

LST lateral spinothalamic tract; lateral spreading tumor; left sacrotransverse [fetal position]; life-sustaining treatment

LSTAT life support for trauma and trans-port

LSTL laparoscopic tubal ligation

LSU lactose-saccharose-urea [agar]; life support unit

LSV lateral sacral vein; left subclavian vein; lesser saphenous vein; Lone Star virus; longitudinal sound velocity

LSVC left superior vena cava

LSVT large scale vocabulary test; left saphenous vein thrombophlebitis

LSWA large amplitude slow wave activity

LT heat-labile toxin; laboratory technol-ogy/technologist; laminar tomography; Laplace transform; left; left thigh; left thoracic; less than; lethal time; leukotriene; Levin tube; levothyroxine; light; line ter-mination; long-term; low temperature; lumbar traction; lymphocytic thyroiditis; lymphocytotoxin; lymphotoxin; syphilis [lues] test

L-T3 L-triiodothyronine

L-T4 L-thyroxine

Lt left; light; low tension

LTA leukotriene A; lipoate transacetylase; lipotechoic acid; local tracheal anesthesia; long-term archives; lost-time accident

L-TAP Lipid Treatment Assessment Project

LTAS lead tetra-acetate Schiff

LTB larparoscopic tubal banding; laryngo-tracheobronchitis; leukotriene B

LTBI latent tuberculosis infection

LTC large transformed cell; leukotriene C; lidocaine tissue concentration; long-term care; lysed tumor cell

L1TC level 1 trauma center

LTCF long-term care facility

LTCIC, LTC-IC long-term culture-initiating cell

LTCS low transverse cervical section

LTD Laron-type dwarfism; laterodorsal tegmental [nucleus]; leukotriene D; long-term [cortical] depression; long-term disability

LTE laryngotracheoesophageal; leuko-triene E

LT-ECG long-term electrocardiography

LTF lactotransferrin; lateral tegmental field; lipotropic factor; lymphocyte-transforming factor
LTFU lost to follow-up
LTG lamotrigine; long-term goal; low-tension glaucoma
LTH lactogenic hormone; local tumor hyperthermia; low temperature holding; luteotropic hormone
LTI lupus-type inclusions
LTK laser thermokeratoplasty; leukocyte tyrosine kinase
Lt lat left lateral
LTLT low-temperature, long-time [pasteurization]
LTM long-term memory
LTN lateral telangiectatic nevus
LTNP long-term non-progressor
LTO₂ long-term oxygen therapy
LTOT long-term oxygen therapy
LTP laryngotracheoplasty; lateral thigh perforator; Learning Technologies Project; leukocyte thromboplastin; lipid transfer protein; long-term potentiation; L-tryptophan
LTPA leisure-time physical activity
LTPP lipothiamide pyrophosphate
LTR laryngotracheal reconstruction; location transactivating region; long terminal repeat
LTRA leukotriene receptor antagonist; long-term repopulating ability
LTS laboratory tests; least trimmed squares [method]; long-term survival; long-term survivor
LTST low-temperature stabilization technology
LTT lactose tolerance test; leucine tolerance test; limited treadmill test; lymphocyte transformation test
LTV lung thermal volume
LTW Leydig-cell tumor in Wistar rat
LTX liver transplantation
LU left upper [limb]; loudness unit; Lupron; lytic unit
Lu lutetium
L&U lower and upper
LUC large unstained cell; luciferase
LUCL lateral ulnar collateral ligament
LUE left upper extremity
LUF lesion underdose factor [radiosurgery]; luteinized unruptured follicle

LUFS luteinized unruptured follicle syndrome
LUKV Lukuni virus
LUL left upper eyelid; left upper limb; left upper lobe; left upper lung
Lumb lumbar
LUMD lowest usual maintenance dose
LUMO lowest unoccupied molecular orbital
LUMPS liver unit management protocol system
LUO left ureteral orifice
LUOQ left upper outer quadrant
LUP left ureteropelvic; low urethral pressure
LUPV left upper pulmonary vein
LUQ left upper quadrant
LURD living unrelated donor
LUS laparoscopic ultrasound; lower uterine segment
LUSB left upper scapular border; left upper sternal border
LUT look-up table
LUTO lower urinary tract obstruction
LUV large unilamellar vesicle
LUZ left upper zone
LV laryngeal vestibule; latent virus; lateral ventricle; lecithovitellin; left ventricle, left ventricular; Lentivirus, lentivirus; leucovorin; leukemia virus; leukosis virus; live vaccine; live virus; low voltage; low volume; lumbar vertebra; lung volume; lyssavirus
Lv brightness or luminance
Lv leave
LVA left ventricular aneurysm; left vertebral artery
LVAD left ventricular assist device
LV_ap apical aspect of left ventricle
L-variant a defective bacterial variant that can multiply on hypertonic medium
LVAS left ventricular assist system
LV_bas lateral basilar left ventricle
LVBP left ventricular bypass pump
LVC low-viscosity cement
LVCS low vertical cesarean section
LVD left ventricular dysfunction
LVd latent viroid; left ventricle, distal [electrode]
LVDD left ventricular diastolic dimension
LVDd left ventricular diastolic dimension; left ventricular dimension in end-diastole
LVDI left ventricular dimension

LVDP left ventricular developed pressure; left ventricular diastolic pressure

LVDT linear variable differential transformer

LVDV left ventricular diastolic volume

LVE left ventricular ejection; left ventricular enlargement

LVED left ventricular end-diastole

LVEDA left ventricular end-diastolic area

LVEDC left ventricular end-diastolic circumference

LVEDD left ventricular end-diastolic diameter; left ventricular end-diastolic dimension

LVEDI left ventricular end-diastolic volume index

LVEDP left ventricular end-diastolic pressure

LVEDV left ventricular end-diastolic volume

LVEF left ventricular ejection fraction

LVEJT left ventricular ejection time

LVEP left ventricular end-diastolic pressure

LVESD left ventricular end-systolic dimension

LVESV left ventricular end-systolic volume

LVESVI left ventricular end-systolic volume index

LVET left ventricular ejection time; low volume eye test

LVETI left ventricular ejection time index

LVF left ventricular failure; left ventricular function; left visual field; low-voltage fast; low-voltage foci

LVFP left ventricular filling pressure

LVFT$_2$ left ventricular slow filling time

LVFW left ventricular free wall

LVG left ventriculogram

LVH large vessel hematocrit; left ventricular hypertrophy

LVI left ventricular insufficiency; left ventricular ischemia

LVID left ventricular internal dimension

LVIDd left ventricle internal dimension in diastole

LVID$_d$ left ventricular internal dimension in end-diastole

LVIDs left ventricle internal dimension in systole

LVID$_s$ left ventricle internal dimension in end-systole

LVIV left ventricular inflow volume

LVL left vastus lateralis

LVLG left ventrolateral gluteal

LVM left ventricular mass; left ventricular mass index

LVMF left ventricular minute flow

LV$_{mid}$ midanterior left ventricle

LVN Laguerre-Volterra network [artificial neural network]; lateral ventricular nerve; lateral vestibular nucleus; Licensed Visiting Nurse; Licensed Vocational Nurse

LVO left ventricle outflow

LVOH left ventricle outflow [tract] height

LVOT left ventricular outflow tract

LVOTG left ventricular outflow tract gradient

LVOTO left ventricular outflow tract obstruction

LVOV left ventricular outflow volume

LVP large volume parenteral [infusion]; left ventricular pressure; levator veli palatini; lysine-vasopressin

LVp left ventricle, proximal [electrode]

LVPFR left ventricular peak filling rate

LVP$_{max}$ maximum left ventricular pressure

LVP$_{min}$ minimum left ventricular pressure

LVPW left ventricular posterior wall

LVQ learning vector quantization

LVR loviride

LVRD left ventricular replacement device

LVRS lung volume reduction surgery

LVS laryngovideostroboscopy; left ventricular strain; live vaccine strain

LVs left ventricular system

LVSEMI left ventricular subendocardial myocardial ischemia

LVSI left ventricular systolic index

LVSO left ventricular systolic output

LV-SO left ventricular site of origin

LVSP left ventricular systolic pressure

LVST lateral vestibulospinal tract

LVSV left ventricular stroke volume

LVSW left ventricular stroke work

LVSWI left ventricular stroke work index

LVT left ventricular tension; levetiracetam; lysine vasotonin

LVV left ventricular volume; Le Veen valve; live varicella vaccine; live varicella virus

LVW left ventricular wall; left ventricular work

LVWI left ventricular work index

LVWM left ventricular wall motion
LVWT left ventricular wall thickness
LW lacerating wound; lateral wall; Lee-White [method]
L&W, L/W living and well
Lw lawrencium
LWA low weight for age
LWBS leaving [hospital] without being seen
LWCT Lee-White clotting time
LWK large white kidney
LWP lateral wall pressure
LWS Lowry-Wood syndrome
LX local irradiation; lower extremity; lymphatic metastases cannot be assessed [TNM (tumor-node-metastasis) classification]
Lx latex
Lx larynx; lower extremity; lux
L-XRF L x-ray fluorescence
LXT left exotopia

LY lactoalbumin and yeastolate [medium]; lymphocyte
Ly a T-cell antigen used for grouping T-lymphocytes into different classes
LYDMA lymphocyte-detected membrane antigen
LYES liver yang exuberance syndrome
LYG lymphomatoid granulomatosis
LYM lymph nodes
Lym, lymph lymphocyte, lymphocytic
LyNeF lytic nephritic factor
Lyo lyophilized
LYP lactose, yeast, and peptone [agar]; lower yield point
LYS, Lys lysine; lysodren
lys lysine
LySLk lymphoma syndrome leukemia
Lyso-PC lysophosphatidyl phosphatidylcholine
lytes electrolytes
LYZ lysozyme
LZM, Lzm lysozyme

M

M blood factor in the MNS blood group system; chin [Lat. *mentum*]; concentration in moles per liter; death [Lat. *mors*]; dullness [of sound, Lat. *mutitas*]; macerate; macroglobulin; macroscopic magnetization vector; magnetization; magnification; male; malignant; married; masculine; mass; massage; maternal contribution; matrix; mature; maximum; mean; meatus; median; mediator; medical; medicine; medium; mega; megohm; membrane; memory; mental; mesial; metabolite; metanephrine; metastases; meter; methionine; methotrexate; *Micrococcus*; Microspora; minim; minute; mitochondria; mitosis; mix, mixed, mixture; mobility; molar [permanent tooth]; molar [solution]; molarity; mole; molecular; moment of force; monkey; monocyte; month; morgan; morphine; mother; motile; mouse; mucoid [colony]; mucous; multipara; murmur [cardiac]; muscle; muscular response to an electrical stimulation of its motor nerve [wave]; *Mycobacterium*; *Mycoplasma*; myeloma or macroglobulinemia [component]; myopia; strength of pole; thousand [Lat. *mille*]

M- mega- [10^6]

M0 leukemia with large granular blasts and negative myeloperoxidase [Franco-American-British (FAB) classification]; no distant tumor metastases [TNM (tumor-node-metastasis) classification]; no metastases [TNM (tumor-node-metastasis) classification]; no tumor metastases [TNM (tumor-node-metastasis) classification]

M1 breast tumor, no distant metastases [TNM (tumor-node-metastasis) classification]; distant metastases [TNM (tumor-node-metastasis) classification]; distant tumor metastases [TNM (tumor-node-metastasis) classification]; leukemia with poorly differentiated myeloblasts [Franco-American-British (FAB) classification]; primary motor area

1M, 2M, 3M, 4M, 5M first, second, third, fourth, fifth metatarsal [head]

M_1 mitral component [first heart sound]; mitral first [sound]; myeloblast; slight dullness

MI, M-I first meiotic metaphase

M2 breast tumor, distant metastases [TNM (tumor-node-metastasis) classification]; leukemia with myeloblasts with differentiation and Auer rods [Franco-American-British (FAB) classification]

2-M 2-microglobulin

M_2 dose per square meter of body surface; marked dullness; promyelocyte

MII, M-II second meiotic metaphase

M3 leukemia with hypergranular promyelocytes and multiple Auer rods [Franco-American-British (FAB) classification]

3-M [syndrome] initials for Miller, McKusick, and Malvaux, who first described the syndrome

M/3 middle third

M_3 absolute dullness; myelocyte at the 3rd stage of maturation

M4 leukemia monoblastic differentiation [Franco-American-British (FAB) classification]

M_4 myelocyte at the 4th stage of maturation

M5 monoblastic leukemia [Franco-American-British (FAB) classification]

M_5 metamyelocyte

M6 erythroleukemia with dyserythropoiesis and megaloblastosis [Franco-American-British (FAB) classification]

M_6 band form in the 6th stage of myelocyte maturation

M7 megakaryoblastic leukemia [Franco-American-British (FAB) classification]

M_7 polymorphonuclear neutrophil

M/10 tenth molar solution

M/100 hundredth molar solution

m electron rest mass; electromagnetic moment; magnetic moment; magnetic quantum number; male; mass; median; melting [temperature]; metastable; meter; milli-; minim; minimum; minute; molality; molar [deciduous tooth]; mutated

m^{-1} per meter

m^2 square meter

m^3 cubic meter

m_s spin quantum number

μ see *mu*

MA macrophage aggregate; malignant arrhythmia; management and administration; mandelic acid; Martin-Albright [syndrome]; masseter; Master of Arts; maternal age; matrix; maximum amplitude; mean arterial; mechanical activity; medial amygdaloid [nucleus]; medical assistance; medical audit; medical authorization; megaampere; megaloblastic anemia; megestrol acetate; membrane antigen; menstrual age; mental age; mentum anterior [fetal position]; metatarsus adductus; meter-angle; methacrylic acid; microadenoma; microagglutination; microaneurysm; microscopic agglutination; Miller-Abbott [tube]; milliampere; mitochondrial antibody; mitogen activation; mitotic apparatus; mixed agglutination; mobile agent; moderately advanced; monoamine; monoarthritis; monoclonal antibody; motor area; movement artifacts; moving average; multiple action; muscle activity; mutagenic activity; myelinated axon; myoclonic absences

MA-104 embryonic rhesus monkey kidney cells

MA-111 embryonic rabbit kidney cells

MA-163 human embryonic thymus cells

MA-184 newborn human foreskin cells

M/A male, altered [animal]; mood and/or affect

Ma mass of atom

mA, ma milliampere; meter-angle

mÅ milliangstrom

ma milliampere

μA microampere

MAA macroaggregated albumin; maleylacetoacetic acid; Medical Assistance for the Aged; melanoma-associated antigen; methacrylic acid; microphthalmia (or anophthalmos) with associated anomalies; moderate aplastic anemia; monoarticular arthritis

MAAC maximum allowable actual charges

MAACL Multiple Affect Adjective Check List

MAAGB Medical Artists Association of Great Britain

MAAP multiple arbitrary amplicon profiling

MAAS Multicenter Anti-Atherosclerosis Study; Multicenter Antiatheroma Study

MAB, MAb, mAB monoclonal antibody

m-AB *m*-aminobenzamide

MABIS Munich and Berlin Infarction Study

MABP mean arterial blood pressure

Mabs, mABs, mAbs monoclonal antibodies

MAC MacConkey [broth]; magnetic authentication code; major ambulatory category; malignancy-associated changes; maximum allowable concentration; maximum aerobic capacity; maximum allowable cost; medical alert center; membrane attack complex; message authentication code; midarm circumference; minimum alveolar concentration; minimum antibiotic concentration; mitral anular calcium; modulator of adenylate cyclase; monitored anesthesia care; multiaccess catheter; *Mycobacterium avium* complex

MACAS Marburg Cardiomyopathy Study

MacCAT-CR MacArthur Competence Assessment Tool for Clinical Research

MACDP Metropolitan Atlanta Congenital Defects Program

MACE main adverse coronary event; major adverse cardiac events; major cardiac event; Mayo Asymptomatic Carotid Endarterectomy [trial]

MAC-ei minimum alveolar concentration-endotracheal intubation

MACEmed Middleware Architecture Committee for Education in Medicine

macer maceration

MACH machine activity [UMLS]; Mortality Assessment in Congestive Heart Failure [study]

mAChR muscarinic acetylcholine receptor

MacMV Maclura mosaic virus

MACR mean axillary count rate

mACR muscarinic acetylcholine receptor

macro macrocyte, macrocytic; macroscopic

MACS maximum aortic cusp separation; Multicenter Acquired Immunodeficiency Syndrome (AIDS) Cohort Study; myristoylated alanine-rich protein kinase C substrate

MACT maximum achievable control technology

MACTAR McMaster-Toronto arthritis and rheumatism [questionnaire]

MACV Machupo virus

MAD major affective disorder; mandibulo-acral dysplasia; master accession database; maximum allowable dose; mean axis direction; median absolute deviation; methylandrostenediol; mind-altering drug; minimum average dose; mitotic arrest defective; mucosal atomization device; multiple autoimmune disorder; myoadenylate deaminase

mAD, MADA muscle adenylate deaminase; myoadenylate deaminase

MADAM Moexipril as Antihypertensive Drug after Menopause [study]

mADAM mouse A disintegrin and A metalloprotease

MadCAM mucosal addressin cell adhesion molecule

MADD Mothers Against Drunk Driving; multiple acyl-CoA dehydrogenase deficiency

MADDS monoacetyldiaminodiphenylsulfone

MADGE microliter array diagonal gel electrophoresis

MADIT Multicenter Automatic Defibrillator Implantation Trial

MADIT/CES Multicenter Automatic Defibrillator Implantation Trial Cost/Effectiveness Study

MADPA Medicaid Antidiscriminatory Drug Pricing and Patient Benefit Restoration Act

MADRS Medicare Automated Data Retrieval System; Montgomery-Asberg Depression Rating Scale

MADT morphology alteration and disintegration test

MADU methylaminodeoxyuridine

MADV Madrid virus

MAE mean absolute error; medical air evacuation; medication administration error; 2-methylaminoethanol; moves all extremities; multilingual aphasia examination; myoclonic astatic epilepsy

MAF macrophage activation factor; macrophage agglutinating factor; maximum atrial fragmentation; minimum audible field; mouse amniotic fluid

MAFD manic affective disorder

MAFF Ministry of Agriculture, Fisheries and Food [UK]

MAFH macroaggregated ferrous hydroxide

MAFI Medic Alert Foundation International

MAG mercaptoacetyltriglycerine; multitumor aberrant growth; myelin-associated glycoprotein

Mag magnesium

mAg minor antigen

mag, magn large [Lat. *magnus*]; magnification

mag cit magnesium citrate

MAGE melanoma antigen

MAGF male accessory gland fluid

MAggF macrophage agglutination factor

MAGIC Magnesium in Cardiac Arrest [trial]; Magnesium in Coronaries [trial]; microprobe analysis generalized intensity correction; mouth (or mucosal) and genital ulceration with inflamed cartilage [syndrome]

MAGICA Magnesium in Cardiac Arrhythmia [trial]

MAGP microfibril-associated glycoprotein

MAGPIE Magnesium Sulfate Compared with Placebo in Pre-Eclampsia [study]

MAGUK membrane-associated guanylate kinase

MAGV Maguari virus

MagV mag virus

mAH, mA-h milliampere-hours

MAHA microangiopathic hemolytic anemia

MAHH malignancy-associated humoral hypercalcemia

MAHI, MAHIV medically acquired human immunodeficiency virus

MAHST Multicenter Austrian Hemodilution Stroke Trial

MaHV Macropodid herpesvirus

MAI microscopic aggregation index; movement assessment of infants; multilevel assessment instrument; *Mycobacterium avium* infection; *Mycobacterium avium-intracellulare*

MAIDS mouse acquired immunodeficiency syndrome

MAIESTRO The Michael Reese Hospital-Institute of Technology Expert System for Stroke

MAIN medication-induced, autoimmune, infectious, and neoplastic [diseases associated with antiphospholipid antibodies]

MAIPA monoclonal antibody-specific immobilization of platelet antigens

MAIR-IR multiple attenuated internal reflexion infrared [spectroscopy]

MAIS manual axial in-line stabilization; mild androgen insensitivity syndrome

MAJIC Mayo Japan Investigation on Chronic Total Occlusion

MAKA major karyotypic abnormality

MAL malemide; midaxillary line; motor activity log

Mal malate; malfunction; malignancy

mal malaise; male; malposition

Mal-BSA maleated bovine serum albumin

MALD matrix-assisted laser desorption

MALDI matrix-assisted laser desorption/ionization

MALDI-MS matrix-assisted laser desorption/ionization mass spectrometry

MALDI-TOF matrix-assisted laser desorption/ionization time-of-flight

MALG Minnesota antilymphoblast globulin

MALiMET Master List of Medical Indexing Terms

MALLS multi-angle laser light scattering

MALS magnetic alignment and light scattering

MALT male, altered [animal]; mucosa-associated lymphoid tissue; Munich Alcoholism Test

MALTOMA mucosal associated lymphoid tissue lymphoma

MALV Malakal virus

MAM median age at menarche; metabolically active mass; methylazoxymethanol

mam milliampere-minute; myriameter

M+Am compound myopic astigmatism

6-MAM monoacetyl-morphine

MAMA medical application multimedia authoring; monoallelic mutation analysis; monoclonal anti-malignin antibody; Mothers Against Misuse and Abuse

MAM Ac methylazoxymethanol acetate

MAMC mean arm muscle circumference

mA-min, ma-min milliampere-minute

Mammo mammogram, mammography

MAN metropolitan area network

MAN, Man mannose

man manipulate

MANA mannosidase alpha

MANB mannosidase beta

ManBP mannan-binding protein

mand mandible, mandibular

MANET mobile ad-hoc network

manifest manifestation

manip manipulation

MANOVA multivariate analysis of variance

MAN-6-P mannose-6-phosphate

MANU manufactured object [UMLS]

MANV Manzanilla virus

MAN/WAN metropolitan area network/wide area network

MAO Master of the Art of Obstetrics; maximal acid output; monoamine oxidase

MAOA monoamine oxidase A

MAOB monoamine oxidase B

MAOI monoamine oxidase inhibitor

MAOUSSC Model of Assistance and Orientation of a User within a System of Coding

MAP malignant atrophic papulosis; mandibular angle plane; maturation-activated protein; maximal aerobic power; maximum a posteriori; mean airway pressure; mean aortic pressure; mean arterial pressure; Medical Audit Program; megaloblastic anemia of pregnancy; memory algorithm processor; mercapturic acid pathway; methyl acceptor protein; methylacetoxy-progesterone; methylaminopurine; microtubule-associated protein; minimum audible pressure; mitogen-activated protein; modified atmosphere packaging; moment angle plotter; monophasic action potential; motor [nerve] action potential; mouse antibody production; multiphasic algorithmic protocol; multiple antigen peptide; muscle action potential; mussel adhesive protein

MAPA muscle adenosine phosphoric acid

MAPC migrating action potential complex

MAPCA major aorto-pulmonary collateral artery

MAPE mean absolute percentage error

MAPF microatomized protein food

MAPHY Metoprolol Atherosclerosis Prevention in Hypertension [study]

MAPI microbial alkaline protease inhibitor; Millon Adolescent Personality Inventory

MAPK mitogen-activated protein kinase

MAPK-K mitogen-activated protein kinase kinase

MAPKP mitogen-activated protein kinase phosphatase

MAPP multiple asynchronous parallel processing

MAPPET Management Strategy and Prognosis of Pulmonary Embolism Trial

MAPREC mutant analysis by polymerase chain reaction and restriction enzyme cleavage

MAPS Make a Picture Story [test]; Micro-AIDS Processing System; Multidimensional Affect and Pain Survey; Multivessel Angioplasty Prognosis Study

MAPT microtubule-associated protein tau

MAPV Mapputta virus; mean area-peak value

MAR main admissions room; marasmus; marrow; matrix attachment region [genomic sequencing]; maximal aggregation ratio; mean atrial rate; medication administration record; microanalysis reagent; minimal angle resolution; mixed antiglobulin reaction; multiple aberration region; multivariate autoregressive [model]

mar margin; marker [chromosome]

MARAV Maraba virus

MARC machine-readable catalog; machine-readable cataloging; Multicenter Asthma Research Collaboration; multifocal and recurrent choroidopathy

MARCKS myristoylated alanine-rich protein C kinase substrate

MarHV Marmomid herpesvirus

MARIAC Magnetic Resonance Image Analysis Research Centre [UK]

MarMV Maracuja virus

MARS magnetic anchor retinal stimulation; medical archival system; Medical Article Record System; methionyl-transfer ribonucleic acid synthetase; Mevinolin Atherosclerosis Regression Study; Missouri Automated Radiology System; mobile autonomous robot software; molecular adsorbent recirculating system; molecular adsorbents system; Monitored Atherosclerosis Regression Study; mouse antirat serum; multivariate adaptive regression spline [algorithm]

MARSA methicillin-aminoglycoside-resistant *Staphylococcus aureus*

MAR/SAR matrix attachment region/scaffold attachment region [genomic sequencing]

MART multiplicative algebraic reconstruction technique

MARV Marburg virus

MARVIN Multi-Agent Robot Vagabond on Information Networks

mar(X) marker X [chromosome]

MAS macrophage activation syndrome; magic angle spinning; Manifest Anxiety Scale; marker-assisted selection; maximum average score; McCune-Albright syndrome; meconium aspiration syndrome; medical administrative services; medical advisory service; medical audit study; meiosis activation sterol; mesoatrial shunt; milk-alkali syndrome; milliampere-second; minor axis shortening; mitral aortic septum; mobile arm support; monoclonal antibodies; Morgagni-Adams-Stokes [syndrome]; motion analysis system; motor assessment scale; multiagent system; multiple access server [telemedicine]; myoclonic astatic seizures

mA-s, mas milliampere-second

MASA Medical Association of South Africa; mental retardation-aphasia-shuffling gait-adducted thumbs [syndrome]; mutant allele specific amplification

masc masculine; mass concentration

MASCIS Multicenter Animal Spinal Cord Injury Study

MASER microwave amplification by stimulated emission of radiation

MASH mobile Army surgical hospital; multiple automated sample harvester

MASK Medical Anatomy Segmentation Kit

MASS Medicine, Angioplasty, or Surgery Study

mass massage

massc mass concentration

MAST Managing Anticoagulation Services Trial; Michigan Alcohol Screening Test; military antishock trousers; motion artifact suppression technique

mast mastectomy; mastoid

MAST-E Multicentre Acute Stroke Trial-Europe

MAST-I Multicenter Acute Stroke Trial-Italy

MASU mobile Army surgical unit

MAT manual arts therapist; master of arts in technology; mean absorption time; medial axis transform; medical assistance team [emergency medicine]; medical augmentation team; methionine adenosyltransferase; microagglutination test; minimal access technique; multifocal atrial tachycardia; multiple agent therapy

Mat, mat maternal [origin]; mature

MATC maximum allowable toxicant concentration

MATCH Matching Alcoholism Treatment to Client Heterogeneity

MatD maternal disomy

MatDp maternal duplication

MATE Medicine vs Angiography for Thrombolytic Exclusions [trial]

mat gf maternal grandfather

mat gm maternal grandmother

MATH Modern Approach to Treatment of Hypertension [study]

MATIS Mathematics Tools Integration System

MATSA Marek-associated tumor-specific antigen

MATTIS Multicenter Aspirin and Ticlopidine Trials after Intracoronary Stenting

MATTUS Minimal Access Therapy Training Unit Scotland

MATV Matucare virus

MAU multi-attribute utility [model]

MAUS Mammography Attitudes and Usage Study

MAUT multi-attribute utility theory

MAV mechanical auditory ventricle; minimal alveolar ventilation; minimum apparent viscosity; movement arm vector; myeloblastosis-associated virus

MAVD mixed aortic valve disease

MAVERIC Midlands Trial of Empirical Amiodarone vs Electrophysiological Guided Intervention and Cardioverter Implant in Ventricular Arrhythmias

MAVIS mobile artery and vein imaging system

MAVR mitral and aortic valve replacement

max maxilla, maxillary; maximum

MaxDu maximum duration

MaxEP maximum esophageal pressure

MAYV Mayaro virus

MB Bachelor of Medicine [Lat. *Medicinae Baccalaureus*]; buccal margin; General

Modeling Bayesian Fitting [program]; isoenzyme of creatine kinase containing M and B subunits; mammillary body; Marsh-Bender [factor]; maximum breathing; medulloblastoma; megabyte; mesiobuccal; methyl bromide; methylene blue; microbiological assay; muscle balance; multibacillary; myocardial band

Mb megabase; megabit; million bases; mouse brain; myoglobin

mb millibar

μ_B Bohr magneton

μb microbar

MBA methylbenzyl alcohol; methyl bovine albumin

MBAC Member of the British Association of Chemists

MBAR myocardial beta adrenergic receptor

mbar millibar

μbar microbar

MBAS methylene blue active substance

MBB modified barbiturate buffer

MBBG metabromobenzylguanidine

MBBS Medicinae Baccalaureus/Bachelor of Surgery [British doctoral degree]

MBC male breast cancer; maximal bladder capacity; maximal breathing capacity; memory B cell; metastatic breast cancer; methyl-1-(butylcarbamoyl)-2-benzimidazole-carbamate; methylthymol blue complex; microcrystalline bovine collagen; minimum bactericidal concentration; moving blood cells

MB-CK creatine kinase isoenzyme containing M and B subunits

MBCL monocytoid B-cell lymphoma

MbCO carbon monoxy myoglobin

MBCR Molecular Biology Computational Resource

MBD Marchiafava-Bignami disease; maximum bactericidal dilution; metabolic bone disease; methylene blue dye; methyl-binding domain; minimal brain damage; minimal brain dysfunction; Morquio-Brailsford disease

MBDG mesiobuccal developmental groove

MBE medium below elbow [cast]

MBEC mouse brain endothelial cell

MBF medullary blood flow; mesenteric blood flow; muscle blood flow; myocardial blood flow

MBFC medial brachial fascial compartment

MBFLB monaural bifrequency loudness balance

MbFV mite-borne filamentous virus

MBG Marburg [disease]; mean blood glucose; morphine-benzedrine group [scale]

MBH medial basal hypothalamus

MBH₂ reduced methylene blue

MBHI Millon Behavioral Health Inventory

MBHO managed behavioral healthcare organization

MBI Maslach Burnout Inventory; maximum blink index

MBK methyl butyl ketone

MBL Marine Biological Laboratory; menstrual blood loss; minimum bactericidal level

MBLA methylbenzyl linoleic acid; mouse-specific bone-marrow-derived lymphocyte antigen

MbLV mite-borne latent virus

MBM meat and bone meal [see BSE]; mineral basal medium

MBNOA Member of the British Naturopathic and Osteopathic Association

MBO management by objective; mesiobucco-occlusal

MBO₂ oxymyoglobin

MBOV Mboke virus

MBP major basic protein; maltose-binding protein; management by policy; mannose-binding protein; mean blood pressure; melitensis, bovine, porcine [antigen from *Brucella bovis, B. melitensis,* and *B. suis*]; mesiobuccopulpal; myelin basic protein

MBPM modified backward Prony method [spectral analysis of heart sounds]

MBPS multigated blood pool scanning

Mbps megabits per second; myeloblastic syndrome

MBq megabecquerel

MBR methylene blue, reduced

MBRT methylene blue reduction time

MBS Martin-Bell syndrome; media broadband service

MBSA methylated bovine serum albumin

MBSI multi-channel blind system identification

MBT mercaptobenzothiazole; mixed bacterial toxin; myeloblastin

MBTA modeling better treatment advice

MBTH 3-methyl-2-benzothiazoline hydrazone

MBTI Myers-Briggs type indicator

MBVT Munich and Berlin Trial for Sustained Ventricular Tachyarrhythmias

MC mass casualties; mast cell; Master of Surgery [Lat. *Magister Chirurgiae*]; maximum concentration; Medical Corps; medium chain; medullary cavity; medullary cyst; megacoulomb; melanocortin; melanoma cell; menstrual cycle; Merkel cell; mesiocervical; mesocaval; metacarpal; methyl cellulose; microcephaly; microcholecystectomy; microcirculation; microscopic colitis; midcapillary; mineralocorticoid; mini-catheterization; minimal change; mitomycin C; mitotic cycle; mitral commissurotomy; mixed cellularity; mixed cryoglobulinemia; monkey cell; mononuclear cell; mucous cell; musculocutaneous; myocardial channeling; myocarditis

M/C male, castrated [animal]

M-C mineralocorticoid

M&C morphine and cocaine

Mc megacurie; megacycle

M_c mitral closure

mC millicoulomb

mc millicurie

μC microcoulomb

μc microcurie

MCA major coronary artery; Maternity Center Association; mean cell [surface] area; medical care administration; Medicines Control Agency [UK]; methylcholanthrene; microchannel architecture; middle cerebral artery; monoclonal antibody; mucinlike carcinoma-associated antigen; multichannel analyzer; multiple congenital anomaly

MCAB monoclonal antibody

MCAD medium chain acyl-CoA dehydrogenase

MCAF monocyte chemotactic and activating factor

MCA/MR multiple congenital anomaly/mental retardation [syndrome]

MCAO middle cerebral artery occlusion

MCAR mixed cell agglutination reaction

MCARE managed care

MCAS middle cerebral artery syndrome

MCAT medical chemical advisory team; medical college admission test; middle cerebral artery thrombosis; Multimedia Cardiac Angiogram Tool; myocardial contrast appearance time

MCAV Macaua virus

MCB master cell bank; membranous cytoplasmic body; monochlorobimane

McB McBurney [point]

mCBF mean cerebral blood flow

MCBIT Munich Coronary Bypass Intervention Trial

MCBM muscle capillary basement membrane

MCBR minimum concentration of bilirubin

MCBS Medicare Current Beneficiary Survey [database]

MCBV minimum conditional bias/variance

MCBW mass casualty biological weapon

MCC mean corpuscular hemoglobin concentration; measles control campaign; medial cell column; Medical Council of Canada; medical information communication controller; metacarpal-carpal [joints]; metacerebral cell; metastatic cord compression; microcalcification cluster; microcrystalline collagen; midstream clean catch [urine]; minimum complete-killing concentration; mucocutaneous candidiasis; mutated in colorectal cancer [gene]

MC-C metacarpo-carpal [joint]

MCCA Medicare Catastrophic Care Act; Medicare Catastrophic Coverage Act

MCCD minimum cumulative cardiotoxic dose

MCCI medical care component of the consumer price index; medical cost control initiative

MCCPI medical care component of the consumer price index

MCCU mobile coronary care unit

MCD magnetic circular dichroism; mastcell degranulation; mean cell diameter; mean central dose; mean corpuscular diameter; mean of consecutive differences; Medicaid competition demonstration; medical concepts dictionary; medullary collecting duct; medullary cystic disease; metacarpal cortical density; minimal cerebral dysfunction; minimal change disease;

multiple carboxylase deficiency; muscle carnitine deficiency

MCDI Minnesota Child Development Inventory

MCDK multicystic dysplastic kidney

MCDNP medullary cystic disease/nephrolithiasis disease

MCDP mast cell degranulating peptide

MCDU mercaptolactate-cysteine disulfiduria

MCE maximum credible event; medical care evaluation; military clinical engineering; multicystic encephalopathy; multiple cartilaginous exostosis; myocardial contrast echocardiography

MCES medical care evaluation study; multiple cholesterol emboli syndrome

MCF macrophage chemotactic factor; median cleft face; medium corpuscular fragility; method conversion factor; microcomplement fixation; mink cell focus-forming; mononuclear cell factor; myocardial contraction force

MCFA medium-chain fatty acid; miniature centrifugal fast analyzer

MCFP mean circulating filling pressure

MCFSR mean circumferential fiber shortening rate

MCG magnetocardiogram; membrane cell graft; membrane coating granule; monoclonal gammopathy

mcg microgram

MCGC metacerebral giant cell

MCGF mast cell growth factor

MCGN mesangiocapillary glomerulonephritis; minimal change glomerulonephritis; mixed cryoglobulinemia with glomerulonephritis

MCGNX mesangiocapillary glomerulonephritis, X-linked

MCH Maternal and Child Health; mean corpuscular hemoglobin; medical college hospital; melanin-concentrating hormone; mucous cell hyperplasia; muscle contraction headache

MCh Master of Surgery [Lat. *Magister Chirurgiae*]; methacholine

mc-h, mch millicurie-hour

μch microcurie-hour

MCHB Maternal and Child Health Bureau

MCHC maternal/child health care; mean corpuscular hemoglobin concentration; mean corpuscular hemoglobin count

MChD Master of Dental Surgery

MCHgb mean corpuscular hemoglobin

MChir Master in Surgery [Lat. *Magister Chirurgiae*]

MChOrth Master of Orthopaedic Surgery

MChOtol Master of Otology

MCHR Medical Committee for Human Rights

mc-hr millicurie-hour

μC-hr microcurie-hour

MCHS Maternal and Child Health Service

MCI mean cardiac index; methicillin; mild cognitive impairment; molecular connectivity index; mucociliary insufficiency; multiple casualty incident; muscle contraction interference

MCi megacurie

mCi millicurie

μCi microcurie

MCICU medical coronary intensive care unit

MCID minimum clinically important difference

M-CIDI Münich Composite International Diagnostic Interview

MCi-hr millicurie-hour

μCi-hr microcurie-hour

MCINS minimal change idiopathic nephrotic syndrome

MCK multicystic kidney

MCKD multicystic kidney disease

MCL Macintosh common lisp; mantle-cell lymphoma; maximum containment laboratory; maximum contaminant level; medial collateral ligament; midclavicular line; midcostal line; minimal change lesion; mixed culture, leukocyte; modified chest lead; most comfortable loudness; mucocutaneous leishmaniasis; multiple cutaneous leiomyomata; myeloid cell leukemia

MCLC medial collateral ligament complex

MCLNS, MCLS mucocutaneous lymph node syndrome

MClSci Master of Clinical Science

MCM medical core metadata; methylmalonic coenzyme A mutase; minimum capacitation medium; multi-chip module; multicompartmental model

MCMC Markov Chain Monte Carlo [method]

MCMI Millon Clinical Multiaxial Inventory

MCMM Monte Carlo multiple minimum [search method]

MCMV murine cytomegalovirus

MCN maternal child nursing; minimal change nephropathy; mixed cell nodular [lymphoma]

MCNS minimal change nephrotic syndrome

MCO managed care organization; medical care organization; multichannel option [computer-assisted surgery]; multicystic ovary

MCommH Master of Community Health

mcoul millicoulomb

μcoul microcoulomb

MCOV Marco virus; modified covariance

MCP major capsid protein; maximum closure pressure; maximum contraction pattern; medical command physician; melanocortin receptor; melphalan, cyclophosphamide, and prednisone; membrane cofactor protein; metacarpophalangeal; metoclopramide; mitotic-control protein; monocyte chemotactic protein; Monte Carlo[computer] program; mucin clot prevention

MCP-1 monocyte chemotactic protein-1

MCPA Member of the College of Pathologists, Australasia

MCPH metacarpophalangeal

MCPJ metacarpophalangeal joint

MCPP metacarpophalangeal pattern profile; metacarpophalangeal profile; metachlorophenylpiperazine

MCPPP metacarpophalangeal pattern profile plot

MCPS Member of the College of Physicians and Surgeons

Mcps megacycles per second

MCPT Monte Carlo photon transport

MCQ multiple-choice question

MCR Medical Corps Reserve; melanocortin receptor; message competition ratio; metabolic clearance rate; myotonia congenita, recessive type

5-MCR 5-methylchrysene

mcr minor breakpoint cluster region

MCRA Member of the College of Radiologists, Australasia

MCRD monolithic controlled release device [cardiac pacing]

MCRE mother-child relationship evaluation

MCRglc cerebral metabolic rate for glucose

MCRI Multifactorial Cardiac Risk Index

MCS malignant carcinoid syndrome; managed care system; massage of the carotid sinus; Meharry Cohort Study; medical computing services; mesocaval shunt; method of constant stimuli; methylcholanthrene [induced] sarcoma; microculture and sensitivity; middle coronary sinus; Miles-Carpenter syndrome; Minnesota Coronary Survey; moisture-control system; multicenter study; multiple chemical sensitivity; multiple cloning site; multiple combined sclerosis; myocardial contraction state

MC & S microscopy, culture, and sensitivity

mc/s megacycles per second

MCSA Moloney cell surface antigen

MCSD minimum clinically significant difference

MCSDS Marlowe-Crowne Social Desirability Scale

MCSDT Minnesota Coronary Survey Dietary Trial

MCSF, (M)-CSF macrophage colony-stimulating factor

MCSP Member of the Chartered Society of Physiotherapists

mCSP melanoma-specific chondroitin sulfate proteoglycan

MCSPG melanoma-specific chondroitin sulfate proteoglycan

McSPI Multicenter Study of Perioperative Ischemia

MCSW male commercial sex worker

MCT manual cervical traction; mean cell thickness; mean cell threshold; mean circulation time; mean corpuscular thickness; medial canthal tendon; medium-chain triglyceride; medullary carcinoma of thyroid; medullary collecting tubule; microtoxicity test; microwave coagulation therapy; microwave computed tomography; minimal common tagset; multiple compressed tablet

μCT micro-computed tomography

MCTC metrizamide computed tomography cisternography

MCTD mixed connective tissue disease

MCTF mononuclear cell tissue factor

MC/TF multiple choice/true-false

MCU malaria control unit; maximum care unit; micturating cystourethrography; motor cortex unit; multipoint control unit

MCUG micturating cystogram

MCV Malvaceous chlorosis virus; mean cell volume; mean clinical value; mean contour value; mean corpuscular volume; measles-containing vaccine; median cell volume; molluscum contagiosum virus; motor conduction velocity; myelocytomatosis virus

MCx main circumflex [artery]

MD Doctor of Medicine [Lat. *Medicinae Doctor*]; magnesium deficiency; main duct; maintenance dose; major depression; malate dehydrogenase; malignant disease; malrotation of duodenum; manic-depressive; Mantoux diameter; Marek disease; maternal deprivation; maximum dose; mean deviation; Meckel diverticulum; mediastinal disease; medical department; Medical Design [brace]; mediodorsal; medium dosage; mendelian dominant gene; Ménière disease; meningococcal disease; Menkes disease; mental deficiency; mental depression; mesiodistal; methyldifluoroarsine; Miller-Dieker [syndrome]; Minamata disease; minimum dose; mitral disease; mixed diet; moderate disability; molecular diagnostics; molecular dynamics; monocular deprivation; movement disorder; multi-drug [therapy]; multiple deficiency; muscular dystrophy; mutual information; myelodysplasia; myocardial damage; myocardial disease; myotonic dystrophy

Md mendelevium

md median

MDA malondialdehyde; manual dilation of anus; mass drug administration; methylene dianiline; 3,4-methylenedioxyamphetamine; minimal deviation adenocarcinoma; monodehydroascorbate; motor discriminative acuity; Mullerian duct anomaly; multivariant discriminant analysis; mutation detection enhancement; right mentoanterior [fetal position]

MDa megadalton

MDAC multiple dose activated charcoal; multiplying digital-to-analog converter

MDACC M.D. Anderson Cancer Center

MDAD mineral dust airway disease

MDAP Machover Draw-A-Person [test]

MDB medulloblastoma; mental deterioration Battery

MDBDF March of Dimes Birth Defect Foundation

MDBK Madin-Darby bovine kidney [cell]

MDC macrophage-derived chemokine; major diagnostic categories; metalloprotease disintegrin cysteine [-rich protein]; Metoprolol in Dilated Cardiomyopathy [trial]; minimum detectable concentration; monocyte-depleted mononuclear cell; Multicenter Dilated Cardiomyopathy [trial]

mDC mature dendritic cell

MDCK Madin-Darby canine kidney

MDCR Miller-Dieker [syndrome] chromosome region

MDCT multi-detector computerized tomography

MDCV Mojui Dos Campos virus

MDD major depressive disorder; mean daily dose; medical data dictionary; medical device directives; monitored drug dictionary

MDDC monocyte-derived dendritic cell

MDDL medical device data language

MDDS Malmö Diet and Disease Study; medical diagnostic decision support [system]

MDE major depressive episode; minimum defibrillation energy; molecular distance edge

MDEBP mean daily erect blood pressure

MDEG mammalian degenerin

MDentSc Master of Dental Science

MDEV medical device [UMLS]

MDF mean dominant frequency; myocardial depressant factor

MDFA multiple developmental field anomalies

MDFC multidirectional flow chamber

MDFD map-dot-fingerprint dystrophy

MDG mean diastolic gradient; methyladenine deoxyribonucleic acid glycosylase

MDGF macrophage-derived growth factor

MDH malate dehydrogenase; medullary dorsal horn

MDHR maximum determined heart rate

MDHV Marek disease herpesvirus

MDI manic-depressive illness; metered dose inhaler; methylene diphenyl diisocyanate; Michelson Doppler imager; multiple daily injection; multiple document interface; multiple dosage insulin; Multiscore Depression Inventory

MDIA multidimensional interaction analysis

MDI-A metered-dose inhaler with aerochamber

MDI-DED metered-dose inhaler with delivery enhancement device

MDIPT Multicenter Diltiazem Postinfarction Trial

MDIS medical diagnostic imaging support; medical diagnostic imaging system

MDIT mean disintegration time

MDK midkine

MDL minimum description length; minimum detection limit

MDLIS molecular diagnostic laboratory information system

MDLS Miller-Dieker lissencephaly syndrome

MDM medical decision making; mid-diastolic murmur; minor determinant mix [penicillin]; monocyte-derived macrophage

MDMA methylenedioxymethamphetamine

MD-MPH Doctor of Medicine-Master of Public Health [combined degree in medicine and public health]

MDMU medical devices for military use

mdn median

MDNB mean daily nitrogen balance; metadinitrobenzene

MDNCF monocyte-derived neutrophil chemotactic factor

MDNV Maiden virus

MDO minimum detectable object

MDOPA, mdopa methyldopa

MDOV Monte Dourado virus

MDP manic-depressive psychosis; maximum diastolic potential; maximum digital pulse; methylene diphosphate; microsomal dipeptidase; minimum distending pressure; muramyldipeptide; muscular dystrophy, progressive; right mentoposterior [fetal position]

MDPD maximum daily permissible dose

MD-PhD combined degree in medicine and science

MDPIT Multicenter Diltiazem Postinfarction Trial

MDPK myotonic dystrophy protein kinase

MDQ memory deviation quotient; Menstrual Distress Questionnaire; minimum detectable quantity

MDR median duration of response; medical device reporting; minimum daily requirement; multidrug resistance

mdr multidrug resistance

MDRD Modification of Diet in Renal Disease [study]

MDRE multidrug-resistant *Enterococcus*

MDREF multidrug-resistant enteric fever

MDRP multidrug resistance protein

MDRS Mattis Dementia Rating Scale

MDRSP multidrug-resistant *Streptococcus pneumoniae*

MDR TB multidrug resistance in tuberculosis

MDR-TB multidrug-resistant tuberculosis

MDRV Mill Door virus

MdRV *Musca domestica* reovirus

MDS Master of Dental Surgery; maternal deprivation syndrome; medical data screening; medical data source; medical data system; medical device system; mesonephric duct system; micro-dilution system; milk drinker's syndrome; Miller-Dieker syndrome; minimum data set; monophasic damped sine; Mood Disorders Service [database]; morpheme database; multidimensional scaling; myelodysplastic syndrome; myocardial depressant substance

MDS+ minimum data set (plus)

MDS/AML myelodysplastic syndrome and acute myeloblastic leukemia

MDSBP mean daily supine blood pressure

MDSC muscle-derived stem cell

MD/SC multidrug/short course

MDS-HCACP minimum data set home care assessment clients protocol

MDSO mentally disturbed sex offender

MDSP multiple diagnostic services program

MDSS medical decision support system

MDT mast [cell] degeneration test; mean dissolution time; median detection threshold; multidisciplinary team; multidrug therapy; right mentotransverse [fetal position]

MDTP multidisciplinary treatment plan

MDTR mean diameter-thickness ratio

MDUO myocardial disease of unknown origin

MDV Main Drain virus; Marek disease virus; mean dye [bolus] velocity; mucosal disease virus; multidose vial

MDW monophasic defibrillation waveform

MDX Medical Internet Exchange

MDY month, date, year

Mdyn megadyne

ME macular edema; malic enzyme; manic episode; maximum effort; maximum entropy; median eminence; medical education; medical examiner; meningoencephalitis; mercaptoethanol; metabolic energy; metabolic equivalent; metabolism; metamyelocyte; microembolism; microenvironment; middle ear; mouse embryo; mouse epithelial [cell]; muscle examination; myalgic encephalomyelitis; myoclonic epilepsy; myo-electric; myoepithelial

M/E myeloid/erythroid [ratio]

M+E, M&E monitoring and evaluation

2-ME 2-mercaptoethanol

Me menton; methyl

μE microelectrode

MEA male-enhanced antigen; Medical Exhibition Association; mercaptoethylamine; monoethanolamine; multi-electrode array [catheter-mounted]; multiple endocrine abnormalities; multiple endocrine adenomatosis

MEA-I multiple endocrine adenomatosis type I

3MeA 3-methyladenine

MEAC Measles Elimination Advisory Committee [Australia]

mEAD monophasic action potential early afterdepolarization

MEADOW Method Alternative: Distal Occlusion and Wash-out in Saphenous Vein Graft [study]

MEANS modular electrocardiogram analysis system

meas measurement

MEAP multiphasic environmental assessment procedure

MEAV Meaban virus

MEB Medical Evaluation Board; muscle-eye-brain [disease]

MeB methylene blue

ME-BH medial eminence of basal hypothalamus

MEBS muscle-eye-brain syndrome

MeBSA methylated bovine serum albumin

MEC mammary epithelial cell; median effective concentration; middle ear canal; middle ear cell; minimum effective concentration; mobile examination center

mec meconium

MECA methylcholanthrene

MeCCNU methylchloroethylcyclohexyl-nitrosourea [semustine]

MECG mixed essential cryoglobulinemia

MECP methyl-CpG-binding protein

MECTA mobile electroconvulsive therapy apparatus

MECY methotrexate and cyclophosphamide

MED median erythrocyte diameter; medical, medication, medicine; medical electronic desktop; Medical Entities Dictionary; minimum effective dose; minimum erythema dose; multiple epiphyseal dysplasia

MED$_{50}$ median effective dose for mild cognitive impairment of the exposed population

med medial; median; medication; medicine, medical; medium

MEDAC multiple endocrine deficiency, Addison's disease, and candidiasis [syndrome]

MEDAL Medical Algorithms [project]

MED-ART Medical Automated Records Technology

MEDAS medical emergency decision assistant system

MEDCEN medical center

MEDCOM medical command

MEDDAC medical department activity

MedDRA medical dictionary of drug regulatory activities

MedDX medical diagnosis

MEDEVAC, Medevac medical evacuation

MEDEX, Medex extension of physician [Fr. *médicin extension*]

MEDIC multi-echo data image combination

medic military medical corpsman [Lat. *medicus*]

Medi-Cal Medicaid in California

MEDICO Medical International Cooperation

MEDICS Medway Integrated Care Support [project]

MED-IDDM multiple epiphyseal dysplasia-insulin dependent diabetes mellitus [syndrome]

MEDIGATE Medical Examination Direct Iconic and Graphic Augmented Test Entry

MEDIHC Military Experience Directed Into Health Careers

MedIndEx medical indexing expert

MEDINFO medical informatics

MEDIPP medical district-initiated planning program

MEDIPRO medical district-initiated peer review organization

MEDIS-DC Medical Information System Development Center [Japan]

MEDIX medical data interchange

MED-LAN medical center with local area network

MedLAN Medical Local Area Network [UK]

MEDLARS Medical Literature Analysis and Retrieval System [NLM information system]

MedLEE Medical Language Extraction and Encoding [system]

MEDLINE MEDLARS Online

MEDPAR medical provider analysis and review

MEdREP Medical Education Reinforcement and Enrichment Program

MEDRIS Medical Records Interface or Input System

MEDS minimum emergency data set

meds medications

MEDScD Doctor of Medical Science

MEDSTATS Medical Statistics Expert System

Med-surg medicine and surgery

medSYNDIKATE Synthesis of Distributed Knowledge Acquired from Medical Text

Med Tech medical technology, medical technologist

MED-TEP Medical Treatment Effectiveness Program

MEDTUTOR microcomputer-based tutorial [for MEDLARS]

MEE measured energy expenditure; methylethyl ether; middle ear effusion; multilocus enzyme electrophoresis

MEES medical element engineering and simulation

MEF maximal expiratory flow; middle ear fluid; midexpiratory flow; migration enhancement factor; mouse embryo fibroblast

MEF₅₀ mean maximal expiratory flow

MEFR maximal expiratory flow rate

MEFV maximal expiratory flow volume

MEG magnetoencephalogram, magnetoencephalography; megakaryocyte; Megestrol; mercaptoethylguanidine; multifocal eosinophilic granuloma

MeG methylguanine

meg megacycle; megakaryocyte; megaloblast

Meg-CSA megakaryocyte colony-stimulating activity

MEGD minimal euthyroid Graves disease

mEGF mouse epidermal growth factor

MegMV Megakepasma mosaic virus

MEGS Montefiore endovascular graft system

Megs maternally expressed genes

MEGX monoethylglycinexylidide

mEH membrane-bound epoxide hydrolase

MEHP Metoprolol in Elderly Hypertensive Patients [study]

MEI master encounter index; maximally exposed individual; Medicare economic index

MEIA microparticle enzyme immunoassay

MEII minimum essential information infrastructure

MEK methylethylketone

MEL metabolic equivalent level; miniature electromechanical latch; mouse erythroleukemia

mel melena; melanoma

MELAS mitochondrial encephalomyopathy, lactic acidosis, and stroke-like symptoms [syndrome]

MEL B melarsoprol

MELC murine erythroleukemia cell

mel-CSPG melanoma-specific chondroitin sulfate proteoglycan

MELODHY Metoprolol Low Dose in Hypertension [study]

MELV Melao virus

MEM macrophage electrophoretic mobility; malic enzyme, mitochondrial; minimal Eagle medium; minimal essential medium

memb membrane, membranous

MEME Metathesaurus Enhancement and Maintenance Environment [UMLS]

MEM-FBS minimal essential medium with fetal bovine serum

MEMR multiple exostoses-mental retardation [syndrome]

MEMRs middle ear muscle reflexes

MEMS medication event monitoring system; micro-electromechanical system

MEN meningitis; multiple endocrine neoplasia

MEN-I multiple endocrine neoplasia, type I

men meningeal; meningitis; meniscus; menstruation

MEND Medical Education for National Defense

MENG magnetoenterography

MENT maximum entropy [algorithm]

ment mental, mentality

MENTOR Medtronic Wiktor Hepamed Stent Trial

MEO malignant external otitis

5-MeODMT 5-methoxy-*N*,*N*-dimethyltryptamine

MeOH methyl alcohol

MEOS microsomal ethanol oxidizing system

MEP maximum expiratory pressure; mean effective pressure; mepiridine; minimum error point; mitochondrial encephalopathy; molecular electrostatic potential; motor end-plate; motor evoked potential

mep meperidine

6-MeP 6-mercaptopurine

MEPAS mobility-assist for paralyzed, amputee, and spastic patients

MEPC miniature end-plate current

6-MeP-dR 6-mercaptopurine deoxyriboside

M-Epi epicardium and M regions

MEPP miniature end-plate potential

MEPS Medical Expenditure Panel Survey

MEPS-IC Medical Expenditure Panel Survey-Insurance Component

mEQ, mEq, meq milliequivalent

mEq/L milliequivalents per liter

MER mean ejection rate; medical emergency room; Merck Index Online; methanol extraction residue; micro-electrode recording; murmur/energy ratio

MERB Medical Examination and Review Board

MERCATOR Multicenter European Research Trial with Cilazapril after Angioplasty to Prevent Transluminal Coronary Obstruction and Restenosis

MERG macular electroretinogram

MERIT Medical Records, Images, Texts Information Exchange

MERIT-HF Metoprolol Controlled-release Randomised Intervention Trial in Heart Failure

MERRF myoclonus epilepsy with ragged red fibers [syndrome]

MERRLA myoclonus epilepsy-ragged red fibers-lactic acidosis [syndrome]

MERS Multiagency Electronic Regulatory Submission

MES maintenance electrolyte solution; maximal electroshock; maximal electroshock seizures; microembolic signal; Minitran Efficacy Study; multiple endocrine syndrome; myoelectric signal

Mes mesencephalon, mesencephalic

MESA Marshfield Epidemiologic Study Area; myoepithelial sialadenitis

Mesc mescaline

MESCH Multi-Environment Scheme

MESF molecules of equivalent soluble fluorochrome

MeSH Medical Subject Headings

MESNA [sodium 2-]mercaptoethanesulfonate

MESOR midline estimating statistic of rhythm

MesPGN mesangial proliferative glomerulonephritis

MESS mangled extremity severity score

MEST mouse ear swelling test

MESV murine embryonic stem-cell virus

MET maximal exercise test; metabolic equivalent of the task; metastasis, metastatic; methionine; midexpiratory time; modality examination terminal; multistage exercise test

Met methionine

met metallic [chest sounds]; methionine

META medical editors trial accounting; medical editors trial amnesty; Metathesaurus [UMLS]; 3-methacryloyloxyethyl trimellitate anhydride

Meta Metathesaurus [UMLS]

metab metabolic, metabolism

metas metastasis, metastatic

Met-Enk methionine-enkephalin

METEOR managing end-to-end operations

METH methicillin

Meth methedrine

meth methyl

Met-Hb methemoglobin

MeTHF methyltetrahydrofolic acid

Met-hGH *N*-methionyl recombinant human growth hormone

MetMb metmyoglobin

METR miniature electronic temperature recorder

METS Medical Equipment Technical Society; metabolic equivalents [of oxygen consumption]

mets metastases

METT maximum exercise tolerance test

MEU maximum expected utility

MEV maximum exercise ventilation; mevalonate; minimal excursionary ventilation; murine erythroblastosis virus

MeV measles virus; megaelectron volts

mev megaelectron volts

MEWD, MEWDS multiple evanescent white dot [syndrome]

MEXIS Metoprolol and Xamoterol Infarction Study

MF magnetic field; magnification factor; maximal force; mean field; meat free; medium frequency; megafarad; membrane filler; merthiolate-formaldehyde [solution]; metacarpal fusion; microfibril; microfilament; microflocculation; microscopic factor; mid frequency; midcavity forceps; mitochondrial fragments; mitogenic factor; mitomycin-fluorouracil; mitotic figure; mucosal fluid; multifactorial; multiplication factor; mutation frequency; mycosis fungoides; myelin figure; myelofibrosis; myocardial fibrosis; myofibrillar

M&F male and female; mother and father

M:F, M/F male:female [ratio]

Mf maxillofrontale

mF millifarad

mf microfarad; microfilaria

μF, μf microfarad

MFA master of fine arts [degree]; mean field annealing [imaging]; metabolic flux analysis; monofluoroacetate; multifocal functional autonomy; multiple factor analysis

MFAQ Multidimensional Functional Assessment Questionnaire

MFAT multifocal atrial tachycardia

MFB medial forebrain bundle; metallic foreign body; multiple feedback

MFC mean fluorescence channel; medical follow-up clinic; Microsoft Foundation Classes; minimal fungicidal concentration

MFCM Master, Faculty of Community Medicine

MFCV muscle fiber conduction velocity

MFD mandibulofacial dysostosis; mid-forceps delivery; milk-free diet; minimum fatal dose; multiple fractions per day

mfd microfarad

MFG magnetic field gradient; minimum-distance frontal gyrus

MFH malignant fibrous histiocytoma

MFH-B malignant fibrous histiocytoma of bone

MFHom Member of the Faculty of Homeopathy

MFI male factor infertility; malleable facial implant; mean fluorescence intensity; multi-facility integration

MFID multielectrode flame ionization detector

M-FISH multiplex fluorescence in situ hybridization

MFL myofibril

m flac membrana flaccida [Lat.]

MFLOPS, Mflops megaflops [million floating points per second]

MFM magnetic force microscopy

MFO medium frequency oscillator; mixed function oxidase

MFOM Master, Faculty of Occupational Medicine

MFP monofluorophosphate; myofascial pain

M-FPIA monoclonal fluorescence polarization immunoassay

MFPR multifetal pregnancy reduction

MFR mean flow rate; mucus flow rate

MFS Marfan syndrome; Medicare fee schedule

MFSS Medical Field Service School

MFST Medical Field Service Technician

MFT multifocal atrial tachycardia; muscle function test

MFTA molecular field topology analysis

MFUN molecular function [UMLS]

MFUS Manitoba Follow-up Study

MFV maximal flow-volume [loop]

MFW multiple fragment wounds

MG maintenance goal; Marcus Gunn [pupil]; margin; mean gradient; medial gastrocnemius [muscle]; membranous glomerulonephritis; menopausal gonadotropin; mesiogingival; methylglucoside; methylguanidine; monoclonal gammopathy; monoglyceride; mucous granule; muscle group; myasthenia gravis; myoglobin

M3G morphine-3-glucuronide

Mg magnesium

m^{7G} 7-methylguanosine

mg milligram

μg microgram [JCAHO unapproved abbreviation]

mγ milligamma

μγ microgamma

MGA master of general administration; medical gas analyzer; melengestrol acetate; 3-methylglutaconicaciduria

MgATP magnesium adenosine triphosphate

MGB medial geniculate body; myoglobin

MGBG methylglyoxal-bis-(guanylhydrazone)

MGC Mammalian Gene Collection; medical genetics center; medical genetics clinic; megacolon; minimal glomerular change

MgC magnocellular neuroendocrine cell

MGCE multifocal giant cell encephalitis

MGCN megalocornea

MGCR meningioma chromosome region

MGCRB Medicare Geographic Classification Review Board

MGD maximal glucose disposal; mixed gonadal dysgenesis; Microbial Germplasm Database; Mouse Genome Database; multiglandular disease

mg/dl milligrams per deciliter

MGDS Member in General Dental Surgery

MGEIR Mouse Gene Expression Information Resource

MGES multiple gated equilibrium scintigraphy

MGF macrophage growth factor; maternal grandfather

MGG May-Grünwald-Giemsa [staining]; molecular and general genetics; mouse gammaglobulin; multinucleated giant cell

MGGH methylglyoxal guanylhydrazone

MGH Massachusetts General Hospital

mgh milligram-hour

MGI magnetically guided intubation

MGIT mycobacterial growth indicator tube

mg/kg milligrams per kilogram

μg/kg micrograms per kilogram

MGL minor glomerular lesion

MgI myoglobin

mg/L milligrams per liter

μg/L micrograms per liter

mGluR metabotropic glutamate receptor

MGM maternal grandmother; meningioma

mgm milligram

MGMA Medical Group Management Association

MGMT methylguanine-deoxyribonucleic acid methyltransferase

MGN medial geniculate nucleus; membranous glomerulonephritis

MGP marginal granulocyte pool; marginating granulocyte pool; membranous glomerulonephropathy; mucin glycoprotein

MGR modified gain ratio; multiple gas rebreathing

mgr milligram

MGS metric gravitational system; modified Gram-Schmidt orthogonalization

MGSA malignant growth stimulatory activity

MGT medical guideline technology; multiple glomus tumors

MGUS monoclonal gammopathies of undetermined significance

MGW magnesium sulfate, glycerin, and water

mGy milligray

μGy microgray

MH malignant histiocytosis; malignant hyperpyrexia; malignant hypertension; malignant hyperthermia; mammotropic hormone; mannoheptulose; marital history; medial hypothalamus; medical history; melanophore-stimulating hormone; menstrual history; mental health; mental hygiene; moist heat; monosymptomatic hypochondriasis; murine hepatitis; mutant hybrid; *Mycobacterium haemophilum*; myohyoid

mH millihenry

μH microhenry

MHA major histocompatibility antigen; May-Hegglin anomaly; Mental Health Association; methemalbumin; microangiopathic hemolytic anemia; microhemagglutination; middle hepatic artery; mixed hemadsorption; Mueller-Hinton agar

MHAM multiple hamartoma

MHAQ Modified Health Assessment Questionnaire

M-HART Montreal Heart Attack Readjustment Trial

MHA-TP microhemagglutination-*Treponema pallidum*

MHB maximum hospital benefit; Mueller-Hinton base

MHb methemoglobin; myohemoglobin

MHBSS modified Hank balanced salt solution

MHC major histocompatibility complex; mental health care; mental health center; mental health clinic; myosin heavy chain

MHCS Mental Hygiene Consultation Service

MHCU mental health care unit

MHD maintenance hemodialysis; mean hemolytic dose; mental health department; minimization of hypersurface distance; minimum hemolytic dilution; minimum hemolytic dose

MHDI Minnesota Health Data Institute

MHDP methylene hydroxydiphosphonate

MHDPS Mental Health Demographic Profile System

M-HEART Multi-Hospital Eastern Atlantic Restenosis Trial

MHFT Munich Mild Heart Failure Trial

MHG metropolitan health group

MHHP Minnesota Heart Health Program

MHHS Minnesota Heart Health Survey

MHI malignant histiocytosis of intestine; Mental Health Index; Mental Health Inventory; minor head injury

MHIQ McMaster health index questionnaire

MHL medial hypothalamic lesion

MHLC Multidimensional Health Locus of Control

MHLS metabolic heat load stimulator

MHN massive hepatic necrosis; Mohs hardness number; morbus hemolyticus neonatorum

MHO microsomal heme oxygenase

mho reciprocal ohm, siemens unit [ohm spelled backwards]

MHP hemiplegic migraine; maternal health program; medical center health plan; 1-mercuri-2-hydroxypropane; metropolitan health plan; monosymptomatic hypochondriacal psychosis; multi-skilled health practitioner

MHPA mild hyperphenylalaninemia

MHPG 3-methoxy-4-hydroxyphenyl-glycol

MHR major histocompatibility region; malignant hyperthermia resistance; maternal heart rate; maximal heart rate; methemoglobin reductase

MHRI Mental Health Research Institute

MHS major histocompatibility system; malignant hyperthermia in swine; malignant hyperthermia syndrome; malignant hypothermia susceptibility; Milan hypertensive [rat]; Minnesota Heart Survey; modified hybrid sign; multiple health screening; multihospital system

MHSA microaggregated human serum albumin

MHSS Military Health Services System

MHT mixed hemagglutination test

MHTS Multiphasic Health Testing Services

MHV magnetic heart vector; middle hepatic vein; mouse hepatitis virus; murine hepatitis virus

MHW mental health worker

MHx medical history

MHyg Master of Hygiene

MHz megahertz

MI magnetic-guided intubation; maturation index; medical illustrator; medical informatics; medical inspection; melanophore index; membrane integrity; menstruation induction; mental illness; mental institution; mercaptoimidazole; mesioincisal; metabolic index; microinvasion; microsatellite instability; migration index; migration inhibition; mild irritant; minimally invasive; mitotic index; mitral incompetence; mitral insufficiency; mononucleosis infectiosa; morphology index; motility index; mutual information; myocardial infarction; myocardial ischemia; myoinositol

mi mile

MIA missing in action

MIAMI Metoprolol in Acute Myocardial Infarction [study]

MIAS Mammographic Image Analysis Society

MIAs multi-institutional arrangements; medically indigent adults

MIB management information base; Medical Impairment Bureau; Medical Information Bureau; minimally invasive biopsy

MIBG, mIBG metaiodobenzylguanidine

MIBI methoxyisobutyl isonitrile

MIBiol Member of the Institute of Biology

MIBK methylisobutyl ketone

MIBT methyl isatin-beta-thiosemicarbazone

MIC maternal and infant care; maximum inhibitory concentration; mean inhibitory concentration; medical intensive care; Medical Interfraternity Conference; methyl isocyanate; microinvasive carcinoma; microscopy; minimal inhibitory concentration; minimal isorrheic concentration; minocycline; model immune complex; mononuclear inflammatory cell; morphologic, immunologic and cytogenic

MICAB minimally invasive coronary artery bypass surgery

MICABG minimally invasive coronary artery bypass graft

MICAM maturation index for colostrum and mature milk

MICC mitogen-induced cellular cytotoxicity

MICCAI Medical Image Computing and Computer-Assisted Intervention

MICG macromolecular insoluble cold globulin

MICN mobile intensive care nursing

MICOL Multicenter Italian Study of Cholesterol

MICR methacholine inhalation challenge response

MICRA Medical Injury Compensation Reform Act

MICRO Medical Information Collecting Robot

micro microcyte, microcytic; microscopic

microbiol microbiology

microCi microcurie

microg microgram

MICRO-HOPE Microalbuminuria, Cardiovascular and Renal Outcomes-Heart Outcomes Prevention Evaluation

MICS Myocardial Infarction Cost Study

MICST Ministry of Industry, Commerce, Science, and Technology [Canada]

MICT mobile intensive care technician

MICU medical intensive care unit; mobile intensive care unit

MICUP management of intensive care unit and patients minimum

MicV micropia virus

MID maximum inhibiting dilution; mesioincisodistal; midinfarct dementia; minimum infective dose; minimum inhibitory dose; minimum irradiation dose; multiinfarct dementia; multiple indicator dilution; multiple ion detection

mid middle

MIDA myocardial ischemia dynamic analysis

MIDAS medical image display and analysis system; Medical Information Data Analysis System; metal ion–dependent adhesion site; microphthalmia–dermal aplasia–sclerocornea [syndrome]; Multicenter Isradipine Diuretic Atherosclerosis Study; Myocardial Infarction Data Acquisition System [study]

MIDCAB minimally invasive direct coronary artery bypass [surgery]

MIDI musical instrument digital interface

MIDS Management Information Decision System

midsag midsagittal

MIDSPAN Middle-aged Span-of-Life Study

MIDV Middelburg virus

MIEMIS model for investment and evaluation of medical information system

MIF macrophage inhibitory factor; melanocyte[-stimulating hormone]-inhibiting factor; maximum inspiratory flow or force; merthiolate-iodine-formaldehyde [method]; microimmunofluorescence; midinspiratory flow; midline interhemispheric fusion; migration-inhibiting factor; mixed immunofluorescence; müllerian inhibiting factor

MIFC merthiolate-iodine-formaldehyde concentration

MIFR maximal inspiratory flow rate

MIG measles immune globulin; Medicare Insured Groups; message implementation guideline; Mitochondria Interest Group

MIg malaria immunoglobulin; measles immunoglobulin; membrane immunoglobulin

mIg membrane-anchored immunoglobulin [Ig]

mIgM membrane-anchored immunoglobulin M

MIGT multiple inert gas elimination technique

MIH Master of Industrial Health; migraine with interval headache; minimal intermittent heparin [dose]; moderate induced hypothermia

MIHA minor histocompatibility antigen

MIHR Management of Intellectual Property in Health Research and Development

MIIO minimally invasive intraoperative osteosynthesis

MIKA minor karyotype abnormalities

MIKE mass-analyzed ion kinetic energy

MIL mean intercept length analysis

MILESTONE Multicenter Iloprost European Study on Endangeitis

MILIS Multicenter Investigation of the Limitations of Infarct Size

MILP mitogen-induced lymphocyte proliferation

MILS medication information leaflet for seniors

MILT medical laboratory technician

MILT-AD medical laboratory technician-associate degree

MILT-C medical laboratory technician-certificate

MIM Mendelian Inheritance in Man; message information model; Multilateral Initiative in Malaria

MIMC multivane intensity modulation compensator

MIME multipurpose Internet mail extension

MIMIC multivane intensity modulation compensation

MIMOSA medical image management in an open system architecture

MIMR minimal inhibitor mole ratio

MIMS medical information management system; medical inventory management system; Migraine and Myocardial Ischemia Study

MIMyCa maternally inherited disorder with adult-onset myopathy and cardiomyopathy

MIN medial interlaminar nucleus; medical information network; multiple intestinal neoplasia

min mineral; minim; minimum, minimal; minor; minute

μin microinch

MINA monoisonitrosoacetone

MinDu minimum duration

MINIA monkey intranuclear inclusion agent

MINPHIS Made in Nigeria Primary Healthcare and Hospital Information System

MINSAT minimum cost satisfactibility

MINT Myocardial Infarction with Novastan and Tissue Plasminogen Activator Study

MINV Minnal virus

MIO metal-induced oxidation; minimum identifiable odor; modular input/output

MiO microorchidism

MION monocrystalline iron oxide

MIOP magnetic iron oxide particle

MIOS Myocardial Infarction Onset Study

MIP macrophage inflammatory protein; major intrinsic protein; maximum inspiratory pressure; maximum intensity pixel; maximum intensity projection; mean incubation period; mean intravascular pressure; Medical Informatics Programme [Singapore]; middle interphalangeal [joint]; minimal inspiratory pressure; minimally invasive procedure

mIP minimum intensity projection

mip macrophage infectivity promoter

MIPA macrophage inflammatory protein alpha

MIPB macrophage inflammatory protein beta

MIPcor coronary maximum intensity projection

MIPO minimally invasive plate osteosynthesis

MIPP maximum intensity pixel projection

MIPPO minimally invasive percutaneous plate osteosynthesis

MIPS Martinsried Institute of Protein Sequences; mean index procedure sum; millions of instructions per second; Munich Information Center for Protein Sequences; myocardial isotope perfusion scan

MIR main immunogenic region; multiple isomorphous replacement

MIRACL myocardial ischemia reduction with aggressive cholesterol lowering

MIRC microtubuloreticular complex

MIRD medical internal radiation dose

MIRL medical imaging research laboratory; membrane inhibitor of reactive lysis

MIRMO Medical Information Resources Management Office

MIRON Medical Information Resources on the Net [UK]

MIRP myocardial infarction rehabilitation program

MIRRACLE Myocardial Infarction Risk Recognition and Conversion of Life-threatening Events into Survival [trial]

MIRS mean index resuscitation sum

MIRSA Multicenter International Randomized Study of Angina Pectoris

MIRU myocardial infarction research unit

MIRV Mirim virus

MIS management information system; manager of information system; medical information service; medical information system; meiosis-inducing substance; minimally invasive surgery; motor index score; müllerian inhibiting substance

MiSAD Milan Study on Atherosclerosis and Diabetes

MISC multi-interface sensor controlled

misc miscarriage; miscellaneous

MISCHF management to improve survival in congestive heart failure

MISG modified immune serum globulin

MISHAP microcephalus-imperforate anus-syndactyly-hamartoblastoma-abnormal lung lobulation-polydactyly [syndrome]

MISI multiple input single input

MISJ Medical Instrument Society of Japan

MISNES Multicenter Italian Study on Neonatal Electrocardiography [ECG] and Sudden Infant Death Syndrome

MISS medical image sharing system; Medical Interview Satisfaction Scale; minimally invasive spinal surgery; Modified Injury Severity Scale

MIST Management of Influenza in the Southern Hemisphere Trials; Medical Information Service by Telephone; Mibefradil Ischemia Suppression Trial; minimally invasive surgery and intervention technology; Multicenter Isradipine Salt Trial

MIT magnetic induction tomography; male impotence test; marrow iron turnover; Massachusetts Institute of Technology; mean input time; melodic intonation therapy; metabolism inhibition test; miracidial immobilization test; mitomycin; monoiodotyrosine

mit mitral

MITF microphthalmia-associated transcription factor

MITI Myocardial Infarction Triage and Intervention [Project]

MITIS Modular Integrated Transplant Information System

MITO mitomycin

Mito C mitomycin C

MITRA Maximal Individual Therapy in Acute Myocardial Infarction

MITT Myers introduction to type; minimally invasive thermal therapy

mIU milli-international unit; one-thousandth of an international unit

μIU one-millionth of an international unit

MIVD mobile interactive videodisk

MIWC mercurial insensitive water channel

mix, mixt mixture

MJ Machado-Joseph [disease]; marijuana; megajoule

mJ, mj millijoule

μJ microjoule

MJA mechanical joint apparatus

MJAD Machado-Joseph Azorean disease

MJD Machado-Joseph disease; Mseleni joint disease

MJI Moral Judgment Interview

MJRT maximum junctional recovery time

MJT Mead Johnson tube

MK megakaryocyte; monkey kidney; myokinase

Mk monkey

mkat millikatal

μkat microkatal

mkat/L millikatals per liter

MKB medical knowledge [data]base; megakaryoblast

MKC monkey kidney cell

MKF MEDLINE Knowledge Finder

m-kg meter-kilogram

MKHS Menkes kinky hair syndrome

MkK monkey kidney

MkL megakaryoblastic leukemia

MKMD Molecular Knowledge of Metabolic Diseases [database]

MKP monobasic potassium phosphate

MKS, mks meter-kilogram-second

MKSAP medical knowledge self-assessment program

MKT mean kinetic temperature

MKTC monkey kidney tissue culture

MKV killed measles vaccine

ML Licentiate in Medicine; Licentiate in Midwifery; malignant lymphoma; marked latency; markup language; maximum likelihood; medial lemniscus; median load; medio-lateral; mesiolingual; middle lobe; midline; molecular layer; motor latency; mucolipidosis; mucosal leishmaniasis; multiple lentiginosis; muscular layer; myeloid leukemia

ML I, II, III, IV mucolipidosis I, II, III, IV

M/L monocyte/lymphocyte [ratio]

M-L Martin-Lewis [medium]

mL millilambert; milliliter

ml milliliter

μL microliter

MLA left mentoanterior [fetal position]; Medical Library Association; mesiolabial; monocytic leukemia, acute

mLa millilambert

MLAA Medical Library Assistance Act

MLAB Multilingual Aphasia Battery

MLAC minimum local anesthetic concentration

MLAEB midlatency auditory evoked potential

MLAEP midlatency auditory evoked potential

MLaI mesiolabioincisal

MLAP mean left atrial pressure

MLaP mesiolabiopulpal

MLB micro-laryngobronchoscopy; monoaural loudness balance

MLb macrolymphoblast

MLBP mechanical low back pain

MLBPNN multilayer back propagation neural network

MLBW moderately low birthweight

MLC minimum lethal concentration; mixed leukocyte culture; mixed ligand chelate; mixed lymphocyte concentration; mixed lymphocyte culture; morphine-like compound; multilamellar cytosome; multileaf collimator; myelomonocytic leukemia, chronic; myosin light chain

MLCCHF Multicenter Lisinopril Captopril Congestive Heart Failure [study]

MLCK myosin light chain kinase

MLCN multilocular cystic nephroma

MLCO Member of the London College of Osteopathy

MLCP myosin light-chain phosphatase

MLCQ Modified Learning Climate Questionnaire

MLCT metal-to-ligand charge transfer

MLD manual lymph drainage; masking level difference; mean luminal diameter; median lethal dose; metachromatic leukodystrophy; minimal lesion disease; minimal luminal diameter; minimum lethal dose

MLD$_{50}$ median lethal dose

mL/dL milliliters per deciliter

MLE maximum likelihood estimation; maximum likelihood estimator

MLEE multilocus enzyme electrophoresis

MLEI most likely exposed individual

MLEL malignant lymphoepithelial lesion

MLEM, ML-EM maximum likelihood expectation maximization [imaging]

MLF medial longitudinal fasciculus; morphine-like factor

MLFF multilayer feed forward

MLG mesiolingual groove; mitochondrial lipid glycogen

MLGN minimal lesion glomerulonephritis

ML-H malignant lymphoma, histiocytic

MLI mesiolinguoincisal; mixed lymphocyte interaction

MLL mixed lineage leukemia; multi-level logistic

mL/L milliliters per liter

MLLT1 mixed lineage leukemia translocated to 1

MLLT2 mixed lineage leukemia translocated to 2

MLM map of local minima; medical logic module

MLN manifest latent nystagmus; membranous lupus nephropathy; mesenteric lymph node; motilin

MLNS minimal lesion nephrotic syndrome; mucocutaneous lymph node syndrome

MLO medio-lateral oblique; mesiolinguoocclusal; *Mycoplasma*-like organism

MLP left mentoposterior [fetal position]; match list position; maximum lifespan potential; medical language processing; mesiolinguopulpal; microsomal lipoprotein; midlevel practitioner; multilayer perception; multilocus probe

ML-PDL malignant lymphoma, poorly differentiated lymphocytic

MLR mean length response; middle latency response; mineralocorticoid receptor; mixed lymphocyte reaction; multilinear regression; multivariate linear regression

MLRD microgastria-limb reduction defects [association]

MLRS multiple launch rocket system [chemical warhead]

MLS maximum length sequence; maximum likelihood estimator; mean lifespan; median life span; median longitudinal section; microphthalmia-linear skin defects [syndrome]; middle lobe syndrome; mouse leukemia virus; multilevel scheme; multiple line scan; myelomonocytic leukemia, subacute

MLS-ART multilevel scheme algebraic reconstruction scheme

MLSB migrating long spike burst

MLSI multiple line scan imaging

MLT left mentotransverse [fetal position]; mean latency time; median lethal time; medical laboratory technician

MLT-AD medical laboratory technician-associate degree

MLT(ASCP) Medical Laboratory Technician certified by the American Society of Clinical Pathologists

MLTC mixed leukocyte-trophoblast culture; mixed lymphocyte tumor cell

MLT-C medical laboratory technician-certificate

MLTI mixed lymphocyte target interaction

MLU mean length of utterance

MLV Moloney leukemia virus; Mono Lake virus; multilaminar vesicle; murine leukemia virus

MLVAR amphotropic receptor for murine leukemia virus

MLVDP maximum left ventricular developed pressure

mlx millilux

MM macromolecule; Maëlzels metronome; major medical [insurance]; malignant melanoma; manubrium to malleus; Marshall-Marchetti; Master of Management; mathematical morphology; medial malleolus; mediastinal mass; medical management; megamitochondria; melanoma metastasis; meningococcal meningitis; menstrually related migraine; metastatic melanoma; methadone maintenance; minimal medium; mismatched; molecular mechanics; morbidity and mortality; mucous membrane; multiple model; multiple myeloma; muscularis mucosae; myeloid metaplasia; myelomeningocele

M&M morbidity and mortality

mM millimolar; millimole; mini-MEDLINE [database]

mm methylmalonyl; millimeter; mucous membrane; muscles

mm² square millimeter

mm³ cubic millimeter

mμ millimicron

μM micromole, micromolar

μm micrometer; micromilli-

μ/μ mass attenuation coefficient

MMA mastitis-metritis-agalactia [syndrome]; medical management analysis; medical materials account; methylmalonic acid; methylmethacrylate; middle meningeal artery; minor morphologic aberration; monomethyladenosine; monomethylarsonic acid

MMAA mini-microaggregates of albumin

MMAD median aerodynamic diameter

MMAP mean maternal arterial blood pressure

MMAS Massachusetts Male Aging Study; modified motor assessment scale

MMATP methadone maintenance and aftercare treatment program

MMC Materials Microcharacterization Collaboratory; mechanical myocardial channeling; migrating myoelectric complex; minimum medullary concentration; mitomycin C; mucosal mast cell

mμc millimicrocurie

μμC micromicrocurie [picocurie]

MMCO Medicaid managed care organization

MMD mass median diameter; minimum morbidostatic dose; moyamoya disease; myotonic muscular dystrophy

MMDB Molecular Modeling Database [NLM]

MMDDI mutual molecular dataset diversity index

MMDTSD multiscale morphological derivative transform-based singularity detector

MME mini mental examination; M-mode echocardiography; mobile medical equipment; mouse mammary epithelium

MMED Master of Medicine

MMEF maximum midexpiratory flow

MMEFR maximum midexpiratory flow rate

MMEP microcephaly-microphthalmia-electrodactyly-prognathism [syndrome]; multimicroelectrode plate

MMF maxillomandibular fixation; maximum midexpiratory flow; mean maximum flow; Member of the Medical Faculty

μμF micromicrofarad [picofarad]

MMFF Merck molecular force field [algorithm]

MMFR maximum midexpiratory flow rate; maximal midflow rate

MMFV maximum midrespiratory flow volume

MMG mean maternal glucose

mμg millimicrogram

μmg micromilligram [nanogram]

μμg micromicrogram [picogram]

MMH monomethylhydrazine

mmHg millimeters of mercury

μmHg micrometer of mercury

mmH₂O millimeters of water

MMI macrophage migration inhibition; man-machine interface; master member index; maximum medical improvement; methylmercaptoimidazole; mucous membrane irritation

MMIF macrophage migration inhibitory factor

MMIH megacystis-microcolon-intestinal hypoperistalsis [syndrome]

MMIHS megacystis-microcolon-intestinal hypoperistalsis syndrome

MMIRG Multicenter Myocardial Ischemia Research Group

MMIS Medicaid management information system

MML medical markup language; Moloney murine leukemia; monomethyllysine; myelomonocytic leukemia

mM/L millimoles per liter

MMLV Moloney murine leukemia virus; Montana myotis leukoencephalitis virus

MMM see 3-M [syndrome]; marginal metallophilic macrophage; microsome-mediated mutagenesis; myelofibrosis with myeloid metaplasia; myelosclerosis with myeloid metaplasia

μmm micromillimeter [nanometer]

μmμ meson

MMMF man-made mineral fibers

MMMM megalocornea-macrocephaly-motor and mental retardation [syndrome]

MMMSE Modified Mini-Mental Status Exam

MMMT malignant mixed müllerian tumor

MMN mismatch negativity; morbus maculosus neonatorum; multiple mucosal neuroma

MMNC marrow mononuclear cell

MMNCB multifocal motor neuropathy with conduction block

MMNN multi-modular neural network

MMO medical management office; methane monooxygenase

MMOA maxillary mandibular odontectomy alveolectomy

MMOB Molecular Modeling Database

M-mode motion mode

MMoL myelomonoblastic leukemia

mmol millimole

μmol micromole, micromolar

mmol/L millimoles per liter

MMP matrix metalloproteinase; maximum maintained pressure; muscle mechanical power

4-MMPD 4-methoxy-*m*-phenylenediamine

MMPI matrix metalloproteinase inhibitor; Minnesota Multiphasic Personality Inventory

MMPNC Medical Maternal Program for Nuclear Casualties

mmpp millimeters partial pressure

MMPR methylmercaptopurine riboside

MMPS Medicare Mortality Predictor System

MMR mass miniature radiography; masseter muscle rigidity; maternal mortality rate; measles-mumps-rubella [vaccine]; megalocornea-mental retardation [syndrome]; mild mental retardation; mobile mass x-ray; mono-methylrutin; multimodal reasoning; myocardial metabolic rate

MMRB mouth-to-mouth rescue breathing

MMRS Mosoriot Medical Record System

MMS mass mammographic screening; Master of Medical Science; methyl methane sulfonate; Mini-Mental State

mμs millimicrosecond

MMSA Master of Midwifery, Society of Apothecaries

MMSc Master of Medical Science

MMSE mini-mental status examination

mm/sec millimeters per second

MMSP malignant melanoma of soft parts

mm st muscle strength

MMT alpha-methyl-*m*-tyrosine; manual muscle test; microcephaly-mesobrachydactyly-tracheoesophageal fistula [syndrome]; mouse mammary tumor

MMTA methylmetatyramine

MMTB multimedia textbook [computer-associated radiology]

MMTP methadone maintenance treatment program

MMTT Multicenter Myocarditis Treatment Trial

MMTV mouse mammary tumor virus

MMU medical maintenance unit; mercaptomethyl uracil

mmu millimass unit

MMuLV Moloney murine leukemia virus

MMV mandatory minute ventilation; mandatory minute volume; Medicines for Malaria Venture [WHO]

MMVD mixed mitral valve disease

MMVF man-made vitreous fiber

MMVT monomorphic ventricular tachycardia

MMWR Morbidity and Mortality Weekly Report

MMWV modulated Morlet wavelet transform vector sum

MN a blood group in the MNSs blood group system; malignant nephrosclerosis; Master of Nursing; median nerve; meganewton; melena neonatorum; melanocytic nevus; membranous nephropathy; membranous neuropathy; mesenteric node; metanephrine; micronucleated; micronucleus; midnight; mononuclear; motor neuron; mucosal neurolysis; multinodular; myoneural

M&N morning and night

Mn manganese; monocyte

mN micronewton; millinormal

mn modal number

μN nuclear magneton

MNA maximum noise area

MNAP mixed nerve action potential; multineuron acquisition processor

MNB mannosidase beta; murine neuroblastoma

5-MNBA 5-mercapto-2-nitrobenzoic acid

MNBCCS multiple nevoid basal-cell carcinoma syndrome

MNC mononuclear cell

MNCV median nerve conduction velocity; motor nerve conduction velocity

MND minimum necrosing dose; minor neurological dysfunction; modified neck dissection; motor neuron disease

MNER multichannel neural ensemble recording

mng morning

MNG/CRD/DA multinodular goiter/cystic renal disease/digital anomalies [syndrome]

MNGIE myo-, neuro-, gastrointestinal encephalopathy

MNH maternal and neonatal health

MNJ myoneural junction

MNK Menkes syndrome

MNL marked neutrophilic leukocytosis; maximum number of lamellae; mononuclear leukocyte

MN/m² meganewtons per square meter

mN/m millinewton per meter

MNMS myonephropathic metabolic syndrome

MNNG *N*-methyl *N'*-nitro-*N*-nitrosoguanidine

MNP mononuclear phagocyte

MNPJSS Misener Nurse Practitioner Job Satisfaction Scale

MNPV multiple nucleopolyhedrovirus

MNR marrow neutrophil reserve; multiple nucleoside resistance

MNRH may not require hospitalization

MNS medial nuclear stratum; Melnick-Needles syndrome; Milan normotensive [rat]

Mn-SOD manganese-superoxide dismutase

MNSs a blood group system consisting of groups M, N, and MN

MNTBV Manitoba virus

MNTD maximum nontoxic dose

MNTV Minatitlan virus

MNU *N*-methyl-*N*-nitrosourea

MO macroorchidism; manually operated; Master of Obstetrics; Master of Osteopathy; medical officer; mesio-occlusal; metastases, zero; mineral oil; minute output; modeling object; molecular orbital; monofunctional; mono-oxygenase; month; morbid obesity

MO₂ myocardial oxygen [utilization]

Mo Moloney [strain]; molybdenum; monoclonal

M_o mitral opening

MΩ megohm

mo mode; month; morgan

mΩ milliohm

μ_o permeability of vacuum

μΩ microhm

MOA monoamine oxidase

MoA mechanism of action

MoAb monoclonal antibody

MOANS Mayo's Older Americans Normative Studies

MOAT multispecific organic anion transporter

MOB mobility [scale]

mob, mobil mobility, mobilization

MOBS Moebius syndrome

MOBV methylhydroxy-benzovesamicol; Mobala virus

MOC maximum oxygen consumption; metronidazole, omeprazole, clarithromycin; multiple ocular coloboma

MOCA 4,4'-methylene-bis(2-chloroaniline)

MOCHA Multicenter Oral Carvedilol in Heart Failure Assessment

MOCV molluscum contagiosum virus

MOD magnetic optic disk; maturity-onset diabetes; Medical Officer of the Day; mesio-occlusodistal

mod moderate, moderation; modification

MODE 3-methoxy-*o*-demethyl-encainide

MODED microcephaly-oculo-digito-esophageal-duodenal [syndrome]

modem modulator/demodulator

MOD/F multiple organ dysfunction/failure

MODM maturity-onset diabetes mellitus

MODS medically oriented data system; multiple-organ dysfunction syndrome

MODV Modoc virus

MODY maturity-onset diabetes of the young

MOF marine oxidation/fermentation; meta object facility; methotrexate, Oncovin, fluorouracil; multiple organ failure

MoF moment of force

MOFE multiple organ failure in the elderly

MOFS multiple organ failure syndrome

MOG myelin-oligodendrocyte glycoprotein

MO&G Master of Obstetrics and Gynaecology

MOH Medical Officer of Health; Ministry of Health

MOHSAIC Missouri Health Strategic Architectures and Information Cooperative

MOI master object index; maximum oxygen intake; mechanism of injury; multiplicity of infection

moi multiplicity of infection

MOIVC membranous obstruction of the inferior vena cava

MOJUV Moju virus

MOKV Mokola virus

MOL method of limits; molecular

mol mole; molecular, molecule

molc molar concentration

molfr mole fraction

mol/kg moles per kilogram

mol/L moles per liter

mol/m³ moles per cubic meter

mol/s moles per second

mol wt molecular weight

MOM milk of magnesia; mucoid otitis media

MoM multiples of the median

MOMA 3,4-methylenedioxidemethylamphetamine; methylhydroxymandelic acid

MOMEDA mobile medical data [European Union]

MoMLV, Mo-MLV Moloney murine leukemia virus

MOMO macrosomia-obesity-macrocephaly-ocular abnormalities [syndrome]

MO-MOM mineral oil and milk of magnesia

MOMP major outer membrane protein

MOMS multiple organ malrotation syndrome

Mo-MSV Moloney murine sarcoma virus

MOMX macroorchidism-marker X chromosome [syndrome]

MON Mongolian [gerbil]

MONET multiwavelength optical network

MONICA monitoring trends and determinants in cardiovascular diseases

mono monocyte; mononucleosis

MONT montelukast

MOOW Medical Officer of the Watch

MOP major organ profile; medical outpatient; memory organization packet

8-MOP 8-methoxypsoralen

MOPD microcephalic osteodysplastic primordial dwarfism

MOPEG 3-methoxy-4-hydroxyphenylglycol

MOPFC medial and orbital prefrontal cortex

MOPP mechlorethamine, Oncovin, procarbazine, prednisone; mission-oriented protective posture [clothing]

MOPS 3-morpholino-propanesulfonic acid

MOPV monovalent oral poliovirus vaccine; Mopeia virus

Mor, mor morphine

MORAC mixed oligonucleotides primed amplification of complementary deoxyribonucleic acid

MORC Medical Officers Reserve Corps

MORD magnetic optical rotatory dispersion

MORFAN mental retardation-pre- and post-natal overgrowth-remarkable face-acanthosis nigricans [syndrome]

morphol morphology

mort, mortal mortality

MORV Moriche virus

MOS mechanism of stroke deducer; medial orbital sulcus; medical outcomes study; metal oxide sensor; microsomal ethanol-oxidizing system; mitral opening snap; Moloney murine sarcoma; myelofibrosis osteosclerosis

mOs milliosmolal

mos mosaic

MOSA Medical Officers of School Association [UK]

MOSES Morbidity and Mortality after Stroke-Eprosartan vs Nitrendipine for Secondary Prevention [study]

MOSF multiple organ system failure

MOSFET metal oxide semiconductor field effect transistor

mOsm milliosmol

mOsm, MOsm milliosmole

mOsm/kg milliosmoles per kilogram

MOST Mode Selection Trial; mother of super twins

MOSV Mossuril virus

MOT mouse ovarian tumor

Mot, mot motor

MOTA Manitoba oculo-tricho-anal [syndrome]

MOTNAC Manual of Tumor Nomenclature and Coding

MOTSA multiple overlapping thin slab acquisition [technique]

MOTT medical observation type table; mycobacteria other than tuberculosis

MOU memorandum of understanding

MOUS multiple occurrence of unexplained symptoms

MOV metal-oxide varistor; minimal occlusive volume; molluscum-like poxvirus

MoV mottle virus

MOVC membranous obstruction of inferior vena cava

MoVd mottle viroid

MOVIES Monongahela Valley Independent Elders Survey

MOX moxalactam

MP macrophage; maintained protocol; malignant pyoderma; matrix protein; mean pressure; mechanical processing; median posterior; megapascal; melphalan and prednisone; melting point; membrane potential; menstrual period; mentum posterior; mercaptopurine; mesenteric panniculitis; mesial pit; mesiopulpal; metacarpophalangeal; metalloprotease; metal particulate [magnetic tape]; metaphalangeal; metatarsophalangeal; methylphosphonate; methylprednisolone; Mibelli porokeratosis; middle phalanx; moist pack; moment preserving; monophasic; monophosphate; motion profile; motor potential; mouthpiece; movement protein; mucopolysaccharide; multiparous; multiprogrammable pacemaker; muscle potential; mycoplasmal pneumonia; myocardial perfusion

3-MP 3-mercaptopropionate

M6P mannose-6-phosphate

6-MP 6-mercaptopurine

8-MP 8-methylpsoralen

M&P managerial and professional [staff]

mp millipoint; melting point

μP microprocessor

MPA main pulmonary artery; master of public administration; mean pulmonary arterial [pressure]; medial preoptic area; Medical Procurement Agency; medroxyprogesterone acetate; mercaptopropionic acid; metaphosphoric acid; methylprednisolone acetate; microscopic polyarteritis; micropipette aspiration; minor physical anomaly; multiple project assurance

MPa megapascal

μPa micropascal

M-PACT Mayo-Physician Alliance for Clinical Trials

MPAP mean pulmonary arterial pressure

MPAS mild periodic acid Schiff [reaction]

mPa/s millipascal per second

M-PATHY Multicenter Pacing Therapy for Hypertrophic Cardiomyopathy; Multicenter Study of Pacing Therapy for Hypertrophic Cardiomyopathy

MPB male pattern baldness; meprobamate; microdissected paraffin block

MPC marine protein concentrate; marker for prostatic cancer; maximum permissible concentration; mean plasma concentration; meperidine, promethazine, and chlorpromazine; metallophthalocyanine; metapyrocatechase; minimum mycoplasmacidal concentration; model predictive control

MPCA microbial pest control agent

MPCh medio-posterior choroidal

MPCO micropolycystic ovary syndrome

MPCP mean pulmonary capillary pressure

MPCUR maximum permissible concentration of unidentified radionucleotides

MPD main pancreatic duct; matched peripheral dose; maximum permissible dose; mean population doubling; membrane potential difference; minimal perceptible difference; minimal phototoxic dose; multiparametric color composite display; multiple personality disorder; myeloproliferative disease; myofascial pain dysfunction

MPDS mandibular pain dysfunction syndrome; medical priority dispatch service; myofascial pain dysfunction syndrome

MPE malignant proliferation of eosinophils; maximum permissible exposure; maximum possible error; Medicaid program evaluation; most probable event

MPEAK multispeak [speech-coding strategy]

MPEC multipolar electrocoagulation

MPED minimum phototoxic erythema dose

MPEH methylphenylethylhydantoin

MPEP Model Performance Evaluation Program [CDC]

MPF maturation promoting factor; mean power frequency; minimally processed foods; M-phase [mitosis] promoting factor

MPG magnetopneumography; mercapto-propionylglycine; methyl green pyronine; 3-methylpurine deoxyribonucleic acid glycosylase; monthly prescribing guide

MPGM monophosphoglycerate mutase

MPGN membranoproliferative glomerulonephritis

MPGR multiple planar gradient recalled

MPH macroporous hydrogel; male pseudohermaphroditism; Master of Public Health; microtiter plate hybridization; milk protein hydrolysate

MPharm Master of Pharmacy

MPHD multiple pituitary hormone deficiencies

mphot milliphot

MPHR maximum predicted heart rate

MPhysA Member of Physiotherapists' Association

MPI mannose phosphate isomerase; master patient index; maximum permitted intake; maximum point of impulse; message-passing interface; multidimensional pain inventory; Multiphasic Personality Inventory; myocardial perfusion imaging

MPI-I/O message passing interface-input/output

MPIP Multicenter Postinfarction Program

MPJ metacarpophalangeal joint

MPKC management problem-knowledge coupler

MPKUCS Maternal Phenylketonuria Collaborative Study

MPKV Maprik virus

MPL maximum permissible level; melphalan; mesiopulpolingual; myeloproliferative leukemia

MPLa mesiopulpolabial

MPLS multiprotocol label switching

MPLV myeloproliferative leukemia virus

MPM malignant papillary or pleural mesothelioma; medial pterygoid muscle; minor psychiatric morbidity; mortality probability model; multiple primary malignancy; multipurpose meal

MPME (5R,8R)-8-(4-*p*-methoxy-phenyl)-1-piperazynylmethyl-6-methylergolene

MPMP 10[(1-methyl-3-piperidinyl)-methyl]-1OH-phenothiazine

MPMT Murphy punch maneuver test

MPMV, M-PMV Mason-Pfizer monkey virus

MPN most probable number

MPNST malignant peripheral nerve sheath tumor

MPO maximum power output; minimal perceptible odor; myeloperoxidase

MPOA medial preoptic area

MPOD myeloperoxidase deficiency

MPOV M'Poko virus

MPP massive peritoneal proliferation; massively parallel processor; methyl phenylpyridinium; medical personnel pool; mercaptopyrazide pyrimidine; metacarpophalangeal profile; myelin protein, peripheral

MPPCD Multifactorial Primary Prevention of Cardiovascular Diseases

mppcf millions of particles per cubic foot of air

MPPEC mean peak plasma ethanol concentration

MPPG microphotoelectric plethysmography

MPPH *p*-tolylphenylhydantoin

MPPN malignant persistent positional nystagmus

MPPT methylprednisolone pulse therapy; mucin-producing pancreatic tumor

MPP$_v$ mean portal vein peak velocity

MPQ McGill Pain Questionnaire

MPQ-SF McGill Pain Questionnaire-Short Form

MPR mannose 6-phosphate receptor; marrow production rate; massive pre-retinal retraction; maximum pulse rate; multiplanar reconstruction; multiplanar reformation [MRI data on computer screen]; multiplanar reformatting; myeloproliferative reaction; myocardial perfusion reserve

MP-RAGE magnetization-prepared rapid gradient-echo

MP-RAGE-WE magnetization-prepared rapid gradient echo-water excitation

MPRD cation-dependent mannose 6-phosphate receptor

mPRF medial pontine reticular formation

MPRG Multicenter Postinfarction Research Group

MPRO mental process [UMLS]

MPRV Mapuera virus

MPS hereditary giant platelet syndrome; meconium plug syndrome; medial premotor system; Member of the Pharmaceutical

Society; methylprednisolone; microbial profile system; mononuclear phagocyte system; Montreal platelet syndrome; movement-produced stimulus; mucopolysaccharide, mucopolysaccharidosis; multidimensional pain scale; multiphasic screening; mushroom poisoning site [database, Italy]; myocardial perfusion scintigraphy; myofascial pain syndrome

MPS I mucopolysaccharidosis I

MPS-I-H mucopolysaccharidosis I, Hurler type

MPS-I-S mucopolysaccharidosis I, Scheie type

MPS II mucopolysaccharidosis II

MPS III mucopolysaccharidosis III

MPS IIIA mucopolysaccharidosis III, type A

MPS IIIB mucopolysaccharidosis III, type B

MPS IIIC mucopolysaccharidosis III, type C

MPS IIID mucopolysaccharidosis III, type D

MPS IV mucopolysaccharidosis IV

MPS IVA mucopolysaccharidosis IV, type A

MPS IVB mucopolysaccharidosis IV, type B

MPS V mucopolysaccharidosis V

MPS VI mucopolysaccharidosis VI

mps meters per second

m-PSA mutated prostate-specific antigen

MPS-H/I-S mucopolysaccharidosis, Hurler-Scheie type

MPSoSIS mucopolysaccharidosis

MPSS methylprednisolone sodium succinate; Music Performance Stress Survey

MPSV myeloproliferative sarcoma virus

MPsyMed Master of Psychological Medicine

MPT mean peak torque; Michigan Picture Test; multiple particle tracking

MPTP 1-methyl-4-phenyl-1,2,3,6-tetrahydropyridine

MPT-R Michigan Picture Test, Revised

MPU Medical Practitioners Union

MPV main portal vein; mean platelet volume; mitral valve prolapse

MpV *Micromonas pusilla* virus

MPVP mean pulmonary venous pressure

MPXV monkeypox virus

MPZ myelin protein, zero

mpz millipièze

MQ memory quotient; motor quotient

M-Q move-quality [descriptor]

MQC microbiologic quality control

MQFD medical quality function deployment

MQIS Medicare quality indicator system

MQL Medical Query Language [computer]

MQNB ^{11}C-labeled methylquinuclidinyl benzylate

MQOV Mosqueiro virus

MQSM molecular quantum similarity measures

MQSPR model-based quantitative structure-property relationship

MR Maddox rods; magnetic resistance; magnetic resonance; mandibular reflex; mannose-resistant; may repeat; measles and rubella; medial raphe; medial rectus [muscle]; medical record; medical release; medium range; megaroentgen; mental retardation; metabolic rate; metathesaurus relational file [UMLS]; methemoglobin reductase; methyl red; mineralocorticoid receptor; mitral reflux; mitral regurgitation; modulation rate; molar refraction; mortality rate; mortality ratio; multicentric reticulohistiocytosis; multiregression; muscarinic receptor; muscle receptor; muscle relaxant; myocardial revascularization

M&R measure and record

M/R measles/rubella [vaccine]

M₂R muscarinic cholinergic receptor

M₂R muscarinic cholinergic receptor

MR4 Malaria Research and Reference Reagent Resource Center

Mr relative molar mass

M$_r$ relative molecular mass

mR, mr milliroentgen

m/r mass attenuation coefficient; modified release [pills]

μR, μr microroentgen

MRA magnetic resonance angiography; main renal artery; marrow repopulation activity; medical record analysis or analyst; medical records administrator; mesenteric resistance artery; mid right atrium; multivariate regression analysis

MRAB machine-readable archives in biomedicine

MRAC model reference adaptive control

mrad millirad

MRAP alpha-2-macroglobulin receptor-associated protein; maximal resting anal pressure; mean right atrial pressure

MRAS main renal artery stenosis

MRB multiply resistant bacteria

MRBC monkey red blood cell; mouse red blood cell

MRBF mean renal blood flow

MRC magnetic resonance cholangiography; maximum recycling capacity; Medical Registration Council; Medical Research Council; Medical Reserve Corps; methylrosaniline chloride; modular robot control

MRCAS medical robotics and computer-assisted surgery

MRC/BHF Medical Research Council, British Heart Foundation Heart Protection Study

MRC CFAS Medical Research Council [UK] Cognitive Function and Ageing Study

MR-CISS magnetic resonance-constructive interference in steady state

MRCNS methicillin-resistant coagulase-negative staphylococci

MRCOA Medical Research Council [UK] Trial in Older Adults

MRCP magnetic resonance cholangiopancreatography; movement-related cortical potential

MRD magnetic resonance diffusion; maximum rate of depolarization; measles-rindenpest-distemper [virus group]; medical records department; minimal reacting dose; minimal renal disease; minimal residual disease

mrd millirutherford

MRDD mentally retarded/developmentally disabled [person]

MRDI medical records document imaging

MR-DTI magnetic resonance diffusion tensor imaging

MRE magnetic resonance elastography; maximal resistive exercise; maximal respiratory effectiveness; Microbiological Research Establishment, Porton [UK]

MREC mismatch repair enzyme cleavage

MREI mean rate ejection index

mrem millirem

mrep milliroentgen equivalent physical

MRF Markov random field; medical record file; melanocyte-[stimulating hormone]-releasing factor; mesencephalic reticular formation; midbrain reticular formation; mitral regurgitant flow; moderate renal failure; monoclonal rheumatoid factor; müllerian regression factor; muscle regulatory factor

mRF monoclonal rheumatoid factor

MRFC mouse rosette-forming cell

MRFIT Multiple Risk Factor Intervention Trial

MRFM magnetic resonance force microscopy

MRFT modified rapid fermentation test

MRH melanocyte-stimulating hormone-releasing hormone; multicentric reticulohistiocytosis

MRHA mannose-resistant hemagglutination

mrhm milliroentgens per hour at one meter

MRI machine-readable identifier; magnetic resonance imaging; magnetic resonance interferometry; medical records information; medical re-engineering initiative; Medical Research Institute; moderate renal insufficiency

M-RIA monoclonal radioimmunoassay

MRIF melanocyte[-stimulating hormone] release-inhibiting factor

MRIH melanocyte[-stimulating hormone] release-inhibiting hormone

MRIPHH Member of the Royal Institute of Public Health and Hygiene

MRISM magnetic resonance imaging simulation

MRK Mayer-Rokitansky-Küster [syndrome]

MR-K mannose-resistant *Klebsiella*-like [hemagglutinin]

MRKH Mayer-Rokitansky-Küster-Hauser [syndrome]

MRL Malaria Reference Laboratory [UK]; maximum residue limit; medical records librarian; Medical Research Laboratory

MRM magnetic resonance mammography; modified radical mastectomy

MRMIB Managed Risk Medical Insurance Board

MRMT Minnesota Rate of Manipulation Test

MRN magnetic resonance neurography; malignant renal neoplasm; medical record number

mRNA messenger ribonucleic acid

mRNA/R messenger ribonucleic acid receptor

mRNP messenger ribonucleoprotein

MRO master reference oscillator; medical review officer; minimal recognizable odor; muscle receptor organ

MROD Medical Research and Operations Directorate

MRP mean resisting potential; medical reimbursement plan; medical removal protection; multidrug resistance-associated protein; mutual recognition process

MR-PET Magnetic Resonance vs Positron Emission Tomography [for detection of myocardial viability, study]

MRR marrow release rate

MRS magnetic resonance spectroscopy; Mania Rating Scale; medical receiving station; medical record summary; Melkersson-Rosenthal syndrome

MRSA methicillin-resistant *Staphylococcus aureus*

MRSD mental retardation-skeletal dysplasia [syndrome]

MRSE methicillin-resistant *Staphylococcus epidermidis*

MRSH Member of the Royal Society of Health

MRSI magnetic resonance spectroscopy imaging

MRSO metathesaurus relational source [UMLS]

MRSX X-linked mental retardation

MRT magnetic resonance tomography; maximum relaxation time; median range score; median reaction time; median recognition threshold; median relapse time; medical radiation technology/technologist; medical records technician; medical response team; methyltryptophan; milk ring test; muscle response test

MRTS message routing and translation system

MRU magnetic recognition unit; magnetic resonance urography; meningococcal reference unit; mass radiography unit; minimal reproductive unit; *Mycobacterium* reference unit

MR/UR Medical Review and Utilization Program

MRV magnetic resonance venography; mammalian orthoreovirus; minute respiratory volume; Mitchell river virus; mixed respiratory vaccine

MRVI mixed virus respiratory infection

MRVP mean right ventricular pressure; methyl red, Voges-Proskauer [medium]

MRW multi-resolution wavelet

MRWT multiresolution wavelet transform

MRX mental retardation, X-linked

MRXA X-linked mental retardation-aphasia syndrome

MRXS mental retardation, X-linked, syndrome

MS Maffuci syndrome; magnesium sulfate [JCAHO unapproved abbreviation]; maladjustment score; mandibular series; mannose-sensitive; Marfan syndrome; margin of safety; Marie-Strümpell [syndrome]; mass spectrometry; Master of Science; Master of Surgery; maternal serum; mean score; mean square [statistics]; mechanical stimulation; Meckel syndrome; mediastinal shift; medical services; medical staff; medical student; medical supplies; medical survey; melanonychia striata; Menkes syndrome; menopausal syndrome; mental status; Meretoja syndrome; metabolic syndrome; microscope slide; Microsporida; midseptal; minimal support; mitral sounds; mitral stenosis; mobile surgical [unit]; modal sensitivity; moderately susceptible; modified sphygmomanometer; molar solution; molecular substitution; Mongolian spot; morning stiffness; morphine sulfate [JCAHO unapproved abbreviation]; morpho-syntactic; mosaic virus; motile sperm; mucosubstance; Münchausen syndrome; multiple sclerosis; muscle shortening; muscle strength; musculoskeletal; myelosarcoma; myoclonic seizures

3MS modified mini-mental state examination

MS I, II, III, IV medical student—first, second, third, and fourth year

Ms murmurs; microsphere

ms millisecond; morphine sulfate

m/s meters per second

m/s² meters per second squared

µs microsecond

MSA magnetic resonance angiography; major serologic antigen; major soluble antigen; male-specific antigen; mammary serum antigen; mannitol salt agar; medical savings account; Medical Services Administration; membrane stabilizing action; membrane-stabilizing activity; metropolitan statistical area; microsomal anti-antibody; mitotic spindle apparatus; molecular shape analysis; morphological sequential approach; mouse serum albumin; multiple sequence alignment [proteins]; multiple system atrophy; muscle sympathetic activity; myosis-specific antibody

MSAA multiple sclerosis-associated agent

MSAD multiple scan average dose

MSAEFI Monitoring System for Adverse Events Following Immunisation [UK]

MSAFP, MS-AFP maternal serum alpha-fetoprotein

MSAM master of science in administrative medicine

MSAN medical student's admission note

MSAP mean systemic arterial pressure

MSB Master of Science in Bacteriology; mid-small bowel; most significant bit

MSBC maximum specific binding capacity

MSBLA mouse-specific B lymphocyte antigen

MSC magnitude-squared coherence; major septic complication; marrow stromal cell; Medical Service Corps; Medical Staff Corps; mesenchymal stem cell; midsystolic click; Multimedia SuperCorridor; multispecialty clinic

MSc Master of Science

MScD Master of Dental Science

MScMed Master of Science in Medicine

MScN Master of Science in Nursing

MSCP mean spherical candle power

MSCU medical special care unit

MSD Material Safety Data [Occupational Safety Service]; mean square deviation; mean square displacement; membrane-spanning domain; midsagittal diameter; mild sickle cell disease; most significant digit; multiple sulfatase deficiency; musculoskeletal dynamic [system]

MSDC Mass Spectrometry Data Centre [UK]

MSDI Martin Suicide Depression Inventory

MS-DOS Microsoft Disk Operating System

MSDS material safety data sheet

MSE mean squared error; medical screening examination; medical support equipment; mental status examination; mental status expert; muscle-specific enolase

mse mean square error

MSEA Medical Society Executives Association

msec millisecond

m/sec meters per second

μsec microsecond

MSEL Materials Science and Engineering Laboratory; myasthenic syndrome of Eaton-Lambert

MSEP mean square error of prediction

MSER mean systolic ejection rate

MSES medical school environmental stress

MSF macrophage slowing factor; macrophage spreading factor; malignant senescent forgetfulness [Alzheimer disease]; meconium-stained fluid; Médicins sans Frontières [Doctors without Borders]; Mediterranean spotted fever; melanocyte-stimulating factor; modified sham feeding; multiple sequence format [molecular genetics]

MSG molecular supergraph; monosodium L-glutamate; motion-sensitizing gradient

MSGQ medical student graduation questionnaire

MSGV mouse salivary gland virus

MSH medical self-help; melanocyte-stimulating hormone; melanophore-stimulating hormone; message header; Multicenter Study of Hydroxyurea

MSHA mannose-sensitive hemagglutination; Mine Safety and Health Administration

MSHIF melanocyte-stimulating hormone-inhibiting factor

MSHR melanocyte-stimulating hormone receptor

MSHRF melanocyte-stimulating hormone-releasing factor

MSHRH melanocyte-stimulating hormone-releasing hormone

M-SHRSP malignant stroke-prone spontaneously hypertensive rat

MSHSC multiple self-healing squamous carcinoma

MSHT Mount Sinai Hypertension Trial

MSHyg Master of Science in Hygiene

MSI magnetic source imaging; medium-scale integration

MSIC mechanically sensitive ion channels
MSIE Microsoft Internet Explorer
MSIM medical systems infrastructure modernization
MSIS multi-state information system
MSJ meatal stapedial joint
MSK medullary sponge kidney; Memorial Sloan-Kettering; mitogen-activated S6 kinase; musculoskeletal
MSKCC Memorial Sloan-Kettering Cancer Center
MSKP Medical Sciences Knowledge Profile
MSL midsternal line; multiple symmetric lipomatosis
MSLA morpho-synthetic lexical ambiguity; mouse-specific lymphocyte antigen
MSLL multifocal signal loss lesion
MSLR mixed skin cell-leukocyte reaction
MSLS Marinesco-Sjögren-like syndrome
MSLT Multicenter Selective Lymphadenectomy Trial; multiple sleep latency test
MSM medium-size molecule; men who have sex with men; midsystolic murmur; mineral salts medium
MSMA monosodium methanearsonate
MSMAID machine, suction, monitor, airway equipment, intravenous line, drugs [for bronchoscopy]
MSMB microseminoprotein beta
MSMI Multicenter Study of Myocardial Ischemia
MS/MS tandem mass spectrophotometry
MSN main sensory nucleus; Master of Science in Nursing; mildly subnormal; moesin
MSNet Mass Spectrometry Network
MSO management services organization; medial superior olive; medical staff organization
MSOF multiple systems organ failure
MSOP medical school objectives project
MSP macrophage stimulating protein; maximum squeeze pressure; median sagittal plane; Medicare secondary payer; microseminoprotein; Münchausen syndrome by proxy
msp muscle spasm
MSPB microseminoprotein beta
MSPGN mesangial proliferative glomerulonephritis
MSPH Master of Science in Public Health
MSPhar Master of Science in Pharmacy

MSPN medical student's progress note
MSPQ Modified Somatic Perception Questionnaire
MSPS myocardial stress perfusion scintigraphy
MSPV Malpais Spring virus
MSQ mental status questionnaire; Minnesota satisfaction questionnaire
MSR macrophage scavenger receptor; magnetically shielded room; Member of the Society of Radiographers; mitro-steno regurgitation; monosynaptic reflex; muscle stretch reflex
MSRI mixed serotonin reuptake inhibitor
MSRPP Multidimensional Scale for Rating Psychiatric Patients
MSRT Minnesota Spatial Relations Test
MSS Marinesco-Sjögren syndrome; Marshall-Smith syndrome; massage; Medical Superintendents' Society; Medicare Statistical System; mental status schedule; minor surgery suite; motion sickness susceptibility; mucus-stimulating substance; multiple sclerosis susceptibility; muscular subaortic stenosis
mss massage
MSSA methicillin-sensitive *Staphylococcus aureus*
MSSE multiple sclerosis self-efficacy scale; multiple self-healing squamous epithelioma
MSSG multiple sclerosis susceptibility gene
MSSMI Multicenter Study of Silent Myocardial Ischemia
MSSVD Medical Society for the Study of Venereal Diseases
MST maximal stimulation test; mean survival time; mean swell time; mercaptopyruvate sulfurtransferase; Montenegro skin test; multiple subpial transections; myeloproliferative syndrome, transient
M-Step maximization step
MSTh mesothorium
MSTI multiple soft tissue injuries
MSTP Medical Scientist Training Program [NIH]; medical student training program
MSTS Musculoskeletal Tumor Society
MsTT microsphere encapsulated tetanus toxoid
MSU maple sugar urine; maple syrup urine; medical studies unit; midstream specimen of urine; mid-stream urine;

monosodium urate; myocardial substrate uptake

MSUD maple syrup urine disease

MSurg Master of Surgery

MSV maximum sustained level of ventilation; mean scale value; mean spatial velocity; Moloney sarcoma virus; monkey sarcoma virus; Muir Springs virus; murine sarcoma virus

mSv millisievert

MSVC maximal sustained ventilatory capacity

MSW male sex worker; Master of Social Welfare; Master of Social Work; medical social worker; multiple stab wounds

MSWYE modified sea water yeast extract

MT magnetization transfer; malaria therapy; malignant teratoma; mammary tumor; mammilothalamic tract; manual traction; Martin-Thayer [plate, medium]; mastoid tip; maximal therapy; mechanotransduction; medial thalamus; medial thickness; medical technologist; medical therapy; melatonin; membrana tympani; mesangial thickening; metallothionein; metatarsal; Metathesaurus [UMLS]; methoxytryptamine; methyltransferase; methyltyrosine; microtome; microtomography; microtubule; mid-trachea; minimal touch; minimum threshold; mitochondrial toxicity; Monroe tidal drainage; more than; motor threshold; movement time; multi-input threshold; multiple tics; Muir-Torre [syndrome]; multitest [plate]; mural thrombus or thrombosis; muscles and tendons; muscle test; music therapy; *Mycobacterium tuberculosis*

M-T macroglobulin-trypsin

M&T *Monilia* and *Trichomonas*

Mt megatonne; *Mycobacterium tuberculosis*

mt mitochondrial

3-MT 3-methoxytyramine

MTA malignant teratoma, anaplastic; medical technical assistant; medical technology assessment; medullary type adenocarcinoma; metatarsus adductus; multithreaded architecture; myoclonic twitch activity

mTA meta-tyramine

MTAC mass transfer area coefficient

MTACR multiple tumor-associated chromosome region

MTAD membrana tympana auris dextrae

MTAL medullary thick ascending limb

MTAP methylthioadenosine phosphorylase

MTAS membrana tympana auris sinistrae

MT(ASCP) Medical Technologist certified by the American Society of Clinical Pathologists

MTase methyltransferase

MTB methylthymol blue; Michelin tire baby [syndrome]; *Mycobacterium tuberculosis*

Mtb *Mycobacterium tuberculosis*

MTBE meningeal tick-borne encephalitis; methyltertiary butyl ether

MTBF mean time between (or before) failures

MTBM mean time between maintenance

MTBN modifiable temporal belief network

MTBV Marituba virus

MTC magnetization transfer contrast; mass transfer coefficient; maximum tolerated concentration; maximum toxic concentration; medical test cabinet; medical training center; medullary thyroid carcinoma; metatarsocuneiform [joint]; mitomycin C

MTCT mother-to-child transmission

MTD maximum tolerated dose; mean total dose; metastatic trophoblastic disease; Midwife Teacher's Diploma; minimal topological difference; Monroe tidal drainage; multidrug therapy; multiple tic disorder; *Mycobacterium tuberculosis* direct test

MTDDA Minnesota Test for Differential Diagnosis of Aphasia

MT-DN multitest, dermatophytes and *Nocardia* [plate]

mtDNA mitochondrial DNA

MTDT modified tone decay test

MTE main timing event; monophasic truncated exponential

mTERF mitochondrial transcription termination factor

MTET modified treadmill exercise test

MTF maximum terminal flow; medical treatment facility; modulation transfer function

mTF mitochondrial transcription factor

MTg mouse thyroglobulin

MTGA multiple time graphic analysis

MTGua 7-methyl-6-thioguanine
MTGuo 7-methyl-6-thioguanosine
MTH mithramycin
MTh motor threshold
MTHF, mTHF 5,10-methylene tetrahydrofolate
5-MTHF 5-methyl-tetrahydrofolate
MTHFR 5,10-methylene tetrahydrofolate reductase
MTI malignant teratoma, intermediate; maximum tolerable intensity; minimum time interval; model tag image; molecular topological index; moving target indicator
MTL mantle zone lymphoma; medial temporal lobe
MTLE mesial temporal lobe epilepsy
MTLP metabolic toxemia of late pregnancy
MTM Thayer-Martin, modified [agar]; myotubular myopathy
MT-M multitest, mycology [plate]
MT-MMP membrane-type metalloproteinase
MTMX myotubular myopathy, X-linked
MTO medical technical officer; medical transport officer
MTOC microtubule organizing center; mitotic organizing center
MTOP Medical Treatment Outcomes Project
MTOS Major Trauma Outcomes Study
MTP maximum tolerated pressure; medial tibial plateau; median time to progression; metatarsophalangeal; micropayment transfer protocol; microsomal triglyceride transfer protein; microtubule protein
MT1PA metallothionein-1 pseudogene-A
MTPD mean trabecular plate density
MTPJ metatarsophalangeal joint
Mt-PK myotonic protein kinase
MTPS mean trabecular plate separation
MTPT mean trabecular plate thickness
MTQ methaqualone
MTR magnetization transfer ratio; maximum tracking rate [pacemaker]; Meinicke turbidity reaction; 5-methylthioribose; methyltetrahydrofolate:L-homocysteine; *S*-methyltransferase
MTRV Matruh virus
MTS magnetization transfer contrast; mechanical testing machine; Medicare transaction system; menopausal transition; mesial temporal sclerosis; methotrexate; Mohr-Tranebjaerg syndrome; multicellu-

lar tumor spheroid; musculotendinous structure
MTST maximal treadmill stress test
MTT malignant teratoma, trophoblastic; maximal treadmill test; meal tolerance test; mean transit time; methyl-thiazoldiphenyl-tetrazolium; mucous transport time; Myocarditis Treatment Trial
MTU malignant teratoma, undifferentiated; medical therapy unit; methylthiouracil
MtuRRF *Mycobacterium tuberculosis* ribosome recycling factor
MTV mammary tumor virus; metatarsus varus; Mibuna temperate virus; mild tigré virus; mouse mammary tumor virus
MTX methotrexate
MT-Y multitest yeast [plate]
MU megaunit; mescaline unit; methyluric [acid]; monitor unit [radiotherapy]; Montevideo unit; motion unsharpness; motor unit; mouse unit
Mu Mache unit
mU milliunit
mu mouse unit
μ Greek letter *mu*; chemical potential; electrophoretic mobility; heavy chain of immunoglobulin M; linear attenuation coefficient; magnetic moment; mean; micro; micrometer; micron; mutation rate; permeability
μU microunit
MUA manipulation under anesthesia; middle uterine artery; motor unit activity
MUAP motor unit action potential
MUC maximum urinary concentration; mucilage; mucin; mucosal ulcerative colitis
muc mucilage; mucous, mucus
MUCV Mucambo virus
MUD matched unrelated donor; minimum urticarial dose
MUDV Mudjinbarry virus
MUE motor unit estimated
MUFA monounsaturated fatty acids
MUG Massachusetts General Hospital Utility Multi-Programming System [MUMPS] Users Group
MUGA multiple gated acquisition [blood pool scan]
MUGEx multigated blood pool image during exercise
MUGR multigated blood pool image at rest

MuHV Murid herpesvirus

mulibrey muscle-liver-brain-eye nanism or dwarfism

MULO multipurpose overboot

mult multiple

Multi-CSF multi-colony-stimulating factor

MultiODA multivariable optimal discriminant analysis

multip multiparous

MULV Muleshoe virus

MuLV, MuLv murine leukemia virus

MUMPS Massachusetts General Hospital Utility Multi-Programming System

MuMTv murine mammary tumor virus

MUNV Munguba virus

MUN(WI) Munich Wistar [rat]

MUO myocardiopathy of unknown origin

MUP major urinary protein; maximal urethral pressure; motor unit potential

mUPD maternal uniparental disomy [UPD]

MUPIBAC Mupirocin in Prevention of Relapses of Wegener Granulomatosis by Elimination of Nasal Bacterial *Staphylococcus aureus* Carriage

mUPID maternal uniparental isodisomy [UPID]

MUPIT Martinez Universal Perineal Interstitial Template

MURAD Moscow-Ulm Radiation Accident Clinical History Database

MURC measurable undesirable respiratory contaminants

MURCS Müllerian duct aplasia, cervicothoracic somite dysostosis [association]

MurNAc N-acetylmuramate

MURP Master of Urban and Regional Planning

MURV Murre virus; Murutucu virus

MUS mouse urologic syndrome; muscinol

musc muscle, musculature, muscular

MUSCAT MUSIC Criteria for Stent Implantation Using the Controlled Angioplasty Technology Catheter

MUSE medicated uretheral system for erection

MUSIC Measuring the Usability of Systems in Context [radiotherapy]; Multicenter Ultrasound During Stent Implantation in Coronary Arteries [study]; Multicenter Ultrasound Stent in Coronary Artery Disease [study]; Multicentre Ultrasound Study in Coronaries; multiple signal classification

[algorithm]; musculoskeletal intervention center

MUST medical unit, medication use studies; Multicenter Stent Study; Multicenter Stents Ticlodipine [study]; Multicenter Ultrasound Study with Ticlid; Multicenter Unsustained Tachycardia [trial]; Medical Unit Self-Contained and Transportable

MUST-EECP Multicenter Study of Enhanced External Counterpulsation

MUSTIC multisite stimulation in cardiac insufficiency; multisite stimulation in cardiomyopathy

MUSTPAC medical ultrasound 3-dimensional portable with advanced communication

MUSTT Multicentre Unstable Tachycardia Trial; Multicenter Unsustained Tachycardia Trial

MUT mutagen

mut mutation

MUU mouse uterine unit

MuV mumps virus

MUWU mouse uterine weight unit

MUX multiplex

MV maturation value; measles virus; mechanical ventilation; megavolt; methotrexate/vinblastine; microvascular; microvillus; Microvirus, microvirus; minute ventilation; minute virus; minute volume; mitral valve; mixed venous; molar volume; mosaic virus; mottle virus; multivessel; myeloblastosis virus; veterinary physician [Lat. *Medicus Veterinarius*]

Mv mendelevium

mV, mv millivolt

μV microvolt

MVA mechanical ventricular assistance; mevalonic acid; mitral valve area; modified vaccinia virus Ankara; motor vehicle accident

MV · A megavolt-ampere

mV · A millivolt-ampere

MVAD mechanical ventricular assist device

mval millival

MVB manual ventilation bag; microvascular bleeding; multivesicular body

MVC maximum voluntary contraction; model-view controller [interaction scheme]; motor vehicle crash; multivane collimator; muscle vasoconstriction; myocardial vascular capacity

MVD Doctor of Veterinary Medicine; microvascular decompression; microvessel density; mitral valve disease; multivessel coronary disease

MVd mosaic viroid

MVE maximum velocity envelope; mitral valve echo; mitral valve excursion; Murray Valley encephalitis

MVEC microvascular endothelial cell

MVEV Murray Valley encephalitis virus

MVF mitral valve flow

MVH massive vitreous hemorrhage

MVI mitral valve insufficiency; multivalvular involvement; multivitamin infusion

MV-HIS multi-vendor hospital information system

MVK mevalonate kinase

MVL mitral valve leaflet

MVLS mandibular vestibulolingual sulcoplasty

MVM microvillose membrane; minute virus of mice

MVMT movement

MVN medial ventromedial nucleus; microvascular network

MVO maximum venous outflow; mitral valve opening or orifice

MVO2, MVO$_2$ myocardial oxygen consumption

MVOA mitral valve orifice area

mVOC mycological volatile organic compound

MVP microvascular pressure; mitral valve prolapse; Multivitamin and Probucol [trial]

MVPP mustine, vinblastine, procarbazine, prednisone

MVPS Medicare Volume Performance Standards; mitral valve prolapse syndrome

MVP-SC mitral valve prolapse-systolic click [syndrome]

MVPT Motor-Free Visual Perception Test

MVR massive vitreous reaction; microvitreoretinal; minimal vascular resistance; mitral valve replacement

MVS mitral valve stenosis; multivendor service

mV · s millivolt-second

MVSR Monthly Viral Statistics Report

MVT mesenteric venous thrombosis; multiattribute value theory

mvt movement

MVTR moisture vapor transmission rate

MVV maximal voluntary ventilation

MW Mallory-Weiss [syndrome]; masterworker [computing paradigm]; mean weight; megawatt; microwave; middleware; Minot-von Willebrand [syndrome]; molecular weight; multiple-window

mW milliwatt

µW microwatt

MWA moving window averaging

MWAPI M [language] windowing application programmer interface

MWAV Manawa virus

MWB modified whole blood

mWb milliweber

MWCB master working cell bank

MWCO molecular weight cut off

MWD maximum walking distance; microwave diathermy; molecular weight data; molecular weight distribution

MWI modified Williams index

MWL mental workload

m-WMFT modified Wolf motor function test

MWM-L Medical Web Master List [telemedicine]

MWP mean wedge pressure

MWS Marden-Walker syndrome; Moersch-Woltman syndrome

MWSP multi wall stereo projection

MWSR multiple window spatial registration

MWT myocardial wall thickness

6-MWT 6-minute walk test

MWTA Medical Waste Tracking Act

MwV Manawatu virus

MX matrix; metastases not assessed [TNM (tumor-node-metastasis) classification]; methylxanthine

Mx extension of physician [MEDEX]; maxwell; metastases not assessed [TNM (tumor-node-metastasis) classification]

MXA morphometric x-ray absorptiometry

MXIP maximum inspiratory pressure

MXV Mexico virus

M$_{xy}$ transverse magnetization

My myopia; myxedema

my mayer

MYBC myosin-binding protein C

MYBH myosin-binding protein H

MYBP myosin-binding protein

MycDB The *Mycobacterium* Database [Stockholm]

Myco *Mycobacterium*
Mycol mycology, mycologist
MyD myotonic dystrophy
MYEL myelogram
Myel myelocyte
myel myelin, myelinated
MYF myogenic factor
MyG myasthenia gravis
MYH heavy chain myosin
MYHC heavy chain cardiac myosin
MYHCA heavy chain cardiac myosin alpha
MYKV Mykines virus
MYL light chain myosin

MyMD myotonic muscular dystrophy
MYO myoglobin
Myop myopia
MYW modified Yule-Walker [autoregressive technique]
MYX myoxoma
MYXV myxoma virus
MZ mantle zone; mezlocillin; monozygotic
M_z longitudinal magnetization
m/z mass-to-charge ratio
MZA monozygotic twins raised apart
MZM marginal zone macrophage
MZT monozygotic twins raised together

N

N asparagine; Avogadro number; blood factor in the MNS blood group system; loudness; nasal; nasion; nausea; negative; neomycin; neper; nerve; neuraminidase; neurology; neuropathy; neutron number; newton; nicotinamide; nifedipine; nitrogen; nodule; normal [solution]; nucleocapsid; nucleoprotein; nucleoside; nucleus; number; number in sample; number of molecules; number of neutrons in an atomic nucleus; population size; radiance; refractive index; signal size; spin density

N0 no breast tumor regional lymph nodes metastases [TNM (tumor-node-metastasis) classification]

0.02N fiftieth-normal [solution]

0.1N tenth-normal [solution]

0.5N half-normal [solution]

N1 breast tumor metastases to ipsilateral axillary lymph nodes [TNM (tumor-node-metastasis) classification]; normal subject

N I–XII, N 1–12 first to twelfth cranial nerves

2N double-normal [solution]

N2 breast tumor metastases to ipsilateral axillary lymph nodes attached to each other or to other structures [TNM (tumor-node-metastasis) classification]

N/2 half-normal [solution]

N3 breast tumor metastases to ipsilateral internal mammary lymph nodes [TNM (tumor-node-metastasis) classification]

N/10 tenth-normal [solution]

N/50 fiftieth-normal [solution]

n amount of substance expressed in moles; born [Lat. *natus*]; haploid chromosome number; index of refraction; nerve; neuter; neutron; neutron night; number density; normal; nostril [Lat. *naris*]; number; number of density of molecule; principal quantum number; refractive index; rotational frequency; sample size

n- nano- [10^{-9}]

2n haploid chromosome; diploid

3n triploid

4n tetraploid

ν see *nu*

NA Avogadro constant or number; nalidixic acid; Narcotics Anonymous; network administrator; neuraminidase; neurologic age; neutralizing antibody; neutrophil antibody; nicotinic acid; Nomina Anatomica; non-A [hepatitis virus]; nonadherent; noradrenalin; not admitted; not applicable; not available; nuclear antibody; nucleic acid; nucleoside analogue; nucleus ambiguus; numerical aperture; nurse's aide; nursing assistant; nursing auxiliary

N/A not applicable

Na Avogadro number

nA nanoampere

NAA *N*-acetyl aspartate; naphthaleneacetic acid; neutral amino acid; neutron activation analysis; neutrophil aggregation activity; nicotinic acid amide; no apparent abnormalities

NAACCR North American Association of Central Cancer Registries

NAACLS National Accrediting Agency for Clinical Laboratory Sciences

NAACOG Nurses Association of the American College of Obstetricians and Gynecologists

NAA/Cr *N*-acetyl aspartate/creatine [ratio]

NA-AAF *N*-acetoxy-*N*-acetylaminofluorene

NAAP *N*-acetyl-4-amino-phenazone

NAAQS national ambient air quality standard

NAB novarsenobenzene; neutralizing antibody

NABP National Association of Boards of Pharmacy

NABPLEX National Association of Boards of Pharmacy Licensing Examination

NAC *N*-acetylcysteine; National Asthma Center; National Audiovisual Center; neuroimaging analysis center; Noise Advisory Council

NaC sodium channel

NACCHO National Association of County and City Health Officials

NACCT North American Congress of Clinical Toxicology

NaC/DEG sodium channel and degenerin

NACDS North American Clinical Dermatological Society

NACED National Advisory Council on the Employment of the Disabled

nAch nicotinic acetylcholine

NAcHPZ 4-*N*-acetyl hydrazinophthalazin-1-one

nAChR nicotinic acetylcholine receptor

NACHRI National Association of Children's Hospitals and Related Institutions

NACI New Applications for Coronary Interventions [registry]; New Approaches to Coronary Interventions [registry]

NACI DCA New Approaches to Coronary Interventions [registry] Directional Coronary Atherectomy [study]

NACNEP National Advisory Council for Nursing Education and Practice

NACOR National Advisory Committee on Radiation

NACPTAR North American Cerebral Percutaneous Transluminal Angioplasty Registration [study]

Nacq number of acquisitions

NACS neonate adaptive capacity to stimulus

NACSAP National Alliance Concerned with School-Age Parents

NACT National Alliance of Cardiovascular Technologists

NAD neutrophil actin dysfunction; new antigenic determinant; nicotinamide adenine dinucleotide; nicotinic acid dehydrogenase; no abnormal discovery; no active disease; no acute distress; no apparent distress; no appreciable disease; normal axis deviation; not done; nothing abnormal detected

NAD⁺ oxidized nicotinamide adenine dinucleotide [NAD]

NaD sodium dialysate

NADA New Animal Drug Application

NADABA *N*-adenoxyldiaminobutyric acid

NaDC sodium dicarboxylate cotransporter

NADG nicotinamide adenine dinucleotide glycohydrolase

NADH reduced nicotinamide adenine dinucleotide

NADL National Association of Dental Laboratories

NaDodSO₄ sodium dodecyl sulfate

NADP nicotinamide adenine dinucleotide phosphate

NADP⁺ oxidized form of nicotinamide adenine dinucleotide phosphate

NADPH reduced nicotinamide adenine dinucleotide phosphate

NADR National Acquired Immunodeficiency Syndrome [AIDS] Demonstration Research; noradrenalin

NADS National Alcohol and Other Drugs Survey [Canada]

NAE net acid excretion

NaE, Naₑ exchangeable body sodium

NaE1ATP sodium-enzyme-adenosine triphosphate [ATP] complex

NAEL no adverse effect level

NAEMD National Academy of Emergency Medical Dispatch

NAEMSP National Association of Emergency Medical Services Physicians

NAEMT National Association of Emergency Medical Technicians

NAEP National Asthma Education Program

NAEPP National Asthma Education and Prevention Program

NaERC sodium efflux rate constant

NAF nafcillin; National Amputation Foundation; National Ataxia Foundation; net acid flux; neural adaptive filter

NAFD Nager acrofacial dysostosis

NAFEC National Association of Freestanding Emergency Centers

NAFTA North American Free Trade Agreement

NAG *N*-acetyl-D-glucosaminidase; narrow-angle glaucoma; nonagglutinable

NAGA *N*-acetyl-alpha-D-galactosaminidase

NAGO neuraminidase and galactose oxidase

NAGS *N*-acetylglutamate synthetase

NAH 2-hydroxy-3-naphthoic acid hydrazide

NAHA National Association of Health Authorities

NAHC National Advisory Heart Council

NAHCS National Association of Health Center Schools

NAHDO National Association of Health Data Organizations

NAHG National Association of Humanistic Gerontology

NAHI National Athletic Health Institute

NAHMOR National Association of Health Maintenance Organization Regulators

NAHPA National Association of Hospital Purchasing Agents

NAHQ National Association for Healthcare Quality

NAHSA National Association for Hearing and Speech Action

NAHSE National Association of Health Services Executives

NAHU National Association of Health Underwriters

NAHUC National Association of Health Unit Clerks-Coordinators

NAHV non-A hepatitis virus

NAI National Aeronautics and Space Administration [NASA] Astrobiology Institute; net acid input; no accidental injury; no acute inflammation; nonadherence index

NAIC National Association of Insurance Commissioners

NAIP National Association of Inpatient Physicians; neuronal apoptosis inhibitory protein

NAIR nonadrenergic inhibitory response

Na,K-ATPase sodium-potassium adenosine triphosphatase

NAL nonadherent leukocyte; Novell Applications Launcher

NALD neonatal adrenoleukodystrophy

NALT nasal-associated lymphoid tissue

NAM *N*-acetylmuramic acid; natural actomyosin

NAMA National Association of Methadone Advocates

NAMCIC National Academic Medical Center Information Consortium

NAMCS National Ambulatory Medical Care Survey

NAME National Association of Medical Examiners; nevi, atrial myxoma, myxoid neurofibroma, ephelides [syndrome]

NAMH National Association for Mental Health

NAMI National Alliance for the Mentally Ill

NAMIS Nifedipine Angina Myocardial Infarction Study

NAMN nicotinic acid mononucleotide

NAMP National Alliance for Mental Patients

NAMRU Navy Medical Reserve Unit

NANA *N*-acetyl neuraminic acid

NANB non-A, non-B [hepatitis]

NANBH non-A, non-B hepatitis

NANBHV non-A, non-B hepatitis virus

NANBNC non-A, non-B, non-C [hepatitis virus]

NANC nonadrenergic noncholinergic

NAND not-and

NANDA North American Nursing Diagnosis Association

NAOO National Association of Optometrists and Opticians

NAOP National Alliance for Optional Parenthood

NAP nasion, point A, pogonion [convexity or concavity of the facial profile]; nerve action potential; network access point; neurotoxin-associated protein; neutrophil-activating peptide; neutrophil alkaline phosphatase; nodular adrenocortical pathology; nucleic acid phosphatase; nucleosome assembly protein

NAPA *N*-acetyl-*p*-aminophenol; *N*-acetyl procainamide

NAPCA National Air Pollution Control Administration

NAPDP National Association of Prepaid Dental Plans

NAPE *N*-acyl-phosphatidylethanolamine

NaPG sodium pregnanediol glucuronide

NAPH naphthyl; National Association of Public Hospitals; nicotinamide adenine dinucleotide phosphate

NAPHSIS National Association for Public Health Statistics and Information Systems

NAPHT National Association of Patients on Hemodialysis and Transplantation

NAPL nucleosome assembly protein-like

NAPM National Association of Pharmaceutical Manufacturers

NAPN National Association of Physicians' Nurses

NAPNAP National Association of Pediatric Nurse Associates and Practitioners

NAPNES National Association for Practical Nursing Education and Services

NAPP nerve agent pyridostigmine pretreatment

NAPPH National Association of Private Psychiatric Hospitals

NAPPS nerve agent pyridostigmine pretreatment set

NAPQI *N*-acetyl-*p*-benzoquinone imine

NAPT National Association for the Prevention of Tuberculosis

NAQAP National Association of Quality Assurance Professionals

NAR nasal airway resistance; National Association for Retarded [Children, Citizens]; no action required

NARA Narcotics Addict Rehabilitation Act; National Association of Recovered Alcoholics

NARAL National Abortion Rights Action League

NARC narcotic; National Association for Retarded Children; nucleus arcuatus

NARCF National Association of Residential Care Facilities

narco narcotic, narcotic addict; drug enforcement agent

NARD National Association of Retail Druggists

NARES nonallergic rhinitis-eosinophilia syndrome

NARF National Association of Rehabilitation Facilities

NARIC National Rehabilitation Information Center

NARL no adverse response level

NARMA nonlinear autoregressive moving average [model]

NARMAX nonlinear autoregressive moving average with exogenous [input]

NARMH National Association for Rural Mental Health

NARP neuropathy-ataxia-retinitis pigmentosa [syndrome]

NARS National Acupuncture Research Society

NARSAD National Alliance for Research on Schizophrenia and Depression

NARSD National Alliance for Research on Schizophrenia and Depression

NARX nonlinear autoregressive model with exogenous input

NAS Narcotics Assistance Section; nasal; National Academy of Sciences; National Association of Sanitarians; neonatal airleak syndrome; network-attached storage; neuroallergic syndrome; neurobehavioral assessment scale [sedation scoring]; no abnormality seen; no added salt; non-*albicans* species; normalized alignment score; Normative Aging Study

NASA National Aeronautics and Space Administration

NASBA nucleic acid sequence-based amplification

NASCET North American Symptomatic Carotid Endarterectomy Trial

NASCIS National Acute Spinal Cord Injury Study

NASD National Association of Schools of Dance

NASE National Association for the Study of Epilepsy

NASEAN National Association for State Enrolled Assistant Nurses

NASH *N*-acryloxysuccinimide

NASHS National Adolescent Student Health Survey

NaSIMM National Study of Internal Medicine Manpower

NASM Naval Aviation School of Medicine

NAS-NRC National Academy of Science-National Research Council

NASPE North American Society for Pacing and Electrophysiology

NASPE/BPEG North American Society of Pacing and Electrophysiology [NASPE]-British Pacing and Electrophysiology Group [BPEG] pacemaker coding

NASS National Accident Sampling System; North American Spine Society

NASV Nasoule virus

NASW National Association of Social Workers

NAT *N*-acetyltransferase; natal; nateglinide; neonatal alloimmune thrombocytopenia; network address translation; no action taken; nonaccidental trauma; nucleic acid testing

Nat native; natural

NaT sodium tartrate

NATCO North American Transplant Coordinator Organization

Natr sodium [Lat. *natrium*]

NATSAL National Survey of Sexual Attitudes and Lifestyles [UK]

NAVAPAM National Association of Veterans Affairs Physician Ambulatory Care Managers

NAVEL naloxone, atropine, Valium, epinephrine, lidocaine

NAVL nerve, artery, vein, lymphatic

NAZC neutrophil azurocidin

NB nail bed; naïve Baues [algorithm]; needle biopsy; neuro-Behçet [syndrome]; neuroblastoma; neurometric battery; new Ballard [score]; newborn; nitrous oxide-barbiturate; normoblast; note well [Lat. *nota bene*]; nutrient broth

nb newborn; note well [Lat. *nota bene*]

NBA neuron-binding activity

NBAC National Bioethics Advisory Committee

NBAT neutral and basic amino acid transporter

NBC network based computing; non-battle casualty; nuclear, biological, chemical

NBCC National Board of Certified Counselors; nevoid basal cell carcinoma

NBCCS nevoid basal cell carcinoma syndrome

NBCIE nonbullous congential ichthyosiform erythroderma

NBCOT National Board for Certification in Occupational Therapy

NBC-PC nuclear, biological, chemical protective cover

NBCRS nuclear, biological, chemical reconnaissance system

NBD neurogenic bladder dysfunction; no brain damage; nucleotide-binding domain

NBF no breast feeding; nucleotide-binding fold

NBI neutrophil bactericidal index; no bone injury; non-battle injury

NBIC neonatal bedside interface controller

NBICU newborn intensive care unit

NBL neuroblastoma

NBM no bowel movement; normal bone marrow; normal bowel movement; nothing by mouth

nBM nucleus basalis of Meynert

nbM newborn mouse

nbMb newborn mouse brain

NBME National Board of Medical Examiners; normal bone marrow extract

NBMPR nitrobenzylmercaptopurine riboside

NBMPR-P nitrobenzylmercaptopurine riboside phosphate

NBN newborn nursery

NBO non-bed occupancy

NBOME National Board of Osteopathic Medicine Examination

NBP needle biopsy of prostate; neoplastic brachial plexopathy; no bone pathology; nonbacterial prostatitis; nucleic acid binding protein

NBPME National Board of Podiatric Medicine Examiners

NBRT National Board for Respiratory Therapy

NBS *N*-bromosuccinimide; National Bureau of Standards; neuroblastoma supressor; nevoid basal cell carcinoma syndrome; newborn bovine serum; Nijmegen breakage syndrome; no bacteria seen; normal blood serum; normal bowel sounds; normal brain stem; nystagmus blockage syndrome

NBSS [Canadian] National Breast Screening Study

NBT nitroblue tetrazolium; non-tumor-bearing; normal breast tissue

NBTE nonbacterial thrombotic endocarditis

NBTNF newborn, term, normal, female

NBTNM newborn, term, normal, male

NBT PABA *N*-benzoyl-L-tyrosyl paraaminobenzoic acid

NBTS National Blood Transfusion Service

n-Bu *n*-butyl

NBV Nelson Bay orthoreovirus

NBW normal birth weight

NC continuous nebulization; nasal cannula; nasal clearance; natural cytotoxicity; near card; neck complaint; neonatal cholestasis; nephrocalcinosis; nerve conduction; neural crest; neurocysticercosis; neurologic check; nevus comedonicus; night call; nitrocellulose; no casualty; no change; no charge; no complaints; noise criterion; noncardiac; noncirrhotic; noncontributory; normal cell; normal control [group]; normocephalic; normocytoplasmic; nose clamp; nose cone; not completed; not cultured; nucleocapsid; nucleo-cytoplasmic; nurse counselor; nursing coordinator

N:C, N/C nuclear-cytoplasmic ratio

nC nanocoulomb

nc nanocurie; not counted

NCA National Certification Agency; National Council on Aging; National Council on Alcoholism; neurocirculatory asthenia; neutrophil chemotactic activity; nodulocystic acne; noncompartmental analysis; noncontractile area; nonspecific cross-reacting antigen; nuclear cerebral angiogram

NCa normal calcium [diet]

n-CAD negative coronoradiographic documentation

NCADI National Clearinghouse for Alcohol and Drug Information

NCAE National Council for Alcohol Education

NC-AFM non-contact mode atomic force microscopy

NCAH National Commission on Allied Health

NCAI National Coalition for Adult Immunization

NCAM neural cell adhesion molecule

NCAMI National Committee Against Mental Illness

NCAMLP National Certification Agency for Medical Laboratory Personnel

NcAMP nephrogenous cyclic adenosine monophosphate

N-CAP Nifedipine Gastrointestinal Therapeutic System Circadian Anti-Ischemic Program

NC/AT normal cephalic atraumatic

NCATS Nursing Child Assessment Teaching Scale

NCBA National Caucus on Black Aged

NCBF noncovalent bond finder

NCBI National Center for Biotechnology Information [NLM]

NCC National Certifying Corporation; New Computational Challenges Program; [National Science Foundation]; noncoronary cusp; nursing care continuity

ncc noncoronary cusp

NCCAM National Center for Complementary and Alternative Medicine

NCCAOM National Certification Commission for Acupuncture and Oriental Medicine

NCCDC National Center for Chronic Disease Control

NCCDPHP National Center for Chronic Disease Prevention and Health Promotion

NCCEA Neurosensory Center Comprehensive Examination for Aphasia

NCCH National Council of Community Hospitals

NCCIP National Center for Clinical Infant Program

NCCLS National Committee for Clinical Laboratory Standards

NCCLVP National Coordinating Committee on Large Volume Parenterals

NCCMHC National Council for Community Mental Health Centers

NCCN National Comprehensive Cancer Network

NCCPA National Commission on Certification of Physician Assistants

NCCRA National Colorectal Cancer Research Alliance

NCCS National Coalition for Cancer Survivorship

NCCT noncontrast computed tomography

NCCTG North Central Cancer Treatment Group

NCCU newborn convalescent care unit

NCD National Commission on Diabetes; National Council on Drugs; neurocirculatory dystonia; nitrogen clearance delay; noncommunicable disease; normal childhood disorder; not considered disabling

NCDA National Council on Drug Abuse

ncDCIS noncomedo-type ductal carcinoma in situ

NCDS National Child Development Study

NCDV Nebraska calf diarrhea virus

NCE Na^+/Ca^{2+} exchange; negative contrast echocardiography; new chemical entity; nonconvulsive epilepsy; normochromatic erythrocyte

NCEH National Center for Environmental Health

NCEP National Center for Environmental Protection; National Cholesterol Education Program

NCEPOD National Confidential Enquiry into Peri-Operative Deaths [study]

NCES National Childhood Encephalopathy Study [UK]; Netherlands Cost-Effectiveness Study

NCF neutrophil chemotactic factor

NCFA Narcolepsy and Catalepsy Foundation of America

NCF(C) neutrophil chemotactic factor (complement)

NCG nanochannel glass

NCH National Claims History [Medicare data file]; nursing care hours

NCHC National Council of Health Centers

NCHCA National Commission for Health Certifying Agencies

NCHCT National Center for Health Care Technology; noncontrast helical computed tomography

NCHD National Claims History Database

NCHECR National Centre in Human Immunodeficiency Virus [HIV] Epidemiology and Clinical Research [Australia]

NCHGR National Center for Human Genome Research

NCHLS National Council of Health Laboratory Services

NCHPD National Council on Health Planning and Development

NCHS National Center for Health Statistics

NCHSR National Center for Health Services Research

NCI National Cancer Institute; noncriterion ischemic [animal]; nuclear contour index; nursing care integration

nCi nanocurie

NCIB National Collection of Industrial Bacteria

NCIC National Cancer Institute of Canada

NCIC CTG National Cancer Institute of Canada Clinical Trial Group

NCID National Center for Infectious Diseases

NCI DIS 2D National Cancer Institute Drug Information System for 2-dimensional substructure searching

NCIH National Council for International Health

NCIMB National Collection of Industrial and Marine Bacteria [UK]

NCIPC National Center for Injury Prevention and Control

NCIRS National Cancer Incidence Reporting System [Canada]; National Centre for Immunisation Research and Surveillance [Australia]

NC-IUB Nomenclature Committee of the International Union of Biochemistry

NCJ needle catheter jejunostomy

NCKHEkg note chemistry and hematology, laboratory values, and electrocardiographic findings

NCL neuronal ceroid-lipofuscinosis; noncoronary leaflet; nucleolin

NCLEX-RN National Council Licensure Examination for Registered Nurses

NCM nailfold capillary microscopy; nurse case manager

N/cm² newtons per square centimeter

NCMC natural cell-mediated cytotoxicity

NCMH National Committee for Mental Health

NCMHI National Clearinghouse for Mental Health Information

NCMI National Committee Against Mental Illness

NCN National Cardiovascular Network; National Council of Nurses

NCNR National Center for Nursing Research

NCO/CIC National Coordinating Office for Computing, Information, and Communication

NCoR, N-CoR nuclear receptor compressor

NCP neuro-cybernetic prosthesis [neurostimulator]; Nijmegen Classification of Pain; noncollagen protein

N-CPAP, n-CPAP nasal continuous positive airway pressure

NCPDP National Council on Prescription Drug Programs

NCPE noncardiac pulmonary edema

NCPF National Collection of Pathogenic Fungi [UK]; noncirrhotic portal fibrosis

NCPI National Clearinghouse for Primary Care Information

NCPIM National Commission to Prevent Infant Mortality

NCPP National Collaborative Perinatal Project

NCPPB National Collection of Plant Pathogenic Bacteria

NCQA National Committee for Quality Assurance

NCR National Research Council; neutrophil chemotactic response; no carbon required; noncoding region; normotensive control rat; nuclear/cytoplasmic ratio

NCRND National Committee for Research in Neurological Diseases

NCRP National Council on Radiation Protection [and Measurements]

NCRR National Center for Research Resources

NCRSP National Congenital Rubella Surveillance Programme [UK]

NCRV National Committee for Radiation Victims

NCS National Collaborative Study; neocarcinostatin; nerve conduction study;

neurocutaneous syndrome; newborn calf serum; no concentrated sweets; non-coronary sinus; noncircumferential stenosis; nystagmus compensation syndrome

NCSA National Center for Supercomputer Applications; National Computational Science Alliance

NCSBN National Council of State Boards of Nursing

NCSE nonconvulsive status epilepticus

NCSI number of combined spherical irradiation

NCSN National Council for School Nurses

NCT neural crest tumor

NCTC National Cancer Tissue Culture; National Collection of Type Cultures [UK]

NCTR National Center for Toxicological Research

NCV nerve conduction velocity; noncholera vibrio

NCVHS National Committee on Vital and Health Statistics

NCVIA National Childhood Vaccine Injury Act

NCVS nerve conduction velocity study

NCX sodium-calcium exchanger

NCYC National Collection of Yeast Cultures [UK]

ND Doctor of Naturopathy; nasal deformity; natural death; Naval Dispensary; neonatal death; neoplastic disease; neurologic deficit; neuropsychological deficit; neurotic depression; neutral density; new drug; Newcastle disease; newly dead; no data; no disease; nondetectable; nondiabetic; nondiagnostic; nondisabling; normal delivery; normal development; Norrie disease; nose drops; not detected, not determined; not diagnosed; not done; nurse's diagnosis; nutritionally deprived

N/D no defects; not done

N&D nodular and diffuse

N$_D$, n$_D$ refractive index

Nd neodymium

n$_D$ refractive index

NDA National Dental Association; New Drug Application; no data available; no detectable activity; no detectable antibody

NDAC not data accepted

NDATUS National Drug and Alcoholism Treatment Unit Survey

NDBA *N*-nitrosodibutylamine

NDC National Data Communications; national drug classification; National Drug Code; National Drug Council; Naval Dental Clinic; nicotine dependence center; nondifferentiated cell

NDCD National Drug Code Directory

NDCG Nursing Development Conference Group

NDD no dialysis days

NDDIC National Digestive Disease Information Clearinghouse

NDDG National Diabetes Data Group

NDE near-death experience; nondestructive evaluation; nondiabetic extremity

NDEC nursing diagnosis extension and classification

NDEKF node-decoupled extended Kalman filtering

NDEV Ndelle virus

NDF neutrophil diffraction factor; new dosage form; no diagnostic findings; no disease found

NDFDA nonadecafluoro-*n*-decanoic acid

NDGA nordihydroguaiaretic acid

NDHPCCB non-dihydropyridine calcium channel blocker

NDHS National Diet-Heart Study

NDI nephrogenic diabetes insipidus

NDIC National Diabetes Information Clearinghouse

NDIR nondispersive infrared analyzer

NDM naturalistic decision making

NDMA nitrosodimethylamine

NDMR nondepolarizing muscle relaxant

nDNA nuclear deoxyribonucleic acid

NDNQI National Database of Nursing Quality Indicators

NDP net dietary protein; nucleoside diphosphate

NDPK nucleoside diphosphate kinase

NDPKA nucleoside diphosphate kinase A

NDPKB nucleoside diphosphate kinase B

NDR neonatal death rate; normal detrusor reflex

NDRC National Defense Research Committee

NDRF endothelium-derived relaxing factor

NDRI National Disease Research Interchange

NDS Naval Dental School; neurologic deficit score; new drug submission; normal dog serum; Novell Directory Services

NDSB Narcotic Drugs Supervisory Board
NDSSC National Dietary Survey of School Children
NDST *N*-deacetylase *N*-sulfotransferase
NDT neurodevelopmental treatment; noise detection threshold; nondestructive test, nondestructive testing
NDTI National Disease and Therapeutic Index
NDTM National Database of Telemedicine [UK]
NDUV Ndumu virus
NDV Newcastle disease virus; Nyando virus
NDVI normalized difference vegetation index
Nd/YAG, Nd-YAG neodymium-yttrium-aluminum garnet
NE national emergency; nausea and emesis; necrotic enteritis; necrotizing enterocolitis; neonatal encephalopathy; nephropathia epidemica; nerve ending; nerve excitation; neuroendocrine; neuroendocrinology; neuroepithelium; neurological examination; neutropenic enterocolitis; neutrophil elastase; niacin equivalent; no effect; no excision; no excitation; no exposure; nocturnal exacerbation; nonelastic; nonendogenous; noninvasive evaluation; norepinephrine; not elevated; not enlarged; not equal; not evaluated; not examined; not exposed; nuclear extract; nurse executive; nutcracker esophagus
Ne neon
NEA neoplasm embryonic antigen; no evidence of abnormality
NEAR National Emergency Airway Registry
NEAS nonerythroid alpha spectrin
NEAT Neurohumoral Effects in Acute Myocardial Infarction of Trandolapril [study]; non-exercise activity thermogenesis
NEB nebulin; neuroendocrine body; neuroepithelial body
NEC National Electrical Code; necrotizing enterocolitis; neuroendocrine cell; neuroendocrine convertase; no essential changes; non-effect concentration; nonesterified cholesterol; not elsewhere classified or classifiable; nursing ethics committee
NECHI Northeastern Consortium for Health Information

NECR noise-effective count rate
NECT non-enhanced computed tomography
NED no-effect dose; no evidence of disease; no expiration date; normal equivalent deviation
NEDEL no epidemiologically detectable exposure level
NEDSS National Electronic Disease Surveillance System
NEDV North End virus
NEE needle electrode examination
NEEE Near East equine encephalomyelitis
NEEP negative end-expiratory pressure
NEET Nordic Enalapril Exercise Trial
NEF, NeF nephritic factor
NEFA nonesterified fatty acid
NEFH heavy polypeptide of neurofilament protein
NEFL light polypeptide of neurofilament protein
NEFM medium polypeptide of neurofilament protein
neg negative
NEGF neurite growth-promoting factor
NEHE Nurses for Environmental Health Education
NEI National Eye Institute
NEISS National Electronic Injury Surveillance System
NEJ neuroeffector junction
NEJM New England Journal of Medicine
NEL non-effect level
NeLH National Electronic Library for Health [UK]
NEM nemaline; *N*-ethylmaleimide; no evidence of malignancy
nem nutritional milk unit [Ger. *Nahrungs Einheit Milch*]
NEMA National Eclectic Medical Association
nema nematode
NEMAS Nursing Education Modular Authoring System
NEMC-PCR New England Medical Center Posterior Circulation Registry
NEMD nonspecific esophageal motor dysfunction
NEMS nine equivalents of nursing manpower use score
Neo neomycin; neoplasm or neoplastic
neo neoarsphenamine

NEP needle exchange program; negative expiratory pressure; nephrology; neutral endopeptidase; no evidence of pathology

nep nephrectomy

NEPA National Environmental Policy Act

Neph nephron; nephritis; nephrosis

NEPHGE nonequilibrated pH gradient electrophoresis

NEPV Nepuyo virus

NEQ noise equivalent quantum

NEQAS National External Quality Assessment Scheme [for blood coagulation, UK]

NERHL Northeastern Radiological Health Laboratory

NER no evidence of recurrence; nucleotide excision repair

NERD no evidence of recurrent disease; non-erosive reflux disease

ner nervous

NERO noninvasive evaluation of radiation output

NERSC National Energy Research Supercomputer Center

NES night eating syndrome; not elsewhere specified

NESH Network for Ecosystem Sustainability and Health

NESO Northeastern Society of Orthodontists

NESP novel erythrocyte stimulating protein; Nurse Education Support Program

NEST Nuclear Emergency Search Team

NET nasoendotracheal tube; nerve excitability test; neuroectodermal tumor; neuroendocrine tumor; norepinephrine transporter

NETI nasotracheal endotracheal intubation

NETRHA North-East Thames Regional Health Authority [study]

NETS National Eye Trauma System; Network for Employers for Traffic Safety

NETT National Emphysema Treatment Trial

NETV Netivot virus

NEU, Neu neuraminidase

neu neurilemma

NeuN neuronal nucleus

neur, neuro, neurol neurology, neurological, neurologist

neuropath neuropathology

neut neuter, neutral; neutrophil

NEVADA Numerical Evaluation of Variance and Dependence Simulation

NEWDILTIL New Diltiazem vs Tildiem [study]

NEXT New European XT Stent Registry

NEXUS National Emergency X-radiography Utilization Study

NEY neomycin egg yolk [agar]

NEYA neomycin egg yolk agar

NF nafcillin; National Formulary; nephritic factor; neurofibromatosis; neurofilament; neutral fraction; neutrophilic factor; noise factor; normal flow; not filtered; not found; nuclear factor; nucleolar frequency [number of nucleoli per 100 nuclei]

nF nanofarad

NF1 neurofibromatosis type I; neurofibromin gene; nuclear factor 1

NF2 neurofibromatosis type II

NFA National Fire Academy; near-fatal asthma; nuclear factor A

NFAIS National Federation of Abstracting and Indexing Services

NFAR no further action required

N-FAS neurogenic fetal akinesia sequence

NFAT, NF-AT nuclear factor of activated T [cells]

NFATp pre-existing subunit of nuclear factor of activated T [cells]

NFB National Foundation for the Blind; nonfermenting bacteria

NFBM normalized fractional brownian motion

NFC National Fertility Center

NFCE near-fatal choking episode

NFCS Nationwide Food Consumption Survey

NFD neurofibrillary degeneration

NFDR neurofaciodigitorenal [syndrome]

NFE nonferrous extract

NFH heavy polypeptide of neurofilament protein; nonfamilial hematuria

NFI near field imaging

NFIC National Foundation for Ileitis and Colitis

NFID National Foundation for Infectious Diseases

NFIRS National Fire Incident Reporting System

NFJ Naegeli-Franceschetti-Jadassohn [syndrome]

NFK nuclear factor kappa

NFKB, NF-kB, NF-κB nuclear factor κB [of pre-B cell]

NFL nerve fiber layer; neurofilament protein, light polypeptide

NFLD nerve fiber layer defect

NFLPN National Federation of Licensed Practical Nurses

NFM neurofilament protein, medium polypeptide

NFMD National Foundation for Muscular Dystrophy

NFND National Foundation for Neuromuscular Diseases

NFNID National Foundation for Non-Invasive Diagnostics

NFNS, NF-NS neurofibromatosis-Noonan syndrome

NFP natural family planning; no family physician; not-for-profit [hospital]; nurse-family partnership

NFS National Fertility Study; [computer] network file system; neural foraminal stenosis; no fracture seen

NFT neurofibrillary tangle; no further treatment

NFTD normal full term delivery

NFTT neurogenic failure to thrive

NFW nursed fairly well

NFX nuclear factor X

NG nasogastric; *Neisseria gonorrhoeae*; neoplastic growth; new growth; nitroglycerin; nodose ganglion; no growth; not given

N/G nasogastric

Ng *Neisseria gonorrhoeae*

ng nanogram

NGA nutrient gelatin agar

NGAST Nimodipine German-Austrian Stroke Trial

NGAV Ngaingan virus

NGBE neuraminidase/beta-galactosidase expression

NGC National Guidelines Clearinghouse [database]; nerve guidance conduit; nucleus reticularis gigantocellularis

NgCAM neuron glial cell adhesion molecule

NGF nerve growth factor

NGFA nerve growth factor alpha

NGFB nerve growth factor beta

NGFG nerve growth factor gamma

NGFIA nerve growth factor-induced clone A

NGFIC nerve growth factor-induced clone C

NGFR nerve growth factor receptor

NGGR nonglucogenic/glucogenic ratio

NGI Next Generation Internet; nuclear globulin inclusions

NGIX next generation Internet exchange points

NGL neutral glycolipid

ng/mL nanograms per milliliter

NGO nongovernmental organization

NGOV Ngoupe virus

NGPA nursing grade point average

NGR narrow gauze roll; nasogastric replacement

NGS next generation software; normal goat serum

NGSA nerve growth stimulating activity

NGSF nongenital skin fibroblast

NGSVd *Nicotiana glutinosa* stunt viroid

NGT nasogastric tube; nominal group technique; normal glucose tolerance

NGU nongonococcal urethritis

NGVL National Gene Vector Laboratories

NH natriuretic hormone; Naval Hospital; neonatal hemochromatosis; neonatal hepatitis; neurologically handicapped; nocturnal hypoventilation; node of His; nonhuman; nursing home

N(H) proton density

NHA National Health Association; National Hearing Association; National Hemophilia Association; nonspecific hepatocellular abnormality; nursing home administrator

NHAAP National Heart Attack Alert Program

NHAMCS National Hospital Ambulatory Medical Care Survey

NHANES National Health and Nutrition Examination Survey

NHB National Health Board

NHBCD non-heart-beating cadaver donor

NHBE normal human bronchial epithelial [cell]

NHBPCC National High Blood Pressure Coordinating Committee

NHBPEP National High Blood Pressure Education Program

NHC National Health Council; neighborhood health center; neonatal hypocalcemia; nonhistone chromosomal [protein]; nursing home care

NHCMQ multistate nursing home case-mix and quality
NHCP nonhistone chromosomal protein
NHCS National Health Care Survey
NHD non-Hodgkin disease; normal hair distribution
NHDC National Hansen's Disease Center
NHDF neonatal human dermal fibroblast; normal human diploid fibroblast
NHDL non–high-density lipoprotein
NHDS National Health Data System; National Hospital Discharge Survey
NHE National Health Expenditure; nonhemolytic enterotoxin; sodium-hydrogen exchanger
NHE 1, 2, 3, 4, 5, 6 sodium-hydrogen exchangers, isoforms 1 to 6
NHEFS National Epidemiologic Follow-up Study
NHES National Health Examination Survey
NHF National Health Federation; National Heart Foundation [Australia]; National Hemophilia Foundation; non-immune hydrops fetalis; normal human fibroblast
NHG normal human globulin
NHGB net hepatic glucose balance
NHGJ normal human gastric juice
NHGRI National Human Genome Research Institute
NHH neurohypophyseal hormone
NHHCS National Home and Hospice Care Survey
NHI National Heart Institute; nuclear hepatobiliary imaging
NHIC National Health Information Council [Canada]
NHIF National Head Injury Foundation
NHIS National Health Interview Survey
NHIS-YRB National Health Interview Survey-Your Risk Behavior
NHK normal human kidney
NHL nodular histiocytic lymphoma; non-Hodgkin lymphoma
NHLA National Health Lawyers Association
NHLBI National Heart, Lung and Blood Institute
NHLBI II National Heart, Lung and Blood Institute Type II [coronary intervention study]

NHLBI-ICD National Heart, Lung and Blood Institute Implantable Cardioverter Defibrillator [trial]
NHLBI-PTCA National Heart, Lung and Blood Institute Percutaneous Transluminal Coronary Angioplasty [registry]
NHLBITS National Heart, Lung and Blood Institute Twin Study
NHLI National Heart and Lung Institute [NIH]
NHML non-Hodgkin malignant lymphoma
NHMRC National Health and Medical Research Council [Australia]
NHP National Hypertension Project [Egypt]; nonhemoglobin protein; nonhistone protein; normal human pooled plasma; Nottingham Health Profile; nursing home placement
NHPC National Health Planning Council
NHPF National Health Policy Forum
NHPIC National Health Planning Information Center
NHPP nonhomogeneous poison processes
NHPPD nursing hours per patient day
NHPPN National Health Professions Placement Network
NHQRA Nursing Home Quality Reform Act
NHR net histocompatibility ratio
NHRA Nursing Home Reform Act
NHRC National Health Research Center
NHS Nance-Horan syndrome; Nasu-Hakola syndrome; National Health Service [UK]; National Hospice Study; natural history; normal horse serum; normal human serum; Nurses' Health Study
NHS-1 First Natural History Study [of congenital heart defects]
NHS-2 Second Natural History Study [of congenital heart defects]
NHSAS National Health Service Audit Staff
NHSC National Health Service Corps
NHS CCC National Health Service Centre for Coding and Classification [UK]
NHSIA National Health Service [NHS] Information Authority [UK]
NHSR National Hospital Service Reserve
NHSTD National Health Service Training Division [UK]
NHT nonpenetrating head trauma

NHTSA National Highway Traffic Safety Administration

NHVR normalized hepatic vascular resistance

NI neuraminidase inhibition; neurological improvement; neutralization index; no information; noise index; noninducible; not identified; not isolated; nursing informatics; nucleus intercalatus

NIA National Institute on Aging; nephelometric inhibition assay; neuroleptic-induced akathisia; niacin; no information available; Nutritional Institute of America

nia niacin

NIAAA National Institute on Alcohol Abuse and Alcoholism

NIADDK National Institute of Arthritis, Diabetes, Digestive and Kidney Diseases

NIAID National Institute of Allergy and Infectious Diseases

NIAMDD National Institute of Arthritis, Metabolism, and Digestive Diseases

NIAMS National Institute of Arthritis, Musculoskeletal and Skin Diseases

NIAP National Information Assurance Partnership

NIB National Institute for the Blind

NIBP noninvasive blood pressure [monitoring]

NIBSC National Institute for Biological Standards and Control

NIC National Informatics Center; neonatal intensive care; network interface card; neurogenic intermittent claudication; neurointensive care; newborn intensive care; nursing interim care; nursing interventions classification

NICD National Information Center on Deafness

NICET National Institute of Certification in Engineering Technologies

NICHCY National Information Center for Children and Youth with Disabilities

NIC-HFH Nephrology Information Center at Henry Ford Hospital

NICHHD National Institute of Child Health and Human Development

NICHSR National Center on Health Services Research

NICOLE Nisoldipine in Coronary Artery Disease in Leuven

NICT new information and communication technology

NICU neonatal intensive care unit; neurointensive care unit; neurological intensive care unit; neurosurgical intensive care unit; nonimmunologic contact urticaria

NID National Immunization Day; nidogen; no identifiable disease; nonimmunological disease; not in distress; number of intervals to fulfill detection [of ventricular fibrillation]

NIDA National Institute of Drug Abuse

NIDCD National Institute of Deafness and Other Communication Disorders

NIDCR National Institute of Dental and Craniofacial Research

NIDD non-insulin-dependent diabetes

NIDDK National Institute of Diabetes and Digestive and Kidney Diseases

NIDDM non-insulin-dependent diabetes mellitus

NIDDY non-insulin-dependent diabetes in the young

NIDM National Institute for Disaster Mobilization

NIDR National Institute of Dental Research

NIDRR National Institute on Disability and Rehabilitation Research

NIDS nonionic detergent soluble

NIDSEC Nursing Information and Data Set Evaluation Center

NIEHS National Institutes of Environmental Health Sciences

NIEPS noninvasive electrophysiological study

NIH neointimal hyperplasia

NIHAS Northern Ireland Health and Activity Survey

NIF negative inspiratory force; neutrophil immobilizing factor; nonintestinal fibroblast

Nig non-immunoglobulin

nig black [Lat. *niger*]

NIGMS National Institute of General Medical Sciences

NIH National Institutes of Health

NIHL noise-induced hearing loss

Ni-Hon-San Nipponese in Honolulu and San Francisco [comparative cardiovascular disease rate in Japanese-Americans living in Honolulu and San Francisco]

NIHR National Institute of Handicapped Research

NIHS National Institute of Hypertension Studies

NIH-SS NIH Stroke Scale

NII National Information Infrastructure; National Insurance Institute

NIIC National Injury Information Clearinghouse

NII-HIN National Information Infrastructure-Health Information Network

NIIS National Institute of Infant Services

NIL noise interference level

NILT Nursing Intervention Lexicon and Toxonomy

NIMBY not in my backyard

NIMH National Institute of Mental Health

NIMP National Intern Matching Program

NIMR National Institute for Medical Research

NIMS National Infant Mortality Surveillance

NINCDS National Institute of Neurological and Communicative Disorders and Stroke

NINCDS/ADRDA National Institute of Neurological and Communicative Diseases and Stroke/Alzheimer's Disease and Related Disorders Association

NINDB National Institute of Neurological Diseases and Blindness

NINDS National Institute of Neurological Disorders and Stroke

NINDS-TPAST National Institute of Neurological Disorders and Stroke-Tissue Plasminogen Activator Stroke Trial

NIOSH National Institute for Occupational Safety and Health

NIOSHTIC National Institute for Occupational Safety and Health Technical Information Center

NIP National Immunization Program; negative inspiratory pressure; nipple; no infection present; no inflammation present; nonimmigrant patient

NIP AAm *N*-isopropylacrylamide

NIPALS nonlinear iterative partial least square

NIPH National Institute of Public Health

NIPPV noninvasive positive pressure ventilation

NIPS neuroleptic-induced Parkinson syndrome; noninvasive programmed [heart] stimulation

NIPTS noise-induced permanent threshold shift

NIR near infrared; New Intravascular Rigid Stent Trial

nIR non-insulin-resistance

NIRA nitrite reductase; Nursing Incentives Reimbursement Award

NIRB non-institutional review board

NIRCA nonisotopic ribonuclease cleavage assay

NIRD nonimmune renal disease

NIRMP National Intern and Resident Matching Program

NIRNS National Institute for Research in Nuclear Science

NIRS near-infrared spectroscopy; normal inactivated rabbit serum

NIRVANA NIR Primo Stent Vascular Advanced North America [trial]

NIS nationwide inpatient sample; National Immunization Survey; near-infrared intracranial spectroscopy; network information system; *N*-iodosuccinimide; no inflammatory signs; nursing information system

NI-SIG nursing informatics special interest group

NISO National Information Standards Organization

NISSO Netherlands Institute for Social Sexological Research

NIST National Institute of Standards and Technology [Department of Commerce]

NIT National Intelligence Test; Nutrition Intervention Trial

NITA National Telecommunications and Information Administration

NITD noninsulin-treated disease

nit nitrous

nitro nitroglycerin

NIV nodule-inducing virus; noninvasive ventilation

NIW nursing intensity weights

NIWG Nursing Informatics Workshop Group

NJ nasojejunal; neighbor joining

nJ nanojoule

NJLV Naranjal virus

NJPC National Joint Practice Commission

NK Commission on [Anatomical] Nomenclature [Ger. *Nomenklatur Kommission*]; natural killer [cell]; neurokinin; not known

n/k not known

NK2 neurokinin 2

NKA neurokinin A; no known allergies

nkat nanokatal

NKB neurokinin B

NKC nonketotic coma

NKCA natural killer cell activity

NKCF natural killer cytotoxic factor

NKDA no known drug allergies

NKE sodium [Na$^+$]/potassium [K$^+$] exchange

NKFA no known food allergies

NKH nonketogenic hyperglycemia; nonketotic hyperosmotic

NKHA nonketotic hyperosmolar acidosis

NKHS nonketotic hyperosmolar syndrome; normal Krebs-Henseleit solution

NKN neurokinin

NKNA neurokinin A

NKNAR neurokinin A receptor

NKNB neurokinin B

NKOV Nkolbisson virus

NKP North Karelia Project

NKSF natural killer cell stimulatory factor

NKTR natural killer triggering receptor

NL natural language; neural lobe; neutral lipid; no direct link [UMLS]; nodular lymphoma; normal; normal libido; normal limits

nL nanoliter

nl normal [value]

NLA National Leukemia Association; neuroleptoanesthesia; normal lactase activity

nLAG nuclear localized β-galactosidase

NLANR National Laboratory for Applied Network Research

NLB needle liver biopsy

NLD nasolacrimal duct; necrobiosis lipoidica diabeticorum

NLDL normal low-density lipoprotein

NLE neonatal lupus erythematosus

Nle norleucine

NLEA Nutrition Labeling and Education Act

NLF nasolabial fold; neonatal lung fibroblast; nonlactose fermentation

NLG natural language generation

NLH nodular lymphoid hyperplasia

NLK neuroleukin

NLL nonlymphoblastic leukemia

NLLS nonlinear least squares

NLM National Library of Medicine; noise level monitor

NLMC nocturnal leg muscle cramp

NLMS National Longitudinal Mortality Study

nLMS normalized least mean square

NLN National League of Nursing; no longer needed

NLNE National League for Nursing Education

NLP natural language processing; neurolinguistic programming; no light perception; nodular liquefying panniculitis; normal light perception; normal luteal phase

NLS Names Learning Test; National Longitudinal Surveys [database]; neonatal lupus syndrome; Neu-Laxova syndrome; nonlinear least squares; normal lymphocyte supernatant; nuclear localization signal

NLSC National Longitudinal Survey of Children [Canada]

NLSCY National Longitudinal Survey of Children and Youth [Canada]

NLSQ nonlinear least square

NLT normal lymphocyte transfer; not later than; not less than; novel liver-specific transporter protein; nucleus lateralis tuberis

nlt not later than; not less than

NLTCS National Long Term Care Survey

NL2SOL nonlinear least square algorithm

NLUS natural language understanding system

NLX naloxone; nephrolithiasis, X-linked

NM near-miss; neomycin; neuromedical; neuromedin; neuromuscular; neuronal microdysgenesis; neuronal mode; neutrophil migration; nictitating membrane; nitrogen mustard; nocturnal myoclonus; nodular melanoma; nodules with microcalcifications; nonmotile; normetanephrine; not malignant; not measurable, not measured; not mentioned; not motile; nuclear medicine; [technologist in] nuclear medicine; nurse manager; nurse/midwife

N-m newton-meter

N&M nerves and muscles; night and morning

N/m newtons per meter

N × m newton meters
N/m² newtons per square meter
nM nanomolar
nm nanometer; night and morning [Lat. *nocte et mane*]
NMA National Malaria Association; National Medical Association; neurogenic muscular atrophy; *N*-nitroso-*N*-methylalanine
nMA nondominant motor area
NMAC National Medical Audiovisual Center
NM(ASCP) Technologist in Nuclear Medicine certified by the American Society of Clinical Pathologists
NMB neuromedin B; neuromuscular blockade; neuromuscular blocking; neuromuscular blocker/blocking [drug, agent]
NMBA neuromuscular blocking agent
NMBR neuromedin B receptor
NMC National Medical Care; Naval Medical Center; neuromuscular control; nonmotor condition; nucleus reticularis magnocellularis
NMCC nasal mucociliary clearance
NMCES National Medical Care Expenditure Survey
NMCUES National Medical Care Utilization and Expenditure Survey
NMD neuromyodysplasia; neuronal migration disorder
NMDA *N*-methyl-D-aspartate
NMDAR *N*-methyl-D-aspartate receptor
NmDG *N*-methyl-D-glutamine
NMDS Nursing Minimum Data Set
NMDSN Nursing Minimum Data Set for the Netherlands
NME National Medical Enterprises; neuromyeloencephalopathy
NMEP neurogenic motor evoked potential
NMES National Medical Expenditure Survey [database]; neuromuscular electrical stimulation
NMF *N*-methylformamide; National Medical Fellowship; National Migraine Foundation; nonmigrating fraction
NMFF Northwestern Medical Faculty Foundation
NMFI National Master Facility Inventory
NMHCA National Mental Health Consumers' Association
NMI no mental illness; normal male infant

NMIHS National Maternal and Infant Health Survey
NMIS nursing management information system
NMJ neuromuscular junction
NML nodular mixed lymphoma
NMM nodular malignant melanoma
NMMDS nursing management minimum data set
NMN nicotinamide mononucleotide; normetanephrine
NMNRU National Medical Neuropsychiatric Research Unit
nmol nanomole
nmol/L nanomoles per liter
NMOR nemadione oxidoreductase; *N*-nitrosomorpholine
NMOS N-type metal oxide semiconductor
NMP normal menstrual period; nuclear matrix protein; nucleoside monophosphate
NMPC nonlinear model predictive control
NMPCA nonmetric principal component analysis
NMPTP *N*-methyl-4-phenyl-1,2,3,6-tetrahydropyridine
NMR national medical resources; neonatal mortality rate; nictitating membrane response; nuclear magnetic resonance
NMRC NeuroMuscular Research Center
NMRD nuclear magnetic relaxation dispersion
NMRDC Naval Medical Research and Development Command
NMRI Naval Medical Research Institute; nuclear magnetic resonance imaging
NMRL Naval Medical Research Laboratory
NMRS nuclear magnetic resonance spectroscopy
NMRU Naval Medical Research Unit
NMS Naval Medical School; neuroleptic malignant syndrome; neuromuscular spindle; *N*-methylscopolamine; normal mouse serum; Norwegian Multicenter Study
N · m/s newton meters per second
NMSC nonmelanoma skin cancer
NMSE normalized mean square error
NMSIDS near-miss sudden infant death syndrome

NMSS National Multiple Sclerosis Society; National Mycobacterial Surveillance System [Australia and New Zealand]

NMT neuromuscular tension; neuromuscular transmission; N-methyltransferase; N-myristoyltransferase; no more than; nuclear medicine technology or technologist

NMTCB Nuclear Medicine Technology Certification Board

NMTD nonmetastatic trophoblastic disease

NMTS neuromuscular tension state; nuclear matrix-targeting signal

NMU neuromuscular unit; nitrosomethylurea

NMV New Minto virus

NN nearest neighbor; neonatal; neural network or net; neuronavigation; nevocellular nevus; normal nutrition; normally not notifiable; nourished; nuclear/nuclear [ratio]; nurse's notes

N/N normocytic/normochromic [anemia]

nN nanonewton

nn nerves; new name [Lat. *nomen novum*]

NN-A nearest neighbor algorithm

NNAS neonatal narcotic abstinence syndrome

NNC National Nutrition Consortium

NND neonatal death; New and Nonofficial Drugs; nonspecific nonerosive duodenitis

NNDC National Naval Dental Center

NNDSS National Notifiable Diseases Surveillance Scheme [Australia and New Zealand]

NNE neonatal necrotizing enterocolitis; nonneuronal enolase; normalized noise energy

NNEB National Nursery Examination Board

NNG nonspecific nonerosive gastritis

NNH number needed to harm

NNHS National Nursing Home Survey

NNI noise and number index

NNIS National Nosocomial Infection Surveillance

NNIWG National Nursing Informatics Work Group

NNJ neonatal jaundice

NNK neural network Kubicek [equation]

NNLIT North Norwegian Lidocaine Intervention Trial

NN/LM National Network of Libraries of Medicine

NNM neonatal mortality

NNMC National Naval Medical Center

NNMT nicotinamide N-methyltransferase; Norwegian Nifedipine Multicenter Trial

NNN Novy-MacNeal-Nicolle [medium]

NNNMU N-nitroso-N-methylurethane

NNO no new orders

nNOS neuronal nitric oxide synthase

n nov new name [Lat. *nomen novum*]

NNP neonatal nurse practitioner; nerve net pulse

NNQ number needed to quit

NNR New and Nonofficial Remedies

NNRTI nonnucleoside reverse transcriptase inhibitor

NNS neural network Sramek [equation]; nicotine nasal spray; nonneoplastic syndrome

NNS III Third Nationwide Nutritional Survey [China, 1992]

NNT nuclei nervi trigemini; number needed to treat

NNU neonatal unit

NNWI Neonatal Narcotic Withdrawal Index

NO narcotics officer; nitric or nitrous oxide; none obtained; nonobese; nurse's office

No nobelium

No, no number [Lat. *numero*]

NOA National Optometric Association; nitro-L-arginine

NOABX no antibiotics

NOAEL no observed adverse effect level

NOAH New York Online Access to Health

NOAPP National Organization of Adolescent Pregnancy and Parenting

N$_{obs}$ number of observations

NOBT nonoperative biopsy technique

NOC N-nitroso compound; not otherwise classified; nursing outcomes classification

NOCDQ nursing organizational climate description questionnaire

NOD Naito-Oyanagi disease; National Organization on Disability; nodular melanoma; nonobese diabetic [mouse]; notify of death

NOE naso-orbital-ethmoid [fracture]; nuclear Overhauser effect

NOEC no observed effect concentration

NOEL no observed effect level

NOES National Occupational Exposure Survey

NOESY nuclear Overhauser effect spectroscopy

NOF National Osteopathic Foundation; National Osteoporosis Foundation

NOFT nonorganic failure-to-thrive

NOHS National Occupational Hazards Survey

NOII nonocclusive intestinal ischemia

NOK next of kin

NOL nitric oxide level

NOLAV Nola virus

nom dub a doubtful name [Lat. *nomen dubium*]

NOMI nonocclusive mesenteric infarction

NONMEM nonlinear mixed effects model

non-REM non-rapid eye movement [sleep]

NOP not otherwise provided for

NOPHN National Organization for Public Health Nursing

NOR Neurologic Outcome Research; noradrenaline; normal; nortriptyline; nucleolar organizer region

NORA Nordic Research on Aging

NORASEPT North American Sepsis Trial

NORC National Opinion Research Center

NORD National Organization for Rare Disorders

NORDIL Nordic Diltiazem [study]

NORDUnet Nordic Countries Network

NOR-EPI norepinephrine

norleu norleucine

NORM naturally occurring radioactive material

norm normal

NORML National Organization for the Reform of Marijuana Laws

NORV Northway virus

NOS network operating system; nitric oxide synthetase; non-organ-specific; not on staff; not otherwise specified

NOs nitric oxide synthetase

NOSAC nonsteroidal anti-inflammatory compound

NOSER Newton's one-step error reconstructor

NOSIC Neurologic Outcome Scale for Infants and Children

NOSIE Nurses' Observation Scale for Inpatient Evaluation

NOSTA Naval Ophthalmic Support and Training Activity

NOT nocturnal oxygen therapy

NOTB National Ophthalmic Treatment Board

NOTT Nocturnal Oxygen Therapy Trial

NOV Nodamura virus; Novantrone

nov n new name [Lat. *novum nomen*]

NOVS National Office of Vital Statistics

nov sp new species [Lat. *novum species*]

NOW network of workstations

NOWIS North Wurttemberg Infarction Study

NO$_x$ nitrogen oxide

NP 4-hydroxy-3-nitrophenylacetyl; nasopharynx, nasopharyngeal; natriuretic peptide; near point; necrotizing pancreatitis; neonatal-perinatal; nerve palsy; neuritic plague; neuropathic pain; neuropathology; neuropeptide; neurophysin; neuropsychiatry; new patient; newly presented; Niemann-Pick [disease]; nitrogen-phosphorus; nitrophenol; nitroprusside; no pain; no pressure; nonpalpable; nonparalytic; nonpathogenic; nonphagocytic; nonpracticing; no progress or progression; normal plasma; normal pressure; nosocomial pneumonia; not palpable; not perceptible; not performed; not pregnant; not present; not protected; nucleoplasmic; nucleoprotein; nucleoside phosphorylase; nurse practitioner; nursed poorly; nursing procedure; proper name [Lat. *nomen proprium*]

N-P need-persistence

Np neper; neptunium; neurophysin

np nucleotide pair

NPA nasopharyngeal airway; nasopharyngeal aspirate; National Pharmaceutical Association; National Pituitary Agency; near point accommodation; negative predictive accuracy; Nurse Practice Act

NPa nail-patella [syndrome]

nPA lanoteplase

NPACI National Partnership for Advanced Computational Infrastructure

NPA-NIHHDP National Pituitary Agency-National Institutes of Health Hormone Distribution Program

N$_{par}$ number of parameters

NPAT nonparoxysmal atrial tachycardia

NPB nodal premature beat; nonprotein bound

NPBF nonplacental blood flow

NPBV negative pressure body ventilator

NPC nasopharyngeal carcinoma; near point of convergence; neuroparacoccidioidomycosis; nodal premature contractions; nonparenchymal [liver] cell; nonphysician clinician; nonproductive cough; nucleus of posterior commissure; nursing protocol consultant

NPCa nasopharyngeal carcinoma

NPCP National Prostatic Cancer Project; non-*Pneumocystis carinii* pneumonia

NPCRDC National Primary Care Research and Development Centre [UK]

NP cult nasopharyngeal culture

NPD narcissistic personality disorder; natriuretic plasma dialysate; negative pressure device; Niemann-Pick disease; nitrogen-phosphorus detector; nonpathologic diagnosis; normal protein diet

NPDB National Practitioner Data Bank

NPDC neurofibromatosis-pheochromocytoma-duodenal carcinoid [syndrome]

NPDL nodular poorly differentiated lymphocytic

NPDR nonproliferative diabetic retinopathy

NPE neurogenic pulmonary edema; neuropsychologic examination; no palpable enlargement; normal pelvic examination

NPF nasopharyngeal fiberscope; National Parkinson Foundation; National Pharmaceutical Foundation; National Provider File; National Psoriasis Foundation; neuronal population function; no predisposing factor

NPFT Neurotic Personality Factor Test

NPGA niched Pareto algorithm

NPH nephrophthisis; neutral protamine Hagedorn (insulin) [not used anymore]; normal pressure hydrocephalus; nucleus pulposus herniation

NPHCE national personal health care expenditures

NPHDO Nadroparin Posthospital Discharge in Orthopedy [study]

NPHE natural phenomenon [UMLS]

NP HRF nasal pool histamine-releasing factor

NPHS National Population Health Survey [Canada]; Northwick Park Heart Study

NPhx nasopharynx

NPI Narcissistic Personality Inventory; National Provider Identifier; neuropsychiatric institution; neuropsychiatric

inventory; no present illness; nuclear polymorphism index; nucleoplasmic index

NPIC neurogenic peripheral intermittent claudication

NPII Neonatal Pulmonary Insufficiency Index

NPIP *N*-nitrosopiperidine

NPJT nonparoxysmal atrioventricular junctional tachycardia

NPK neuropeptide K

nPKC novel protein kinase C

NPL National Physics Laboratory; neoproteolipid

NPM nonpacemaker [cells]; nothing per mouth

NPN neural Petri net; nonprotein nitrogen

NPO nothing by mouth [Lat. *nil per os*]; nucleus preopticus

NPO/HS nothing by mouth at bedtime [Lat. *nil per os hora somni*]

NPOS nurses professional orientation scale

NPP nitrophenylphosphate; normal pool plasma; nucleus tegmenti pedunculopontinus

NPPase nucleotide pyrophosphatase

NPPC Nursing Professional Practice Council

NPPE negative pressure pulmonary edema

NPPH nucleotide pyrophosphohydrolase

NPPNG nonpenicillinase-producing *Neisseria gonorrhoeae*

NP polio nonparalytic poliomyelitis

NPPV noninvasive positive-pressure ventilation

NPR net protein ratio; normal pulse rate; nucleoside phosphoribosyl

NPRL Navy Prosthetics Research Laboratory

NPS nail-patella syndrome; nasopharyngeal secretion; National Pharmaceutical Stockpile; neonatal progeroid syndrome; noise power spectrum

NPSA normal pilosebaceous appartus

NPSH nonprotein sulhydryl [group]

NPT nasal provocation test; neoprecipitin test; nocturnal penile tumescence; normal pressure and temperature; sodium phosphate transport

NPTR National Pediatric Trauma Registry

NPU net protein utilization

NPUI nursing process utilization inventory

NPV negative predictive value; negative pressure value; negative pressure ventilation; net present value; nuclear polyhidrosis virus; nucleus paraventricularis

NPY neuropeptide Y

NPYR neuropeptide Y receptor; nitrosopyrrolidine

N pyr nitrosopyrrolidine

NQA nursing quality assurance

NQMI non-Q-wave myocardial infarction

NQO NAD(P)H:quinone oxidoreductase

4NQO 4-nitroquinoline 1-oxide

NQR nuclear quadruple resonance; reduced nicotinamide adenine dinucleotide [NADH] quinine reductase

NR do not repeat [Lat. *non repetatur*]; nerve root; neural retina; neutral red; noise reduction; no radiation; no reaction; no recurrence; no refill; no report; no respiration; no response; no result; nonmatch response; nonreactive; nonrebreathing; nonresponder; nonretarded; normal range; normal reaction; normotensive rat; not readable; not recorded; not reported; not resolved; nurse; nursing [service]; nutrition ratio; Reynold's number

N/R not remarkable

N$_R$ Reynold's number

NR50 neutral red 50%

nr near

NRA nitrate reductase; nucleus retroambigualis

NRASMC neonatal rat aortic smooth muscle cell

NRB nonrejoining break; nursing reference base

NRBC National Rare Blood Club; normal red blood cell; nucleated red blood cell

NRbc nucleated red blood cell

NRC National Red Cross; National Research Council [Canada]; National Response Center; normal retinal correspondence; not routine care; Nuclear Regulatory Commission

NRCAM National Resource for Cell Analysis and Modeling

NrCAM neuron glial cell-related cell adhesion molecule

NRCC National Registry in Clinical Chemistry; National Research Council of Canada

NRCL nonrenal clearance

NRDL Naval Radiological Defense Laboratory

NREH normal renin essential hypertension

NREM nonrapid eye movement [sleep]

NREMT National Registry of Emergency Medical Technicians

NREMT-P nationally registered emergency medical technician-paramedic

NREN National Aeronautics and Space Administration [NASA] Research and Education Network

NRF Neurosciences Research Foundation; normal renal function

NRFC nonrosette-forming cell

NRFD not ready for data

NRG nursing resources grouping

NRGC nucleus reticularis gigantocellularis

NRH nodular regenerative hyperplasia

NRHA National Rural Health Association

NRHS National Runners' Health Study

NRI nerve root involvement; nerve root irritation; nonrespiratory infection

NRICR National Registry of Inhospital Cardiopulmonary Resuscitation

NRIV Ngari virus

NRK normal rat kidney

NRL nucleus reticularis lateralis

NRM National Registry of Microbiologists; normal range of motion; nucleus reticularis magnocellularis

NRMI National Registry of Myocardial Infarction

NRMP National Resident Matching Program

NRMSE normalized root mean square error

nRNA nuclear ribonucleic acid

nRNP nuclear ribonucleoprotein

NROM normal range of motion

NRP nucleus reticularis parvocellularis

NRPB National Radiological Protection Board

NRPC nucleus reticularis pontis caudalis

NRPG nucleus reticularis paragigantocellularis

NRR net reproduction rate

NRRC National Rotavirus Reference Centre [Australia]

NRRL Northern Regional Research Laboratory

NRS Neurobehavioral Rating Scale; normal rabbit serum; normal reference serum; Norman-Roberts syndrome; numerical rating scale

NRSA National Research Service Award [NIH]

NRSCC National Reference System in Clinical Chemistry

NRSCL National Reference System for the Clinical Laboratory

NRSFPS National Reporting System for Family Planning Services

NRT near-real time; networking research team; nicotine replacement therapy; nucleus reticularis thalami

NRTI nucleoside reverse transcriptase inhibitor

NRU neutral red uptake; nursing research unit

NRV nucleus reticularis ventralis

NRVR normalized renal vascular resistance

NS natural science; Neosporin; nephrosclerosis; nephrotic syndrome; nervous system; Netherton syndrome; neurological surgery, neurosurgery; neurosecretion, neurosecretory; neurosyphilis; neurotic score; nodular sclerosis; noise to signal [ratio]; nonsmoker; nonspecific; nonstimulation; nonstructural; nonsymptomatic; Noonan syndrome; normal saline [solution]; normal serum; normal sodium [diet]; Norwegian scabies; no sample; no sequelae; no shear; nosocomial sinusitis; no specimen; not seen; not significant; not specified; not sufficient; not symptomatic; nuclear sclerosis; nursing services; Nursing Sister

N/S noise to signal [ratio]; normal saline [solution]

Ns nasospinale; nerves

ns nanosecond; nonspecific; no sequelae; no specimen; not significant; nylon suture

NSA National Stroke Association; Neurological Society of America; Niger seed agar [culture medium]; normal serum albumin; no salt added; no significant abnormality; no significant anomaly; number of signals averaged

nsa no salt added

NSABP National Surgical Adjuvant Breast and Bowel Project

NSAD no signs of acute disease

NSAE non-serious adverse event; nonsupported arm exercise

NSAI nonsteroidal anti-inflammatory [drug]

NSAIA nonsteroidal anti-inflammatory agent

NSAID nonsteroidal anti-inflammatory drug

NSAM Naval School of Aviation Medicine

NSAS National Survey of Ambulatory Surgery

NSC neurosecretory cell; no significant change; nonservice connected; non–small cell; nonspecific suppressor cell; normal child with short stature

nsc nonservice connected; no significant change

NSCC National Society for Crippled Children

NSCD nonservice connected disability

NSCLC non-small-cell lung cancer

NSCS night shift call system

NSCT National Society of Cardiovascular Technologists

NSD *N*-acetylneuraminic acid storage disease; Nairobi sheep disease; neonatal staphylococcal disease; neurosecretory dysfunction; night sleep deprivation; nominal single dose; nominal standard dose; normal standard dose; no significant defect; no significant deficiency; no significant deviation; no significant difference; no significant disease; normal spontaneous delivery

NSDV Nairobi sheep disease virus

NSE neuron-specific enolase; nonspecific esterase; normal saline enema

nsec nanosecond

NSEP needle and syringe exchange program; nuclease-sensitive element protein

NSERC Natural Sciences and Engineering Research Council [Canada]

NSF National Science Foundation; National Service Framework; nodular subepidermal fibrosis

NSFNET National Science Foundation (NSF) [Computer] Network

NSFTD normal spontaneous full-term delivery

NSG neurosecretory granule

nsg nursing

NSGA nondominated sorting genetic algorithm

NSGC National Society of Genetic Counselors

NSGCT nonseminomatous germ cell tumor

NSGCTT nonseminomatous germ-cell tumor of the testis

NSG Hx nursing history

NSGI nonspecific genital infection

NSH National Society for Histotechnology

NSHD nodular sclerosing Hodgkin disease

NSHG National Study of Health and Growth

NSHL non-syndromic hearing loss

NSHPT neonatal severe hyperparathyroidism

NSI negative self-image; neurosensory impairment; no signs of infection/inflammation; non-syncytium-inducing

NSICU neurosurgical intensive care unit

NSIDS near sudden infant death syndrome

NSILA nonsuppressible insulinlike activity

NSILP nonsuppressible insulinlike protein

NSIVCD nonspecific intraventricular conduction delay

NSJ nevus sebaceus of Jadassohn

NSK nonsquamous keratin

NSM neurosecretory material; neurosecretory motor neuron; nonantigenic specific mediator; nutrient sporulation medium

N · s/m² newton seconds per square meter

NSMR National Society for Medical Research

NSN nephrotoxic serum nephritis; nicotine-stimulated neurophysin

NSNA National Student Nurse Association

NSND nonsymptomatic and nondisabling

NSO Neosporin ointment; nucleus supraopticus; Nursing Standard Online

NSP neuron specific protein; neurotoxic shellfish poisoning; nonstructural protein; nuclear shuttle protein; nurse scheduling problem

NSPB National Society for the Prevention of Blindness

NSPH neonatal severe hyperparathyroidism

NSPN neurosurgery progress note

NSPORT nurse-sensitive patient outcome research team

NSQ Neuroticism Scale Questionnaire; not sufficient quantitiy

NSR nasal septal reconstruction; nonspecific reaction; normal sinus rhythm; no sign of recurrence; not seen regularly

NSR/M no sign of recurrence or metastases

NSS Nordic Sleep Survey; normal saline solution; normal size and shape; not statistically significant; nutrition support services

NSSQ Norbeck social support questionnaire

NSSTT nonspecific ST and T [wave]

NST neospinothalamic [tract]; nonshivering thermogenesis; nonstress test; nutritional support team

NSTC National Science and Technology Council

NSTEMI non-ST segment elevation myocardial infarction

NSTI necrotizing soft tissue infection

NST-ICF nonstationary ionic channel current fluctuations

NSTT nonseminomatous testicular tumor

NSU neurosurgical unit; nonspecific urethritis

NSurg neurosurgery, neurosurgeon

NSV nonspecific vaginitis/vaginosis

NSVD normal spontaneous vaginal delivery

NSVR normalized systemic vascular resistance

NSVT nonsustained ventricular tachycardia

NSX neurosurgical examination

nsy nursery

NT nasotracheal; neotetrazolium; neurotensin; neurotoxin; neurotrophic; neutralization test; nicotine tartrate; nontender; nontumoral; normal temperature; normal tissue; normotensive; nortriptyline; not tested; N-terminal [fragment]; nourishment taken; nuchal translucency; nuclear transfer; nucleation time; nucleotidase; nucleotide; numbness and tingling

NT-3 neurotrophin 3

5'NT 5'-nucleotidase

Nt amino terminal

nt nucleotide

N&T nose and throat

NTA natural thymocytotoxic autoantibody; nitrilotriacetic acid; Nurse Training Act
NTAB nephrotoxic antibody
NTAV Ntaya virus
NTBR not to be resuscitated
NTC neotetrazolium chloride
NTCC National Type Culture Collection
NTCP noninvasive transcutaneous cardiac pacing; normal tissue complication probability
NTCT negative temperature-coefficient thermistor
NTD neural tube defect; nitroblue tetrazolium dye; noise tone difference; 5′-nucleotidase
NTE neuropathy target esterase; neurotoxic esterase; no toxic effect level; not to exceed
NTF neurotrophic factor; normal throat flora
NTFOM normal tissue complication-based figure-of-merit
NTG nitroglycerin; nitrosoguanidine; nontoxic goiter; normal triglyceridemia
NTGO nitroglycerin ointment
Nth normothermia
NTHH nontumorous, hypergastrinemic hyperchlorhydria
NTHi nontypable *Haemophilus influenzae*
NTI nonthyroid illness
NTIA National Telecommunications and Information Administration
NTIG nontreated immunoglobulin
NTIS National Technical Information Service
NTKR neurotrophic tyrosine kinase receptor
NTL near-total laryngectomy; non-thoracotomy lead [cardioverter-defibrillator]; nortriptyline; no time limit
NTLI neurotensin-like immunoreactivity
NTM nontuberculous mycobacteria
NTMI nontransmural myocardial infarction
NTN nephrotoxic nephritis
NTNH nontoxic, nonhemagglutinating [protein]
NTO nontarget organism
NTON National Transparent Optical Network
NTOS neurogenic thoracic outlet syndrome

NTP narcotic treatment program; National Toxicology Program; nitroprusside; nonthrombopenic purpura; normal temperature and pressure; 5′-nucleotidase; sodium nitroprusside
NT&P normal temperature and pressure
NTR negative therapeutic reaction; nitroreductase; nontranslated region; normotensive rat; nutrition
ntr nutrition
NTRC National Toxins Research Center
NTS nasotracheal suction; nephrotoxic serum; neurotensin; nicotine transdermal system; nontropical sprue; nucleus tractus solitarius
NTT nearly total thyroidectomy
NTU Navy Toxicology Unit
N-TUL internal tumescent ultrasound liposculpture
NTV nerve tissue vaccine
NTVR normal transvalvular regurgitation
nt wt net weight
NTX naltrexone
NTZ normal transformation zone
NU name unknown
nU nanounit
nu nude [mouse]
ν Greek letter *nu*; degrees of freedom; frequency; kinematic velocity; neutrino
NUAPS National Unstable Angina Pectoris Study
NUBS nonuniform rational B-spline
NUC nonspecific ulcerative colitis; sodium urate crystal
Nuc nucleoside
nuc nucleated
NUCARE nursing care research
nucl nucleus
NUD nonulcer dyspepsia; nursing utilization database
NUG necrotizing ulcerative gingivitis
NUGV Nugget virus
NUI number user identification
nullip nulliparous
νm nanometers
NUMA nonuniform memory access; nuclear mitotic apparatus
numc number concentration
NUPV nucleopolyhedrovirus
NURB Neville upper reservoir buffer
Nut nutrition
NUV near ultraviolet

NV nausea and vomiting; necrosis virus; negative variation; neovascularization; next visit; nonveteran; normal value; Norwalk virus; not vaccinated; not venereal; not verified; not volatile
N&V nausea and vomiting
Nv naked vision
nv new variant
NVA near visual acuity
NVB neurovascular bundle
NVCA National Venereology Council of Australia
nvCJD new variant Creutzfeldt-Jakob disease
NVD nausea, vomiting, and diarrhea; neck vein distention; neovascularization of the disk; neurovesicle dysfunction; nonvalvular disease; normal vaginal delivery; no venereal disease; Newcastle virus disease; number of vessels diseased
N/V/D nausea, vomiting, diarrhea
NVE native valve endocarditis
NVG neovascular glaucoma; night vision goggles; nonventilated group
NVIm *N*-vinyl imidazole
NVL no visible lesion
NVM neovascular membrane; nonvolatile matter
NVP nevirapine; *N*-vinyl pyrrolidone
NVPO National Vaccine Program Office
NVS neurologic vital signs
NVSS normal variant short stature
NVTS normal volunteer telephone screening
NW naked weight; nasal wash
nW nanowatt
NWB nonweightbearing

NWCL New World cutaneous leishmaniasis
NWDA National Wholesale Druggists Association
NWM nucleotide weight matrix
NWR normotensive Wistar rat
NWTS National Wilms' Tumor Study
NX naloxone; no evidence of lymph node metastases [TNM (tumor-node-metastasis) classification]; no evidence of breast tumor lymph node metastases [TNM (tumor-node-metastasis) classification]
Nx no evidence of lymph node metastases [TNM (tumor-node-metastasis) classification]; no evidence of breast tumor lymph node metastases [TNM (tumor-node-metastasis) classification]
NXG necrobiotic xanthogranuloma
ny, nyst nystagmus
NYAV Nyabira virus
NYC New York City [medium]
NYD not yet diagnosed; not yet discovered
NYHA New York Heart Association
NYHAFC New York Heart Association Functional Class
NYMV Nyamanini virus
NYQAS New York Quality Assurance System
NYV New York virus
NZ neutral zone; normal zone
NZB New Zealand black [mouse]
NZC New Zealand chocolate [mouse]
NZO New Zealand obese [mouse]
NZR New Zealand red [rabbit]
NZV New Zealand virus
NZW New Zealand white [mouse]

O blood type in the ABO blood group; eye [Lat. *oculus*]; nonmotile strain of microorganisms [Ger. *ohne Hauch*]; no response [pacemaker]; objective findings; observed frequency in a contingency table; obstetrics; obvious; occipital electrode placement in electroencephalography; occiput; occlusal; [doctor's] office; often; ohm; old; opening; operator; operon; opium; oral, orally; orange [color]; orderly respirations [anesthesia chart]; ortho-; orthopedics; osteocyte; other; output; ovine; oxygen; pint [Lat. *octarius*]; respirations [anesthesia chart]; zero

O$_2$ both eyes; diatomic oxygen; molecular oxygen

O$_3$ ozone

O125 nonmucinous ovarian tumor antigen

o eye [Lat. *oculus*]; opening; ovary transplant; pint [Lat. *octarius*]; see *omicron*

ō negative; without

o see *omicron*

Ω see *omega*

ω see *omega*

OA [o]esophageal atresia; obstructive apnea; occipital artery; occipito-anterior; occiput anterior; occupational asthma; octanoic acid; ocular albinism; old age; okadaic acid; oleic acid; on admission or arrival; open appendectomy; opiate analgesia; ophthalmic artery; opsonic activity; optic atrophy; oral airways; oral alimentation; organic anion; orotic acid; osteoarthritis; osteoarthrosis; ovalbumin; ovarian antibody; overall assessment; Overeaters Anonymous; oxalic acid

O&A observation and assessment

O$_2$a oxygen availability

OAA Old Age Assistance; Older Americans Act; Opticians Association of America; oxaloacetic acid

OAAD ovarian ascorbic acid depletion

OAAS observer's assessment alertness/sedation scale

OAAV ovine adeno-associated virus

OAdV ovine adenovirus

OAdV-A, B, C ovine adenoviruses A, B, C

OAB old age benefits

OABP organic anion binding protein

OA/BVM oral airway/bag-valve-mask

OAC omeprazole, amoxicillin, clarithromycin

OACT occupational activity [UMLS]

OAD obstructive airway disease; organic anionic dye

OADC oleate-albumin-dextrose-catalase [medium]

OAE otoacoustic emission

OAF off-axis factor; off-axis ratio [radiotherapy]; open air factor; osteoclast activating factor

OAFNS oculo-auriculofrontonasal syndrome

OAG open angle glaucoma

OAH ovarian androgenic hyperfunction

OAIS Outcomes and Information Set

OAISO overaction of the ipsilateral superior oblique

OAK Kjer optic atrophy

OALF organic acid labile fluid

OALL ossification of anterior longitudinal ligament

OAM Office of Alternative Medicine [NIH]; outer acrosomal membrane

OAP Office of Adolescent Pregnancy; old age pension, old age pensioner; ophthalmic artery pressure; osteoarthropathy; oxygen at atmospheric pressure; precocious osteoarthrosis

OAPP Office of Adolescent Pregnancy Programs

OAR organ at risk; Ottawa ankle rule

OARS older Americans resources and services; Optimal Atherectomy Restenosis Study

OAS old age security; oral allergy syndrome; osmotically active substance

OASD ocular albinism-sensorineural deafness [syndrome]

OASDHI Old Age, Survivors, Disability and Health Insurance

OASDI Old Age Survivors and Disability Insurance

OASI Old Age and Survivors Insurance

OASIS Older Adults Service and Information System; Organization to Assess Strategies for Ischemic Syndromes; Outcome and Assessment Information Set

OASP organic acid soluble phosphorus

OAstV ovine astrovirus

OAT *O*-acetyltransferase; Ochanomizu Aspirin Trial; Open Artery Trial; organic anion transporter; ornithine aminotransferase

OATL ornithine aminotransferase-like

OATR organism attribute [UMLS]

OAV oculoauriculovertebral [dysplasia]

OAVS oculo-auriculovertebral syndrome

OAVD oculoauriculovertebral dysplasia

OAW oral airways

OB obese [mouse]; obese, obesity; objective benefit; obliterative bronchiolitis; obstetrics, obstetrician; occult bacteremia; occult bleeding; olfactory bulb; oligoclonal band

O&B opium and belladonna

ob obese [mouse]

OBAD optimal biologically active dose

OBB own bed bath; oriented bounding boxes

OBD organic brain disease

OBCAM opioid-binding cell adhesion molecule

OBE Office of Biological Education

OBET odor-baited entry trap

OBF organ blood flow

OBG, ObG obstetrics and gynecology, obstetrician-gynecologist

OBGS obstetrical and gynecological surgery

OB-GYN, ob-gyn obstetrics and gynecology, obstetrician-gynecologist

obj objective

obl oblique

OBMT omeprazole, bismuth, metronidazole, tetracycline

OBOV Obodhiang virus

OBP odorant-binding protein; ova, blood, parasites [in stool]

OBR obesity gene receptor

OBRA Omnibus Reconciliation Act

OBS obesity; obstetrical service; organic brain syndrome

Obs observation, observed; obstetrics, obstetrician

obs obsolete

Obst obstetrics, obstetrician

obst, obstr obstruction, obstructed

OB-US obstetrical ultrasound [examination of the fetus]

OC obstetrical conjugate; occlusocervical; oesophageal candidiasis; office call; on call; only child; optic chiasma; oral contraceptive; orbicularis oculi [muscle]; order communication [system]; original claim; organ culture; orofacial cleft; outer canthal [distance]; ovarian cancer; oxygen consumed

O&C onset and course

OCA octylcyanoacrylate; oculocutaneous albinism; olivopontocerebellar atrophy; oral contraceptive agent

OCa ovarian carcinoma

OCAD occlusive carotid artery disease

O₂cap oxygen capacity

OCB obsessive-compulsive behavior

OCBAS Optimal Coronary Balloon Angioplasty vs Stent [trial]; Optimal Coronary Balloon Angioplasty with Provisional Stenting vs Primary Stent [trial]

OCBF outer cortical blood flow

OCC object-centered coordinate [method]; oculocerebrocutaneous [syndrome]; operable case based reasoning [CBR]-oriented case; optimum care committee; oral cholecystography; original component complexes

occ occasional; occiput, occipital; occlusion, occlusive; occupation; occurrence

occas occasional

OCCI oblique clear corneal incision

occip occiput, occipital

occl occlusion, occlusive

OCCPR open chest cardiopulmonary resuscitation

OccTh occupational therapy, occupational therapist

occ ther occupational therapist or therapy

occup occupation, occupational

occup Rx occupational therapy

OCCV object-centered coordinate [OCC] values

OCD obsessive compulsive disorder; Office of Child Development; Office of Civil Defense; osteochondritis dissecans; ovarian cholesterol depletion; oxygen cost diagram

OCDD octachlorodibenzo-*p*-dioxin

OCF occipito-frontal [circumference]

OCG omnicardiogram; oral cholecystogram

OCH oral contraceptive hormone

OCHAMPUS Office of Civilian Health and Medical Programs of the Uniformed Services [database]

OCHS Office of Cooperative Health Statistics

OCIS Oncology Clinical Information System

OCLC Ohio Computer Library Center; online computer library center

OCM oral contraceptive medication

OCN oculomotor nucleus; oncology certified nurse; osteocalcin

OCOA Online Cytogenetics of Animals

OCP octacalcium phosphate; ocular cicatricial pemphigoid; Onchocerciasis Control Programme [Africa]; oral case presentation; oral contraceptive pill

OC&P ova, cysts, and parasites

OCPD obsessive compulsive personality disorder

OCPE office of clinical practice evaluation

OCR oculocardiac reflex; oculocerebrorenal [syndrome]; optical character reader; optical character recognition

oCRF ovine corticotropin-releasing factor

OCRG oxycardiorespirography

oCRH ovine corticotropin-releasing hormone

OCRL oculocerebrorenal [syndrome] of Lowe

OCRM OpenGALEN Common Reference Model

OCRS oculocerebrorenal syndrome

OCS occipital condyle syndrome; Ondine's curse syndrome; open canalicular system; oral contraceptive steroid; order communication system; outpatient clinic substation; Oxford Cholesterol Study

OCSD oculocraniosomatic disease

OCSI orthostatic change in shock index

OCSP Oxfordshire Community Stroke Project

OCT object classification test; optical coherence tomography; optimal cutting temperature; oral cavity tumor; oral contraceptive therapy; organic cation transporter; ornithine carbamoyltransferase; orthotopic cardiac transplantation; outer canthal distance; oxytocin challenge test

O-CT ortho-computed tomography

OCTD overlap connective tissue disease

OCTM open cavity tympanomastoidectomy

OCU observation care unit

OCV ordinary conversational voice

OD Doctor of Optometry; object dictionary; obtained absorbance; occipital dysplasia; occupational dermatitis; occupational disease; oculodynamic; Ollier disease; on duty; once a day; open drop [anesthesia]; optical density; optimal dose; originally derived; out-of-date; outside diameter; overdose, overdosage; right eye [Lat. *oculus dexter*]

O-D obstacle-dominance

OD-1 Organ Disease 1 [coronary atherosclerosis multicenter study]

OD-2 Organ Disease 2 [cerebrovascular atherosclerosis multicenter study]

O₂D oxygen delivery

ODA office document architecture; open document architecture; overall disease assessment; right occipitoanterior [fetal position, Lat. *occipito-dextra anterior*]

ODB opiate-directed behavior

ODBC open database connectivity

ODC oritidine decarboxylase; ornithine decarboxylase; oxygen dissociation curve

Odc ornithine decarboxylase

ODCP ornithine decarboxylase pseudogene

ODD oculodentodigital [dysplasia]; oppositional defiant disorder; osteodental dysplasia

OD'd overdosed [drug]

ODE Office of Device Evaluation [of FDA]; ordinary differential equation

ODED oculo-digito-esophago-duodenal [syndrome]

ODES Oslo Diet and Exercise Study

ODFR oxygen-derived free radical

ODIF office document interchange format

ODISY Online Deaconess Information System

ODM ophthalmodynamometer, ophthalmodynamometry

ODN oligodeoxyribonucleotide

ODOD oculo-dento-osseous dysplasia

Odont odontogenic

ODP offspring of diabetic parents; open distributed processing; right occipitoposterior [fetal position, Lat. *occipito-dextra posterior*]

ODPHP Office of Disease Prevention and Health Promotion

ODQ on direct questioning

ODRV Odrenisrou virus

ODS organized delivery system; original dataset; osmotic demyelination syndrome
ODSG ophthalmic Doppler sonogram
ODT oculodynamic tract; right occipito-transverse [fetal position, Lat. *occipito-dextra transversa*]
ODTS organic dust toxic syndrome
ODU optical density unit
OE on examination; organization engine [database]; orthopedic examination; otitis externa; out-stationed enrollment
O/E observed/expected [ratio]
O&E observation and examination
Oe oersted
OEE osmotic erythrocyte enrichment; outer enamel epithelium
OEF oil immersion field; oxygen extraction fraction
O₂EI oxygen extraction index
OEIS omphalocele, exstrophy, imperforate anus, spinal defects [complex]
OEL occupational exposure limit
OELM optimal external laryngeal manipulation
OEM object exchange model; opposite ear masked; original electronic manufacturer
OEP operational effectiveness program
OEPA Onchocerciasis Elimination Program for the Americas
OER osmotic erythrocyte [enrichment]; oxygen enhancement ratio
O₂ER oxygen extraction ratio
OERP Office of Education and Regional Programming
OERR order entry and results reporting
OE/RR online physician's order entry and results reporting
OES oral esophageal stethoscope; optical emission spectroscopy
oesoph esophagus [oesophagus]
OET oral endotracheal tube; oral esophageal tube
O₂Ext oxygen extraction
OF occipitofrontal; opacity factor; open field [test]; optical fundus; orbital fracture; orbitofrontal; osmotic fragility; osteitis fibrosa; output factor; oxidation-fermentation
O/F oxidation-fermentation
OFA oncofetal antigen
OFAGE orthogonal field alternation gel electrophoresis

OFBM oxidation-fermentation basal medium
OFC occipitofrontal circumference; optical flow constraint [equation]; orbitofacial cleft; osteitis fibrosa cystica
OFCTAD occipito-facio-cervico-thoraco-abdomino-digital dysplasia
OFD object-film distance; occipital frontal diameter; oro-facial-digital [syndrome]
ofd object-film distance
Off official
OFHA occipitofrontal headache
OFI open and flexible learning
OFM orofacial malformation
OFNE oxygenated fluorocarbon emulsion [delivery system]
OFS optical file system
OFTT organic failure to thrive
OFUN organism function [UMLS]
OG obstetrics and gynecology; occluso-gingival; 1-*O*-octyl-beta-ᴅ-glucopyranoside; oligodendrocyte; optic ganglion; orange green; orogastric; [protective] overgarment
O&G obstetrics and gynecology
OGC oculogyric crisis
OGD [o]esophago-gastro-duodenoscopy
OGDH oxoglutarate dehydrogenase
OGF ovarian growth factor; oxygen gain factor
OGH ovine growth hormone
OGI oxygen-glucose index
OGJ [o]esophagogastric junction
OGS oxygenic steroid
OGTT oral glucose tolerance test
OGZN organization [UMLS]
OH hydroxycorticosteroid; obstructive hypopnea; occipital horn; occupational health; occupational history; oligomer hybridization; open heart [surgery]; ortho-static hypotension; osteopathic hospital; out of hospital; outpatient hospital
17-OH 17-hydroxycorticosteroid
OHA oral hypoglycemic agents
OHAHA ophthalmoplegia-hypotonia-ataxia-hypacusis-athetosis [syndrome]
OHB₁₂ hydroxycobalamin
O₂Hb oxyhemoglobin
OHC occupational health center; outer hair cell; Oxford Haemophilia Centre
5-OHC 5-hydroxycysteine
OHCA out-of-hospital cardiac arrest
OH-Cbl hydroxycobalamin

OHCC hydroxycalciferol; out-of-home child care

OHCOB hydroxycobalamin

OHCS hydroxycorticosteroid

OHD hydroxylase deficiency; hydroxy-vitamin D; Office of Human Development; Ondine-Hirschsprung disease; organic heart disease

1,25(OH)₂D₃ 1,25-dihydroxyvitamin D₃ [calcium transport]

25-OH-D 25-hydroxyvitamin D

OHDA hydroxydopamine

8-OH-dG 8-hydroxy-2′-deoxyguanosine

16-OH-DHAS 16-alpha-hydroxydehy-droepiandrosterone sulfate

8-OH-DPAT 8-hydroxy-2-(di-*n*-propyl-amino)tetralin

OHDS Office of Human Development Services

OHE other hospital employee

OHF Omsk hemorrhagic fever

OHFA hydroxy fatty acid

OHFT overhead frame trapeze

OHFV Omsk hemorrhagic fever virus

OHI Occupational Health Institute; operative hypertension indicator; oral hygiene index; Oral Hygiene Instruction

OHIAA hydroxyindoleacetic acid

OHIPD Office of Health Information Programs Development

OHI-S Oral Hygiene Instruction-Simpli-fied

OHL oral hairy leukoplakia

OHMO Office of Health Maintenance Organizations

OHN occupational health nurse; optical nerve head

OHP hydroxyprogesterone; hydroxypro-line; occupational health plan; Oregon Health Plan; oxygen under high pressure

17-OHP 17-hydroxyprogesterone

OHPCC Office of High Performance Computing and Communications

OHR occupational health research; Office of Health Research

OHS obesity hypoventilation syndrome; occipital Horn syndrome; occupational health and safety; occupational health service; ocular histoplasmosis syndrome; open heart surgery; Oslo Hypertension Study; ovarian hyperstimulation syndrome

OHSD hydroxysteroid dehydrogenase

OHSR Office of Human Subject Research [NIH]

OHSS ovarian hyperstimulation syndrome

OHT ocular hypertension; orthotopic heart transplantation; Oslo Heart Trial

OHTA Office of Health Technology Assessment

5-OHU 5-hydroxyuracil

OI obturator internus; occasional insom-nia; opportunistic infection; opsonic index; orgasmic impairment; orientation inven-tory; orthoiodohippurate; osteogenesis imperfecta; ouabain insensitivity; oxygen intake

O-I outer and inner

OIC organized indigenous caregiving; osteogenesis imperfecta congenita

OID object identifier; optimal immuno-modulating dose; Organism Identification Number; oxygen insufflation device

OIF observed intrinsic frequency; oil immersion field; open internal fixation; Osteogenesis Imperfecta Foundation

OIG Office of the Inspector General

OIH Office of International Health; orthoiodohippurate; ovulation-inducing hormone

OILD occupational immunologic lung disease

oint ointment

OIP organizing interstitial pneumonia

OIR Office of Information Resources; Office of International Research

OIS object information system; organ injury scale; Oslo Ischemia Study; out-patient information system

OIT organic integrity test

OITAV Oita virus

OJ orange juice

OKC odontogenic keratocyst

OKHV Okhotskiy virus

OKN optokinetic nystagmus

OKOV Okola virus

OKR optokinetic response; Ottawa knee rules

OKS optokinetic stimulus

OKT ornithine ketoacid amino-transferase

OL open label(ed)

ol left eye [Lat. *oculus laevus*]

OLA left occipitoanterior [fetal position, Lat. *occipito-laeva anterior*]; oligonucleo-tide ligation assay

OLAP online analytical processing

OLAS oligoisoadenylate synthetase

OLB olfactory bulb; open liver biopsy; open lung biopsy

OLBx open lung biopsy

OLC ouabain-like compound

OLD obstructive lung disease; orthochromatic leukodystrophy

OLDMEDLINE Old MEDLARS Online [NLM database of 1960–1965 citations]

OLE object linking and embedding

olf olfactory

OLFR olfactory receptor

OLH ovine lactogenic hormone

oLH ovine luteinizing hormone

OLI octree level index

OLIDS open loop insulin delivery system

OLIV Olifantsvlei virus

OLMC online medical control

OLP left occipitoposterior [fetal position, Lat. *occipito-laeva posterior*]

OLR otology, laryngology, and rhinology

ol res oleoresin

OLRx orthotopic liver transplantation

OLS ordinary least square; ouabain-like substance

OLT left occipitotransverse [fetal position]; orthotopic liver transplantation

OLVV Oliveros virus

OM obtuse marginal [artery]; obtuse mental; occipitomental; occupational medicine; ocular movement; oculomotor; operations manager [database]; Osborne Mendel [rat]; osteomalacia; osteomyelitis; osteopathic manipulation; otitis media; outer membrane; ovulation method

OMA object management architecture

OMAC otitis media, acute catarrhal

OMAS occupational maladjustment syndrome

OMB obtuse marginal branch; Office of Management and Budget

OMC office of managed care; orientation-memory-concentration [test]

OMCH Office of Maternal and Child Health

OMCT Orientation-Memory-Concentration Test

OMD ocular muscle dystrophy; oculomandibulodyscephaly; orbital maxillary disjunction; organic mental disorder; oromandibular dystonia

OMDB object microdatabase

OME office of medical examiner; otitis media with effusions

OMEGA Ottawa-Madison electron gamma algorithm

Ω Greek capital letter *omega*; ohm

ω Greek lowercase letter *omega*; angular velocity

OMERACT Outcome Measures in Rheumatoid Arthritis Clinical Trial

OMFAQ older Americans resources and services (OARS) multidimensional functional assessment questionnaire

OMG object management group; oligodendrocyte-myelin glycoprotein; osteopathic medical school graduate

OMGE Organisation Mondiale de Gastro-Enterologie

OMGP oligodendrocyte-myelin glycoprotein

OMH Office of Mental Health

OMI office of medical investigator; old myocardial infarction

OMIA Online Mendelian Inheritance in Animals [database]

o Greek letter *omicron*

OMIM Online Mendelian Inheritance in Man [database]

OML orbitomental line

OMN oculomotor nerve

OMNI Organizing Medical Networked Information [UK]

OMOV Omo virus

OMP olfactory marker protein; oligonucleoside methylphosphonate; ornithine monophosphate; orotidine-5′-monophosphatase; outer membrane protein

OMPA octamethyl pyrophosphoramide; otitis media, purulent, acute

OmpA, ompA outer membrane protein A

OMPC, OMPCh otitis media, purulent, chronic

OmpF, ompF outer membrane protein F

OMR oligomycin-resistant; online medical record

OMRT Ontario Association of Medical Radiation Technologists

OMS occupational medical services; organic mental syndrome; otomandibular syndrome

OM&S osteopathic medicine and surgery

OMSA otitis media, suppurative, acute

OMSC otitis media secretory (or suppurative) chronic

OMT object modeling technique; ocular microtremor; *O*-methyltransferase; ophthalmic medical technician or technologist; osteopathic manipulative therapy

OMV outer membrane vesicle

OMVC open mitral valve commissurotomy

ON occipitonuchal; office nurse; olfactory nucleus; onlay; optic nerve; orthopedic nurse; osteonecrosis; osteonectin; overnight

ONAC Office of Noise Abatement and Control

ONC oncogene; oncology; open network communication; Orthopaedic Nursing Certificate; over-the-needle catheter

OND Ophthalmic Nursing Diploma; orbitonasal dislocation; other neurological disorders

ONE [computer-assisted] otoneurological expert system

ONG optic nerve glioma

ONMRS onychotrichodysplasia-neutropenia-mental retardation syndrome

ONNV o'nyong-nyong virus

ONP operating nursing procedure; orthonitrophenyl

ONPG *o*-nitrophenyl-beta-D-galactopyranoside

ONS Oncology Nursing Society

ONSA Organization for Nucleotide Sequencing and Analysis

ONTG oral nitroglycerin

ONTR orders not to resuscitate

OO object-oriented; oophorectomy; orbicularis oculi [muscle]

O&O on and off

OOA object-oriented analysis; outer optic anlage

OOB out of bed

OODB object-oriented database

OODBMS object-oriented database management system

OOG optic oculography

OOH out-of-hospital

OOH/CA out-of-hospital cardiac arrest

OOHRT object-oriented health care terminology respository

OOLR ophthalmology, otology, laryngology, and rhinology

OOM, oom oogonial metaphase

OOMM object-oriented matrix model

OOP object-oriented programming

OOR out-of-room

OORR orbicularis oculi reflex response

OOSE object-oriented software engineering

OOSS Outpatient Ophthalmic Surgery Society

OOW out of wedlock

OOWS objective opiate withdrawal scale

OP occipitoparietal; occipitoposterior; occiput posterior; octapeptide; olfactory peduncle; opening pressure; operation, operative; operative procedure; ophthalmology; opponens pollicis; optic neuritis; organophosphate; oropharynx; orthostatic proteinuria; osmotic pressure; osteoporosis; outpatient; ovine prolactin

O&P ova and parasites

O/P outpatient

Op ophthalmology; opisthocranion

op operation; operator

OPA oligonucleoside phosphoramidate; open procurement agency; optic atrophy; organ procurement agency; oropharyngeal airway; outcome and process assessment

OPALS Ontario Prehospital Advanced Life Support [study]

op-amp operational amplifier

OPB outpatient basis

OPC oculopalatocerebral [syndrome]; oligonucleotide purification cartridge; outpatient clinic; overall performance category

OPCA olivopontocerebellar atrophy

OPCAB off-pump coronary artery bypass

OPCD olivopontocerebellar degeneration

OPCOS oligomenorrheic polycystic ovary syndrome

OPCRIT operational criteria

OPCS Office of Population Censuses and Surveys [UK]

OPD obstetric prediabetic; optical path difference; otopalatodigital [syndrome]; outpatient department; outpatient dispensary; *o*-phenylenediamine

o-PDA *o*-phenylenediamine

O'p-DDD mitotane

OpDent operative dentistry

OPDG ocular plethysmodynamography

OPDS otopalatodigital syndrome

OPF oligo[poly(ethylene glycol) fumarate]

OPG ocular pneumoplethysmography; orthopantomogram; oxypolygelatin
opg opening
OPH obliterative pulmonary hypertension; ophthalmia; organic phosphate
OPH, Oph ophthalmology; ophthalmoscopy, ophthalmoscope
Oph A ophthalmic artery
OPHC Office of Prepaid Health Care
OphD Doctor of Ophthalmology
OPHS Office of Public Health and Science
Ophth ophthalmology
OPI oculoparalytic illusion; Omnibus Personality Inventory
OPIDN organophosphate-induced delayed neuropathy
OPIDP organophosphate-induced delayed polyneuropathy
OPIM other potentially infectious material
OPK object processing kernal; optokinetic
OPL other party liability; outer plexiform layer; ovine placental lactogen
OPLINK Ohio Public Library Information Network
OPLL ossification of posterior longitudinal ligament
OPM occult primary malignancy; Office of Personnel Management; ophthalmoplegic migraine
OPMD oculopharyngeal muscular dystrophy
OPMSS Olestra Postmarketing Surveillance Study
OPN ophthalmic nurse; osteopontin
OPO Organ Procurement Organization
OPP osmotic pressure of plasma; oxygen partial pressure
opp opposite
OPPA vincristine, procarbazine, prednisone, Adriamycin
OPPG oculopneumoplethysmography
OPRD opiate receptor delta
OPRK opiate receptor kappa
OPRR Office for Protection from Research Risks
OPPS outpatient prospective payment system
OPRT orotate phosphoribosyltransferase
OPRTase orotate phosphoribosyltransferase
OPS operations; optical position sensor; optimal parameter search [algorithm];

osteoporosis-pseudolipoma syndrome; outpatient service; outpatient surgery
OPSA ovarian papillary serous adenocarcinoma
OpScan optical scanning
OPSEC operations security
OPSI overwhelming postsplenectomy infection
OPSR Office of Professional Standards Review
OPT oligonucleoside phosphorothioate; *o*-phthaldialdehyde; optimization [method]; outpatient; outpatient treatment
opt best [Lat. *optimus*]; optics, optician
OPTHD optimal hemodialysis
OPTICUS Optimization with Intracoronary Ultrasound to Reduce Stent Restenosis [trial]
OPTIMAAL Optimal Trial in Myocardial Infarction with Angiotensin II Antagonist Losartan
OPTIME Outcomes of a Prospective Trial of Intravenous Milrinone for Exacerbations [of chronic heart failure]
OPTIME CHF Outcomes of a Prospective Trial of Intravenous Milrinone for Exacerbations of Chronic HeartFailure
OPTN organ procurement and transplant network
OPUS Orbofiban in Patients with Unstable Coronary Syndromes [study]
OPV oral polio vaccine; ovine papillomavirus
OPV 1, 2 ovine papillomaviruses 1, 2
OPWL opiate withdrawal
OQAQ Overview Quality Assessment Questionnaire
OR a logical binary relation that is true if any argument is true, and false otherwise; [o]estrogen receptor; odds ratio; oil retention [enema]; oligomer of resveratrol; open reduction; operating room; optic radiation; oral rehydration; orbicularis oris [muscle]; orosomucoid; orthopedic; orthopedic research; ouabain-resistant; outwardly rectifying [current]; oxidized radical
O-R oxidation-reduction
O$_R$ rate of outflow
Or orbitale
ORA opiate receptor agonist

ORACLE Overview of the Role of Antibiotics in Curtailing Labor and Early Delivery [trial]

ORALABX oral antibiotics

ORANS Oak Ridge Analytical System

ORB object request broker

ORBIT Oral Glycoprotein IIb/IIIa Receptor Blockade to Inhibit Thrombosis [trial]

ORBC ox red blood cell

ORC oculo-reno-cerebellar [syndrome]; origin recognition complex

ORCA open record for care

orch orchitis

ORCHIDS Office Records Charts Information Data System

OR$_{Cl}$ outwardly rectifying chloride current

ORD optical rotatory dispersion; oral radiation death

ORDS Office of Research, Demonstration, and Statistics

ORE oil retention enema

OREF Orthopedic Research and Education Foundation

ORESTES open reading expressed sequence tags

ORF open reading frame

OR&F open reduction and fixation

orf open reading frame

ORFV orf virus

Org, org organic

ORGM organism [UMLS]

ORH order header

ORI Office of Research Integrity [NIH]

ORIA Office of Radiation and Indoor Air

ORIF open reduction with internal fixation

ORIS ophthalmic retrobulbar injection simulator

oriT origin of transfer

ORIV Oriboca virus

OrJ orange juice

ORL otorhinolaryngology

ORLS Oxford Record Linkage Study

ORM object relational mapping; Office of Research and Methodology; orosomucoid; other regulated material; oxygen ratio monitor

ORMC oxygen ratio monitor controller

ORN olfactory receptor neuron; operating room nurse; orthopedic nurse

Orn ornithine

ORNL Oak Ridge National Laboratory

ORO oil red O

OR$_O$ observed odds ratio

OROS oral osmotic

OROV Oropouche virus

ORUV 1, 2, 3, 4 Orungo viruses 1, 2, 3, 4

ORP operating room personnel; oxidation-reduction potential

ORPM orthorhythmic pacemaker

ORR objective response rate

ORS olfactory reference syndrome; oral rehydration solution; oral surgery, oral surgeon; Orthopaedic Research Society; orthopedic surgeon, orthopedic surgery; oxygen radical scavengers

ORSA osteoclast resorption stimulating activity; oxacillin-resistant *Staphylococcus aureus*

ORT object relations technique; operating room technician; oral rehydration therapy

OR$_T$ true odds ratio

orth, ortho orthopedics, orthopedic

ORW Osler-Rendu-Weber [syndrome]

ORXV Oriximina virus

ORYX outcome research yields excellence

OS left eye [Lat. *oculus sinister*]; object oriented; occipitosacral; occupational safety; office surgery; oligosaccharide; Omenn syndrome; opening snap; open source; open splenectomy; operating system; Opitz syndrome; oral surgery; ordinal scale; organ-specific; orthognathic surgery; orthopedic surgeon, orthopedic surgery; Osgood-Schlatter [disease]; osteogenic sarcoma; osteosarcoma; osteosclerosis; ouabain sensitivity; overall survival; oxygen saturation

Os osmium

OSA obstructive sleep apnea; Office of Services to the Aging; Optical Society of America; ovarian sectional area

OSACA Osaka Follow-Up Study for Ultrasonographic Assessment of Carotid Atherosclerosis

OSAI organism-specific antibody index

OSAS obstructive sleep apnea syndrome

OSBP oxysterol binding protein

OSC on-scene coordinator

osc oscillation

OSCAR Olive Oil, Safflower Oil, Canola Oil and Rapeseed Oil [dietary study]; online survey, certification and reporting system

OSCC oral squamous cell carcinoma

OSCE objective structured clinical examination

OS-CS osteopathia striata-cranial sclerosis [syndrome]

OSDAT Oslo Study Diet and Antismoking Trial

OS-EM ordered-subsequent expectation maximization

OSF open software foundation; organ system failure; osteoclast-stimulating factor; outer spiral fiber; overgrowth stimulating factor

OSF/DCE open software foundation/distributed computing environment

OSG Office of the Surgeon General

OSGi open services gateway initiative

OSHA Occupational Safety and Health Administration

OSH Act Occupational Safety and Health Act of 1970

OsHV ostreid herpesvirus

OSI open systems interconnection [reference model]

OSIRIS Open Study of Infants at High Risk or with Respiratory Insufficiency: the Role of Surfactants; Optimization Study of Infarct Reperfusion Investigated by ST-Monitoring

OSLER objectively structured long examination record

OSM ovine submaxillary mucin; oxygen saturation meter

Osm osmosis, osmolarity

osm osmole; osmosis, osmotic

OSMED otospondylometaphyseal dysplasia

Osm/kg osmoles per kilogram

Osm/L osmoles per liter

osmol osmole

OSMT Ontario Society of Medical Technologists

O-SP O-specific polysaccharide

OspA outer surface protein A

OSQL object structure query language

OSRC osteosarcoma

OSRD Office of Scientific Research and Development

OSS osseous; over-the-shoulder strap

oss osseous

OSSAV Ossa virus

OST object sorting test; Office of Science and Technology; Ottawa Stroke Trial

osteo osteoarthritis; osteomyelitis; osteopathy

OSTI Optimal Stent Implantation [trial]

OSTP Office of Science and Technology Policy

OSUK Ophthalmological Society of the United Kingdom

OSV observable state variable

OT objective test; oblique talus; occlusion time; occupational therapist, occupational therapy; ocular tension; office therapy; old term (in anatomy); old tuberculin; olfactory threshold; on treatment; optic tract; orientation test; original tuberculin; ornithine transcarbamylase; orotracheal; orthopedic treatment; otolaryngology; otology; oxytocin; oxytryptamine

Ot otolaryngology

OTA ochratoxin A; occupational therapy assistant; Office of Technology Assessment; ornithine transaminase; orthotoluidine arsenite

OTC ornithine transcarbamylase; oval target cell; ovarian tissue culture; over-the-counter; oxytetracycline

OTCD ornithine carbamoyltransferase deficiency

OTD oculotrichodysplasia; oral temperature device; organ tolerance dose

OTE optically transparent electrode

OTF octamer-binding transcription factor; optical transfer function; oral transfer factor; outpatient treatment file [database]

OTFC oral transmucosal fentanyl citrate

OTI ovomucoid trypsin inhibitor

OTM orthotoluidine manganese sulfate

OTO otology; otorhinolaryngology

Otol otology, otologist

OTPS other than personal services

OTR Ovarian Tumor Registry; Occupational Therapist, Registered

OTReg Occupational Therapist, Registered

OTS *n*-octadecyltrichlorosilane; occipital temporal sulcus; optical tracking system; orotracheal suction

OTSG Office of the Surgeon General

OTSMD Ornithine Transcarbamoylase Structure and Mutation Database

OTT orotracheal tube

OTU olfactory tubercle; operational taxonomic unit

OTW over the wire
OTZ oxathiozolidine
OU observation unit; Oppenheimer-Urbach [syndrome]
ou both eyes together [Lat. *oculi unitas*]
OUAV Ouango virus
OUB ouabain
OUBIV Oubi virus
OUBR ouabain resistance
OULQ outer upper left quadrant
OUME operative unit of medical herpetology
OUR oxygen uptake rate
OURQ outer upper right quadrant
OURS Oxford University Research Study; oxygen utilization rate study
OURV Ourem virus
OUS overuse syndrome
OUTCLAS Outpatient Coronary Low-profile Angioplasty Study
OUTI other urinary tract infections
OV oculovestibular; office visit; oncovirus; osteoid volume; outflow volume; ovalbumin; ovary; overventilation; ovulation
Ov ovary
ov ovum
OVA ovalbumin
ova ovariectomy
OVC ovarian cancer
OVD occlusal vertical dimension; ophthalmological viscosurgical device
OvDF ovarian dysfunction
OvHV ovine herpesvirus
OVLT organum vasculosum of the lamina terminalis
OVRV Oak-Vale virus
OVSF orthogonal variable spreading factor [telemedicine]
OVSMC ovine vascular smooth muscle cell

OVX ovariectomized
OW outcome washing; once weekly; open wedge; outer wall; oval window; overweight
O/W, o/w oil in water
OWCL Old World cutaneous leishmaniasis
OWI Office of Worksite Initiatives
OW/O overweight and obesity
o/w/o oil in water/oil
OWR Osler-Weber-Rendu [syndrome]; ovarian wedge resection
OWS outerwear syndrome
OX optic chiasma; oxacillin; oxalate; oxide; orthopedic examination; oxytocin
Ox oxygen
ox oxidized
OXA oxaprotiline
OXCHECK Oxford and Collaborators Health Check [trial]
OXIPHOS oxidative phosphorylation
OxLDL, Ox-LDL oxidized low-density lipoprotein
OXMIS Oxford Myocardial Infarction Incidence Study
Oxo oxanosine
8oxoA 8-oxoadenine
8oxoG 8-oxoguanine
OXP oxypressin
OXPHOS oxidative phosphorylation
OXT oxytocin
OXTR oxytocin receptor
OXY oxytocin
OXY, oxy oxygen
OYE old yellow enzyme
OYS Oslo Youth study
oz ounce
oz ap, oz apoth apothecaries' ounce (US)
oz t, oz tr troy ounce (UK)

P

P an electrocardiographic wave corresponding to a wave of depolarization crossing the atria; by weight [Lat. *pondere*]; father [Lat. *pater*]; near [Lat. *proximum*]; near point [Lat. *punctum proximum*]; pain; parietal electrode placement in electroencephalography; parity; part; partial pressure; *Pasteurella*; paternal; patient; penicillin; penta- [10^{15}]; percent; percussion; perforation; permeability; peta-; pharmacopeia; phenophthalein; phenylalanine; phosphate group; phosphorus; physiology; pig; pint; placebo; plan; plasma; *Plasmodium*; *Pneumocystis*; point; poise; poison, poisoning; polarity; polarization; pole; polymyxin; pons; population; porcelain; porcine; porphyrin; position; positive; posterior; postpartum; power; precipitin; precursor; prednisone; premolar; presbyopia; pressure; primary; primipara; probability; product; progesterone; prolactin; proline; promoter; properdin; propionate; protein; *Proteus*; proximal; *Pseudomonas*; psychiatry; pulmonary; pulse; pupil; radiant power; significance probability [value]; simple programmable [pacemaker]; sound power; weight [Lat. *pondus*]

P₁ first parental generation; pulmonic first sound

P₂ pulmonic second sound

P₃ proximal third

P³ primary prevention project

P-50 oxygen half-saturation pressure

P₉₀ 90 percentile [statistics]

p120 phosphoprotein 120 (kDa)

p atomic orbital with angular momentum quantum number 1; freeze preservation; the frequency of the more common allele of a pair; momentum; papilla; pathological; phosphate; pico-; pint; pond; pressure; probability; proton; pulse; pupil; short arm of chromosome; sound pressure

p- para

p̄ after [L. *post*]

p24 HIV antigen

Π see *pi*

π see *pi*

φ see *phi*

ψ see *psi*

PA panic attack; pantothenic acid; paralysis agitans; paranoia; parathion; passive aggressive; pathology; patient's advocate; peak amplitude; performance assessment; periarteritis; peridural artery; periodic acid; periodontal abscess; pernicious anemia; perpetual asymmetry; phakicaphakic; phenylalkylamine; phosphatidic acid; phenylalanine; phosphoarginine; photoallergy; phthalic anhydride; physical abuse; physician advisor; physician assistant; pituitary-adrenal; plasma adsorption; plasma aldosterone; plasminogen activator; platelet adhesiveness; platelet aggregation; platelet-associated; plicatic acid; polyamine; polyarteritis; polyarthritis; post-aural; posteroanterior; prealbumin; preadipocyte; preamplifier; predictive accuracy; pregnancy-associated; presents again; pressure augmentation [respiration]; primary aldosteronism; primary amenorrhea; primary anemia; prior to admission; proactivator; proanthocyanidin; procainamide; professional association; prolonged action; propionic acid; prostate antigen; protective antigen; proteolytic action; prothrombin activity; protrusio acetabuli; pseudoaneurysm; *Pseudomonas aeruginosa*; psychoanalysis; psychogenic aspermia; pulmonary arterial [pressure]; pulmonary artery; pulmonary atresia; pulpoaxial; puromycin aminonucleoside; pyruvic acid; pyrrolizidine alkaloid; yearly [Lat. *per annum*]

P-A posteroanterior

P(A) probability of event A

P&A percussion and auscultation

P_A alveolar pressure; atrial pressure; paternal allele; partial pressure of arterial fluid

PA3 Atrial Pacing Peri-Ablation for Paroxysmal Atrial Fibrillation [trial]

Pa acellular pertussis [vaccine]; atrial pressure; pascal; pathologist, pathology; prealbumin; protactinium; *Pseudomonas aeruginosa*; pulmonary arterial [pressure]

pA picoampere

pa through the anus [Lat. *per anum*]; yearly [Lat. *per annum*]

PAA partial agonist activity; phenylacetic acid; phosphonoacetic acid; physical abilities analysis; plasma angiotensinase activity; polyacrylamide; polyacrylic acid; polyamino acid; pyridine acetic acid

PAAI personal access and alert interface [telemedicine]

pAAM polyacrylamide

P(A−a)O₂ $P(A-a)O_2$ alveolar-arterial oxygen pressure difference

PAAS panic and anticipatory anxiety scale

PAB para-aminobenzoate; performance assessment battery; pharmacologic autonomic block; poly(A)-binding [protein]; premature atrial beat; purple agar base

Pab abdominal pressure

pAb polyclonal antibody

PABA, pABA para-aminobenzoic acid

PABD predeposit autologous blood donation

PABP poly A binding protein; pulmonary artery balloon pump

PABV percutaneous aortic balloon valvuloplasty

PAC paclitaxel; P1 artificial chromosome; papular acrodermatitis of childhood; parent-adult-child; pericarditis-arthropathy-camptodactyly [syndrome]; phenacetin, aspirin, and caffeine; physical activity [scale]; plasma aldosterone concentration; platelet-associated complement; Policy Advisory Committee; preadmission certification; premature atrial contraction; product of ambulatory care; pulmonary artery catheterization

pac pachytene

PACAP pituitary adenylate cyclase activating polypeptide

PAC-A-TACH Pacemaker Atrial Tachycardia [trial]

PACC primary ambulatory care center; promoting aphasics' communicative competence

PACCO Pulmonary Artery Catheterization and Clinical Outcomes [study]

PACCS Prospective Army Coronary Calcium Study

PACE Pacing and Clinical Electrophysiology; paired basic amino acid cleaving enzyme; Partnership in Active Continuous Education; Patient Care Expert [artificial intelligence nursing decision support]; people with arthritis can exercise [program]; personalized aerobics for cardiovascular enhancement; population-adjusted clinical epidemiology; Prevention with Low-dose Aspirin of Cardiovascular Diseases in the Elderly [study]; primary ambulatory care and education; Program of All-inclusive Care for the Elderly; pulmonary angiotensin I converting enzyme

PACI Partnership for Advanced Computational Infrastructure

PACIFIC potential angina class improvement from intramyocardial channels

PACK Prevention of Atherosclerotic Complications with Ketanserin [study]

PACNS primary angiitis of the central nervous system

PA_CO PA_{CO} mean alveolar gas volume

P_ACO₂ P_{ACO_2} partial pressure of carbon dioxide in alveolar gas

P_aCO₂ P_{aCO_2} partial pressure of carbon dioxide in arterial blood

PACP pulmonary alveolar-capillary permeability; pulmonary artery counterpulsation

PACS picture archiving and communication system; postoperative atrial fibrillation in cardiac surgery

PACS DB picture archiving and communication system data base

PACST Putney Auditory Comprehension Screening Test

PACT papillary carcinoma of thyroid; Philadelphia Association of Clinical Trials; Plasminogen Activator Angioplasty Compatibility Trial; Plasminogen Activator Coronary Angioplasty Trial; precordial acceleration tracing; Prehospital Application of Coronary Thrombolysis [study]; prepaid accountable care term; prescription analyses and cost; Prospective Acute Coronary Syndrome Trial; Pro-urokinase in Acute Coronary Thrombosis [study]

PACU postanesthetic care unit

PACV Pacui virus

PACWP pulmonary arterial capillary wedge pressure

PAD pain and distress; patient surface axis depth; percutaneous abscess drainage; percutaneous automated discectomy; peripheral artery disease; phenacetin, aspirin, and desoxyephedrine; photon absorption densitometry; practitioners accessing data; primary affective disorder; psychoaffective disorder; public access to defibrillation;

pulmonary artery diastolic; pulsatile assist device; pulsed amperometric detection

PAD-I Public Access Defibrillation I [trial]

PADL personal activities of daily living

PADP pulmonary artery diastolic pressure

PADPRP, pADPRP polyadenosine diphosphate–ribose polymerase

PADS patient archiving and documentation system

PADUA progressive augmentation by dilating the urethra anterior

PAdV 1–3, 4, 5 porcine adenoviruses 1–3, 4, 5

PAdV-A, B, C porcine adenoviruses A, B, and C

PADyC passive arm with dynamic constrains [computer-assisted surgery]

PAE paradoxical air embolism; postanoxic encephalopathy; post-antibiotic effect; progressive assistive exercise

PAEC porcine aortic endothelial cell

paed [*paediatrics, paediatric*] pediatrics, pediatrics

PAEDP pulmonary artery end-diastolic pressure

PAEP progestagen-associated endometrial protein

PAES popliteal artery entrapment syndrome

PAF paroxysmal atrial fibrillation; peroxisomal assembly factor; phosphodiesterase-activating factor; plain abdominal film; platelet-activating factor; platelet-aggregating factor; pollen adherence factor; population-attributable fractions; premenstrual assessment form; progressive autonomic failure; pulmonary arteriovenous fistula; pure autonomic failure

PA&F percussion, auscultation, and fremitus

PAFA priority based assessment of foot additives

PAF-A platelet-activating factor of anaphylaxis

PAFAC Prevention of Atrial Fibrillation After Cardioversion [study]

PAFAH platelet-activating factor acetylhydrolase

PAFAMS Pan-American Federation of Associations of Medical Schools

PAFD percutaneous abscess and fluid drainage; pulmonary artery filling defect

PAFI platelet-aggregation factor inhibitor

PAFIB paroxysmal atrial fibrillation

PAFIT Paroxysmal Atrial Fibrillation Italian Trial

PAFP pre-Achilles fat pad

PAFra platelet-activating factor receptor antagonist

PAFT Propafenone Atrial Fibrillation Trial

PAG periaqueductal gray [matter]; polyacrylamide gel; pregnancy-associated globulin; proliferation-associated gene; proximal anastomosis graft; pulmonary arteriography

pAg protein A-gold [technique]

PAGA proliferation-associated gene A

PAGE perfluorocarbon-associated gas exchange; polyacrylamide gel electrophoresis

PAGE-IEF polyacrylamine gel electrophoresis–isoelectric focusing [electrophoresis]

PAGIF polyacrylamide gel isoelectric focusing

PAGMK primary African green monkey kidney

PAGOD pulmonary hypoplasia-hypoplasia of pulmonary artery-agonadism-omphalocele/diaphragmatic defect-dextrocardia [syndrome]

PAH para-aminohippurate; phenylalanine hydroxylase; polycyclic aromatic hydrocarbon; predicted adult height [by Bayley-Pinneau]; pulmonary alveolar hypoventilation; pulmonary artery hypertension; pulmonary artery hypotension

PAHA para-aminohippuric acid; procainamide-hydroxylamine

PAHO Pan-American Health Organization

PAHP *p*-aminoheptanoylphenone

PAHV Pahayokee virus

PAHVC pulmonary alveolar hypoxic vasoconstrictor

PAI pain assessment inventory; partial androgen insensitivity; pathogenicity island; patient assessment instrument; perforating arterial infarction; plasminogen activator inhibitor; platelet accumulation index

PAI-1 plasminogen activator inhibitor 1

PAI-2 plasminogen activator inhibitor 2

PAIC procedures, alternatives, indications, and complications

PAICS phosphoribosylaminoimidazole carboxylase

PAID problem areas in diabetes [scale]

PAIDS paralyzed academic investigator's disease syndrome; pediatric acquired immunodeficiency syndrome

PAIg platelet-associated immunoglobulin

PAIgG platelet-associated immunoglobulin G

PAIMS Plasminogen Activator Italian Multicenter Study

PAIN pyoderma gangrenosum, aphthous stomatitis, inflammatory eye disease, erythema nodosum [disorders associated with inflammatory bowel disease]

PAIRS Pain and Impairment Relationship Scale

P$_{airway}$ airway pressure

PAIS partial androgen insensitivity syndrome; phosphoribosylaminoimidazole synthetase; Pravastatin in Acute Ischemic Syndromes [study]; psychosocial adjustment to illness scale

PAIS-SR psychosocial adjustment to illness scale-self reported

PAIVS Pulmonary Atresia with Intact Ventricular Septum [collaborative study]

PAJ paralysis agitans juvenilis

PAK p21-activated kinase; pancreas after kidney [transplantation]

PAKY percutaneous access to kidney

PAKY-RCM percutaneous access to kidney–remote center of motion [computer-assisted surgery]

PAL paradox advanced [computer] language; pathology laboratory; peptidyl-alpha-hydroxyglycine alpha-amidating lysine phase alteration plane; physical activity level; pointer to text application language; posterior assisted levitation [cataract surgery]; posterior axillary line; product of activated lymphocytes; pyogenic abscess of the liver

pal palate

PALA *N*-(phosphonacetyl)-L-aspartate

PALP placental alkaline phosphatase

palp palpation, palpate

palpi palpitation

PALS parietolateral lymphocyte sheath; Patient Advocacy and Liaison Service; pediatric advanced life support; prison-acquired lymphoproliferative syndrome

PALV Palyam virus

PAM pancreatic acinar mass; penicillin aluminum monostearate; peptidylglycine alpha-amidating monooxygenase; phenylalaline mustard; physical agent modality; physical archive manager [database element]; *p*-methoxyamphetamine; postauricular myogenic; potassium-aggravated myotonia; pralidoxime; pre-arrest morbidity [index]; pregnancy-associated α-macroglobulin; primary amebic meningoencephalitis; principles of ambulatory medicine; professions allied to medicine; pulmonary alveolar macrophage; pulmonary alveolar microlithiasis; pulse amplitude modulation; pyridine aldoxime methiodide

PAMC pterygoarthromyodysplasia congenita

2-PAM Cl 2-pralidoxime chloride

PAMD primary adrenocortical micronodular dysplasia

PAME preanesthesia medical examination; primary amebic meningoencephalitis

PAMI Primary Angioplasty in Myocardial Infarction [trial]

PAMIE physical and mental impairment of function evaluation

PAMI-No SOS Primary Angioplasty in Myocardial Infarction with No Surgery on Site

PAMP pulmonary artery mean pressure

PAMR progressively automated medical record

PAMV Pampa virus

PAN periarteritis nodosa; periodic alternating nystagmus; peroxyacylnitrate; personal area network; polyarteritis nodosa; positional alcohol nystagmus; puromycin aminonucleoside

pan pancreas, pancreatic, pancreatectomy

Panc pancreas or pancreatic

P-ANCA perinuclear anti-neutrophilic cytoplasmic antibody

PAND primary adrenocortical nodular dysplasia

PANDA Paediatric Asthma Education of a New Multidose Dry Powder Inhaler [study]

PANDAS pediatric autoimmune neuropsychiatric disorders associated with streptococcal infection

PANE pediatric ambulance needs evaluation

PANI polyanilide

PANS puromycin aminonucleoside

PANSS Positive and Negative Syndrome Scale

PAO peak acid output; periacetabular osteotomy; peripheral airway obstruction; plasma amine oxidase; polyamine oxidase; pulmonary artery occlusion; pustulotic arthroosteitis

PAO$_2$ alveolar oxygen partial pressure

PAo airway opening pressure; ascending aortic pressure; pulmonary artery occlusion pressure

PaO$_2$ partial arterial oxygen tension

PAO$_2$/FIO$_2$, PaO$_2$/FiO$_2$ ratio of alveolar partial pressure of oxygen to fraction of inspired air

PAOD peripheral arterial occlusive disease; peripheral arteriosclerotic occlusive disease

Pao, max peak airway pressure

PAOP *p*-aminooctanoylphenone; pulmonary artery occlusion pressure

PaOP pulmonary artery occlusion pressure

PAP pancreatitis-associated protein; Papanicolaou [test]; papaverine; passive-aggressive personality; password authentication protocol; patient assessment program; peak airway pressure; phosphoadenosine phosphate; peroxidase antibody to peroxidase; peroxidase-antiperoxidase [method]; placental acid/alkaline phosphatase; poly A polymerase; positive airway pressure; primary atypical pneumonia; prostatic acid phosphatase; pulmonary alveolar proteinosis; pulmonary artery pressure; purified alternate pathway

Pap Papanicolaou test

pap papilla

PAPC paraxial protocadherin

PAPF platelet adhesiveness plasma factor

papova papilloma-polyoma-vacuolating agent [virus]

PAPP para-aminopropiophenone; pregnancy-associated plasma protein

PAPPA pregnancy-associated plasma protein A

PAPPC pregnancy-associated plasma protein C

PAPR powered air purifying respirator

PAPS 3′-phosphoadenosine-5′-phosphosulfate; primary antiphospholipid antibody syndrome

Paps papillomas

Pap sm Papanicolaou smear

PAPUFA physiologically active polyunsaturated fatty acid

pa-pv pulmonary arterial pressure-pulmonary venous pressure

PAPVC partial anomalous pulmonary venous connection

PAPVD partial anomalous pulmonary venous drainage

PAPVR partial anomalous pulmonary venous return

PAQ patient asked questions; Personal Attitudes Questionnaire

PAQLQ Pediatric Asthma Quality of Life Questionnaire (PAQLQ)

PAR parent in semantic hierarchy [UMLS]; participating provider; passive avoidance reaction; percentage abnormal results; perennial allergic rhinitis; photosynthetically active radiation; Physical Activity Recall [Questionnaire]; physiological aging rate; plain abdominal radiograph; platelet aggregation receptor; platelet aggregate ratio; Policy, Action, and Rational Drug Use [WHO]; population-attributable risk; postanesthesia recovery; postanesthesia [recovery] room; posterior wall or aortic root; primary angioplasty research; Program for Alcohol Recovery; proximal alveolar region; pseudoautosomal region; pulmonary arteriolar resistance

PAR% population-attributable risk percent

par paraffin; paralysis

PARA, Para, para number of pregnancies producing viable offspring

para paraplegic; parathyroid, parathyroidectomy

para 0 nullipara

para I primipara

para II secundipara

para III tripara

para IV quadripara

PARADIGM Platelet Aggregation Receptor Antagonist Dose Investigation for Perfusion Gain in Myocardial Infarction [study]

PARADISE Platelet IIb/IIIa Antagonism for the Reduction of Acute Coronary

Events Dose Investigation and Safety Evaluation [study]

PARAGON Platelet IIb/IIIa Antagonist for the Reduction of Acute Coronary Syndrome Events in a Global Organization Network [study]

parasit parasitology; parasite, parasitic

parasym parasympathetic

PARAT Prevention of Arterial Restenosis Angiographic Trial

PARC Palo Alto Research Center; Pan-African Rinderpest Campaign

PARCO parallel computing

parent parenteral

pArg poly-L-arginine

PARIS Peripheral Artery Radiation Investigational Study; Persantine Aspirin Reinfarction Study

PARK Postangioplasty Restenosis Ketanserin [study]; Prevention of Angioplasty Reocclusion with Ketanserin

parox paroxysm, paroxysmal

PARP poly(adenosine diphosphate ribose) polymerase

PARR postanesthesia recovery room

PARS Personal Adjustment and Role Skills Scale

PART Prevention of Atherosclerosis with Ramipril Therapy [trial]; Probucol Angioplasty Restenosis Trial

PART-1 Predictors of Atherosclerosis Risk and Thrombosis [trial]

PART-2 Predictors of Atherosclerosis Risk and Thrombosis [trial]

PARTNER Peripheral Arterial Disease Response to Taprostene with New Established Response Criteria [trial]

PARTNERS Primary Care Access to Resources, Training, Networks, Education, and Research Services

PARTY prevent alcohol and risk-related trauma in youth

PARU postanesthetic recovery unit

PARV Parana virus

ParVox Parallel Volume Rendering System for Scientific Visualization [trial]

PAS para-aminosalicylate; Paragon Elective or Acute Stent [trial]; Parent Attitude Scale; patient administration system; patient appointments and scheduling; periodic acid-Schiff [reaction]; peripheral anterior synechia; persistent atrial standstill; Personality Assessment Scale;

photoacoustic spectroscopy; phosphatase acid serum; physician-assisted suicide; Polish Amiodarone Study; posterior airway space; pre-admission screening; predictive accuracy on survival; pregnancy advisory service; premature atrial stimulus; professional activity study; progressive accumulated stress; pulmonary arterial stenosis; pulmonary artery systolic

Pas, Pa · s, Pa × s pascal-second

PASA para-aminosalicylic acid; polymerase chain reaction amplification of specific alleles; primary acquired sideroblastic anemia; proximal articular set angle

PASAR programmable automatic scanning arrhythmia reversion [algorithm]

PASAR-O orthorhythmic programmable automatic scanning arrhythmia reversion [algorithm]

PASARR pre-admission screening and resident review

PASAT Paced Auditory Serial Addition Task

PASB protein-associated strand breaks

PAS-C para-aminosalicylic acid crystallized with ascorbic acid

PASD after diastase digestion

PASE Pacemaker Selection in the Elderly [trial]; physical activity scale for the elderly [evaluation]

PASG pneumatic antishock garment

PASH periodic acid-Schiff hematoxylin; pseudoangiomatous stromal hyperplasia

PASM periodic acid-silver methenamine

PASP pancreas-specific protein; pulmonary artery systolic pressure

PASS personal alerting safety system; Piracetam in Acute Stroke Study; Postarthroplasty Screening Study [for deep venous thrombosis]; Practical Applicability of Saruplase Study; Prehospital Applicability of Saruplase Study

pass passive

pass ROM passive range of motion

PASSOR Physiatric Association for Spine, Sports, and Occupational Rehabilitation

PAST periodic acid-Schiff technique

Past *Pasteurella*

PASTA Percutaneous Ambulatory Stent Trial; polarity altered spectral selective acquisition; Primary Angioplasty vs Stent

Implantation in Acute Myocardial Infarction [trial]

PAstV porcine astrovirus

PASVR pulmonary anomalous superior venous return

PASW personal assistance service worker

PAT Pain Apperception Test; paroxysmal atrial tachycardia; patient; patient domain; penetrating abdominal trauma; phenylaminotetrazole; physical abilities test; picric acid turbidity; platelet aggregation test; Polish Amiodarone Trial; polyamine acetyltransferase; postoperative atrial tachycardia; preadmission assessment team/ test; preadmission testing; predictive ability test; pregnancy at term; psychoacoustic test

pat patella; patent; paternal origin; patient

PATAF Prevention of Arterial Thromboembolism in Nonvalvular Atrial Fibrillation [study]; Primary Prevention of Arterial Thromboembolic Processes in Atrial Fibrillation [trial]

PATAV Pata virus

PATCH planned approach to community health

Pat-CIS patient clinical information system

PatDp paternal duplication

PATE Pravastatin Anti-atherosclerosis Trial in the Elderly; psychodynamic and therapeutic education; pulmonary artery thromboembolism

PATENT Pro-Urokinase and Tissue Plasminogen Activator Enhancement of Thrombolysis [trial]

PATG patient group [UMLS]

PATH pathologic function [UMLS]; pathology, pathological; pituitary adrenotropic hormone; physicians at teaching hospitals

path pathogenesis, pathogenic; pathology, pathological

PATHS Prevention and Treatment of Hypertension Study

Patm atmospheric pressure

PATMAN Patient Workflow Management [system]

Patr pulmonary atresia

PATRIC position and time resolved ion counting

PATS Poststroke Antihypertensive Treatment Study; Prehospital Administration of Tissue Plasminogen Activator Study; Protection Assessment Test System

PAT-SED pseudoachondroplastic dysplasia

PA-T-SP periodic acid-thiocarbo-hydrazide-silver proteinate

PATV Patois virus

PAU phenol-acetic acid-urea

PAUP phylogenic analysis using parsimony

PAUSE Popliteal Artery Ultrasound Examination [study]

PAV percutaneous aortic valvuloplasty; poikiloderma atrophicans vasculare; posterior arch vein; proportional assist ventilation

PaV Pariacoto virus

Pav airway pressure

P$_{ave}$ mean average pressure during inspiration

PAVEC porcine aortic valve endothelial cell

pavex passive vascular exercise

PAVF pulmonary arteriovenous fistula

PAVM pulmonary arteriovenous malformation

PAVNRT paroxysmal atrioventricular nodal reciprocal tachycardia

pAVP plasma arginine vasopressin

PA-VSD pulmonary atresia with ventricular septal defect

PAW peripheral airways; pulmonary artery wedge

P$_{AW}$, Paw airway pressure

PAWP pulmonary arterial wedge pressure

PAWS primary withdrawal syndrome

PAX paired box homeotic [family]

PAZ prednisone/azathioprine

PB British pharmacopeia [*Pharmacopoeia Britannica*]; paraffin bath; paraffin block; paucibacillary; Paul-Bunnell [antibody]; periodic breathing; peripheral blood; peroneus brevis; phenobarbital; phenoxybenzamine phonetically balanced; pinealoblastoma; Polybrene; polymyxin B; premature beat; pressure breathing; protein binding; punch biopsy; pyridostigmine bromide

P$_B$ barometric pressure

P&B pain & burning; phenobarbital and belladonna

Pb body [surface] pressure; lead [Lat. *plumbum*]; phenobarbital; presbyopia

PBA polyclonal B-cell activity; pressure breathing assist; prolactin-binding assay; prune belly anomaly; pulpobuccoaxial

PBAL protected bronchoalveolar lavage

PBB polybrominated biphenyl

Pb-B lead in blood

PBBs polybrominated biphenyls

PBC perfusion balloon catheter; phosphocreatine; peripheral blood cell; point of basal convergence; pre-bed care; primary biliary cirrhosis; progestin-binding complement

PBCC point biserial correlation coefficient

PBCH polymorphic B-cell hyperplasia

PBCL polymorphic B-cell lymphoma

PBCRA progressive bifocal chorioretinal atrophy

PBCV *Paramecium bursaria* chlorella virus

PBD postburn day

PBDE polybrominated diphenyl ether

PBE tuberculin from *Mycobacterium tuberculosis bovis* [Ger. *Perlsucht Bacillen-emulsion*]

PBF pencil beam function [radiotherapy]; peripheral blood flow; placental blood flow; predominant breast feeding; pulmonary blood flow

PBFE peroxisomal bifunctional enzyme

PBFe protein-bound iron

PBG porphobilinogen

PBGD porphobilinogen deaminase

PBGS, PBG-S porphobilinogen synthase

PBH profiling by hybridization; pulling boat hands; pyrenabutyric acid hydrazide

PBHB poly-beta-hydroxybutyrate

PBI parental bonding instrument; penile pressure/brachial pressure index; protein-bound iodine

PbI lead intoxication

PBIgG platelet surface bound immunoglobulin G

PBK phosphorylase B kinase

PBL peripheral blood leukocyte; peripheral blood lymphocyte; problem-based learning

PBLC peripheral blood lymphocyte count; premature birth living child; problem-based learning curriculum

PBLM problem-based learning module

PBLT peripheral blood lymphocyte transformation

PBM peak bone mass; peripheral basement membrane; peripheral blood mononuclear [cell]; placental basement membrane

PBMC peripheral blood mononuclear cell; pharmaceutical benefit management company

PBMNC peripheral blood mononuclear cell

PBMV pulmonary blood mixing volume

PBN alpha-phenyl-*n-tert*-butylnitrone; paralytic brachial neuritis; peripheral benign neoplasm; polymyxin B sulfate, bacitracin, and neomycin

PBNA partial body neutron activation

PBO penicillin in beeswax and oil; placebo

PBP penicillin-binding protein; platelet basic protein; porphyrin biosynthesis pathway; prostate-binding protein; pseudobulbar palsy; pulsatile bypass pump

PBPC peripheral blood progenitor cell; progressive bulbar palsy of childhood

PBPI penile-brachial pulse index

PBPK physiologically based pharmacokinetic [model]

PBPND progressive bulbar palsy with neural deafness

PBPV percutaneous balloon pulmonary valvuloplasty

PBRN practice-based research network

PBS perfusion-pressure breakthrough syndrome; phenobarbital sodium; phosphate-buffered saline; planar beam scan; primer binding site; protected brush specimen; prune belly syndrome; pulmonary branch stenosis

PBSA phosphate buffered saline [solution]

PBSC peripheral blood stem cell

PBSCT peripheral blood stem cell transplantation

PBSP prognostically bad signs during pregnancy

PBT Paul-Bunnell test; phenacetin breath test; piebald trait; profile-based therapy; pulmonary barotrauma

PBT$_4$ protein-bound thyroxine

PBV predicted blood volume; pulmonary blood volume

PBW posterior bite wing

PBX private branch exchange

PBZ personal breathing zone; phenylbutazone; phenoxybenzamine; pyribenzamine

PC avoirdupois weight [Lat. *pondus civile*]; pacinian corpuscle; packed cells; paper chromatography; paracortex; paramyotonia congenita; parent cell; particulate component; partition coefficient; patch clamp; penicillin; penile carcinoma; pentose cycle; peritoneal cell; personal care; personal computer; pharmacology; phase contrast; pheochromocytoma; phosphate cycle; phosphatidylcholine; phosphorylcholine; photoconduction; physicians' corporation; pill counter; piriform cortex; placebo-controlled; plasma concentration; plasma cortisol; plasmacytoma; plasmin complex; plastocyanin; platelet concentrate; platelet count; pneumotaxic center; polycarbonate; polycentric; polyposis coli; poor condition; poor coordination; portacaval; portal cirrhosis; postcoital; posterior cervical; posterior chamber; posterior commissure; posterior cortex; potential complications; preconditioned, preconditioning; precordial; prenatal care; present complaint; primary closure; principal component; printed circuit; procollagen; productive cough; professional corporation; prohormone convertase; prophlogistic corticoid; prostacyclin; prostatic carcinoma; protective cover; protein C; protein convertase; proximal colon; pseudocyst; pubococcygeus [muscle]; pulmonary capillary; pulmonary circulation; pulmonary compliance; pulmonic closure; Purkinje cell; pyloric canal; pyruvate carboxylase

PC1 first principal component

P$_c$ critical pressure

pc parsec; percent; picocurie

p/c presenting complaint

PCA pancreatic carcinoma; para-chloramphetamine; parietal cell antibody; passive cutaneous anaphylaxis; patient care assistant/aide; patient care audit; patient-controlled analgesia; penicillamine; perchloric acid; percutaneous carotid angiography; percutaneous coronary angioplasty; personal care assistant; personal computer advisory; phenylcarboxylic acid; Physicians Corporation of America; plasma catecholamine; polyclonal antibody; porcine coronary artery; porous coated anatomic

[prosthesis]; postconceptional age; portacaval anastomosis; postcoronary [cardiac] arrest; posterior cerebral artery; posterior communicating aneurysm/artery; posterior cricoarytenoid [muscle]; precoronary care area; prehospital cardiac arrest; President's Council on Aging; principal components analysis; procainamide; procoagulant activity; program component area; prostatic carcinoma; protected catheter aspirate; protective concentration level; pyrrolidine carboxylic acid

PcA prostatic adenocarcinoma

PCAD Patent Citation Analysis Database; progression of coronary artery disease

pCAF phasic carotid activation function

PCAPS Primary Care Act Pilot Sites [UK]

PCASSO Patient-Centered Access to Secure System Online

PCAST President's Committee of Advisors on Science and Technology

PCASYS pattern-level classification automation system

PCAT phosphatidylcholine-cholesterol acyltransferase; primary care assessment tool

PCAV Pacora virus

PCB paracervical block; polychlorinated biphenyl; portacaval bypass; postcoital bleeding; printed circuit board; procarbazine

PcB near point of convergence to the intercentral base line [Lat. *punctum convergens basalis*]

PC-BMP phosphorylcholine-binding myeloma protein

PCC Pasteur Culture Collection; percutaneous cecostomy; peripheral cholangiocarcinoma; pheochromocytoma; phosphate carrier compound; plasma catecholamine concentration; platinum-containing compound; pneumatosis cystoides coli; Poison Control Center; precoronary care; premature chromosome condensation; primary care clinic or center; primary care continuum; primary care curriculum; protein C cofactor

PCc periscopic concave

pcc premature chromosome condensation

PCCA polychlorocycloalkane

PCCC pediatric critical care center

PCCF protein C cofactor

PC CLIN-SIM personal computer clinical simulation

PCCM pediatric critical care medicine; primary care case management; primary care case manager

PCCTEA patient-controlled continuous thoracic epidural analgesia

PCCU post-coronary care unit

PCD pacer-cardioverter-defibrillator; papillary collecting duct; paraneoplastic cerebellar degeneration; paroxysmal cerebral dysrhythmia; percutaneous catheter drainage; pervasive developmental disorder; phosphate-citrate-dextrose; plasma cell dyscrasia; polycystic disease; posterior corneal deposits; postmortem cesarean delivery; premature centromere division; primary ciliary dyskinesia; programmable cardioverter-defibrillator; programmed cell death; prolonged contractile duration; pterin-4a-carbinolamine dehydratase; pulmonary clearance delay

PCDC plasma clot diffusion chamber

PCDD Patient Clinical Data Directory; polychlorinated dibenzodioxin

PCDF polychorinated dibenzofuran

PCDS Patient Care Data Set

PCE patient care encounter; perchloroethylene; physical capacity evaluation; pseudocholinesterase; polychromatic erythrocyte

PCEA patient-controlled epidural anesthesia

PCES patient care evaluation study

PCF peripheral circulatory failure; pharyngoconjunctival fever; platelet complement fixation; posterior cranial fossa; potential [gene] coding fragment

pcf pounds per cubic feet

PCFIA particle concentration of fluorescence immunoassay

PCFT platelet complement fixation test

PCG pancreatico-cholangiography; paracervical ganglion; phonocardiogram, phonocardiography; pneumocardiogram; postcentral gyrus; preconditioned conjugate gradient [algorithm]; preventive care group; primate chorionic gonadotropin; pubococcygeus [muscle]

PCH paroxysmal cold hemoglobinuria; patient care hours; polycyclic hydrocarbon

PCHE pseudocholinesterase

PCHI Partners Community Health Care

P²C² HIV Pediatric Pulmonary and Cardiovascular Complications of Human Immunodeficiency Virus Infection [study]; Pediatric Pulmonary and Cardiac Complications of Vertically Transmitted HIV Infection [study]

PCHLS continuous heterogeneous lumped systems

PCI patient classification index; peripheral [computer] component interconnect; percutaneous coronary intervention; pneumatosis cystoides intestinales; prophylactic cranial irradiation; protein C inhibitor; prothrombin consumption index

P/CI physical and chemical indicators

pCi picocurie

PCIC Poison Control Information Center

pCi/L picocuries per liter

PC-IRV pressure-controlled inverted ratio ventilation

PCIS Patient-Care Information System; point-of-care information system; postcardiac injury syndrome

PCK phosphoenolpyruvate carboxykinase; polycystic kidney

PCKD polycystic kidney disease

PCL pacing cycle length; packaging cell line; persistent corpus luteum; plasma cell leukemia; posterior chamber lens; posterior cruciate ligament; primary care loan; proximal collateral ligament

PCLI plasma cell labeling index

PCM paracoccidioidomycosis; patient care management; patient care manager; phase contrast microscopy; primary cutaneous melanoma; process control monitor; protein-calorie malnutrition; protein carboxymethylase

PCMB parachloromercuribenzoate

PCMO Principal Clinical Medical Officer

PCMR Pediatric Cardiomyopathy Registry

PC-MRA phase contrast magnetic resonance angiography

PCMS patient care management system

PCMs patient care management categories

PCMT pacemaker circus movement tachycardia; protein carboxyl methyltransferase

PCMX para-chloro-metoxylenol

PCN parent-child nursing; penicillin; pregnenolone-16α-carbonitrile; primary care network; primary care nursing

PCNA proliferating cell nuclear antigen

PCNB pentachloronitrobenzene

PCNL percutaneous nephrostolithotomy

PCNV postchemotherapy nausea and vomiting; Provisional Committee on Nomenclature of Viruses

PCO parametric clinical observation; patient complains of; polycystic ovary; posterior capsular opacification; predicted cardiac output

P$_{CO}$ partial pressure of carbon monoxide

P$_{CO_2}$, pCO$_2$ partial pressure of carbon dioxide

PCOC Primary Care Organization Consortium

PCOD polycystic ovarian disease

PCOM phase contrast optical method; posterior communicating [artery]

PCON Primary Care Organization Network

PCOS polycystic ovary syndrome

PCOV porcine type C oncovirus

PCP parachlorophenate; patient care plan; pentachlorophenol; 1-(1-phenylcyclohexyl)piperidine; peripheral coronary pressure; persistent cough and phlegm; phencyclidine palmitate; *Pneumocystis carinii* pneumonia; postoperative constrictive pericarditis; primary care physician; primary care provider; prochlorperazine; procollagen peptide; prolylcarboxypeptidase; pulmonary capillary pressure; pulse cytophotometry

PCPA para-chlorophenylalanine; Pest Control Practices Act [Canada]

PCPB procarboxypeptide B

PCPL pulmonary capillary protein leakage

pcpn precipitation

PCPP poly[di(carboxylatophenoxy)phosphazene]

PCPV pseudocowpox virus

PCQ polychloroquaterphenyl

PCR patient contact record; perinatal clinical record; phosphocreatinine; photoconvulsive response; plasma clearance rate; polymerase chain reaction; post-compression remodeling; prehospital care report; principal component regression; protein catabolism rate

PCr phosphocreatine

P$_{Cr}$ plasma creatinine

pcr protein catabolic rate

PCRA percutaneous coronary rotational atherectomy

PCR-DS polymerase chain reaction–direct sequencing

PCR-ELISA polymerase chain reaction–enzyme linked immunosorbent assay

PCR-ISH polymerase chain reaction–in situ hybridization

PCR-MASA polymerase chain reaction–mutant allele specific amplification

PCR-RFLP polymerase chain reaction–restriction fragment length polymorphism

PCR-RH polymerase chain reaction–reverse hybridization

PCRS [sex] partner counseling and referral service

PCR/SSCP polymerase chain reaction–single stranded conformation polymorphism

PCRV Parry Creek virus; polycythemia rubra vera

PCS palliative care service; patient care system; patient classification system; patient-controlled sedation; patterns of care study; pelvic congestion syndrome; pharmacogenic confusional syndrome; portacaval shunt; post-cardiac surgery; postcardiotomy syndrome; postcholecystectomy syndrome; postconcussion syndrome; premature centromere separation; Prevention of Coronary Atherosclerosis Study; primary cancer site; prolonged crush syndrome; proportional counter spectrometry; proximal coronary sinus; pseudotumor cerebri syndrome

pcs preconscious

PCS/ADS patient care system/application development system

PCSM percutaneous stone manipulation

PCSS Perth Community Stroke Study

PCSW personal care service worker

PCT peripheral carcinoid tumor; phase contrast tomography; plasma clotting time; plasmacrit test; plasmacytoma; polychlorinated triphenyl; porphyria cutanea tarda; portacaval transposition; positron computed tomography; postcoital test; primary care team; progesterone challenge test; prothrombin consumption time; proximal convoluted tubule

pCT porcine calcitonin

pct percent

PCTI penetrating cardiac trauma index

PCU pain control unit; palliative care unit; primary care unit; progressive care unit; patient care unit; pulmonary care unit

PCV packed cell volume; polycythemia vera; porcine circovirus; postcapillary venule; pressure-control ventilation

PCV84 parvo-like virus of crabs

PCVC percutaneous central venous catheter

PCV-M polycythemia vera with myeloid metaplasia

PCW pericanalicular web; personal care worker; primary capillary wedge; pulmonary capillary wedge; purified cell walls

PCWP pulmonary capillary wedge pressure

PCx patient's cardex; periscopic convex

PCZ procarbazine; prochlorperazine

PD Doctor of Pharmacy; Dublin Pharmacopoeia; interpupillary distance; Paget disease; pancreas divisum; pancreatic duct; panic disorder; papilla diameter; paralyzing dose; Parkinson disease; parkinsonian dementia; paroxysmal discharge; pars distalis; patent ductus; patient day; pediatric, pediatrics; percentage difference; percutaneous discectomy; percutaneous drain; peritoneal dialysis; personal database; personality disorder; pharmacodynamics; phenyldichlorarsine; phosphate dehydrogenase; phosphate dextrose; photodiode; photosensitivity dermatitis; Pick disease; plasma defect; poorly differentiated; postdischarge; posterior descending; posterior division; postnasal drainage; postural drainage; potential difference; pregnanediol; present disease; pressor dose; prism diopter; problem drinker; program director; progression of disease; progressive disease; proliferative disease; protein degradation; protein diet; proton density; psychotic depression; pulmonary disease; pulpodistal; pulse duplicator; pulse duration; pulsed diastolic; pulsed Doppler [wave]; pupil diameter; pupillary distance; pyloric dilator; pyrimidine dimer

P/D proximal-to-distal [vessel]

2-PD two-point discrimination

Pd palladium; pediatrics

P$_d$ diastolic pressure

PDA patent ductus arteriosus; patient distress alarm; personal digital assistant; poorly differentiated adenocarcinoma;

portable decontamination apparatus; posterior descending artery; pulmonary disease anemia

PdA pediatric allergy

PDAB para-dimethylaminobenzaldehyde

PD-AB-SAAP pulsed diastolic autologous blood selective aortic arch perfusion

PDAP Palmer drug abuse program

PD/AR photosensitivity dermatitis and actinic reticuloid syndrome

PDAY pathological determinants of atherosclerosis in youth

PDAY/RFEHA Pathobiological Determinants of Atherosclerosis in Youth/Risk Factors in Early Human Atherogenesis [study]

PDB Paget disease of bone; paradichlorobenzene; patient's database; phosphorus-dissolving bacteria; preventive dental [health] behavior; Protein Data Bank

PDBu phorbol 12,13-dibutyrate

PDC parkinsonism dementia complex; patient data card; pediatric cardiology; penta-decylcatechol; phosducin; physical dependence capacity; plasma dioxin concentration; preliminary diagnostic clinic; private diagnostic clinic

PdC pediatric cardiology

PDCA plan-do-check-act

PDCD primary degenerative cerebral disease

PD-CSE pulsed Doppler cross-sectional echocardiography

PDD percentage depth dose; pervasive developmental disorder; platinum diamminodichloride [cisplatin]; primary degenerative dementia; primary degenerative disorder; pervasive developmental disorder; pyridoxine-deficient diet

PDDA poly(dimethyldiallylammonium chloride); power-driven decontamination apparatus

PDDD primary degenerative/deformative disorder

PD DNA pyrimidine dimer DNA

PDDNOS pervasive developmental disorder not otherwise specified

PDDP Poincaré dispersed dot plots

PDDR pseudovitamin D–dependent rickets

PDE paroxysmal dyspnea on exertion; partial differential equation; peritoneal dialysis effluent; phosphodiesterase;

physician data entry; progressive dialysis encephalopathy; pulsed Doppler echocardiography

PdE pediatric endocrinology

PDEA phosphodiesterase

PDEAEM poly(diethylaminoethyl methacrylate)

PDEB phosphodiesterase beta

PDEC pancreatic ductal epithelial cell

PDECG platelet-derived endothelial growth [factor]

PD-ECGF platelet-derived endothelial cell growth factor

PDEG phosphodiesterase gamma

PDF parameterized diastolic filling; Parkinson's Disease Foundation; peritoneal dialysis fluid; Portable Document Format; probability density function; pyruvate dehydrogenase

pdf probability density function

PDG parkinsonism-dementia complex of Guam; Pharmacopoeial Discussion Group; phosphogluconate dehydrogenase

PDGA pteroyldiglutamic acid

PDGF platelet-derived growth factor

PDGF-A platelet-derived growth factor A

PDGF-B platelet-derived growth factor B

PDGFR platelet-derived growth factor receptor

PDGFRB platelet-derived growth factor receptor beta

PDGS partial form of DiGeorge syndrome

PD-GXT postdischarge graded exercise test

PDH past dental history; phosphate dehydrogenase; position-of-the-dynamometer-handle [test]; progressive disseminated histoplasmosis; pyruvate dehydrogenase

PDHA pyruvate dehydrogenase alpha

PDHa pyruvate dehydrogenase in active form

PDHB pyruvate dehydrogenase beta

PDHC pyruvate dehydrogenase complex

PdHO pediatric hematology-oncology

PdHV perdicid herpesvirus

PDI pain disability index; periodontal disease index; plan-do integration; portal dose image; psychomotor development index

Pdi, P_{di} transdiaphragmatic pressure

PDIE phosphodiesterase

Pdi$_{max}$ maximum transdiaphragmatic pressure

P-diol pregnanediol

PDIS participatory design of information system

PDK primary duck kidney

PDL pancreatic duct ligation; periodontal ligament; poorly differentiated lymphocyte; population doubling level; progressive diffuse leukoencephalopathy

pdl poundal; pudendal

PDLC poorly differentiated lung cancer

PDLD poorly differentiated lymphocytic-diffuse

PDLL poorly differentiated lymphocytic lymphoma

PDLN poorly differentiated lymphocytic-nodular

PDM point distribution model

PDMS pain data management system; patient data management system; pharmacokinetic drug monitoring service; polydimethylsiloxane

PDN prednisone; private duty nurse

pDNA plasmid deoxyribonucleic acid

PdNEO pediatric neonatology

PdNEP pediatric nephrology

PDP pancreatic duct pressure; papular dermatitis of pregnancy; parallel distributed processing; pattern disruption point; peak diastolic pressure; piperidinopyrimidine; plasma display; platelet-derived plasma; postural drainage and chest percussion; primer-dependent deoxynucleic acid polymerase; Product Development Protocol; programmed data processor; Protein Domain Parser

PDPD prolonged-dwell peritoneal dialysis

PDPDM protein-deficient pancreatic diabetes mellitus

PDPH postdural puncture headache

PDPI primer-dependent deoxynucleic acid polymerase index

PDQ Personality Diagnostic Questionnaire; physician's data query; Premenstrual Distress Questionnaire; prescreening developmental questionnaire; protocol data query

PDR pediatric radiology; peripheral diabetic retinopathy; physical device representation [computer-assisted surgery]; *Physicians' Desk Reference*; postdelivery room; primary drug resistance; proliferative diabetic retinopathy

PdR pediatric radiology

pdr powder

PDRB Permanent Disbility Rating Board

PDRT Portland Digit Recognition Test

PDS pain-dysfunction syndrome; Paris dosimetry system [radiotherapy]; paroxysmal depolarizing shift; patient data system; Patient-Doctor Society; pediatric surgery; penile Doppler study; perfusion defect size; peritoneal dialysis system; personnel decontamination station; plasma-derived serum; polydioxanone sutures; post determination software; predialyzed serum; progressive deterioration scale; proteodermatan sulfate

PdS pediatric surgery

PDSG pigment dispersion syndrome glaucoma

PDSIP Physician-delivered Smoking Intervention Project

PDSRS Panic Disorder Self-Rating Scale

PDT photodynamic therapy; population doubling time

PDTC pyrrolidine dithiocarbamate

PDUF pulsed Doppler ultrasonic flowmeter

PDUFA Prescription Drug User Fee Act

PDUR Predischarge Utilization Review

PDV peak diastolic velocity; phocine distemper virus; plasma-derived vaccine

PDVT proximal deep vein thrombosis

PDW platelet distribution width

PDWA proliferative disease without atypia

PDWHF platelet-derived wound-healing factor

PDYN prodynorphin

PE Edinburgh Pharmacopoeia; pancreatic extract; paper electrophoresis; partial epilepsy; peak ejection; peak error; pelvic examination; penile erection; pericardial effusion; peritoneal exudate; pharyngoesophageal; phase-encoded; phenylethylamine; phenylephrine; phenytoin equivalent; phosphatidyl ethanolamine; photographic effect; photosensitive epilepsy; phycoerythrin; physical education; physical engineering; physical examination; physical exercise; physician extender; physiological ecology; pigmented epithelium; pilocarpine-epinephrine; placental extract; plant engineering; plasma exchange; platinum etoposide; pleural effusion; point of entry; polyethylene; potential energy; powdered extract; preeclampsia; preexcitation; prescription error; present evaluation; pressure equalization; presumptive eligibility; prior to exposure; probable error; processing element; professional engineer; program evaluation; pseudoexfoliation; pulmonary edema; pulmonary embolism; pulmonary embolus; pyrogenic exotoxin

Pe pressure on expiration

PEA patient-controlled epidural anesthesia; pelvic examination under anesthesia; phenylethyl alcohol; phenylethylamine; polysaccharide egg antigen; pulseless electrical activity

PEAAc poly(ethylacrylic acid)

PEACH Physiologic Evaluation After Coronary Hyperemia [trial]

PEAP positive end-airway pressure

PEAR phase encoded artifact reduction

PEARLA pupils equal and react to light and accommodation

PEAS patient education and activation system; possible estuary-associated syndrome

PEAV Peaton virus

PEBG phenethylbiguanide

PEBP patient escorted by police

PEC patient evaluation center; pelvic cramps; peritoneal exudate cell; perivascular epithelioid cell; probability of error in classification; pulmonary ejection click; pyrogenic exotoxin C

PECAM platelet endothelial cell adhesion molecule

PECG pseudo-electrocardiogram

PECHO prostatic echogram

PECS patient evaluation and conference system; pediatrics evaluation in community setting

PECT positron emission computed tomography

PECTE Pulmonary Embolism Colfarit Trial in the Elderly

PECV porcine enteric calicivirus

PECVD plasma-enhanced chemical vapor deposition

PED palmoplantar ectodermal dysplasia; patient examined by doctor; pediatric emergency department; pink-eyed dilution

PED, ped pediatrics

PEDF pigment epithelium-derived factor

PeDS Pediatric Drug Surveillance

PedsQL pediatric quality of life

PEDV porcine epidemic diarrhea virus
PEE phosphate-eliminating enzyme
PEEC pathogen elicited epithelial chemo-attractant
PEEK polyetheretherketone
PEEP positive end-expiratory pressure
PEEP/CPAP positive end-expiratory pressure/continuous positive airway pressure
PEEPrs resistive positive end-respiratory pressure
PEER peer review effectiveness evaluation research
PEF peak expiratory flow; pharyngoepiglottic fold; potential energy function; prediction error filter; Psychiatric Evaluation Form; pulmonary edema fluid
PEFR peak expiratory flow rate
PEFV partial expiratory flow volume
PEG Patient Evaluation Grid; percutaneous endoscopic gastrostomy; pneumoencephalogram, pneumoencephalography; polyethylene glycol
PEG-ADA polyethylene glycol-modified adenine deaminase
PEGASUS Percutaneous Endarterectomy, the Goal of Atherectomy Successfully Guided by Ultrasound [trial]
PEGDA, PEG-DA polyethylene glycol diacrylate
PEGDMA polyethylene glycol dimethacrylate
PEGME polyethylene glycol methyl ether
Pegs paternally expressed genes
PEG-SOD polyethylene glycol superoxide dismutase
PEG-SPA polyethylene glycol succinyl propionate
PEHO progressive encephalopathy-edema-hypsarrhythmia-optic atrophy [syndrome]
PEHPC periodic examination and health promotion center
PeHV percid herpesvirus
PEI Patient Exit Interview; percutaneous ethanol injection; phosphate excretion index; physical efficiency index; polyethyleneimine
PEIRS pathology expert interpretative reporting system
PEJ percutaneous endoscopic jejunostomy
PEK punctate epithelial kerotopathy
PEL peritoneal exudate lymphocyte; permissible exposure limit

PELA peripheral excimer laser angioplasty
PELCA percutaneous excimer laser coronary angioplasty
PELF pulse extremely low frequency
PEM pediatric emergency medicine; peritoneal exudate macrophage; polymorphic epithelial mucin; prescription event monitoring; precordial electrocardiographic monitoring; primary enrichment medium; probable error of measurement; protein energy malnutrition; pulmonary endothelial membrane
PEMA phenylethylmalonamide
PE$_{max}$ maximum expiratory pressure
PEMF pulsed electromagnetic field
PEN pharmacy equivalent name; practitioners entering notes
Pen penicillin
PENK proenkephalin
PEN&PAD practitioners entering notes and practitioners accessing data [system]
PENT phenylethanolamine N-methyl-transferase
Pent pentothal
PEO polyethylene oxide; progressive external ophthalmoplegia
PEO-PBD polyethyleneoxide-polybutadiene
PEO-PLA polyethylene dioxide–polylactic acid
PEP patient education program; Pediatric Education for Paramedics [course]; peptidase; peer evaluation program; phosphoenolpyruvate; pigmentation, edema, and plasma cell dyscrasia [syndrome]; polyestradiol phosphate; pore-forming protein; positive expiratory pressure; postencephalitic parkinsonism; post-ERCP pancreatitis; postexposure prophylaxis; pre-ejection period; protein electrophoresis; Psychiatric Evaluation Profile; pudendal evoked potential
Pep peptidase
PEPA peptidase A; prospective evaluation of prognosis in angina
PEPB peptidase B
PEPC peptidase C
PEPc corrected pre-ejection period
PEPCK phosphoenolpyruvate carboxykinase
PEPD peptidase D
PEPE peptidase E

PEPI pre-ejection period index; Postmenopausal Estrogen-Progestin Intervention [trial]

PEPP Payment Error Prevention Program; positive expiratory pressure plateau; Pregnancy Exposures and Pre-eclampsia Prevention [project]

PEPS peptidase S

PEPT peptide transporter

PEPV penguinpox virus

PER peak ejection rate; periodogram; peritoneum; protein efficiency ratio

per perineal; periodicity, periodic

perc percutaneous

perCP peridinin chlorophyll protein

percus percussion

Perf perfusion or perfusionist

perf perforation

PERFEXT Perfusion, Performance, Exercise Trial

PERG pattern electroretinogram

PERI Psychiatric Epidemiology Research Interview

periap periapical

Perio periodontics

Peritf peritoneal fluid

PERK prospective evaluation of radial keratotomy [protocol]

p-ERK dual phosphorylated extracellular signal–regulated kinase

PERLA pupils equal, react to light and accommodation

PERM Prospective Evaluation of Perfusion Markers [study]

PerNET peripheral neuroectodermal tumor

PERP positive end-respiratory pressure

perp perpendicular

PERRLA pupils equal, round, and reactive to light and accommodation

PERS Patient Evaluation Rating Scale; pediatric emergency rating scale

PERT phenol-enhanced reassociation technique; program evaluation review technique

PERV Perinet virus

PES Patient Escort Service; perceived stress scale; photoelectron spectroscopy; physical examination syndrome; physicians' equity services; polyethylene sulfonate; postextrasystolic; preepiglottic space; preexcitation syndrome; primary empty sella [syndrome]; programmed electrical stimulation; pseudoepileptic seizures; pseudoexfoliation or pseudoexfoliative syndrome; psychiatric emergency services

Pes esophageal pressure

PESDA perfluorocarbon-exposed sonicated dextrose albumin

PESP postextrasystolic potentiation

P$_{es}$/P$_I$max mean esophageal pressure/maximum inspiratory pressure [ratio]

PESS problem, etiology, signs and symptoms

Pess pessary

PEST pesticides [dataset]

PET paraffin-embedded tissue; peak ejection time; peritoneal equilibrium test; polyethylene terephthalate [film]; polyethylene tube; poor exercise tolerance; positron emission tomography; preeclamptic toxemia; pressure equalization tube; privacy-enhancing technique; progressive exercise test; psychiatric emergency team

PET$_{CO_2}$, P$_{ET}$CO$_2$ end-tidal pressure of carbon dioxide

PETH pink-eyed, tan-hooded [rat]

PET-MRI positron emission tomography–magnetic resonance imaging

PETN pentaerythritol tetranitrate

PETQI patient education total quality improvement

petr petroleum

PETRA parameter estimation for the treatment of reactivity application

PETSc portable extensible toolkit for scientific computation

PETT pendular eye-tracking test; positron emission transverse tomography

PETV Petevo virus

PEU plasma equivalent unit

PEUU polyurethane-urea

PEV peak expiratory velocity; positive effect variegation; pseudoenteritis virus

pev peak electron volts

PEV 2–7, 8, 9, 10, 11–13 porcine enteroviruses 2–7, 8, 9, 10, and 11–13

PEV A, B porcine enteroviruses A and B

PEW pulmonary extravascular water

PEWV pulmonary extravascular water volume

PEx physical examination

Pex peak exercise

P$_{ext}$ pressure across external breathing apparatus

PF pair feeding; peak flow; peak frequency; pemphigus foliaceus; perfusion fluid; pericardial fluid; periosteal fibroblast; peritoneal fluid; permeability factor; personality factor; picture-frustration [study]; plantar flexion; plasma factor; plasmapheresis; platelet factor; pleural fluid; power factor; primary fibrinolysin; prostatic fluid; protection factor; pterygoid fossa; pulmonary factor; pulmonary function; Purkinje fiber; purpura fulminans; push fluids; pyrozafurin

P-F picture-frustration [test]

PF$_{1-4}$ platelet factors 1 to 4

Pf *Plasmodium falciparum*

P$_f$ final pressure

pF picofarad

PFA profunda femoris artery; *p*-fluorophenylalanine; phosphonoformate; pulverized fluid ash

PFAS perception of functional ability scale; performic acid-Schiff [reaction]

PFB perflubron; proportion of fed bugs [Chagas disease]

PFC pair-fed control [mice]; patient-focused care; pelvic flexion contracture; perfluorocarbon; perfluorochemical; pericardial fluid culture; persistent fetal circulation; plaque-forming cell

pFc noncovalently bonded dimer of the C-terminal immunoglobulin of the Fc fragment

PFD polyostotic fibrous dysplasia; pseudoinflammatory fundus disease

PFDA perfluoro-decanoic acid

PfDNV *Periplanata fuliginosa* densovirus

PFE pelvic floor exercise

PFFD proximal focal femoral deficiency

PFG peak flow gauge; pulsed-field gel electrophoresis

PFGE pulsed field gel electrophoresis

PFGS phosphoribosyl formylglycinamide synthetase

PFIB perfluoroisobutylene

PFIC progressive familial intrahepatic cholestasis

PFJ patellofemoral joint

PFK phosphofructokinase; 6-phosphofructo-2-kinase

PFKF 6-phosphofructo-2-kinase, fibroblast type

PFKL phosphofructokinase, liver type; 6-phosphofructo-2-kinase, liver type

PFKM phosphofructokinase, muscle type

PFKP phosphofructokinase, platelet type; 6-phosphofructo-2-kinase, platelet type

PFKX 6-phosphofructo-2-kinase X

PFL profibrinolysin

pflops pentaflops [floating points per second]

PFM peak flow meter

PFN partially functional neutrophil; profilin; proximal femoral nail

PFO patent foramen ovale; perfringolysin O; plantar fasciitis orthosis

PFOB perfluorocytylbromide

PFOR pyruvate:ferredoxin oxidoreductase

PFP pentafluorophenol; peripheral facial paralysis; plain film pelvis [x-ray]; platelet-free plasma; pulmonary fibroproliferation

P-FPIA polyclonal fluorescence polarization immunoassay

PFPS patellofemoral pain syndrome

PFQ personality factor questionnaire

PFR parotid flow rate; particulate filter respirator; peak flow rate

PFRC predicted functional residual capacity

PFS patellofemoral syndrome; primary fibromyalgia syndrome; protein-free supernatant; pulmonary function score; pulsatile flow system

PFSH past, family and social history

PFT pancreatic function test; parafascicular thalamotomy; Pick from Thousands [model for coded data]; posterior fossa tumor; prednisone, fluorouracil, and tamoxifen; pulmonary function test

PFTBE progressive form of tick-borne encephalitis

PFTL pulmonary function test laboratory

PFU plaque-forming unit; pock-forming unit

pfu plaque-forming unit

PFUO prolonged fever of unknown origin

PFV physiologic full value

PFWD pain-free walking distance

PG parallel group; parapsoriasis guttata; paregoric; parotid gland; partial gastrectomy; pentagastrin; pepsinogen; peptidoglycan; percutaneous gastrostomy; Pharmacopoeia Germanica; phase gradient [angiography]; phosphate glutamate; phosphatidylglycerol; phosphogluconate; pigment granule; pituitary gonadotropin; plasma glucose; plasma triglyceride;

polygalacturonate; post graft; postgraduate; postprandial glucose; practice guideline; pregnanediol glucuronide; pregnant; progesterone; prolyl hydrolase; propyl gallate; propylene glycol; Prospect Hill [virus]; prostaglandin; proteoglycan; pulse generator [implantable converter-defibrillator]; pyoderma gangrenosum

2PG 2-phosphoglycerate

3PG 3-phosphoglycerate

P$_G$ plasma glucose

Pg nasopharyngeal electrode placement in electroencephalography; gastric pressure; plakoglobin; plasminogen; pogonion; pregnancy, pregnant; pregnenolone

pg parthenogenic; picogram; pregnant

PGA pancreaticogastrostomy; pepsinogen A; phosphoglyceric acid; polyglandular autoimmune [syndrome]; polyglycolic acid; programmable-gain amplifier; prostaglandin A; pteroylglutamic acid

PGA$_{1-3}$ prostaglandins A$_1$ to A$_3$

PGAM monophosphoglycerate mutase

PGAP pilot geriatric arthritis program

PGAS persisting galactorrhea-amenorrhea syndrome; polyglandular autoimmune syndrome

PGAV Pongola virus

PGB progabide; prostaglandin B

PGC progastricin; primordial germ cell

PGCL [nucleus] paragigantocellularis lateralis

PGD phosphogluconate dehydrogenase; phosphoglyceraldehyde dehydrogenase

PGD$_2$ prostaglandin D$_2$

6-PGD 6-phosphogluconate dehydrogenase

PGDH phosphogluconate dehydrogenase

PGDR plasma glucose disappearance rate

PGE platelet granule exract; posterior gastroenterostomy

PGE$_1$ prostaglandin E$_1$

PGE$_2$ prostaglandin E$_2$

PGF phylogenetic footprint

PGF$_{2\alpha}$ prostaglandin F$_{2\alpha}$

PGFT phosphoribosylglycinamide formyltransferase

PGG polyclonal gamma globulin

PGG$_2$ prostaglandin G$_2$

PGH pituitary growth hormone; porcine growth hormone

PGH$_2$ prostaglandin H$_2$

PGHS prostaglandin G/H synthase

PGI phosphoglucose isomerase; potassium, glucose, and insulin

PGI$_2$ prostacyclin [prostaglandin I$_2$]

PGK phosphoglycerate kinase

PGL persistent generalized lymphadenopathy; phosphoglycolipid; 6-phosphogluconolactonase

PGLN periglandular lymph node

PGlyM phosphoglyceromutase

PGM phosphoglucomutase; phosphoglycerate mutase

PGMA phosphoglycerate mutase A

PGMB phosphoglycerate mutase B

PGMDE postgraduate and continuing medical and dental education

pg/mL picograms per milliliter

PGN proliferative glomerulonephritis

PGNA prompt gamma neutron activation

PGO ponto-geniculo-occipital [spike]

PGP phosphoglyceroyl phosphatase; postgamma proteinuria; prepaid group practice; progressive general paralysis

PGP/MIME pretty good privacy/multipurpose Internet Mail Extension

PGPV pigeonpox virus

PGR progesterone receptor; psychogalvanic response

PgR progesterone receptor

PGS peristent gross splenomegaly; Pettigrew syndrome; plant growth substance; polar grid system; postsurgical gastroparesis syndrome; primary generalized seizures; prostaglandin synthetase

PGSI prostaglandin synthetase inhibitor

PGSR phosphogalvanic skin response

PGT preimplantation genetic testing

PGTR plasma glucose tolerance rate

PGTT prednisolone glucose tolerance test

PGU peripheral glucose uptake; postgonococcal urethritis

PGUT phosphogalactose uridyl transferase

PGV proximal gastric vagotomy

PGVS postganglionic vagal stimulation

PGWB psychological general well-being [index]

PGX prostacyclin

PGY postgraduate year

PGYE peptone, glucose yeast extract

PH Pallister-Hall [syndrome]; papillary hyperplasia; parathyroid hormone; partial hepatectomy; partial hysterectomy; passive hemagglutination; past history;

patient's history; persistent hepatitis; personal history; pharmacopeia; pharmacy, pharmacist, pharmaceutical; physical history; porphyria hepatica; posterior heel; posterior hypothalamus; prehospital; previous history; primary hyperoxaluria; primary hyperparathyroidism; prostatic hypertrophy; pseudohermaphroditism; public health; pulmonary hypertension; pulmonary hypoplasia

PH1 primary hyperoxaluria type 1

Ph phantom; pharmacopeia; phenyl; Philadelphia [chromosome]; phosphate

Ph¹ Philadelphia chromosome

pH hydrogen ion concentration

pH₁ isoelectric point

ph phial; phot

PHA passive hemagglutination assay; peripheral hyperalimentation; phenylalanine; phytohemagglutinin; phytohemagglutinin antigen; pseudohypoaldosteronism; public health agency; Public Health Association; pulse-height analyzer

pH_A arterial blood hydrogen tension

pH_a arterial hydrogen ion concentration

PHAC phaclofen

PhAdV pheasant adenovirus

PHAF peripheral hyperalimentation formula

PHAH polyhalogenated aromatic hydrocarbon

PHAL phytohemagglutinin-stimulated lymphocyte

phal phalangeal

PHA-LCM phytohemagglutinin-stimulated leukocyte conditioned medium

PHA-NSP passive hemagglutination to nonstructural protein

PHAP phytohemagglutinin protein

PHAR pharmacologic substance [UMLS]

phar pharmaceutical; pharmacy; pharynx

Phar C pharmaceutical chemist

PHARM Pharmacist in Heart Failure: Assessment, Recommendation and Monitoring [study]

Pharm pharmacy

pharm pharmacist; pharmacology; pharmacopeia; pharmacy

Pharm B Bachelor of Pharmacy [Lat. *Pharmaciae Baccalaureus*]

Pharm D Doctor of Pharmacy [Lat. *Pharmaciae Doctor*]

Pharm M Master of Pharmacy [Lat. *Pharmaciae Magister*]

PHASE prehospital arrest survival evaluation

PHAVER pterygia-heart defects-autosomal recessive inheritance-vertebral defects-ear anomalies-radial defects [syndrome]

PHB polyhydroxybutyrate; preventive health behavior; prohibitin

PhB, Phb Pharmacopoeia Britannica

PHBB propylhydroxybenzyl benzimidazole

PHBQ Physicians' Humanistic Behaviors Questionnaire

PHC personal health costs; posthospital care; premolar hypodontia, hyperhidrosis, [premature] canities [syndrome]; primary health care; Primary Healthcare Center [Sweden]; primary hepatic carcinoma; proliferative helper cell; public health center

PhC pharmaceutical chemist

Ph¹ᶜ Philadelphia chromosome

PHCC primary hepatocellular carcinoma

PHCDM public health computational data model

PHCP prehospital care provider

PHD pathological habit disorder; personal health data; post-heparin plasma diamine oxidase; potentially harmful drug

PhD Doctor of Pharmacy [Lat. *Pharmaciae Doctor*]; Doctor of Philosophy [Lat. *Philosophiae Doctor*]

PHE periodic health examination; phenylephrine

Phe phenylalanine

PhEEM photoemission electron microscopy

PHEI prevention and health evaluation informatics

pHEMA polyhydroxyethyl methacrylate

PHEN phenomenon or process [UMLS]

Phen phentermine

Pheo pheochromocytoma; pheophytin

PhEur Pharmacopeia Europaea

Ph. Eur. U. European Pharmacopoeia unit

PHEX phosphate-regulating gene with homologies to endopeptidase on X chromosome

PHF paired helical filament; personal hygiene facility

PHFB psyllium husk fiber bar

PHFG primary human fetal glia

PhG Graduate in Pharmacy; Pharmacopoeia Germanica

phgly phenylglycine

PHHI persistent hyperinsulinemic hypoglycemia of infancy

PHHP Pawtucket Heart Health Program

PhHV phalacrocoracid herpesvirus

PHI passive hemagglutination inhibition; past history of illness; Personalized Healthcare Information [Internet-based, Malaysia]; personalized health information; phosphine; phosphohexose isomerase; physiological hyaluronidase inhibitor; prehospital index

PhI Pharmacopoeia Internationalis

Phi Partnership in Health Information [UK]

pHi intracellular hydrogen ion concentration; intramucosal hydrogen ion concentration

φ Greek letter *phi*; magnetic flux; osmotic coefficient

PHI-BLST pattern hit initiated basic local alignment search tool

PHICOG Philadelphia Cooperative Group

PHIDIAS laser *ph*otopolymerisation models based on medical *i*maging, a *d*evelopment *i*mproving the *a*ccuracy of *s*urgery

PHIDS Personalized Healthcare Information Delivery System [telemedicine]

PHIHM prehospital invasive hemodynamic monitoring

PHIM posthypoxic intention myoclonus

PHIS personal health information seeking

PhIS pharmacy information system

PHK phosphohexokinase; phosphorylase kinase; postmortem human kidney

PHKA phosphorylase kinase, alpha

PHKB phosphorylase kinase, beta

PHKD phosphorylase kinase, delta

PHKG phosphorylase kinase, gamma

PHL public health laboratory

PHLA postheparin lipolytic activity

PHLOP polymerase-halt-mediated linkage of primers

PHLS Public Health Laboratory Service [UK]

PHM peptide histidine methionine; peptidylglycine alpha-hydroxylating monooxygenase; posterior hyaloid membrane; pulmonary hyaline membrane

PhM Master of Pharmacy [Lat. *Pharmaciae Magister*]; pharyngeal muscle

PhmG Graduate in Pharmacy

PHN paroxysmal noctural hemoglobinuria; passive Heymann nephritis; postherpetic neuralgia; primary healthcare nurse [Australia]; proximal humeral nail; public health nursing, public health nurse

PHO physician-hospital organization

PH₂O partial pressure of water vapor

PHOCUS Primary Health-Oriented Computer Users' System

PhoHV phocid herpesvirus

phos phosphate

PHOX paired mesoderm homeobox [gene]

PHP panhypopituitarism; postheparin phospholipase; prehospital program; prepaid health plan; primary hyperparathyroidism; pseudohypoparathyroidism; psychological health profile

PHPA passive hemolytic plaque assay; *p*-hydroxyphenylacetate

PHPLA *p*-hydroxyphenyllactic acid

pHPPA *p*-hydrophenylpyruvic acid

p-HPPO *p*-hydroxyphenyl pyruvate oxidase

PHPT primary hyperparathyroidism; pseudohypoparathyroidism

pHPT primary hyperparathyroidism

PHPV persistent hyperplastic primary vitreous

PHR parent-held record; peak heart rate; photoreactivity

PHS Partial Hospitalization System; Personal Handphone System [telemedicine]; phenylalanine hydrolase stimulator system; Physicians' Health Study; pooled human serum; posthypnotic suggestion; pseudoprogeria-Hallermann-Streiff [syndrome]; Public Health Service

PHSC pleuripotent hemopoietic stem cell; powdered human stratum corneum

PHS-LAN Personal Handphone System–Local Area Network

PHS-PC Personal Handphone System–Personal Computer

pH-stat apparatus for maintaining the pH of a solution

PHT peak height of tension; phenytoin; portal hypertension; pressure half-time; primary hyperthyroidism; pulmonary hypertension

PhTD Doctor of Physical Therapy

PHTLS prehospital trauma life support

PHTN pulmonary hypertension
PHU population health unit
PHV peak height velocity; perch hyperplasia virus; Prospect Hill virus
PHX pulmonary histiocytosis X
Phx past history; pharynx
PHY pharyngitis; physical; physiology
PHYLLIS Plaque Hypertension Lipid-Lowering Italian Study
PHYS physiologic function [UMLS]; physiology
PhyS physiologic saline [solution]
phys physical; physician
Phys Ed physical education
physio physiology; physiotherapy
Phys Med physical medicine
PHYS-SPEC physician's specialty
PhysPRC Physician's Payment Review Commission
Phys Ther physical therapist or therapy
PHZ phenylhydrazine
PI class I protein; first meiotic prophase; isoelectric point; pacing impulse; package insert; pain intensity; pancreatic insufficiency; parainfluenza; pars intermedia; patient's interest; performance indicator or index; performance intensity; perinatal injury; periodontal index; permeability index; personal injury; personality inventory; phagocytic index; Pharmacopoeia Internationalis; phosphatidylinositol; physically impaired; physiologic index; pineal body; plaque index; plasmin inhibitor; pneumatosis intestinalis; poison ivy; ponderal index; postictal immobility; postinfection; postinfluenza; postinjury; postinoculation; preinduction [examination]; premature infant; prematurity index; preparatory interval; prescribing information; present illness; primary infarction; primary infection; principal investigator; processor interface; product information; proinsulin; prolactin inhibitor; propidium iodide; proportional plus integral; protamine insulin; protease inhibitor; proximal intestine; pulmonary incompetence; pulmonary index; pulmonary infarction; pulsatility index
P₁ inspiratory pressure
P&I pneumonia and influenza
Pi inorganic phosphate; parental generation; pressure in inspiration; protease inhibitor
Pᵢ inorganic phosphate

pI isoelectric point
p-I postinspiratory
pi post-injection
Π Greek capital letter *pi*
π Greek lowercase letter *pi*; the ratio of circumference to diameter, 3.1415926536
PIA photoelectric intravenous angiography; plasma insulin activity; preinfarction angina; Psychiatric Institute of America; *R*-phenylisopropyladenosine
PiAdV pigeon adenovirus
PIAF pharmacologic intervention in atrial fibrillation; prognosis in atrial fibrillation
PIAT Peabody Individual Achievement Test
PIAV Picola virus
PIAVA polydactyly-imperforate anus-vertebral anomalies [syndrome]
PIB periinfarction block
PIBC percutaneous intraaortic balloon counterpulsation [catheter]
PIBIDS, PIBI(D)S photosensitivity-ichthyosis-brittle hair-impaired intelligence-(possibly decreased fertility)-short stature syndrome
PIC pacing in cardiomyopathy; peripherally-inserted indwelling central catheter; Personality Inventory for Children; polymorphism information content; pre-initiation complex [RNA transcription]; pre-injury condition; prior informed consent
PICA percutaneous transluminal coronary angioplasty; Porch Index of Communicative Abilities; posterior inferior cerebellar artery; posterior inferior communicating artery
PICC percutaneous indwelling central venous catheter; peripherally inserted central catheter
PICD primary irritant contact dermatitis
PICFS postinfective chronic fatigue syndrome
PICNIC Pediatric Investigators Collaborative Network on Infections in Canada
PICO Pimobendan in Congestive Heart Failure [study]; population, intervention, comparison and outcome
PiCO₂ partial pressure of carbon dioxide in air
PICS Pacing in Cardiomyopathy Study
PICSO pressure-controlled intermittent coronary sinus occlusion

PICSS Patent Foramen Ovale in Cryptogenic Stroke Study

PICTURE Post-intracoronary Treatment Ultrasound Results Evaluation [study]

PICU pediatric intensive care unit; pulmonary intensive care unit

PICV Pichinde virus

PiCV pigeon circovirus

PID pain intensity difference [score]; patient identification; patient identity; pelvic inflammatory disease; photoionization detector; picture image directory; plasma iron disappearance; postinertia dyskinesia; preimplantation diagnosis; prolapsed/protruded intervertebral disk; proportional integral derivative; proportional integral-differential control

PIDRA portable insulin dosage regulating apparatus

PIDS patient identification service; primary immunodeficiency syndrome

PIDT plasma iron disappearance time

PIE postinfectious encephalomyelitis; preimplantation embryo; prosthetic infectious endocarditis; pulmonary infiltration with eosinophilia; pulmonary interstitial emphysema

PIF paratoid isoelectric focusing variant protein; peak inspiratory flow; photoinhibition factor; proinsulin-free; prolactin-inhibiting factor; prolactin release-inhibiting factor; proliferation-inhibiting factor; prostatic interstitial fluid

PIFG poor intrauterine fetal growth

PIFR peak inspiratory flow rate

PIFT platelet immunofluorescence test

PIG Polaris Investigator Group; polymeric immunoglobulin

PIGA phosphatidylinositol glycan A

pIgA polymeric immunoglobulin A

pIgM polymeric immunoglobulin M

pigm pigment, pigmented

PIGR, PigR polymeric immunoglobulin receptor

PIH periventricular-intraventricular hemorrhage; pheniprazine; phenyl isopropylhydrazine; pregnancy-induced hypertension; prolactin-inhibiting hormone; pseudointimal hyperplasia

PII plasma inorganic iodine; primary irritation index

PIIgG surface IgG

P$_{ij}$ propagation delay

PIIP portable insulin infusion pump

PIIS posterior inferior iliac spine

PI3K, PI-3K phosphatidylinositol-3'-kinase

PIL patient information leaflet

PILBD paucity of interlobular bile ducts

PILL Pennebaker Inventory of Limbic Languidness

PILOT Polish Intramural Low Molecular Weight Heparin Outpatient Stent Trial; Preliminary Investigation of Local Therapy [using porous percutaneous transluminal coronary angioplasty balloons]

PILP postinfarction late potential

PILS Pilsen Longitudinal Study

πm pi meson

PIM penicillamine-induced myasthenia

PI$_{max}$ maximum inspiratory pressure at residual volume

P$_i$max maximum inspiratory pressure

PIMI predictive index for myocardial infarction; psychophysiological interventions in myocardial ischemia

PIMS patient information management system

PIN patient information network; personal identification number; product identification number; prostatic intraepithelial neoplasia

Pin inflow pressure; initial pressure

PINN proposed international nonproprietary name

PINV postimperative negative variation

PIO$_2$ partial pressure of inspired oxygen

PION posterior ischemic optic neuropathy

PIOPED Prospective Investigation of Pulmonary Embolism Diagnosis [database]

PIP paralytic infantile paralysis; peak inflation pressure, peak inspiratory pressure; periodic interim payment; piperacillin; postinfusion phlebitis; pressure inversion point; primary injury prevention; prolactin-inducible protein; proximal interphalangeal [joint]; Psychotic Inpatient Profile; psychosis, intermittent hyponatremia, polydipsia [syndrome]; posterior interphalangeal; probable intrauterine pregnancy

PI-P phosphatidylinositol-4-phosphate

PIP$_2$ phosphatidylinositol 4,5-bisphosphate

Pi/PCr inorganic phosphate/creatine phosphate [ratio]

PIPE persistent interstitial pulmonary emphysema

PIPER Patient Information Projects Register [database, UK]

PIPIDA *p*-isopropylacetanilidoimidodiacetic acid

PIPJ proximal interphalangeal joint

PI-PP phosphatidylinosetol-4,5-biphosphate

PIPS patient information protocol system

PIQ Performance Intelligence Quotient

PIR participant inquiry research; postinhibition rebound; protein information or identification resource

PIRI plasma immunoreactive insulin

PIR-NREF Protein Information or Identification Resource-Nonredundant Reference [database]

PIRS plasma immunoreactive secretion; postinfarction risk stratification

PIRTS patient identification for rotational therapy system

PIRV Pirital virus

PIRYV Piry virus

PIS pharmacy information system; preinfarction syndrome; primary immunodeficiency syndrome; Primary Index Score; Provisional International Standard

pIs isoelectric point

PISA proximal isovelocity surface area

PISA-PED Prospective Investigative Study of Acute Pulmonary Embolism Diagnosis

PISCES percutaneously inserted spinal cord electrical stimulation

PISH polymerase chain reaction–in situ hybridization

PISI pediatric illness severity index

PIT pacing-induced tachycardia; patella inhibition test; pericranial injection therapy; picture identification test; pitocin; pitressin; plasma iron turnover

pit pituitary

PITAC President's Information Technology Advisory Committee

PITC phenylisothiocyanate

PITR plasma iron turnover rate

PIU polymerase-inducing unit; programmed instruction unit

PIV parainfluenza virus; particle image velocity [determination]; polydactyly-imperforate anus-vertebral anomalies [syndrome]; projective image visualization; Puffin Island virus

PIVD protruded intervertebral disk

PIVH peripheral intravenous hyperalimentation; periventricular-intraventricular hemorrhage

PIVKA protein induced by vitamin K absence or antagonism

P/I/X patients, indicators, external bodies

PIXE particle-induced x-ray emission; proton-induced x-ray emission

Pixel picture element

PIXI paternally imprinted X inactivation

PIXV Pixuna virus

PJ pancreatic juice; Peutz-Jeghers [syndrome]

PJB premature junctional beat

PJC premature junctional contractions

pJC Jamestown Canyon virus plasmid

PJM positive joint mobilization

PJP pancreatic juice protein

PJRT permanent junctional reciprocating tachycardia

PJS peritoneojugular shunt; Peutz-Jeghers syndrome

PJT paroxysmal junctional tachycardia

PK penetrating keratoplasty; pericardial knock; pharmacokinetics; pig kidney; Prausnitz-Küstner [reaction]; protein kinase; psychokinesis; pyruvate kinase

Pk peak [rate]

pK negative logarithm of the dissociation constant; plasma potassium

pK′ apparent value of a pK; negative logarithm of the dissociation constant of an acid

pk peck

PKA protein kinase A

PkA prekallikrein activator

pK$_a$ negative logarithm of the acid ionization constant

PKAR protein kinase activation ratio

PKase protein kinase

PKB protein kinase B

PKC Permanente Knowledge Connection; problem-knowledge coupler; protein kinase C

PKCA protein kinase C alpha

PKCB protein kinase C beta

PKCE protein kinase C epsilon

PKCG protein kinase C gamma

PKCSH protein kinase C heavy chain

PKCSL protein kinase C light chain

PKCZ protein kinase C zeta

PKD polycystic kidney disease; proliferative kidney disease
PKD-1 polycystic kidney disease gene-1
PKD-2 polycystic kidney disease gene-2
PKDL post–kala-azar dermal leishmaniasis
PKF phagocytosis and killing function
PKG protein kinase G
PKI potato kallikrein inhibitor; protein kinase inhibitor; public key infrastructure [telemedicine]
PKK plasma prekallikrein
PKL pyruvate kinase, liver type
PKM protein kinase M; pyruvate kinase, muscle
PKN parkinsonism
pkn pseudoknot
PKP penetrating keratoplasty; plakophilin
PK/PD pharmacokinetic/pharmacodynamic [model]
PKPV peacockpox virus
PKR phased knee rehabilitation; Prausnitz-Küstner reaction
Pk/Rr peak respiratory rate
PKS protein kinase sequence
PKT pancreas-kidney transplantation; Prausnitz-Küstner test
PKU phenylketonuria
PKV killed poliomyelitis vaccine
pkV peak kilovoltage
PL *Paenibacillus larvae*; palmaris longus; pancreatic lipase; perception of light; peroneus longus; phospholipase; phospholipid; photoluminescence; placebo; placental lactogen; plantar; plasmalemma; plastic surgery; platelet lactogen; polarized light; posterolateral; preleukemia; programming language; prolactin; prolymphocytic leukemia; pulpolingual; Purkinje layer
3PL 3-point line [algorithm]
Pl poiseuille
P_L transpulmonary pressure
PL/I programming language I (one)
pL picoliter
pl picoliter; placenta; plasma; platelet
PLA peripheral laser angioplasty; phenyl lactate; phospholipase A; phospholipid antibody; placebo therapy; plasminogen activator; platelet antigen; polylactic acid; potentially lethal arrhythmia; procaine/lactic acid; Product License Application; pulp linguoaxial

PLA2 phospholipase A2
PLa pulpolabial
P_La, Pla left atrial pressure
PLAC Pravastatin Limitation in Atherosclerosis in the Coronary Arteries [study]
PLAC-2 Pravastatin, Lipids and Atherosclerosis in the Carotid Arteries [study]
PLAP placental alkaline phosphatase
PLAT plasminogen activator, tissue-type
Plat platelet
PLAU plasminogen activator, urinary
PLAUR plasminogen activator receptor, urokinase type
PLAV Playas virus
PLB parietal lobe battery; phospholamban; phospholipase B; planar lipid bilayer; porous layer bead; posterolateral bundle
PLC phospholipase C; pityriasis lichenoides chronica; primary liver cancer; primed lymphocyte culture; programmable logic controller; proinsulin-like component; protein-lipid complex; pseudolymphocytic choriomeningitis
PLCC primary liver cell cancer
PLCO postoperative low cardiac output
PLCx posterolateral circumflex branch [of coronary artery]
PLD peripheral light detection; phospholipase D; platelet defect; polycystic liver disease; posterior latissimus dorsi [muscle]; potentially lethal damage
PLDH plasma lactic dehydrogenase
PLDR potentially lethal damage repair
PLE paraneoplastic limbic encephalopathy; pleura; protein-losing enteropathy; pseudolupus erythematosus
PLED periodic lateral epileptiform discharge
PLES parallel-line equal space
PLET polymyxin, lysosome, EDTA, thallous acetate [in heart infusion agar]
PLEVA pityriasis lichenoides et varioliformis acuta
PLEXES Pacing Lead Explant with Excimer Sheath [study]
PLF perilymphatic fistula; posterior lung fiber
Plf pleural fluid
PLFD perilunate fracture dislocation
3PLFLS 3-point line fixed least squares [algorithm]
PLFS perilymphatic fistula syndrome

PLG plasminogen; polylactic-co-glycolic acid; poly-DL-lactide/glycolide; L-propyl-L-leucyl-glucinamide

PLGA polylactic-glycolic acid

PlGF placental growth factor

PLGL plasminogen-like

P-LGV psittacosis-lymphogranuloma venereum

PLH placental lactogenic hormone

PLHP personalized lifetime health plan

PIHV pleuronectid herpesvirus

PLI pancreatic lymphocytic infiltration; professional liability insurance

PLIF posterior lumbar interbody fusion

PLISSIT permission to be sexual, limited information, specific suggestions, intensive therapy

PLL peripheral light loss; phase-locked loop; poly-L-lysine; posterior longitudinal ligament; potential loss of life; pressure length loop; prolymphocytic leukemia

PLM percent labeled mitoses; periodic leg movement; plasma level monitoring; polarized light microscopy; Prevention of Mortality with Low-molecular Weight Heparin in Medical Patients [study]

PLMS periodic limb movements during sleep

PLMV posterior leaf mitral valve

PLN peripheral lymph node; phospholamban

PLNA percutaneous lung needle aspiration

PLND pelvic lymph node dissection

PLNT plant

PLO polycystic lipomembranous osteodysplasia

PLOD procollagen-lysine 2-oxoglutarate 5-dioxygenase

PLOSA Physiologic Low-Stress Angioplasty [trial]

PLP *Paenibacillus larvae* subsp. *pulvifaciens*; phospholipid; plasma leukapheresis; polypeptide; polystyrene latex particles; posterior lobe of pituitary [gland]; proteolipid protein; pyridoxal phosphate

PLPH post-lumbar puncture headache

PLR pupillary light reflex

PLS Papillon-Lefèvre syndrome; partial least square; polydactyly-luxation syndrome; Postsurgery Logiparin Study; preleukemic syndrome; primary lateral sclerosis; prostaglandin-like substance; pulmonary leukostasis syndrome

PLSA posterolateral segment [coronary] artery

PLSD protected least significant difference

PLSR partial least-square regression

PLST progressively lowered stress threshold

Pl Surg plastic surgeon or surgery

PLSV Palestina virus

PLT platelet; primed lymphocyte test; primed lymphocyte typing; psittacosis-lymphogranuloma venereum-trachoma [group]

PLTC Partnership for Long Term Care

PLTP phospholipid transfer protein

plumb lead [Lat. *plumbum*]

PLUT Plutchnik [geriatric rating scale]

PLV panleukemia virus; partial liquid ventilation; poliomyelitis live vaccine; panleukopenia virus; phenylalanine, lysine, and vasopressin; posterior left ventricle; puma lentivirus

P$_{LV}$ left ventricular pressure

PLVP peak left ventricular pressure

PLW Prader-Labhart-Willi [syndrome]

PLWA, PLW As person living with acquired immune deficiency syndrome

PLWS Prader-Labhart-Willi syndrome

plx plexus

PLZ phenelzine

PLZF promyelocytic leukemia zinc finger

PM after death [Lat. *post mortem*]; after noon [Lat. *post meridiem*]; mean pressure; pacemaker; pantomography; papilla mammae; papillary muscle; papular mucinosis; partial meniscectomy; particle mass; particulate matter; patient management; pectinate muscle; pectoralis major [muscle]; perinatal mortality; periodontal membrane; peritoneal macrophage; petit mal epilepsy [Fr. *petit mal*]; photomultiplier; physical medicine; plasma membrane; platelet membrane; platelet microsome; pneumomediastinum; poliomyelitis; polymorph [polymorphonuclear leukocyte]; polymorphic; polymyositis; poor metabolizer; porokeratosis of Mibelli; posterior mitral; postmenstrual; postmortem; power management; premarketing [approval]; premenstrual; premolar; premotor; presents mainly; presystolic murmur; pretibial myxedema; preventive maintenance; preventive medicine; primary motivation; process manager [database module]; Prony method [spectral analysis of heart sounds]; prophylactic mastectomy; prostatic massage; protein methylesterase; protocol management; psammomatous meningioma; pterygoid muscle; pubertal macromastia; pulmonary macrophage; pulpomesial; purple membrane

PM₁₀ particulate matter < 10 microns

Pm promethium

pM picomolar

pm picometer

PMA index of prevalence and severity of gingivitis, where P = papillary gingiva, M = marginal gingiva, and A = attached gingiva; papillary, marginal, attached [gingiva]; para-methoxyamphetamine; Pharmaceutical Manufacturers Association; phenylmercuric acetate; phorbol myristate acetate; phosphomolybdic acid; polymethacrylic acid; premarket approval; primary mental abilities; progressive muscular atrophy; pyridylmercuric acetate

PMAA polymethacrylic acid

P(MAA-g-EG) poly [methacrylic acid-grafted-poly (ethylene glycol)]

PMAC Pharmaceutical Manufacturers Association of Canada; phenylmercuric acetate; programmable multi-axis controller

PMAS phenylmercuric acetate

P+ₘₐₓ peak positive pressure

PMB papillomacular bundle; para-hydroxymercuribenzoate; polychrome methylene blue; polymorphonuclear basophil; polymyxin B; postmenopausal bleeding

PMC paramyotonia congenita; patient management category; percutaneous myocardial channeling; phenylmercuric chloride; physical medicine clinic; pleural mesothelial click; premature mitral closure; probability of misclassification; pseudomembranous colitis

Pmc mean circulatory pressure

PMCC product-moment correlation coefficient [Pearson]

PMCH pro-melanin-concentrating hormone

PMCHL pro-melanin-concentrating hormone-like

PMC-RIS patient management category-relative intensity score

PMCS patient management computer stimulation

PMD Pelizaeus-Merzbacher disease; posterior mandibular depth; primary myocardial disease; private medicine doctor; primary physician; programmed multiple development; progressive muscular dystrophy

PMDD premenstrual dysphoric disorder

PMDF proportion of maternal deaths among women of reproductive age

PM/DM polymyositis/dermatomyositis

PMDS peristent müllerian duct syndrome; primary myelodysplastic syndrome

PME pelvic muscle exercise; periodic monitoring examination; phosphomonoester; polymorphonuclear eosinophil; progressive multifocal encephalopathy; progressive myoclonus epilepsy

PMEA 9-(2-phosphomethoxyethyl) adenine

PMEL Pacific Marine Environmental Laboratory

PMF platelet membrane fluidity; progressive massive fibrosis; proton motive force; pterygomaxillary fossa

pmf proton motive force

PMG primary medical group

PMGCT primary mediastinal germ-cell tumor

PMH past medical history; posteromedial hypothalamus

PMHAB Provincial Mental Health Advisory Board [Canada]

PMHR predicted maximum heart rate

PMHx past medical history

PMI pain management inventory; past medical illness; patient master index; patient medication instruction; perioperative myocardial infarction; photon migration imaging; point of maximal impulse; point of maximal intensity; posterior myocardial infarction; postmyocardial infarction; present medical illness; previous medical illness

PMIA *N*-(1-pyrenamethyl)-iodoacetamide

P−ₘᵢₙ peak negative pressure

PMIS postmyocardial infarction syndrome; PSRO Management Information System

PMK pacemaker

PML peripheral motor latency; polymorphonuclear leukocyte; posterior mitral leaflet; progressive multifocal leukodystrophy; progressive multifocal leukoencephalopathy; prolapsing mitral leaflet; promyelocytic leukemia; pulmonary microlithiasis

PMLD Pelizaeus-Merzbacher-like disease

PMLE polymorphous light eruption

PMM pentamethylmelamine; protoplast maintenance medium

PMMA polymethylmethacrylate

PMMIS Program Management and Medical Information System [Medicare]

PMN polymorphonuclear; polymorphonuclear neutrophil; premanufacture notification

PMNC percentage of multinucleated cells; peripheral blood mononuclear cell

PMNG polymorphonuclear granulocyte

PMNL peripheral blood monocytes and polymorphonuclear leukocytes; polymorphonuclear leukocyte

PMNN polymorphonuclear neutrophil

PMNR periadenitis mucosa necrotica recurrens

PMNSG Pravastatin Multinational Study Group

PMO postmenopausal osteoporosis; Principal Medical Officer

pmol picomole

pmol/L picomoles per liter

PMP pain management program; paramagnetic particle; patient management problems; patient management program; patient medication profile; peripheral myelin protein; peroxisomal membrane protein; persistent mentoposterior [fetal position]; previous menstrual period

PMPM, pmpm per member per month

PMPS postmastectomy pain syndrome

PMPY per member per year

PMQ phytylmenaquinone

PMR paper medical record; patient metarecord; percutaneous myocardial revascularization; perinatal mortality rate; periodic medical review; physical medicine and rehabilitation; polymyalgia rheumatica; prior medical record; progressive muscular relaxation; proportionate morbidity/mortality ratio; proton magnetic resonance

PM&R physical medicine and rehabilitation

PMRA Pest Management Regulatory Agency [Canada]

PMRG Pimobendan Multicenter Research Group; Postmastectomy Rehabilitation Group

PMRS physical medicine and rehabilitation service

31P-MRS, ^{31}P-MRS magnetic resonance spectroscopy with phosphorus 31

PMS patient management system; perimenstrual syndrome; periodic movements during sleep; phenazine methosulfate; polydactyly-myopia syndrome; postmarketing surveillance; postmenstrual stress or syndrome; postmeiotic segregation; postmitochondrial supernatant; Pravastatin Multinational Study; pregnant mare serum; premenstrual stress or syndrome, premenstrual symptoms; progressive multiple sclerosis; psychotic motor syndrome

PMSC pediatric medical special care; pluripotent myeloid stem cell

PMSF phenylmethylsulfonyl fluoride

PMSG pregnant mare serum gonadotropin

PMSR peptide methionine sulfoxide reductase

PMT pacemaker modulated tachycardia; parent management training; phenol *O*-methyltransferase; photomultiplier tube; Porteus maze test; premenstrual tension; pyridoxyl-methyl-tryptophan

PMTDI provisional maximum tolerable daily intake

PMTS premenstrual tension syndrome

PMTT pulmonary mean transit time

PMV paramyxovirus; percutaneous mitral balloon valvotomy; prolapse of mitral valve

pMV prolapse of mitral valve

PMVI peak myocardial video intensity

PMVL polymorphic ventricular tachycardia; posterior mitral valve leaflet

pMVL posterior mitral valve leaflet

PMW pacemaker wires; patient management workstation

PMX paired mesoderm homeobox [gene]

PN papillary necrosis; parenteral nutrition; patient note; penicillin; perceived noise; percussion note; periarteritis nodosa; perinatal; peripheral nerve; peripheral neuropathy; Petri net; phrenic nerve; plaque neutralization; pneumonia;

polyarteritis nodosa; polyneuritis; polyneuropathy; polynuclear; positional nystagmus; posterior nares; postnatal; practical nurse; predicted normal; primary nurse; progress note; protease nexin; psychiatry and neurology; psychoneurotic; pyelonephritis; pyridine nucleotide

P&N psychiatry and neurology

P/N positive/negative

P$_{N_2}$ partial pressure of nitrogen

P-5'-N pyridine-5'-nucleosidase

Pn pneumatic; pneumonia

pN positive regional lymph node [TNM (tumor-node-metastasis) classification]

pN0 no regional lymph node metastases

pN1 poorly differentiated myeloblasts

pN1a tumor micrometastases [none larger than 0.2 cm]

pN1b tumor metastases to lymph nodes [larger than 0.2 cm]

pN1bi tumor metastases to 1–3 lymph nodes [from 0.2 to 2.0 cm]

pN1bii tumor metastases to 4 or more lymph nodes [0.2 to 2.0 cm]

pN1biii tumor metastases beyond lymph node capsule [none larger than 2.0 cm]

pN1biv tumor metastases to lymph nodes [larger than 2.0 cm]

pN2 tumor metastases to ipsilateral axillary lymph nodes

pN3 tumor metastases to ipsilateral mammary lymph nodes

pn pain

PNA Paris Nomina Anatomica; peanut agglutinin; pentose nucleic acid; *p*-nitroaniline

P$_{Na}$ plasma sodium

pNA *p*-nitroaniline

pNa plasma sodium

PNAvQ positive-negative ambivalent quotient

PNB perineal needle biopsy; peripheral nerve block; *p*-nitrobiphenyl; premature nodal beat

PNBA *p*-nitrobenzoic acid

PNBT *p*-nitroblue tetrazolium

PNC penicillin; peripheral nucleated cell; pneumotaxic center; premature nodal contracture; primitive neuroendothelial cell

Pnc pneumococcus

PNCA proliferating nuclear cell antigen

PNCG preconditioned nonlinear conjugate gradient [algorithm]

PND paroxysmal nocturnal dyspnea; partial neck dissection; postnasal drainage; postnasal drip; postnatal death; prenatal diagnosis; principal neutralizing determinant; purulent nasal drainage

PNdb perceived noise decibel

PNDS postnasal drip syndrome

PNE peripheral neuroepithelioma; plasma norepinephrine; pneumoencephalography; pseudomembranous necrotizing enterocolitis

PNEM paraneoplastic encephalomyelitis

PNET peripheral neuroepithelioma; primitive neuroectodermal tumor

PNEU, pneu, pneum pneumonia

PNF proprioceptive neuromuscular facilitation

PNG penicillin G

PNH paroxysmal nocturnal hemoglobinuria; polynuclear hydrocarbon

PNHA Physicians National Housestaff Association

PNI peripheral nerve injury; postnatal infection; prognostic nutritional index

PNID Peer Nomination Inventory for Depression

PNK polynucleotide kinase; pyridoxine kinase

PNK(H) pyridoxine kinase, high

PNK(L) pyridoxine kinase, low

PNL peripheral nerve lesion; polymorphonuclear neutrophilic leukocyte

PNLA percutaneous needle lung aspiration

PNM perinatal mortality; peripheral dysostosis, nasal hypoplasia, and mental retardation [syndrome]; peripheral nerve myelin

PNMK pyridine nucleoside monophosphate kinase

PNMR postnatal mortality risk

PNMT phenyl-ethanolamine-*N*-methyltransferase

PNN polynomial neural network; probabilistic neural network

PNO Principal Nursing Officer

p-NO$_2$ *p*-nitrosochloramphenicol

PNP pancreatic polypeptide; paraneoplastic pemphigus; para-nitrophenol; peak negative pressure; pediatric nurse practitioner; peripheral neuropathy; pneumoperitoneum; polyneuropathy; predictive value of negative results; psychogenic nocturnal polydipsia; purine nucleoside phosphorylase

P-NP para-nitrophenol

PNPase polynucleotide phosphorylase

PNPB positive-negative pressure breathing

PNPG α-p-nitrophenylglycerol

PNPP para-nitrophenylphosphate

PNPR positive-negative pressure respiration

PNS paraneoplastic syndrome; parasympathetic nervous system; partial nonprogressive stroke; peripheral nerve stimulation; peripheral nervous system; posterior nasal spine; practical nursing student

PNSA partial negative surface area

PNT partial nodular transformation; patient; picture naming task

Pnt patient

Pnthx pneumothorax

PNU protein nitrogen unit

PNUT portable nursing unit terminal

PNVIm poly-N-vinyl imidazole

PNVX pneumococcal vaccine

Pnx pneumothorax

pNX regional lymph node tumor metastases cannot be assessed [TNM (tumor-node-metastasis) classification]

PNZ posterior necrotic zone

PO parieto-occipital; parietal operculum; period of onset; perioperative; posterior; postoperative; power output; predominant organism; pulse oximetry

PO₂, P$_{O_2}$ partial pressure of oxygen

Po porion

pO₂ partial pressure of oxygen

P$_o$ airway occlusion pressure; open probability; opening pressure

p/o postoperative

POA pancreatic oncofetal antigen; phalangeal osteoarthritis; preoptic area; primary optic atrophy

POADS postaxial acrofacial dysostosis syndrome

POAG primary open-angle glaucoma

POA-HA preoptic anterior hypothalamic area

POB penicillin, oil, beeswax; phenoxybenzamine; place of birth

POBA plain old balloon angioplasty

POBJ physical object [UMLS]

POC particulate organic carbon; persistent organohalogen compound; point of

care; polyolefin copolymer; postoperative care; probability of chance; product of conception; proopiomelanocortin

POCS prescription order communication system; projection onto convex sets

POCT point of care testing

POD peroxidase; place of death; podiatry; polycystic ovary disease; pool of doctors; postoperative day; pouch of Douglas; promyelocytic leukemia oncogenic domain

POD1 first postoperative day

POD2 second postoperative day

PODx preoperative diagnosis

POE pediatric orthopedic examination; physician order entry; point of entry; polyoxyethylene; postoperative endophthalmitis; proof of eligibility

POEA polyoxyethylene amine

POEMS Patient-Oriented Evidence that Matters; polyneuropathy, organomegaly, endocrinopathy, M protein, skin changes [syndrome]

POET physician order entry term

POF pattern of failure; position of function; primary or premature ovarian failure; pyruvate oxidation factor

PofE portal of entry

POFX X-linked premature ovarian failure

POG pediatric oncology group; polymyositis ossificans generalisata

Pog pogonion

POGO percentage of glottic opening

pOH hydroxide ion concentration in a solution

POHI physically or otherwise health-impaired

POHS presumed ocular histoplasmosis syndrome

PoHV pongine herpesvirus

PoHV 1, 2, 3 pongine herpesviruses 1, 2, 3

POI Personal Orientation Inventory; piece of information

PoI Pourcelot Index

poik poikilocyte, poikilocytosis

POIS Parkland On-Line Information Systems

pois poison, poisoning, poisoned

POL physician's office laboratory; physicians' online; Pollution Abstracts; polymerase

Pol polymerase

pol polish, polishing

POLA polymerase alpha

pol-GIK Polish Glucose-Insulin-Kalium [study]

polio poliomyelitis

POLIP polyneuropathy-ophthalmoplegia-leukoencephalopathy-intestinal pseudo-obstruction [syndrome]

POLISH Polish [investigators to evaluate the effect of amiodarone on mortality after myocardial infarction]

Pol-MONICA Polish Monitoring Trends and Determinants in Cardiovascular Diseases [study]

POLONIA Polish-American Local Lovenox NIR Stent Assessment [study]

Poly polymorphonuclear

poly-A, poly(A) polyadenylic acid

poly-C, poly(C) polycytidylic acid

poly(CPH) poly[1,6-bis(*p*-carboxyphenoxy)hexane]

poly-dA, poly(dA) polydeoxyadenylic acid

poly-G, poly(G) polyguanylic acid

poly-I, poly(I) polyinosinic acid

poly-IC, poly-I:C copolymer of polyinosinic and polycytidylic acids

polys polymorphonuclear leukocytes

poly(SA) poly(sebacic anhydride)

poly-T, poly(T) polythymidylic acid

poly-U, poly(U) polyuridylic acid

POM pain on motion; prescription only medicine; purulent otitis media

POMC proopiomelanocortin

POMONA pregnancy and postpartum, osteoporosis, mastectomy rehabilitation, osteoarthritis, nerve pain, athletic injuries

POMP phase-offset multiplanar [pulse sequence in magnetic resonance imaging]; principal outer material protein

POMR problem-oriented medical record

POMS problem-oriented medical synopsis; Profile of Mood States

POMT phenol *O*-methyltransferase

PON paraoxonase; particulate organic nitrogen; Pollution and Toxicology Database

pond by weight [Lat. *pondere*]; heavy [Lat. *ponderosus*]

P-one first parental generation

POOV Poovoot virus

POP diphosphate group; pain on palpation; paroxypropione; persistent occipitoposterior [fetal position]; pituitary opioid peptide; plasma osmotic pressure; plaster of Paris; polymyositis ossificans progressiva; point-of-presence; post office protocol

Pop popliteal; population

POPG population group [UMLS]

POPLINE Population Information Online

poplit popliteal

POPOP 1,4-bis-(5-phenoxazol-2-yl) benzene

POPR pre-operative patient representation

POPS patient outcome plans; postoperative pacing study

pops points of presence

POR patient-oriented research; physician of record; postocclusive oscillatory response; prevalence odds ratio; problem-oriented record

PORC porphyria, Chester type

PORH postoperative reactive hyperemia

PORP partial ossicular replacement prosthesis

PORT Patient Outcomes Research Teams [study]; Pneumonia Outcomes Research Team; postoperative radiation therapy; postoperative respiratory therapy

PORV Porton virus

PoRV porcine rubulavirus

PoRV-C porcine rotavirus Cowden

PoRV-E/DC9 porcine rotavirus DC-9

POS periosteal osteosarcoma; physician order set; point of service; polycystic ovary syndrome; provider of services; psychoorganic syndrome

pos position; positive

POSC problem-oriented system of charting

POSCH Program on Surgical Control of Hyperlipidemia

POSM patient-operated selector mechanism

pOsm plasma osmolality

POSS persistent object storage system; proximal over-shoulder strap

POSSUM Pictures of Standard Syndromes and Undiagnosed Malformations; Physiological and Operative Severity Score for the Enumeration of Morbidity and Mortality [study]

POST posterior; Predictors and Outcomes of Stent Thrombosis [study]

Post, post posterior

POST-CARG postcoronary artery bypass graft

postgangl postganglionic

POST LAT posterolateral
postop, post-op postoperative
Post Pit posterior pituitary [gland]
POT periostitis ossificans toxica; postoperative treatment; precursor onset time
pot potassium; potential
potass potassium
POTS plain old telephone service; postural orthostatic tachycardia syndrome
POTV Potosi virus; Potiskum virus
PoTV porcine torovirus
POU placenta, ovary, and uterus
Pout outflow pressure
POV physician order verification
PoV portal vein
PO₂v venous oxygen pressure
POW Powassan [encephalitis]
powd powder
POWER Patients Online for Wellness, Education and Research
POWV Powassan virus
POX point of exit
PP diphosphate group; emphysema [pink puffers]; near point of accommodation [Lat. *punctum proximum*]; pacesetter potential; palmoplantar; pancreatic polypeptide; paradoxical pulse; paraplatin; parietal pericardium; parietal pulse; partial pressure; perfusion pressure; peritoneal pseudomyxoma; persisting proteinuria; Peyer patches; photoplethysmography; pinprick; placental protein; placenta previa; planned parenthood; plasma pepsinogen; plasmapheresis; plasma protein; plaster of Paris; polypropylene; polystyrene agglutination plate; population planning; posterior papillary; posterior pituitary; postpartum; postprandial; precocious puberty; preferred provider; primapara; primary provider; primer protein; private practice; proactivator plasminogen; protein phosphatase; protoporphyria; protoporphyrin; proximal phalanx; prudent practices [for disposal of chemicals]; pseudomyxoma peritonei; pterygoid process; pulmonary pressure; pulse pressure; pulsus paradoxus; purulent pericarditis; pyrophosphatase; pyrophosphate
P-P prothrombin proconvertin
PP1 protein phosphatase type 1
P-5'-P pyridoxal-5'-phosphate
PP₁ free pyrophosphate
Pp plateau pressure

pp near point of accommodation [Lat. *punctum proximum*]; postprandial; postpartum
p-p peak-to-peak
PPA palpation, percussion, auscultation; pepsin A; phenylpropanolamine; phenylpyruvic acid; Pittsburgh pneumonia agent; plasmid profile analysis; polyphosphoric acid; positive predictive accuracy; posterior margin of pulmonary artery; posterior pulmonary artery; postpartum amenorrhea; postpill amenorrhea; preferred provider arrangement; prescription-pricing authority; primary progressive aphasia; propanolamine; pure pulmonary atresia
PP&A palpation, percussion, and auscultation
PP2A protein phosphatase type 2A
Ppa pulmonary artery pressure
PP2Ac catalytic subunit of protein phosphatase type 2A
PPACK L-propyl-*p*-phenylalanyl-chloromethylketone
PP2A_D dimeric protein phosphatase type 2A
PPAF progressive perivenular alcoholic fibrosis
PPAR peroxisome proliferator activated receptor
PPAS peripheral pulmonary artery stenosis
PPase protein phosphatase
Ppaw pulmonary artery wedge pressure
PPB parts per billion; plasmatic protein binding; platelet-poor blood; pneumococcal pneumonia and bacteremia; positive pressure breathing
PPb postparotid basic protein
ppb parts per billion
PPBP pro-platelet basic protein
PPBS postprandial blood sugar
PPBV Phnom Penh bat virus
PPC patient-physician communication; pentose phosphate cycle; peripheral posterior curve; plasma protein concentration; plasma prothrombin conversion; pneumopericardium; pocket personal computer; posterior parietal cortex; progressive patient care; proximal palmar crease
PP1c protein phosphatase type 1, catalytic subunit
PP2C protein phosphatase type 2C

PPCA plasma prothrombin conversion accelerator; proserum prothrombin conversion accelerator

PPCD polymorphous posterior corneal dystropy

PPCE postproline cleaving enzyme

PPCF peripartum cardiac failure; plasma prothrombin conversion factor

PPCM postpartum cardiomyopathy

PPCRA pigmented paravenous chorioretinal atrophy

PPD packs per day; paraphenylenediamine; percussion and postural drainage; permanent partial disability; phenyldiphenyloxadiazole; postpartum day; primary physical dependence; progressive perceptive deafness; purified protein derivative

PPDS phonologic programming deficit syndrome

PPD-S purified protein derivative-standard

PPD-T purified protein derivative stabilized with Tween

PPE palmoplantar erythrodysesthesia; personal protective equipment; polyphosphoric ester; porcine pancreatic elastase; probabilistic population estimation; pulmonary permeability edema

P_peak peak cycling respiratory pressure

PPES palmar-plantar erythrodysesthesia syndrome

PPET patient-physician encounter table

PPF pellagra preventive factor; phagocytosis promoting factor; phosphonoformate; plasma protein fraction

PPFA Planned Parenthood Federation of America

PPG phonopneumography; photoelectric plethysmography; photoplethysmography; platelet proteoglycan; portal pressure gradient

ppg picopicogram

PPGA postpill galactorrhea-amenorrhea

PPGB protective protein of beta-galactosidase

PPGF polypeptide growth factor

PPGP prepaid group practice

ppGpp 3′-pyrophosphoryl-guanosine-5′-diphosphate

PPH past pertinent history; persistent pulmonary hypertension; phosphopyruvate hydratase; postpartum hemorrhage; primary prevention of hypertension; primary

pulmonary hypertension; protocollagen proline hydroxylase

pph parts per hundred

pphm parts per hundred million

PPHN persistent pulmonary hypertension of the newborn

PPHP pseudopseudohypoparathyroidism

ppht parts per hundred thousand

PPI partial permanent impairment; patient package insert; patient physiological image; permanent pacemaker insertion; post [cardiac] pacing interval; present pain intensity; proton-pump inhibitor; purified porcine insulin

PPi, PP_i inorganic pyrophosphate

PPIase peptidyl-prolyl isomerase

PPID peak pain intensity difference [score]

PPIE prolonged postictal encephalopathy

PPK palmoplantar keratosis; prekallikrein

PPL penicilloyl polylysine; posterior pulmonary leaflet

Ppl intrapleural pressure; pleural pressure

Pplat plateau pressure

PPLO pleuropneumonia-like organism

PPM parts per million; permanent pacemaker; phosphopentomutase; physician practice management; pigmented pupillary membrane; posterior papillary muscle; pulse position modulated

ppm parts per million; pulses per minute

PPMA progressive postmyelitis muscular atrophy

PPMD Provincial Performance Management Database [Canada]

PPMoVd Pigeon pea mosaic mottle viroid

PPMS Performax's Personal Matrix System

PPN partial parenteral nutrition; parameterized Petri net; pedunculopontine nucleus

PPNA peak phrenic nerve activity

PPNAD primary pigmented nodular adrenocortical disease

PPNG penicillinase-producing *Neisseria gonorrhoeae*

PPO platelet peroxidase; preferred provider option; preferred provider organization; protoporphyrin oxidase

P&PO principles and practice of oncology

PPP pain perception profile; palatopharyngoplasty; palmoplantar pustulosis; pentose phosphate pathway; peripheral pulse present; photostimulable phosphor plate;

Pickford projective pictures; platelet-poor plasma; pluripotent progenitor; point-to-point protocol; polyphoretic phosphate; porcine pancreatic polypeptide; portal perfusion pressure; Prospective Pravastatin Pooling [project]; protein phosphatase; purified placental protein

PPPA protein phosphatase alpha

PPPBL peripheral pulses palpable both legs

PPPD pylorus-preserving pancreatoduodenectomy

PPPI primary private practice insurance

PPPMA progressive postpolio muscle atrophy

PPPP porokeratosis punctata palmaris et plantaris

PPP/SLIP point-to-point protocol/serial line internet protocol

PPR patient-provider relationship; percentage of predicted recovery; photoparoxysmal response; physician-patient relation; physician payment reform; posterior primary ramus; Price precipitation reaction

PPr paraprosthetic

PPRC Physician Payment Review Commission

PPRF paramedian pontine reticular formation; pontine perireticular formation; postpartum renal failure

PP1$_{RG}$ protein phosphatase type 1, regulatory subunit

PPRM Portable Patient Record Model

PPROM preterm premature rupture of fetal membranes

PPRV peste-des-petits-ruminants virus

PPRWP poor precordial R-wave progression

PPS Paris Prospective Study; Personal Preference Scale; physician, patient and society [course]; polyvalent pneumococcal polysaccharide; popliteal pterygium syndrome; postpartum sterilization; postperfusion syndrome; postpericardiotomy syndrome; postpolio syndrome; postpump syndrome; prescription preparation system [radiotherapy]; primary acquired preleukemic syndrome; prospective payment system; prospective pricing system; protein plasma substitute; pulse per second

PPSC Play Performance Scale for Children

PPSH pseudovaginal perineoscrotal hypospadias

PP1$_{SR}$ protein phosphatase type 1, sarcoplasmic reticulum

PPSTH population poststimulus time histogram

PPT parietal pleural tissue; partial prothrombin time; parts per thousand; parts per trillion; peak-to-peak threshold; Pfeiffer-Palm-Teller [syndrome]; pedunculopontine tegmental [nucleus]; physical performance test; plant protease test; polypurine tract; postpartum thyroiditis; posterior pelvic tilt; preprotachykinin; pressure pain threshold; pulmonary platelet trapping; pulmonary physical therapy

ppt parts per thousand; parts per trillion; precipitation, precipitate; prepared

pptd precipitated

PPTL postpartum tubul ligation

PPTS pyridinium *p*-toluenesulfonate

PPV *Parapoxvirus*, parapoxvirus; pneumococcal polysaccharide vaccine; porcine parvovirus; positive predictive value; positive pressure ventilation; Precarious Point virus; progressive pneumonia virus; pulmonary plasma volume

PPVr regional pulmonary plasma volume

PPVT Peabody Picture Vocabulary Test

PPVT-R Peabody Picture Vocabulary Test, Revised

PPW patient protective wrap

Ppw pulmonary wedge pressure

PPX protein phosphatase X

PPX1 protein phosphatase X type 1

PPX2 protein phosphatase X type 2

PPY pancreatic polypeptide

PPyV baboon polyomavirus 2

PQ paraquat; parent questionnaire; permeability quotient; physician's questionnaire; plastoquinone; pronator quadratus; pyrimethamine-quinine

pQCT peripheral quantitative computed tomography

PQI process quality improvement

PQOL Perceived Quality of Life [scale]

PQQ pyrroloquinoline quinone

P-QRS QRS P potential [ECG]

PQRST Probucol Quantitative Regression Swedish Trial; provocative and palliative factors, quality of pain, radiation of pain, severity of pain, timing of pain [pain characteristics in low back pain syndrome]

PR by way of the rectum [Lat. *per rectum*]; far point of accommodation [Lat. *punctum remotum*]; palindromic rheumatism; parallax and refraction; partial reinforcement; partial remission; partial response; particulate respirator; peer review; perfusion rate; peripheral resistance; per rectum; phenol red; photoreaction; photoresist; physical rehabilitation; pityriasis rosea; police report; posterior root; postmyalgia rheumatica; postural reflex; potency ratio; preference record; pregnancy; pregnancy rate; preretinal; pressoreceptor; pressure; prevention; Preyer reflex; proctology; production rate; profile; progesterone receptor; progressive relaxation; progressive resistance; progress report; prolactin; prolonged remission; propranolol; prosthion; protective ratio; protein; public relations; pulmonary regurgitation; pulmonary rehabilitation; pulse rate; pulse repetition; pyramidal response

P-R the time between the P wave and the beginning of the QRS complex in electrocardiography [interval]

P&R pelvic and rectal [examination]; pulse and respiration

Pr in prone position; praseodymium; prednisolone; presbyopia; primary; prism; production, productivity; production rate [of steroid hormones]; prolactin; propyl

pr far point of accommodation [Lat. *punctum remotum*]; pair; per rectum; prism

PRA panel-reactive antibody; patient record architecture; percent reactive antibody; phosphoribosylamine; physician recognition award; plasma renin activity; progesterone receptor assay; proximal reference axis [imaging]

prac, pract practice, practitioner

PRACTICAL Placebo-Controlled Randomized ACE Inhibition Comparative Trial in Cardiac Infarction and Left Ventricular Function

PRAGMATIC pregnancy, rheumatoid arthritis, acromegaly, glucose metabolism disorders, mechanical injury, amyloid, thyroid disease, infectious disease, crystals in gout or pseudogout [disorders associated with carpal tunnel syndrome]

PRAGUE Primary Angioplasty After Transfer of Patients from General Community Hospitals to Catheterization Units

with or without Emergency Thrombolytic Infusion [study]

PrA-HPA protein A hemolytic plaque assay

PRAI pattern recognition and artificial intelligence

PRAISE Prospective Randomized Amlodipine Survival Evaluation

PRAMS pregnancy risk assessment monitoring system

PRANN prediction recurrent artificial neural network

PRAS pre-reduced anaerobically sterilized [medium]; pseudo-renal artery syndrome

PRB basic proline-rich protein; Prosthetics Research Board

pRB, pRb retinoblastoma protein

PRBC packed red blood cells; placental residual blood volume

pRB-P phosphorylated form of retinoblastoma protein

PRBS pseudorandom binary sequence

PRBV placental residual blood volume

PRC packed red cells; peer review committee; phase response curve; plasma renin concentration; professional review committee

PRCA pure red cell aplasia

pRCA posterior right coronary artery

PRCCT prospective randomized controlled clinical trial

PRCF peak response coarse frequency

PRCG Polak-Ribiere conjugate gradient [algorithm]

PRCoV porcine respiratory coronavirus

PRCV porcine respiratory coronavirus

PRD partial reaction of degeneration; patient reference dosier; physician relations department; Pitt-Rogers-Danks [syndrome]; postradiation dysplasia

PRDP Provincial Resource Directory Project [Canada]

PRDS Pitt-Rogers-Danks syndrome

PRE photoreacting enzyme; physician's report of examination; pigmented retinal epithelium; preliminary evaluation; preplacement examination; progressive resistive exercise; prospective randomized evaluation; proton relaxation enhancement

pre preliminary; preparation or prepare; pretreatment

pre-AIDS pre-acquired immune deficiency syndrome

pre-amp preliminary amplifier

PRECEDE predisposing, reinforcing, and enabling causes in educational diagnosis and evaluation [model]

precip precipitate, precipitated, precipitation

PRECISE Prospective Randomized Evaluation of Carvedilol in Symptoms and Exercise [trial]

PRED prednisone

PREDICT Prospective Randomized Evaluation of Diltiazem CD Trial

PREFACE Pravastatin-Related Effects Following Angioplasty on Coronary Endothelium [study]

prefd preferred

PREFER patient randomization to either femoral or radial catheterization

preg, pregn pregnancy, pregnant

prelim preliminary

prem premature, prematurity

PreMACE prednisone, methotrexate, Adriamycin, cyclophosphamide, etoposide

PREMIS Prehospital Myocardial Infarction Study

pre-mRNA precursor messenger ribonucleic acid

preop, pre-op preoperative

PREP pattern reversal electrical potential; Physician Review and Enhancement Program

prep, prepd prepare, prepared

Pres resistive pressure

PRESEP Pediatric Rural Emergency System and Education Project

preserv preserve, preserved, preservation

PRESERVE Prospective Randomized Enalapril Study Evaluating Regression of Ventricular Enlargement

PRESS Percutaneous Retroperitoneal Spleno-renal Shunt [study]; point-resolved spectroscopy

press pressure

PREV Pretoria virus

prev prevention, preventive; previous

PREVENT Program in Ex Vivo Vein Graft Engineering via Transfection; Proliferation Reduction Using Vascular Energy Trial; Prospective Randomized Evaluation of the Vascular Effects of Norvasc Trial

PREVMEDU preventive medicine unit

PREZ posterior root entry zone

PRF partial reinforcement; patient report form; peak repetition frequency; perforin; plasma recognition factor; pontine reticular formation; postrepetition frequency [Doppler]; progressive renal failure; prolactin releasing factor; pulse repetition frequency

pRF polyclonal rheumatoid factor

PRFF,TRFF peak [through] response fine frequency

PRFLE Prospective Randomized Flosequinan Longevity Evaluation

PRFM premature rupture of fetal membranes

PRG phleborheography; purge

PRGS phosphoribosylglycineamide synthetase

PRH past relevant history; postrepetition frequency [Doppler]; prolactin releasing hormone

PrH propositus hypoglossi

PRHCIT The Project for Rural Health Communication and Information Technologies [Australia]

PRHHP Puerto Rico Heart Health Program

PRI Pain Rating Index; patient review instrument; phosphate reabsorption index; phosphoribose isomerase; placental ribonuclease inhibitor

P-RIA polyclonal radioimmunoassay

PRIAS Packard radioimmunoassay system

PRICE protection, relative rest, ice, compression, elevation

PRICEMM protection, relative rest, ice, compression, elevation, modalities, medication

PRICES protection, rest, ice, compression, elevation, support [primary treatment of tendinitis and overuse injury]; physician modalities, rehabilitation, injections, cross-training, evaluation, salicylates [secondary treatment of tendinitis and overuse injury]

PRIDE Parents Resource Institute for Drug Education; Platelet Aggregation and Receptor Occupancy with Integrilin-A Dynamic Evaluation [study]; Primary Implantable Defibrillator [study]

PRIH prolactin release-inhibiting hormone

PRIM primase

PRIMA Primary Care Information Across Anglia

PRIME preinversion multiecho; Prematriculation Program in Medical Education; Promotion of Reperfusion by Inhibition of Thrombin During Myocardial Infarction Evaluation [study]; Promotion of Reperfusion in Myocardial Infarction Evolution [study]; Prospective Randomized Ibopamine Mortality Evaluation [study]; Prospective Randomized Study of Ibopamine on Mortality and Efficacy in Heart Failure

PRIME-MD Primary Care Evaluation of Mental Disorders

PRIMEROSE probabilistic rule based on rough sets

PRIMEX primary care extender

PRIMI Prourokinase in Myocardial Infarction [trial]

primip primipara

PRINCE prevention of radiocontrast-induced nephropathy evaluation

PRIND prolonged reversible ischemic neurologic deficit

PRINS primed in situ [labeling]

PRI(S) pain rating intensity score

PRISAM Primary Stenting for Acute Myocardial Infarction [trial]

PRISE Primary Care Sharing the Evidence [UK]

PRISM pediatric risk of mortality; Platelet Receptor Inhibition in Ischemic Syndrome Management [study]

PRISM-PLUS Platelet Receptor Inhibition in Ischemic Syndrome Management in Patients Limited by Unstable Signs and Symptoms [study]

PRISMS Prevention of Relapses and Disability by Interferon Beta-1a Subcutaneously in Multiple Sclerosis [study]

PRIST paper radioimmunosorbent test

PRISTINE Praxilene in Stroke Treatment in Northern Europe [study]

PRK photorefractive keratectomy; primary rabbit kidney

PRKAR protein kinase, cyclic adenosine monophosphate-dependent, regulatory

PRKAR1A protein kinase, cyclic adenosine monophosphate-dependent, regulatory, type 1 alpha

PRKC protein kinase C

PRKCA protein kinase C alpha

PRL, Prl prolactin

PRLR prolactin receptor

PRM phosphoribomutase; photoreceptor membrane; premature rupture of membranes; Primary Reference Material; primidone; protamine

PrM preventive medicine

PRMS percent root mean square

PRMSE percent root mean square error

PRN pertactin; Physicians Research Network; polyradiculoneuropathy; prion; protectin

p.r.n. as needed [Lat. *pro re nata*]

PRNP prion protein

PRNT plaque reduction neutralization test

PRO peer review organization; physician review organization; Professional Review Organization; pronation; protein

Pro proline; prophylactic; prothrombin

pro protein

PROACT Prolyse in Acute Cerebral Thrombolysis Trial; Prourokinase in Acute Cerebral Thromboembolism [trial]; Prourokinase in Acute Thromboembolic Stroke [trial]

ProACT professionally advanced care team

prob probable

PROBE Prospective, Randomized, Open Blinded Endpoint Trial; Prospective, Randomized, Open Trial with Blinded Endpoint Evaluation

PROC protein C

proc proceedings, procedure; process

PROCAM Prospective Cardiovascular Münster Study

PROC GLM general linear model procedure

proct, procto proctology, proctologist; proctoscopy

prod production, product

PROFET Prevention of Falls in the Elderly Trial

prog progress, progressive

progn prognosis

PROGRESS Perindopril Protection Against Recurrent Stroke Study

proGRP pro-gastrin-releasing peptide

PROH propyl-4-hydrolase

PROHB propyl-4-hydrolase, beta

PROLOG Precursor to EPILOG [study]; programming in logic

prolong prolongation, prolonged

PROM passive range of motion; premature rupture of fetal membranes; prolonged rupture of fetal membranes; programmable read only memory; prosthetic range of motion

PROMIS Problem-Oriented Medical Information System

PROMISE Prospective Randomized Milrinone Survival Evaluation [study]

PROMPTOR-FM probabilistic method of prompting for test ordering in family medicine

pron pronator, pronation

PROP propranolol

ProPAC Prospective Payment Assessment Commission

PRO-PBP pro-platelet basic protein

proph prophylactic, prophylaxis

ProPO prophenoloxidase

ProRS propyl transfer ribonucleic acid synthase [RNAse]

PROS Pediatric Research in Office Settings [network]; protein S

pros prostate, prostatic

PROSIT proteinuria screening and intervention

PROSP protein S pseudogene

PROSPECT Proscar Safety Plus Efficacy Canadian Two-Year Study

PROSPER Prospective Study of Pravastatin in the Elderly at Risk

PROST pronuclear stage transfer

PROSTATE Physicians for Rational Ordering and Screening Tests and Therapeutic Effectiveness

prosth prosthesis, prosthetic

PROTECT Perindopril Regression of Vascular Thickening European Community Trial; Prospective Reinfarction in the Thrombolytic Era: Cardizem-CD Trial

PROTO protoporphyrin; protoporphyrinogen

pro-u-PA proenzyme urokinase plasminogen activator

prov provisional

PROVED Prospective Randomized Study of Ventricular Failure and the Efficacy of Digoxin

PROW Protein Review on the Web

prox proximal

PRP photolyase regulatory protein; physiologic rest position; pityriasis rubra pilaris; platelet-rich plasma; polyribosyl

ribitol phosphate; postural rest position; pressure rate product; primary Raynaud phenomenon; progressive rubella panencephalitis; proliferative retinopathy photocoagulation; proline-rich protein; Psychotic Reaction Profile; pulse repetition period

PrP, Prp prion protein

PRPH peripherin

PRPP phosphoribosylpyrophosphate

PRPS prostatic secretory protein

PRP,TRP peak [through] response phase

PRQ personal resources questionnaire

PRR pattern recognition receptor; proton relaxation rate; pulse repetition rate

PrR progesterone receptor

PRRB Provider Reimbursement Review Board

PRRE pupils round, regular, and equal

PRRF paramedian pontine reticular formation

PR-RSV Prague Rous sarcoma virus

PRS Personality Rating Scale; Pierre Robin syndrome; plasma renin substrate; Prieto syndrome; proctorectosigmoidoscopy

PRSIS Prospective Rate Setting Information System

PRT patient record tree; *Penicillium roqueforti* toxin; pharmaceutical research and testing; phosphoribosyl transferase; pivot repeatability test; postoperative respiratory therapy; prospective randomized trial

PrT protein truncation [test]

PRTD proximal renal tubular dysfunction

PRTH pituitary resistance to thyroid hormone

PRTH-C prothrombin time control

PRTN proteinase

PRTS Partington syndrome

PRU peripheral resistance unit

PRUJ proximal radioulnar joint

PRV Paroo River virus; planning organ at risk volume [imaging]; polycythemia rubra vera; pseudorabies virus; posterior right ventricle; python orthoreovirus

PRVC pressure-regulated volume control [respiration]

PRVEP pattern reversal visual evoked potential

PRW polymerized ragweed

PRX pseudoexfoliation

Prx prognosis

prx proximal

PRZF pyrazofurin

PS pacemaker syndrome; pain stimulation; paired stimulation; pancreozymin secretin; paradoxical sleep; paralaryngeal space; paranoid schizophrenia; paraspinal; parasympathetic; Parkinson syndrome; parotid sialography; partial saturation; partial seizure; pathological stage; patient's serum; pediatric site [database, Italy]; pediatric surgery; performing scale [intelligence quotient, IQ]; performance status; periodic syndrome; pferdestärke (German for horsepower); phosphate saline [buffer]; phosphatidyl serine; photosensitivity, photosensitization; photosynthesis; phrenic stimulation; physical status; physiologic saline; phytosterol; pixel size; plastic surgery; polysaccharide; polystyrene; population sample; population spike; Porter-Silber [chromogen]; postcardiotomy shock; posterior synechiae or synechiotomy; posteroseptal; postmaturity syndrome; prescription; precursor state; presenilin; presenting symptom; pressure sore; pressure support; prestimulus; procedural sedation; programmed symbol; prostatic secretion; protamine sulfate; proteasome; protein S; protein synthesis; Proteus syndrome; P selectin; psychiatric; pulmonary sequestration; pulmonary stenosis; pulse sequence; pyloric stenosis

P&S paracentesis and suction

P/S polisher-stimulator; polyunsaturated/saturated [fatty acid ratio]

Ps prescription; *Pseudomonas*; psoriasis

P$_s$ systolic pressure

ps per second; picosecond

PSA pacemaker system analysis; parasternal short axis; pleomorphic salivary gland adenoma; polar surface area; polyethylene sulfonic acid; polysaccharide adhesin; polysialic acid; posterior spinal artery; power spectrum analysis; primary sampling unit; professional services agreement; progressive spinal ataxia; prolonged sleep apnea; prostate specific antigen; protein S alpha; pseudoaneurysm; psoriatic arthritis

PS/A polysaccharide adhesin

Psa systemic blood pressure

PSAAMI Primary Stenting vs Angioplasty in Acute Myocardial Infarction [trial]

PSAC President's Science Advisory Committee

PSACH pseudoachondrodysplasia

PSAD prostate-specific antigen density; psychoactive substance abuse and dependence

PSAG pelvic sonoangiography

PSAGN poststreptococcal acute glomerulonephritis

PSAn psychoanalysis

PSA-NCAM polysialic acid neuronal cell adhesion molecule

PSAP peak systolic aortic pressure; primary public safety answering point; prosaposin; pulmonary surfactant apoprotein

P/SAT pediatric severity assessment

PSB protected specimen brush; protein S beta

PSbetaG, PSBG pregnancy-specific beta-1-glycoprotein

PSC patient services coordination; peripheral stem cell; Plasma Single Nucleotide Polymorphism [SNP] Consortium; pluripotential stem cell; Porter-Silber chromogen; posterior subcapsular cataract; primary sclerosing cholangitis; professional service corporation; prospective studies collaboration; proteasome component; pulse synchronized contractions

PS-CF pancreatic-sufficient cystic fibrosis

PsChE pseudocholinesterase

PSCI Primary Self Concept Inventory

Psci pressure at slow component intercept

PSCM problem space computational model

PSCT peripheral stem cell transplantation

PSD particle size distribution; peptone, starch, and dextrose; percutaneous stricture dilatation; periodic synchronous discharge; phase-sensitive detector; pilonidal sinus disease; poststenosis dilation; pituitary stalk distortion; posterior sagittal diameter; post-stroke depression; postsynaptic density; power spectral density; prevention of significant deterioration; Protein Sequence Database; psychosomatic disease

PSDA Patient Self-Determination Act

PSDES primary symptomatic diffuse esophageal spasm

PSE paradoxical systolic expansion; penicillin-sensitive enzyme; portal systemic encephalopathy; Present State Examination; purified spleen extract

psec picosecond

PSEK progressive symmetrical erythrokeratoderma

PSEN1 presenilin 1 gene

PSEN2 presenilin 2 gene

PSEP post-sexual exposure prophylaxis

pseudo-BTX pseudobatrachotoxin

PSF peak scatter factor; peptide supply factor; point spread function; posterior spinal fusion; prostacyclin stabilizing factor; pseudosarcomatous fasciitis

PSG peak systolic gradient; phosphate, saline, and glucose; polysomnogram; presystolic gallop; pregnancy-specific glycoprotein; programmable sound generator

PSGL P selectin glycoprotein ligand

PSGN poststreptococcal glomerulonephritis

PSH past surgical history; postspinal headache

PsHD pseudoheart disease

PSHV pulmonary syndrome hantavirus

PsHV psittacid herpesvirus

PSI parenting stress inventory; pneumonia severity index; pollutant standard index; posterior sagittal index; problem solving information; prostaglandin synthetic inhibitor; Psychiatric Society for Informatics; psychological services index; psychosomatic inventory; purified photosystem I

psi pounds per square inch

ψ Greek letter *psi*; wave function

psia pounds per square inch absolute

PSI-BLAST position-specific iterated basic local alignment search tool

PSICU pediatric surgical intensive care unit

pSIDS partially unexplained sudden infant death syndrome

PSIFT platelet suspension immunofluorescence test

PSIL percentage signal intensity loss; preferred frequency speech interference level

PSIS posterior sacroiliac spine

PSK protein serine kinase

PSL parasternal line; photostimulable luminescence; potassium, sodium chloride, and sodium lactate [solution]; prednisolone

PSM patient self-management; patient-specific mortality; personal status monitor; polymerase chain reaction [PCR]

mediated–site-directed mutagenesis; presystolic murmur; problem solving method

psm patient-specific mortality

PSMA prostate-specific membrane antigen; proximal spinal muscular atrophy

PSMed psychosomatic medicine

PSMF protein-sparing modified fast

PSMS Physical Self-Maintenance Scale

PSMT psychiatric services management team

PSN provider service network

PSNR peak signal to noise ratio

PSO proximal subungual onychomycosis

PSOM probabilistic self-organizing map

PSP pancreatic spasmolytic peptide; paralytic shellfish poisoning; parathyroid secretory protein; peak systolic pressure; periodic short pulse; phenolsulfonphthalein; phosphoserine phosphatase; photostimulable phosphor plate; positive spike pattern; posterior spinal process; postsynaptic potential; prednisone sodium phosphate; primary spontaneous pneumothorax; progressive supranuclear palsy; prostatic secretory protein; pseudopregnancy; pulmonary surfactant apoprotein

PspA pneumococcal surface protein A

PSPR particle surface plasmon resonance

PSPS secretory pancreatic stone protein

PSPV psittacinepox virus

PSQ Parent Symptom Questionnaire; Patient Satisfaction Questionnaire

PsqO$_2$ subcutaneous tissue oximetry

PSR pain sensitivity range; perspective surface rendering; portal systemic resistance; posteroseptal right atrium; poststreptococcal reactive arthritis; pressure sore risk assessment; proliferative sickle retinopathy; pulmonary stretch receptor

PSRC Plastic Surgery Research Council

PSRO Professional Standards Review Organization

PSS painful shoulder syndrome; pain sensation score; patient scheduling system; patient stimulation stack; performance support system; physiologic saline solution; polystyrene sulfonate; porcine stress syndrome; primary Sjögren syndrome; progressive systemic scleroderma; progressive systemic sclerosis; psoriasis severity scale; Psychiatric Status Schedule; pure sensory stroke

pSS Perceived Stress Scale; primary Sjögren syndrome
PSSE partial saturation spin echo
PSSS perceived stress support scale
PST pancreatic suppression test; paralytic shellfish toxin; paroxysmal supraventricular tachycardia; patient-specific therapy; penicillin, streptomycin, and tetracycline; penoscrotal transposition; peristimulus time; phenolsulfotransferase; platelet survival time; posterior sinus tympani; poststenotic; poststimulus time; prefrontal sonic treatment; protein-sparing therapy; proximal straight tubule
PSTAF Pilsicainide Suppression Trial of Atrial Fibrillation
PSTE phase space time evolution [radiotherapy]
PSTH poststimulus time histogram
PSTI pancreatic secretory trypsin inhibitor
PSTN public switched telephone network [telemedicine]
PSTV potato spindle tuber virus
PSU patient service unit; photosynthetic unit; primary sampling unit
PSurg plastic surgery
PSV papular stomatitis virus; pressure-support ventilation; Punta Salinas virus
pSV simian vacuolating virus plasmid
PSVER pattern shift visual evoked response
PSVT paroxysmal supraventricular tachycardia
PSW primary surgical ward; positive sharp wave; psychiatric social worker
PSWT psychiatric social work training
PSX pseudoexfoliation
Psy psychiatry; psychology
psych psychology, psychological
PSYCHE Psychiatry Educator [computer-assisted instruction]
psychiat psychiatry, psychiatric
psychoan psychoanalysis, psychoanalytical
psychol psychology, psychological
psychopath psychopathology, psychopathological
psychosom psychosomatic
psychother psychotherapy
psy-path psychopathic
Ps-ZES pseudo-Zollinger-Ellison syndrome

PT pain threshold; pancreatic transplantation; parathormone; parathyroid; paroxysmal tachycardia; part time; patient; pericardial tamponade; permanent and total; phage type; pharmacy and therapeutics; phenytoin; phosphorothioate; photophobia; phototoxicity; physical therapy, physical therapist; physical training; physiotherapy; pine tar; plasma thromboplastin; pluridirectional tomography; pneumothorax; polynomial transform; polyvalent tolerance; position tracking; posterior tibial [artery pulse]; posttetanic; posttransfusion; posttransplantation; posttraumatic; premature termination [of pregnancy]; preoperative therapy; preterm; preventive therapy; previously treated; primary tumor; propylthiouracil; protamine; prothrombin time; proton density; pulmonary tuberculosis; pseudotumor; psychometric test; psychotherapy; pulmonary thrombosis; pyramidal tract; temporal plane
P&T permanent and total [disability]; pharmacy and therapeutics
Pt patient; platinum
pT pertussis toxin; postoperative tumor size [TNM (tumor-node-metastasis) classification: **pT0** surgery not done or not applicable, **pT1** no visible tumor tissue, **pT2** less than 1.5 cm remains, **pT3** 1.5 to 5.0 cm remains, **pT4** more than 5.0 cm remains to primary tumors in progressing thickness, and **pTX** no evidence of primary tumor]
pT0 no evidence of primary tumor [TNM (tumor-node-metastasis) classification]
pt part; patient; pint; point
PTA pancreatic transplantation alone; parallel tubular arrays; parathyroid adenoma; peak twitch amplitude; percutaneous transluminal angioplasty; peroxidase-labeled antibody; persistent truncus arteriosus; phosphotungstic acid; physical therapy assistant; plasma thromboplastin antecedent; posttraumatic amnesia; pretreatment anxiety; primitive trigeminal artery; prior to admission; prior to arrival; prothrombin activity
PTAB pterygoalar bar
PTAF platelet activating factor
PTAFR platelet activating factor receptor
PTAH phosphotungstic acid hematoxylin

PTAP purified diphtheria toxoid precipitated by aluminum phosphate

PTAT pure tone average threshold

PTB patellar tendon bearing; polypyrimidine tract binding; prior to birth

PTb pulmonary tuberculosis

PTBA percutaneous transluminal balloon angioplasty

PTBBS peripheral type benzodiazepine binding site

PTBD percutaneous transhepatic biliary drainage; percutaneous transluminal balloon dilatation

PTBE pyretic tick-borne encephalitis

PTBNA protected transbronchial needle aspirate

PTBPD posttraumatic borderline personality disorder

PTBS posttraumatic brain syndrome

PTBW peak torque to body weight

PTC papillary thyroid carcinoma; percutaneous transhepatic cholangiography; phase transfer catalyst; phenothiocarbazine; phenylthiocarbamide; phenylthiocarbamoyl; plasma thromboplastin component; plugged telescopic catheter; posttetanic count; premature termination codon; premature tricuspid closure; prior to conception; prothrombin complex; pseudotumor cerebri

PTCA percutaneous transluminal coronary angiography; percutaneous transluminal coronary angioplasty; pyrrole-2,3,5-tricarboxylic acid

PT(C)A percutaneous transluminal [coronary] angioplasty

PtcCO$_2$ transcutaneous partial pressure of carbon dioxide

PTCDA perylene-tetracarboxylic dianhydride

PTCER pulmonary transcapillary escape rate

PtcO$_2$ transcutaneous oxygen tension

PTCR percutaneous transluminal coronary recanalization or revascularization

PTCRA percutaneous transluminal coronary rotational ablation

PTD percutaneous transluminal dilatation; permanent total disability; personality trait disorder; photothermal deflection; preterm delivery; prior to delivery

PTDS posttraumatic distress syndrome

PTE parathyroid extract; posttraumatic epilepsy; pretibial edema; proximal tibial epiphysis; pulmonary thromboembolism

PTEAM particle total exposure assessment methodology

PTED pulmonary thromboembolic disease

PteGlu pteroylglutamic acid

PTEN pentaerythritol tetranitrate

pter end of short arm of chromosome

PTF patient treatment file; plasma thromboplastin factor; posterior talofibular [ligament]; pre-term formula; proximal tubular fragment

PTFA prothrombin time fixing agent

PTFE polytetrafluoroethylene

PTFNA percutaneous transthoracic fine-needle aspiration

PTFS posttraumatic fibromyalgia syndrome

PTG parathyroid gland; prostaglandin

PTGE prostaglandin E

PTGER prostaglandin E receptor

PTH parathormone; parathyroid; parathyroid hormone; percutaneous transhepatic drainage; phenylthiohydantoin; plasma thromboplastin component; posttransfusion hepatitis

PTHC percutaneous transhepatic cholangiography

PTHL parathyroid hormone-like

PTHLP parathyroid-hormone–like protein

PTH/PTHrP parathyroid hormone/parathyroid hormone–related peptide

PTHR parathyroid hormone receptor

PTHRP, PTHrP parathyroid-hormone-related peptide; parathyroid-hormone-related protein

PTHS parathyroid hormone secretion [rate]

PTHV Pathun Thani virus

PTI pancreatic trypsin inhibitor; penetrating trauma index; persistent tolerant infection; Pictorial Test of Intelligence; placental thrombin inhibitor; pulsatility transmission index

PTK phosphotyrosine kinase; phototherapeutic keratectomy; protein-tyrosine kinase

PTL peritoneal telencephalic leukoencephalomyopathy; pharyngotracheal lumen; plasma thyroxine level; posterior tricuspid leaflet; preterm labor

pTL posterior tricuspid leaflet

PTLA pharyngeal tracheal lumen airway
PTLC precipitation thin-layer chromatography
PTLD posttransplantation lymphoproliferative disorder; prescribed tumor lethal dose
PTLV primate T-lymphotropic virus
PTLV 1, 2, 3 primate T-lymphotropic viruses 1, 2, 3
PTM posterior trabecular meshwork; posttransfusion mononucleosis; posttranslational modification; post-traumatic meningitis; prothymosin; pulse time modulation
P$_{TM}$ transmural pressure
Ptm pterygomaxillary [fissure]
PTMA phenyltrimethylammonium; prothymosin alpha
PTMDF pupils, tension, media, disc, fundus
PTMPY per thousand members per year
PTMR percutaneous transluminal myocardial revascularization
PTMS parathymosin
PTN pain transmission neuron; pleiotrophin; posterior tibial nerve; Prevention Trials Network [NIH]; proximal tibial nail; public telephone network [telemedicine]
pTNM pathological classification of primary tumors, regional nodes and metastases [coding]
PTO Klemperer's tuberculin [Ger. *Perlsucht Tuberculin Original*]
P$_{total}$ total pressure
PTP pancreatic thread protein; pediatric telephone protocol; percutaneous transhepatic portography; phosphotyrosine phosphatase; physical treatment planning; posterior tibial pulse; posttetanic potential; posttransfusion purpura; pretest probability; previously treated patient; protein-tyrosine phosphatase; proximal tubular pressure
Ptp transpulmonary pressure
PTPA phosphotyrosyl phosphatase activator
PTPC protein-tyrosine phosphatase C
PTPG protein-tyrosine phosphatase gamma
PTPI posttraumatic pulmonary insufficiency

PTPinsp inspiratory pressure-time product
PTPM post-traumatic progressive myelopathy
PTPN protein-tyrosine phosphatase, nonreceptor
PTPRA protein-tyrosine phosphatase receptor alpha
PTPRB protein-tyrosine phosphatase receptor beta
PTPRF protein-tyrosine phosphatase receptor F
PTPRG protein-tyrosine phosphatase receptor gamma
PTPS postthrombophlebitis syndrome; 6-pyruvoyl tetrahydropterin synthase
PTPT protein-tyrosine phosphatase, T-cell
PT/PTT prothrombin time/partial thromboplastin time [test]
PTQ parent-teacher questionnaire
PTR patellar tendon reflex; patient termination record; patient to return; peripheral total resistance; plasma transfusion reaction; prothrombin time ratio; psychotic trigger reaction
PTr porcine trypsin
Ptr intratracheal pressure
PTRA percutaneous transluminal renal angioplasty
PT Rep patient's representative
PTRIA polystyrene-tube radioimmunoassay
Ptrx pelvic traction
PTS para-toluenesulfonic acid; pediatric trauma score; postthrombotic syndrome; posttraumatic syndrome; Pressure and Tension Scale; prior to surgery; 6-pyruvoyl tetrahydropterin synthase; patient treatment file
Pts, pts patients
PTSD posttraumatic stress disorder
PTSM Plant, Technology and Safety Management
PTSS posttraumatic stress syndrome
PTT partial thromboplastin time; particle transport time; posterior tibial tendon (transfer); protein truncation test; prothrombin time; pulmonary transit time; pulse transit time
ptt partial thromboplastin time
PTTI penetrating thoracic trauma index
PTU phenylthiourea; propylthiouracil

PTV patient-triggered ventilation; planning target volume; porcine teschovirus; posterior terminal vein; posterior tibial vein; Punta Toro virus

PTV₂ planning target volume 2

PtV pneumotropic virus

PTVT planning target volume tool

PTVV Ponteves virus

PTX palytoxin; pentoxifylline; picrotoxinin; pneumothorax

PTx parathyroidectomy; pelvic traction

Ptx pneumothorax

pTX no evidence of primary tumor [TNM (tumor-node-metastasis) classification]

PTXT pointer to text

PTZ pentylenetetrazol

PU palindromic unit; passed urine; patient unit; pepsin unit; peptic ulcer; perfusion unit; polyurethane; pregnancy urine; 6-propyluracil; prostatic urethra

Pu plutonium; purine; purple

PUA patient unit assistant

pub public

PUBS percutaneous umbilical blood sampling; purple urine bag syndrome

PUC pediatric urine collector; premature uterine contractions

PUCV Puchong virus

PUD peptic ulcer disease; pudendal

PuD pulmonary disease

PUF polyurethane foam; pure ultrafiltration

PUFA polyunsaturated fatty acid

PUF-HAL polyurethane foam-hybrid artificial liver

PUH pregnancy urine hormones

PUI platelet uptake index; posterior urethral injury

PUJO pelvi-ureteric junction obstruction

PUL percutaneous ultrasonic lithotripsy

PUL, pul, pulm pulmonary

PULHEMS physique, upper extremity, lower extremity, hearing and ears, eyes and vision, mental capacity, emotional stability [profile]

PULSES physical condition, upper limb function, lower limb function, sensory component, excretory function, mental and status (or support factors in revised version) [profile]

PUM peanut-reactive urinary mucin

PUMF public use microdata file

PUMP putative metalloproteinase

PUMS patient utility measurement set; permanently unfit for military service

PUN plasma urea nitrogen

PUO pyrexia of unknown origin

PUP previously untreated patient; previously untreated product

pUPID paternal uniparental isodisomy

PUPPP pruritic urticarial papules and plaques of pregnancy

PUR polyurethane

Pur purple

pur purulent

purg purgative

PurR purine repressor

PURSUIT Platelet Glycoprotein IIb/IIIa Underpinning the Receptor for Suppression of Unstable Ischemia Trial; Platelet Glycoprotein IIb-IIIa in Unstable Angina: Receptor Suppression Using Integrilin Therapy

PURV Purus virus

PUT provocative use test; putamen

PUU puumala [virus]

PUUV Puumala virus

PUV posterior urethral valve

PUVA psoralen ultraviolet A-range

PV pancreatic vein; papilla of Vater; papillomavirus; paramyxovirus; parapoxvirus; paraventricular; paravertebral; partial volume; parvovirus; pemphigus vulgaris; peripheral vascular; peripheral vein; peripheral vessel; picornavirus; pityriasis versicolor; plasma viscosity; plasma volume; pneumonia virus; polio vaccine; poliovirus; polycythemia vera; polyoma virus; polyvinyl; portal vein; postvasectomy; postvoiding; poxvirus; predictive value; pressure velocity; pressure-volume [curve]; process variable; progressive vaccinia; pulmonary valve; pulmonary vein

P-V pressure-volume [curve]

P&V pyloroplasty and vagotomy

Pᵥ ventricular pressure

PV-1, 2, 3 human polioviruses 1, 2, 3

Pv *Proteus vulgaris*; venous pressure

PVA Paralyzed Veterans of America; peripheral venous alimentation; polyvinyl acetate; polyvinyl alcohol; pressure volume area

PVₐ pulmonary venous atrial

PVA-C polyvinyl alcohol cryogel

PVAc polyvinyl acetate

PVAd polyvinyladenine

PVALB parvalbumin

PVARP postventricular atrial refractory period

PVB cis-platinum, vinblastine, bleomycin; paravertebral block; pigmented villonodular bundle; premature ventricular beat

PVC peripheral venous catheterization; permanent visual circuit; persistent vaginal cornification; polyvinyl chloride; postvoiding cystogram; predicted vital capacity; premature ventricular complex; premature ventricular contraction; primary visual cortex; pulmonary venous capillaries; pulmonary venous confluence; pulmonary venous congestion

PVCM paradoxical vocal cord motion

PV$_{CO_2}$ partial pressure of carbon dioxide in mixed venous blood

PVD patient very disturbed; peripheral vascular disease; portal vein dilation; posterior vitreous detachment; postural vertical dimension; premature ventricular depolarization; pulmonary valvular dysplasia; pulmonary vascular disease

PVDF polyvinylidene difluoride; polyvinyl diisopropyl fluoride

PVE partial volume effect; premature ventricular extrasystole; prosthetic valve endocarditis

PVE partial volume effect; perivenous encephalomyelitis; periventricular echogenicity; postvaccinial encephalopathy; premature ventricular event; premature ventricular extrasystole; prosthetic valve endocarditis

PV-ECF plasma volume/extracellular fluid [ratio]

PVEM postvaccinial encephalomyelitis

P-VEP pattern visual evoked potential

PVF peripheral visual field; portal venous flow; primary ventricular fibrillation

PVFS postviral fatigue syndrome

PVG periventricular gray matter; pulmonary valve gradient

PVH paraventricular hyperintensity; pulmonary venous hypertension

PVI patient video interview; peripheral vascular insufficiency; perivascular infiltration; positron volume imaging; protracted venous infusion

PVK penicillin V potassium

PVL perivalvular leakage; periventricular leukomalacia; permanent vision loss

PVM parallel virtual machine; pneumonia virus of mice; proteins, vitamins, and minerals

PVMed preventive medicine

PVMR PRODIGY Virtual Medical Record

PVN paraventricular nucleus; predictive value negative

PVNPS post-Viet Nam psychiatric syndrome

PVNS pigmented villonodular synovitis

PVNZ parapoxvirus of red deer in New Zealand

PVO pulmonary venous obstruction

PV$_{O_2}$ partial oxygen pressure in mixed venous blood

PVOD pulmonary vascular obstructive disease; pulmonary veno-occlusive disease

PVP penicillin V potassium; peripheral vein plasma; peripheral venous pressure; polyvinylpyrrolidone; portal venous phase; portal venous pressure; predictive value of positive results; pulmonary vein potential; pulmonary venous pressure

PVP-I polyvinylpyrrolidone-iodine

PVR peripheral vascular resistance; perspective volume rendering; poliovirus receptor; postvoiding residual; pulmonary valve replacement or repair; pulmonary vascular resistance; pulse volume recording

pVR perspective volume rendering [imaging]

PVRI pulmonary vascular resistance index

PVS percussion, vibration, suction; percutaneous vascular surgery; peritoneovenous shunt; persistent vegetative state; persistent viral syndrome; Plummer-Vinson syndrome; poliovirus susceptibility; polyvinyl sponge; premature ventricular systole; programmed ventricular stimulation; pulmonary valvular stenosis

PV$_s$ pulmonary venous systolic

PVST prevertebral soft tissue

PVU Pueblo Viejo virus

PVT paroxysmal ventricular tachycardia; periventricular thalamic [nucleus]; portal vein thrombosis; pressure, volume, and temperature; private patient; psychomotor vigilance task

PVW posterior vaginal wall

PVX potato virus X

PVY potato virus Y

pvz pulverization
PW peristaltic wave; plantar wart; posterior wall [of the heart]; pressure wave; psychological warfare; pulmonary wedge [pressure]; pulsed wave; pulse width
Pw progesterone withdrawal; pulse wave [echocardiography]; whole-cell pertussis [vaccine]
pW picowatt
PWA person with AIDS; pulse wave analysis
PWB partial weight bearing
PWBC peripheral white blood cell
PWBRT prophylactic whole brain radiation therapy
PWBT partial weight-bearing therapy
PWC peak work capacity; physical work capacity
PWCA pure white cell aplasia
PWCR Prader-Willi chromosome region
PWCT perfusion-weighted computed tomography
PWD posterior wall in diastole; printed wiring board
pwd powder
PWDS postweaning diarrhea syndrome
PWDU pulse wave Doppler ultrasound
PWE posterior wall excursion
PWI posterior wall infarct
PWLV posterior wall of left ventricle
PWM pokeweed mitogen; pulse with modulation
pw-MW pre-whitening [of data] multiple window
PWP patient word processing; pulmonary wedge pressure
PWS port wine stain; physician's workstation; Prader-Willi syndrome
PWS/AS Prader-Willi/Angelman syndromes
PWT physician waiting time; posterior wall thickness; pseudo-Winger transform
pwt pennyweight
PWTT pulse wave transit time
PWV pulse wave velocity

PX pancreatectomized; peroxidase; physical examination
Px past history; peroxidase; physical examination; pneumothorax; prognosis
px pancreas, pancreatic
PXA pleomorphic xanthoastrocytoma
PXE pseudoxanthoma elasticum
PXM projection x-ray microscopy; pseudoexfoliation material
PXMP peroxysomal membrane protein
PXS pseudoexfoliation syndrome
PXT piroxantrone
P_{xy} propagation delay
Py phosphopyridoxal; polyoma [virus]; pyridine; pyridoxal
py pack-years [cigarettes]
PYA psychoanalysis
PyC pyogenic culture
PYCR pyrroline-5-carboxylate reductase
PYE peptone yeast extract
PYG peptone-yeast extract-glucose [broth]
PYGM peptone-yeast-glucose-maltose [broth]
PYLL potential years of life lost
PYM psychosomatic
PyNPase pyridine nucleoside phosphorylase
PYP pyrophosphate
Pyr pyridine; pyruvate
PyrP pyridoxal phosphate
PyV *Polyomavirus*, polyomavirus
PZ pancreozymin; phthalazinone; pregnancy zone; proliferative zone; protamine zinc
Pz 4-phenylazobenzylcarbonyl; parietal midline electrode placement in electroencephalography
pz pièze
PZA pyrazinamide
PZ-CCK pabcreozymin-cholecystokinin
PZE piezoelectric
PZI protamine zinc insulin
PZP pregnancy zone protein
PZQ praziquantel
PZT lead zirconate titanate

Q

Q coulomb [electric quantity]; electric charge; flow; 1,4-glucan branching enzyme; glutamine; heat; qualitative; quality; quantity; quart; quartile; Queensland [fever]; query [fever]; question; quinacrine; quinidine; quinone; quotient; radiant energy; reactive power; reaction energy; temperature coefficient; see QRS [wave]

Q$_{10}$ temperature coefficient

Q̇ cardiac output

q electric charge; long arm of chromosome; probability of failure in single trial [statistics]; quart; quintal

QA quality assessment; quality assurance; questions and answers

QAAA quantitative amino acid analysis

QAC quaternary ammonium compound; quinacrine

QACC quality assurance coordination committee

QAF quality adjustment factor

QAHCS Quality of Australian Health Care Study

QA&I quality assessment and improvement

QALD quality-adjusted life days

QALE quality-adjusted life expectancy

QALPACS quality patient care scale

QALY quality-adjusted life year

QAM quality assurance monitoring

QAP quality assurance program or professional; quinine, atabrine, and pamaquine

QA/QC quality assurance and quality control

QAR quantitative autoradiography

QARANC Queen Alexandra's Royal Army Nursing Corps

QARNNS Queen Alexandra's Royal Naval Nursing Service

QAS quality assurance standard

QAUR quality assurance and utilization review

QB whole blood

Q$_B$ total body clearance

Q$_b$ blood flow

QBC query by case

QBIC query by image content

QBV whole blood volume

QC quality characteristics; quality control; quantum computing; quinine colchicine

Qc pulmonary capillary blood flow

QCA quantitative coronary arteriography or angiography

QCID qualitative contingent influence diagram [model]

QCIM Quarterly Cumulative Index Medicus

QCM quartz crystal microbalance

Q$_{co_2}$ carbon dioxide evolution by a tissue

QCP quality care program

QCS Quebec Cardiovascular Study; Quick Confusion Scale

QCT quantitative computed tomography

QD Qi deficiency; quantum dot

Q$_d$ probability of detection

QDE quantum detection efficiency

QDH/SS [protective] quick doff hood/second skin

QDPR quinoid dihydropteridine reductase

QE quantum efficiency

QEA quantitative culture of endotracheal aspirates

QED quantum electrodynamics

QEE quadriceps extension exercise

QEEG, qEEG quantitative electroencephalography

QEF quail embryo fibroblasts

QENF quantifying examination of neurologic function

QEONS Queen Elizabeth's Overseas Nursery Service

QEW quick early warning

QF quality factor; query fever; quick freeze; relative biologic effectiveness

QFCM quantitative fluorescence cytometry

QFD quality function deployment

QFES Quality Feedback Expert System

Q fever query fever

QFFV Queensland fruit fly virus

QFT QuantiFERON tuberculosis test

QGS quantitative gated SPECT [single photon emission computed tomography]

QHDS Queen's Honorary Dental Surgeon

QHFT Quinapril Heart Failure Trial

QHNS Queen's Honorary Nursing Sister

QHP Queen's Honorary Physician

QHS quantitative hepatobiliary scintigraphy; Queen's Honorary Surgeon

QI quality improvement; quality indicator; Quetelet Index

QIDN Queen's Institute of District Nursing

QIN quality improvement network

QIO quality improvement organization

QIP quality improvement project

QISMC Quality Improvement System for Managed Care

QJ quadriceps jerk

QL quality of life

QLE quasi-likelihood estimation

Q-LES-Q Quality of Life Enjoyment and Satisfaction Questionnaire

QLP quality laboratory process

QLQ quality of life questionnaire

QLQ-C quality of life questionnaire-cancer

QLS Quality of Life Scale; quasielastic light-scattering spectroscopy

QLV quasi-linear viscoelastic [model]

QM quality management; quantization matrix; quinacrine mustard

qm every morning [Lat. *quaque mane*]

QMAN query manager

QMB qualified Medicare beneficiary

QMC quantum Monte Carlo

QMF quadrature mirror filter

QMI Q-wave myocardial infarction

QMP Quality Management Program

QMR Quick Medical Reference

QMR-DT Quick Medical Reference-Decision Theoretic

QMR-KAT Quick Medical Reference-Knowledge Acquisition Tool

QMRP qualified mental retardation professional

QMT quantitative muscle test

QMWS quasi-morphine withdrawal syndrome

QN, qn quantitative

qn every night [Lat. *quaque nocte*]

QNB quinuclidinyl benzilate

QNS Queen's Nursing Sister

qns quantity not sufficient

QO$_2$ flow of oxygen

Qo oxygen consumption

Q$_{O_2}$ oxygen quotient; oxygen utilization

Q$_o$ flow at origin

qod every other day [Lat. *quaque altera die*; JCAHO unapproved abbreviation]

qoh every other hour [Lat. *quaque altera hora*]

QOLHS Quality of Life Hypertension Study

qon every other night [Lat. *quaque altera nocte*]

QOL quality of life

QOLI quality of life index

QOLI-P quality of life index-Padilla

QLOQ quality of life questionnaire

QoS quality of service

QP quadrigeminal plate; quality planning; quanti-Pirquet [reaction]

Qp pulmonary blood flow

QPC quadratic phase coupling; quadrigeminal plate cistern; quality of patient care

Qpc pulmonary capillary blood flow

QPCR quantitative polymerase chain reaction

QPD quadrature phase detector

QPEEG quantitative pharmaco-electro-encephalography

QPMV Quail pea mosaic virus

QPV Quokka poxvirus

Qp:Qs pulmonary-to-systemic flow ratio; pulmonic-to-systemic flow ratio

QR quality review; quieting response; quinaldine red; quinone reductase

qr quadriradial; quarter

QRA quantitative risk assessment

QRB Quality Review Bulletin

Q$_{rbc}$ flow of red blood cells

QRFV Quaranfil virus

QRM quality and resource management

QRNG quinoline-resistant *Neisseria gonorrhoeae*

QRP quick response program

QRS in electrocardiography, the complex consisting of Q, R, and S waves, corresponding to depolarization of ventricles [complex]; in electrocardiography, the loop traced by QRS vectors, representing ventricular depolarization [interval]

QRS-ST the junction between the QRS complex and the ST segment in the electrocardiogram [junction]

QRS-T the angle between the QRS and T vectors in vectorcardiography [angle]

qRT-PCR quantitative reverse transcriptase [RT] polymerase chain reaction [PCR]

QRZ wheal reaction time [Ger. *Qaddel Reaktion Zeit*]

QS question screening; quiet sleep

Qs, Q$_s$ systemic blood flow

QSAR quantitative structure-activity relationship

QSART quantitative sudomotor axon reflex testing

QSFR quantitative structure-function relationship

QSM quality assurance and safety of medicine

QSPR quantitative structure-property relationship

QSPV quasistatic pressure volume

Q$_s$Q$_T$ shunted blood to total blood flow [ratio]

QSR quality system regulation

QSS quantitative sacroiliac scintigraphy

QSSR quantitative structure-stability relationship

QST quantitative sensory test

QT cardiac output; Quick test

Q-T in electrocardiography, the time from the beginning of the QRS complex to the end of the T wave [interval]

qt quantity; quart; quiet

QTc, Q-Tc Q-T interval corrected for heart rate

qter end of long arm of chromosome

QTL quantitative trait locus

Q-TWIST quality-adjusted time without symptoms of disease and subjective toxic effects of treatment

Quad quadratic [potential]

quad quadrant; quadriceps; quadriplegic

QUADS Quinapril Australian Dosing Study

QUAL qualitative attribute [UMLS]

qual quality, qualitative

QUAL-PACS quality of patient care system

QUALYs quality-adjusted life years

QUAN quantitative attribute [UMLS]

quant quantity, quantitative

quar quarantine

QUART quadrantectomy, axillary dissection, radiotherapy

QUASAR Quinapril Anti-Ischemia and Symptoms of Angina Reduction [trial]

QUEST Quality, Utilization, Effectiveness, Statistically Tabulated

QUESTAR query estimation and refinement

QUESTT Question the child, Use pain rating scale, Evaluate behavior and physiologic changes, Secure parents' involvement, Take cause of pain into account, Take action and evaluate results [pain assessment in children]

QUEXTA Quantitative Exercise Testing and Angiography [study]

QUICHA quantitative inhalation challenge apparatus

QUIET Quinapril Ischemic Event Trial

QuIC Quality Interagency Coordinating Task Force

QUIN quinolinic acid

quint fifth

QUIS Questionnaire on User Interface Satisfaction

quot quotient

quotid daily, quotidian [Lat. *quotidie*]

QUPV Quailpox virus

QUS quantitative ultrasound

qv which see [Lat. *quod vide*]

QWB quality of well-being [questionnaire, scale, or index]

QYBV Qalyub virus

QYD Qi and Yin deficiency

R

R Behnken unit; Broadbent registration point; any chemical group [particularly an alfyl group]; a conjugative plasmid responsible for resistance to various elements; electrical resistance; in electrocardiography, the first positive deflection during the QRS complex [wave]; far point [Lat. *remotum*]; gas constant; organic radical; race; racemic; radioactive; radiology; radius; ramus; Rankine [scale]; rapid accelerator; rate; rate modulation [pacemaker]; ratio; reaction; Réaumur [scale]; receptor; rectal; rectified; red; registered trademark; regression coefficient; regular; regular insulin; regulator [gene]; rejection factor; relapse; relaxation; release [factor]; remission; remote; reperfusion; repressor; residual tumor [TNM (tumor-node-metastasis) classification]; residue; resistance; respiration; respiratory exchange ratio; respiratory quotient; response; responder; rest; restricted; reverse [banding]; rhythm; ribose; *Rickettsia*; right; Rinne [test]; roentgen; rough [colony]; rub

R′ in electrocardiography, the second positive deflection during the QRS complex

R+ Rinne test positive

R1 first repeat

R2 second repeat

+R Rinne test positive

−R Rinne test negative

°R degree on the Rankine scale; degree on the Réaumur scale

R1, R2, R3, etc. years of resident study

r correlation coefficient; density; radius; ratio; recombinant; regional; ribose; ribosomal; ring chromosome; roentgen; sample correlation coefficient

r² coefficient of determination

ρ see *rho*

R0 residual tumor not assessed [TNM (tumor-node-metastasis) classification]

R1 longitudinal relativity; small residual tumor [TNM (tumor-node-metastasis) classification]

R2 large residual tumor [TNM (tumor-node-metastasis) classification]; transverse relativity

RA radial artery; radioactive; radiographic abstraction; radiographic absorptiometry; ragocyte; ragweed antigen; rapidly adapting [receptors]; reactive arthritis; reciprocal asymmetrical; refractory anemia; refractory ascites; regression analysis; renal artery; renin-angiotensin; repeat action; residual air; retinoic acid; rheumatoid arthritis; right angle; right arm; right atrium; right auricle; risk adjustment; risk assessment; rotation angiography; Roy adaptation [model]

R$_A$ airway resistance

Ra access resistance; radial; radium; radius

rA riboadenylate

ra receptor antagonist

RAA renin-angiotensin-aldosterone [system]; right aortic arch; right atrial appendage

RAAMC Royal Australian Army Medical Corps

RAAMI Randomized Angiographic Trial of Alteplase in Myocardial Infarction; Rapid Administration of Alteplase in Myocardial Infarction [trial]

RAAPI resting ankle-arm pressure index

RAAS Randomized Angiotensin II Receptor Antagonist, Angiotensin-Converting Enzyme Inhibitor Study; renin-angiotensin-aldosterone system

rAAV recombinant adeno-associated virus

RAB remote afterloading brachytherapy

Rab rabbit

RABA rabbit antibladder antibody

RAC rabeprazole, amoxicillin, clarithromycin; Recombinant Deoxyribonucleic Acid [DNA] Advisory Committee; research appraisal checklist

rac racemate, racemic

RACAT rapid acquisition computed axial tomography

RACC receptor-activated calcium channel

RACE ramipril angiotensin-converting enzyme [ACE]; Ramipril Cardioprotective Evaluation [trial]; rapid amplification of complementary deoxyribonucleic acid [cDNA] ends; Rapid Assessment of Cardiac Enzymes

RACGP Royal Australian College of General Practitioners

RACT reasonably available control technology; research activity [UMLS]

RACV relative autonomic conduction velocity

RAD radial artery catheter; radiation absorbed dose; radical; radiography or radiographic; reactive airways disease; receptor affinity distribution; right atrium diameter; right axis deviation; roentgen administered dose

Rad radiology; radiotherapy; radium

rad radiation absorbed dose; radial; radian; radical; radius; root [Lat. *radix*]

RADA rosin amine-D-acetate

RADAI rheumatoid arthritis disease activity index

RADAR rapid assessment of disease activity in rheumatology

RADC Royal Army Dental Corps

RADES randomly amplified differentially expressed sequence

RADES-PCR randomly amplified differentially expressed sequence polymerase chain reaction [PCR]

RADIANCE Randomized Assessment of Digoxin on Inhibitors of Angiotensin-Converting Enzyme [ACE, study]

RADIO radiotherapy

radiol radiology

RADIUS Routine Antenatal Diagnostic Imaging with Ultrasound [trial]

RadLV radiation leukemia virus

RADMOS radiotherapy data management and organization system

RADP right acromiodorsoposterior

RADS reactive airways dysfunction syndrome; retrospective assessment of drug safety

rad/s rad per second; radian per second

rad/s² rad per second squared

rad ther radiation therapy

RADTS rabbit antidog thymus serum

RADTT radiation therapy technologist

RADVIS radiological visualization

RAE right atrial enlargement

RAEB refractory anemia with excess blasts

RAEBiT, RAEB-T refractory anemia with excess blasts in transformation

RAEC rat aortic endothelial cell; rate control vs electrical cardioversion

RAEM refractory anemia with excess myeloblasts

RAF repetitive atrial firing; rheumatoid arthritis factor

RAFMS Royal Air Force Medical Services

RAFT Recurrent Atrial Fibrillation Trial; Rythmol-SR Atrial Fibrillation Trial

RAFW right atrial free wall

RAG radioautography; ragweed; recombinase activating gene; recombination activating gene; [computer-assisted] risk assessment in genetics

RAGE rapid gradient echo; receptor for advanced glycosylation end-products

Ragg rheumatoid agglutinin

RAH regressing atypical histiocytosis; right atrial hypertrophy

RAHM randomly amplified hybridization microsatellite

RAHO rabbit antibody to human ovary

RAHTG rabbit antihuman thymocyte globulin

RaHV ranid herpesvirus

RAI radioactive iodine; radioactive isotope; resident assessment instrument; resting ankle index; right atrial inversion; right atrial involvement

RAID radioimmunodetection; radiolabeled antibody imaging; redundant array of independent disks; redundant array of inexpensive disks

RAIS reflection-absorption infrared spectroscopy

RAITI right atrial inversion time index

RAIU radioactive iodine uptake

RALES Randomized Aldactone Evaluation Study

RALPH renal-anal-lung-polydactyly-hamartoblastoma [syndrome]

RALT routine admission laboratory tests

RAM random-access memory; rapid alternating movements; rectus abdominis muscle; rectus abdominis myocutaneous [flap]; reduced acquisition matrix; research aviation medicine; resistance-associated mutation; resource allocation methodology; right anterior measurement

RAMEDIS Rare Metabolic Diseases

RAMC Royal Army Medical Corps

RAM-FAST reduced acquisition matrix-Fourier acquired steady state

RaMI Ravenna Myocardial Infarction [trial]

RAMIT Ravenna Myocardial Infarction Trial

RAMM remote-access multidimensional microscopy

RAMP radioactive antigen microprecipitin; rate modulated pacing; right atrial mean pressure

RAMPO randomly amplified microsatellite polymorphism

RAMR risk-adjusted mortality rate

RAMT rabbit antimouse thymocyte; right atrial mobile thrombi

RAN random number; remote area nurse [Australia]; resident's admission notes

RANA rheumatoid arthritis nuclear antigen

rANP rat atrial natriuretic peptide

RANTES regulated on activation, T-cell expressed and secreted

RANTTAS Randomized Trial of Tirilazad in Acute Stroke

RAO right anterior oblique; right anterior occipital; rotational acetabular osteotomy

RaONC radiation oncology

RAP rapid atrial pacing; recurrent abdominal pain; regression-associated protein; renal artery pressure; resident assessment protocol; rheumatoid arthritis precipitin; ribonucleic acid [RNA] arbitrarily primed; right atrial pressure

RAPD randomly amplified polymorphic deoxyribonucleic acid [DNA]; relative afferent pupillary defect

RAPDDIP randomly amplified polymorphic deoxyribonucleic acid [DNA] for the diploid cases

RAPDHAP randomly amplified polymorphic deoxyribonucleic acid [DNA] for the haploid cases

RAPID Recombinant Plasminogen Activator Angiographic Phase II International Dose Finding Study; Regional Arizona Prehospital Infarction Diagnosis [study]; Reteplase Angiographic Patency International Dose-Ranging Study

RAPK reticulate acropigmentation of Kitamura

RAPM refractory anemia with partial myeloblastosis

RAPO rabbit antibody to pig ovary

RAP-PCR ribonucleic acid [RNA] arbitrarily primed polymerase chain reaction [PCR]

RAPPORT ReoPro in Acute Myocardial Infarction and Primary Percutaneous Transluminal Coronary Angioplasty Organization and Randomized Trial

RAPS Renfrew and Paisley Study; resident assessment protocols

RAPs radiologists, anesthesiologists, and pathologists

RAPT Ridogrel vs Aspirin Potency Trial

RAR rapidly adapting receptor; rat insulin receptor; retinoic acid receptor; right arm reclining; right arm recumbent

RARA retinoic acid receptor alpha

RARB retinoic acid receptor beta

RARE rapid acquisition with relaxation enhancement; retinoic acid response element

RARG retinoic acid receptor gamma

RARLS rabbit anti-rat lymphocyte serum

RARS refractory anemia with ring sideroblasts

RARTS rabbit anti-rat thymocyte serum

RAS radiologist aid system [digital mammography algorithm]; rapid atrial stimulation; recurrent aphthous stomatitis; reflex activating stimulus; reliability, availability, serviceability; remote access service; renal artery stenosis; renal artery stent; renin-angiotensin system; residency application service; reticular activating system; rheumatoid arthritis serum; rotational atherectomy system; Rokitansky-Aschoff sinus; routine analysis station

RA-S refractory anemia with ringed sideroblasts

ras retrovirus-associated DNA sequence

RASE rapid acquisition spin echo

RASMC rat aortic smooth muscle cell

RASS rheumatoid arthritis and Sjögren syndrome

RAST radioallergosorbent test

RAT repeat action tablet; rheumatoid arthritis test; right anterior trigone

RATG rabbit antithymocyte globulin

RATHAS rat thymus antiserum

RATMAP Rat Genome Database

rAT-P recombinant antitrypsin Pittsburgh

RATx radiation therapy

RAU radioactive uptake; remote access unit [telemedicine]

RAV rheumatoid arthritis virus; Rous-associated virus

RAVC retrograde atrioventricular conduction; Royal Army Veterinary Corps

RAVES Reduced Anticoagulation in Saphenous Vein Graft Stent [trial]; Reduced Anticoagulation Vein Graft Study

RAVLT Rey Auditory Verbal Learning Test

RAW right atrial wall

Raw airway resistance

R$_{Aw}$ airway resistance

RAWP Resource Allocation Working Party

RAWTS ribonucleic acid amplification with transcript sequencing

RAZ razoxane

RB broader semantic relationship [UMLS]; radial basis [imaging]; radiation burn; rating board; rebreathing; reticulate body; retinoblastoma; retrobulbar; right breast; right bronchus; right bundle; rigid bronchoscopy

RB1 The RB1 Gene Mutation Database

Rb retinoblastoma

RBA relative binding affinity; rescue breathing apparatus; right basilar artery; right brachial artery; rose bengal antigen

RBAC role-based access control

RBAP repetitive bursts of action potential

RbAP retinoblastoma-associated protein

RBAS rostral basilar artery syndrome

rBAT related to b$^{0,+}$ amino acid transporter

RBB right bundle branch

RBBB right bundle-branch block

RBBP retinoblastoma binding protein

RBBsB right bundle-branch system block

RBBx right breast biopsy

RBC ranitidine bismuth citrate; red blood cell; red blood count

rbc red blood cell

RBCA risk-based corrective action

RBC-ChE red blood cell cholinesterase

RBCD right border cardiac dullness

rBCG recombinant bacille Calmette-Guérin [vaccine]

RBCM red blood cell mass

RbCoV rabbit coronavirus

RBCV red blood cell volume

RBD recurrent brief depression; relative biological dose; RNA binding domain; right border of dullness

RBE relative biologic effectiveness

RBF radial basis function; regional blood flow; regional bone mass; renal blood flow

RBFN radial basis function network

RBG red blue green [Doppler]

RBI radiographic baseline

RBI-EM rescaled block-iterative expectation maximization [algorithm]

Rb Imp rubber base impression

RBL rat basophilic leukemia; Reid baseline; retinoblastoma-like

RBL-ILD respiratory bronchiolitis with associated interstitial lung disease

RBM ribonucleic acid [RNA] binding motif

rBM reconstituted basement membrane

RBN retrobulbar neuritis

RBNA Royal British Nurses Association

RBNN recurrent backpropagation neural network

RBOW rupture of the bag of waters

RBP retinol-binding protein; riboflavin-binding protein

RBPC cellular retinol-binding protein

RBPI intestinal retinol-binding protein

rBPI recombinant bactericidal/permeability increasing [protein]

RBR risk-based response; rule-based reasoning

RB-RB right bundle to right bundle [depolarization]

RBRVS resource-based relative value scale

RBS random blood sugar; receptor binding site; remote [computer] backup service; Roberts syndrome; Rutherford backscattering

RbSA rabbit serum albumin

RBSL risk-based screening level

RBST rubber-band straightening transform

rBST recombinant bovine somatotropin

RBT resistive breathing training

RBTN rhombotin

RBTNL rhombotin-like

RBUV Rochambeau virus

RBV ribavirin; Rio Bravo virus; right brachial vein

RBW relative body weight

RBZ rubidazone

RC an electronic circuit containing a resistor and capacitor in series; radiocarpal; reaction center; recrystallization; red cell; red cell casts; red corpuscle; Red Cross; referred care; regenerated cellulose; rehabilitation counseling; Renshaw cell; residential care; resistance and compliance; resistive capacity; respiration ceases;

respiratory care; respiratory center; respiratory compensation; rest cure; retention catheter; retrograde cystogram; rib cage; root canal; routine cholecystography

R&C resistance and capacitance

Rc conditioned response; receptor

RCA red cell agglutination; regulator of complement activity; relative chemotactic activity; renal cell carcinoma; replication-competent adenovirus; replication-competent alphavirus; retained cortical activity; right coronary angiography; right coronary artery; rotational coronary atherectomy

RCAMC Royal Canadian Army Medical Corps

rCBF regional cerebral blood flow

rCBV regional cerebral blood volume

RCC radiological control center; rape crisis center; ratio of cost to charges; receptor-chemoeffector complex; red cell cast; red cell concentrate; red cell count; regulator of chromosome condensation; renal cell carcinoma; reverse cumulative curve; right common carotid [artery]; right coronary cusp

RCCM Regional Committee for Community Medicine

RCCP renal cell carcinoma, papillary

RCCS remote clinical communications system

RCCT randomized controlled clinical trial

RCD relative cardiac dullness; robust change detection [algorithm in insulin therapy]

RCDA recurrent chronic dissecting aneurysm

RCDP rhizomelic chondrodysplasia punctata

RCDR relative corrected death rate

RCE reasonable compensation equivalent; Red Coding Engine [software]

RCF red cell ferritin; red cell folate; refractory ceramic fiber; relative centrifugal field/force; ristocetin cofactor

RCG radioelectrocardiography

RCGP Royal College of General Practitioners

RCH rectocolic hemorrhage

RCHF right congestive heart failure

RCHMS Regional Committee for Hospital Medical Services

RCI radiation conformity index; respiratory control index; retrospective cohort incidence

RCIA red cell immune adherence

RCIRF radiologic contrast-induced renal failure

RCIT red cell iron turnover

RCITR red cell iron turnover rate

RCL renal clearance; right coronary leaflet

RCM radial contour model; radiographic contrast medium; red cell mass; reinforced clostridial medium; remacemide; remote center of motion; replacement culture medium; retrospective cohort mortality; right costal margin; Royal College of Midwives

rCMR regional cerebral metabolism rate

rCMRGlc, rCMRglc regional cerebral metabolic rate for glucose

rCMRO$_2$ regional cerebral metabolic rate for oxygen

RCN right caudate nucleus; Royal College of Nursing

RCO right coronary ostium

RCoF ristocetin cofactor

RCOG Royal College of Obstetricians and Gynaecologists

RCoV respiratory coronavirus

RCP radiochemical purity; red cell protoporphyrin; retrocorneal pigmentation; riboflavin carrier protein; Royal College of Physicians

rCP regional cerebral perfusion

rcp reciprocal translocation

RCPath Royal College of Pathologists

RCPG respiratory center pattern generator

RCPH red cell peroxide hemolysis

RCPP recurrent coronary prevention program

rCPP regional cerebral perfusion pressure

RCPSC Royal College of Physicians and Surgeons of Canada

RCPSGlas Royal College of Physicians and Surgeons, Glasgow

RCR relative consumption rate; replication-competent recombinant; replication-competent retrovirus; respiratory control ratio

RCRA Resource Conservation and Recovery Act

rCRF recombinant corticotropin-releasing factor

RCS rabbit aorta-contracting substance; real-time control system; red cell suspension; reference coordinate system; renal collector system; reticulum cell sarcoma; revision control system; right coronary sinus; Royal College of Science; Royal College of Surgeons

RCSE Royal College of Surgeons, Edinburgh

RCSSS resource coordination system for surgical service

RCT radiotherapy and chemotherapy; randomized clinical trial; randomized controlled trial; registered care technologist; retrograde conduction time; root canal therapy; Rorschach content test; rotator cuff tear

rct a marker showing the ability of virulent strains to replicate at 40°C, while vaccine strain shows no replication

rCTB recombinant cholera toxin B

RCTE randomized clinical trial evaluator

RCU respiratory care unit

RCV rabbit calicivirus; recoverin; red cell volume

RCVS Royal College of Veterinary Surgeons

RCWI right cardiac work index

RD radial deviation; radiology department; rate difference; Raynaud disease; reaction of degeneration; registered dietitian; Reiter disease; related donor; relative dose; renal disease; resistance determinant; resistant disease; respiratory disease; resuscitation device; retinal degeneration; retinal detachment; Reye disease; rheumatoid disease; right deltoid; Riley-Day [syndrome]; Rolland-Desbuquois [syndrome]; rubber dam; ruminal drinking; ruptured disk

Rd rate of disappearance

rd rutherford

R&D research and development

RDA rapid epidemiological assessment; recommended daily allowance; recommended dietary allowance; Registered Dental Assistant; representation difference analysis; right dorsoanterior [fetal position]; right ductus arteriosus

RDB random double-blind [trial]; relational database

RDBMS regional database management system; relational database management system

RDBP RD [gene] binding protein

RDBS relational database server

RDB-X random double-blind crossover

RDC research data center; research diagnostic criteria

RDCRD Rare Disease Clinical Research Database

RDD relative depth dose [radiation]

RDDA recommended daily dietary allowance

RDDB Rare Disease Database

RDDP ribonucleic acid-dependent deoxynucleic acid polymerase

RDE receptor-destroying enzyme; remote data entry

RDEB recessively inherited dystrophic epidermolysis bullosa

RDE$_D$ radiation dose required

RDES remote data entry system

RDF rapid dissolution formula

RDFC recurring digital fibroma of childhood

RDG retrograde duodenogastroscopy

RDH Registered Dental Hygienist

RDHBF regional distribution of hepatic blood flow

RDHI research and development health informatics

RDI recommended daily intake; respiratory disturbance index; rupture-delivery interval

RDIC resuscitation device, individual chemical

RDLBBB rate-dependent left bundle-branch block

RDM readmission

RDMS registered diagnostic medical sonographer

rDNA recombinant deoxyribonucleic acid [DNA]

RDOG radiology diagnostic oncology group

RDP right dorsoposterior [fetal position]

RDPA right descending pulmonary artery

RDQ respiratory disease questionnaire

RDR research data repository

RDRP, RdRp ribonucleic acid [RNA]-dependent ribonucleic acid polymerase

RDRS Rapid Disability Rating Scale

RDS Raskin Depression Scale; respiratory distress syndrome; reticuloendothelial depressing substance; rhodanese; slow retinal degeneration

RDT randomized discontinuation trial; retinal damage threshold; routine dialysis therapy

RDW red blood cell distribution width index

RDX radixin

RE radium emanation; random error; reading epilepsy; readmission; rectal examination; reference emitter; reflux esophagitis; regional enteritis; relative effectiveness; renal and electrolyte; resistive exercise; resting energy; restriction endonuclease; reticuloendothelial; retinol equivalent; right ear; right eye

R_E respiratory exchange ratio

R&E research and education

Re rhenium

R_e Reynold number

REA radiation emergency area; radioenzymatic assay; regulatory effectiveness analysis; renal anastomosis; restriction endonuclease analysis; right ear advantage

rea rearrangement

REAB refractory anemia with excess of blasts

REACH research on endothelin antagonism in chronic heart failure; resource utilization in congestive heart failure [studies]

REACT rapid early action in coronary treatment

REAC/TS Radiation Emergency Assistance Center/Training Site

readm readmission

READS restriction enzyme analysis of differentially expressed sequences

REAL Revised European-American Lymphoma [classification]

REALM rapid estimate of adult literacy in medicine

REAP restriction endonuclease analysis of plasmid

REAR renal, ear, anal, and radial [malformation syndrome]

REAS reasonably expected as safe; retained, excluded antrum syndrome

REAT radiological emergency assistance team

REB roentgen-equivalent biological

REC receptor; recombination, recombinant chromosome

rec fresh [Lat. *recens*]; recessive; recombinant chromosome; record; recovery; recurrence, recurrent

RECA recombination protein A

RECAP retrosynthetic combinatorial analysis procedure

recCHO recombinant Chinese hamster ovary

R_{ECF} extracellular fluid resistance

RECG radioelectrocardiography

recip recipient; reciprocal

RECIT Représentation du Contenu Informationel de Testes Médicaux

recon the smallest unit of DNA capable of recombination

recond reconditioned, reconditioning

RECPAM recursive partition and amalgamation

recumb recumbent

RECREATE Rescue of Closed Arteries Treated by Stent for Threatened or Abrupt Closure [study]

recryst recrystallization

rect rectal; rectification, rectified; rectum; rectus [muscle]

Rec Ther recreational therapy

recur recurrence, recurrent

RED radiation experience data; rapid erythrocyte degeneration; repeat expansion detection

red reduction

REDAP rural emergency department approved for pediatrics

RED-LIP Reduction of Lipid Metabolism [study]

redox oxidation-reduction

REDP reduced energy diet program

REDS Retrovirus Epidemiology Donor Study

REDUCE Randomized Double-Blind Unfractionated Heparin and Placebo-Controlled Multicenter Trial; Restenosis Reduction by Cutting Balloon Evaluation [study]

REE rapid extinction effect; rare earth element; resting energy expenditure

REEDS retention of tears, ectrodactyly, ectodermal dysplasia, and strange hair, skin and teeth [syndrome]

REEG radioelectroencephalography

R-EEG resting electroencephalography

ReEND reproductive endocrinology
REEP right end-expiratory pressure
reev re-evaluate
reex re-examine
REF ejection fraction at rest; rat embryo fibroblast; referred; refused; renal erythropoietic factor; restriction endonuclease fingerprinting; right ventricular ejection fraction
ref reference; reflex
Ref-1 redox factor 1
Ref Doc referring doctor
REFI regional ejection fraction image
ref ind refractive index
refl reflex
REFLECT-1 Randomized Evaluation of Flosequinan on Exercise Tolerance-Initial Efficacy Trial
REFLECT-2 Randomized Evaluation of Flosequinan on Exercise Tolerance-Dose Response Study
REFLEX Randomized Evaluation of Flosequinan on Exercise Tolerance [study]; Restenosis Rates with Flexible GFX Stents [study]
Ref Phys referring physician
REFRAD released from active duty
REFSA Randomized European Femoral Stent vs Angioplasty Trial
RefSeq Reference Sequence [NLM database]
REG radiation exposure guide; radioencephalogram, radioencephalography
Reg registered
reg region; regular
regen regenerated, regenerating, regeneration
ReGIS respiration-gated irradiation system
REGRESS Regression Growth Evaluation Statin Study
reg rhy regular rhythm
REGU regulation [UMLS]
regurg regurgitation
REH renin essential hypertension
rehab rehabilitation, rehabilitated
REIN Ramipril Effect in Nephropathy [study]
REL rate of energy loss; recommended exposure limit; resource location; resting expiratory level
rel relative

RELACS Reikjavik experimental light-activated cell sorter
RELANCA relation between antineutrophil cytoplasm autoantibody [ANCA] levels and relapses of ANCA-associated glomerulonephritis and vasculitis
RELAY relayed correlation spectroscopy
RELE resistive exercise of lower extremities
RelTox Relational Toxicology [Project]
REM rapid eye movement; recent-event memory; reticular erythematous mucinosis; return electrode monitor; roentgen-equivalent-man
Rem roentgen-equivalent-man
rem radiation equivalent in man; removal
REMA repetitive excess mixed anhydride
REMAB radiation-equivalent-manikin absorption
REMAIN remission-maintenance [therapy for systemic vasculitis]
REMATCH Randomized Evaluation of Mechanical Assistance in the Treatment of Congestive Heart Failure [study]
REMBRANDT Rather Exciting and Memorable Blind Randomized Assessment of a New Drug on Three Continents
REMCAL radiation-equivalent-manikin calibration
remit remittent
REMO regional emergency medical organization
REMP roentgen-equivalent-man period
REMPAN radiation emergency medical preparedness
REMS rapid eye movement sleep
REMT trigger signal rapid eye movements
REN renal; renin
REn, Ren replication enhancer
RENAAL Reduction of Endpoints in Non-insulin-dependent Diabetes Mellitus with Angiotensin II Antagonist Losartan [trial]
rENaC rat epithelial sodium channel
RENEWAL Randomized Trial of Endoluminal Reconstruction Using the NIR Stent or Wallstent in Angioplasty of Long Segment Disease
REO respiratory enteric orphan [virus]
REOP rural elderly outreach program
REP reepithelialization; repaglinide; replication protein; rest-exercise program; restriction endonuclease profile; retrograde pyelogram; Rochester Epidemiology Project; roentgen equivalent-physical

rep replication; roentgen equivalent-physical

REPA replication protein A

REPAIR Reperfusion in Acute Infarction, Rotterdam [study]

repol repolarization

REPR reproductive

REPS reactive extensor postural synergy

rept let it be repeated

req request, requested

RER renal excretion rate; replication error; respiratory exchange ratio; rough endoplasmic reticulum

RER$_+$ replication error positive

RERC Rehabilitation Engineering Research Center

RERF Radiation Effects Research Foundation

RES radionuclide esophageal scintigraphy; real environment sensing [system]; Reproducibility Echocardiography Study; Rotterdam Elderly Study; reticuloendothelial system

res research; resection; resident; residue; resistance

RESAC Real-Time Expert System for Advice and Control

RESCUE Randomized Evaluation of Salvage Angioplasty with Combined Utilization of Endpoints [trial]

Res Gen Research Genetics [database]

RESIST Restenosis after Intravascular Ultrasound-guided Stenting [study]

RESNA Rehabilitation Engineering Society of North America

RESOLVD, RESOLVED Randomized Evaluation of Strategies for Left Ventricular Dysfunction [study]

resp respiration, respiratory; response

Resp Ther respiratory therapy

REST Raynaud's phenomenon, esophageal motor dysfunction, sclerodactyly, and telangiectasia [syndrome]; regressive electroshock therapy; Restenosis Stent Trial

RESTORE Randomized Efficacy Study of Tirofiban for Outcomes and Restenosis [trial]

RESTT respiratory therapy technician

resusc resuscitation

RET reticular; reticulocyte; retina; retention; retained; right esotropia

ret rad equivalent therapeutic

RETA Registry for the Endovascular Treatment of Aneurysms

retard retardation, retarded

ret cath retention catheter

RETEST retention probability is initially estimated [genome computing]

retic reticulocyte

REU rectal endoscopic ultrasonography

reu radiation effect unit

REV rat encephalomyelitis virus; reticuloendotheliosis virus

ReV regulator of virion

rev reverse; review; revolution

re-x reexamination

Rex regulator x

R$_{ext}$ external resistance [respiration]

RF radial fiber; radiofrequency; rapid filling; readiness field; reading factor; receptive field; regurgitant fraction; Reitland-Franklin [unit]; relative flow; relative fluorescence; release factor; renal failure; replacement fluid; replication factor; replicative form; repopulation factor [radiotherapy]; resistance factor; resonant frequency; respiratory failure; respiratory frequency; reticular formation; retroperitoneal fibromatosis; rheumatic fever; rheumatoid factor; riboflavin; risk factor; root canal filling; rosette formation

R^F rate of flow

Rf [in chromatography] ratio of the distance traveled by solute to the distance traveled by spot of pigment; respiratory frequency; rutherfordium

R$_f$ in paper or thin-layer chromatography, the distance that a spot of a substance has moved from the point of application

rf radiofrequency; rapid filling

rFVIII recombinant factor VIII

RFA radiofrequency ablation; requirements for accreditation; resident functional atlas; right femoral artery; right frontoanterior [fetal position]; risk factor of atherosclerosis

RFB retained foreign body

RFC radiofrequency coil; replication factor C; request for comments; retrograde femoral catheter; rosette-forming cell

RFCA radiofrequency catheter ablation

RFD, RfD reference dose

RFDS Royal Flying Doctors Service [Australia]

RFE relative fluorescence efficiency

RFFIT rapid fluorescent focus inhibition test

rFGF1 recombinant fibroblast growth factor 1 [acidic]

rFGF2 recombinant fibroblast growth factor 2 [basic]

RFH right femoral hernia

RFI radiofrequency interference; recurrence-free interval; renal failure index; request for information

RFIED round femoral inferior epiphysis dysplasia

RFK Richardson-Flory-Kops [mask]

RFL right frontolateral [fetal position]

RFLA rheumatoid-factor-like activity

RFLP restriction fragment length polymorphism

RFLS rheumatoid-factor-like substance

RFLV restriction fragment length variant

Rfm rifampin

RFNA red fuming nitric acid

RFP rapid filling period; recurrent facial paralysis; request for proposal; right frontoposterior [fetal position]

RF-PMR radiofrequency-percutaneous myocardial revascularization [revascularization with radiofrequency energy generator]

RFPS (Glasgow) Royal Faculty of Physicians and Surgeons of Glasgow

RFR rapid fluid resuscitation; refraction

RFS relapse-free survival; renal function study; rotating frame spectroscopy

RFT respiratory function test; right frontotransverse [fetal position]; rod-and-frame test

RFU relative fluorescence unit

RFV right femoral vein; Royal Farm virus

RFW rapid filling wave

RG right gluteal

Rg Rodgers [antigen]

rG regular gene

RgasD relative gas density

RGB red-green-blue [imaging]

RGBMT renal glomerular basement membrane thickness

RGC radio-gas chromatography; remnant gastric cancer; retinal ganglion cell; right giant cell

RGD range-gated Doppler; refractional geometric distortions [imaging]

RGE relative gas expansion

RGEA right gastroepiploic artery

RGH rat growth hormone

RGHBV Ross' goose hepatitis B virus

RGI recovery from growth inhibition

RGL random glucose level

RGM right gluteus medius

rGM-CSF recombinant granulocyte-macrophage colony-stimulating factor

RGN refinement grouper number; Registered General Nurse

RGO reciprocating gait orthosis

RGP retrograde pyelography

RGR relative growth rate

RGS regulation of G_α signaling; Rieger syndrome

RGU regional glucose utilization

RGV Rio Grande virus

RH radiant heat; radiation hybrid; radiological health; reactive hyperemia; recurrent herpes; regulatory hormone; rehabilitation; relative humidity; releasing hormone; renal hemolysis; retinal hemorrhage; reverse hybridization; ribonuclease H; right hand; right-handed [person]; right heart; right hemisphere; right hyperphoria; room humidifier

Rh rhesus [factor]; rhinion; rhodamine; rhodium

Rh+ rhesus positive

Rh− rhesus negative

rh recombinant human; rheumatic

r/h roentgens per hour

RHA Regional Health Authority; relative highest avidity; right hepatic artery

RhA rheumatoid arthritis

RhAG Rh-associated glycoprotein

RHB regional hospital board [UK]; right heart bypass

RHBF reactive hyperemia blood flow

rh-BMP recombinant human bone morphogenetic protein

RHBs Regional Hospital Boards

RHC rad homolog in *Cerevisiae*; resin hemoperfusion column; respiration has ceased; right heart catheterization; right hypochondrium; rural health center

RHCSA Regional Hospitals Consultants' and Specialists' Association

RHD radiological health data; relative hepatic dullness; renal hypertensive disease; rheumatic heart disease

RhD Rhesus factor and D antigen

RHDV rabbit hemorrhagic disease virus

RHDV-AST89 rabbit hemorrhagic disease virus AST89

RHDV-BS89 rabbit hemorrhagic disease virus BS89

RHDV-FRG rabbit hemorrhagic disease virus FRG

RHDV-SD rabbit hemorrhagic disease virus SD

RHDV-V351 rabbit hemorrhagic disease virus V351

rhDNase recombinant human deoxyribonuclease [DNAse]

RHE retinohepatoendocrinologic [syndrome]

RHEED reflection high-energy electron diffraction

rheo rheology

rhEPO recombinant human erythropoietin

rheu, rheum rheumatic, rheumatoid

RHF restricted Hartree-Fock [level]; right heart failure

Rh F rheumatic fever

rhFVIII recombinant human factor 8

rhFSH recombinant human follicle stimulating hormone

RHG right hand grip

rhG-CSF recombinant human granulocyte colony-stimulating factor

rhGH recombinant human growth hormone

rhGM-CSF recombinant human granulocyte macrophage colony-stimulating factor

RHI Rural Health Initiative

RHIA registered health information administrator

RhIG Rh [rhesus] factor immune globulin

rhIGF recombinant human insulin-like growth factor [IGF]

rhIL recombinant human interleukin

RHIN regional health information network

Rhin rhinology

rhino rhinoplasty

RHIT registered health information technician

RHJSC Regional Hospital Junior Staff Committee

RHL recurrent herpes labialis; right hepatic lobe

RHLN right hilar lymph node

rhm roentgens per hour at 1 meter

RHMAP radiation hybrid mapping program

RhMK rhesus monkey kidney

RhMk rhesus monkey

RhMkK rhesus monkey kidney

RHMV right heart mixing volume

RHN Rockwell hardness number

rhnRNP recombinant heterogeneous nuclear ribonucleoprotein

Rh$_{null}$ erythrocytes which fail to express rhesus antigens

RHO rhodopsin; right heeloff

ρ Greek letter *rho*; correlation coefficient; electric charge density; electrical resistivity; mass density; reactivity

RhoGAM Rh$_o$D immune globulin

RHOM rhombosine

RHR renal hypertensive rat; resting heart rate

r/hr roentgens per hour

RHRV relative heart rate variability

RHS radius head subluxation; Ramsay Hunt syndrome; Rapp-Hodgkin syndrome; reciprocal hindlimb-scratching [syndrome]; Richner-Hanhart syndrome; right hand side; right heelstrike

RHSC Royal Hospital for Sick Children

RHSIG Rehabilitation Hospitals Special Interest Group

rhSp1 recombinant human Sp1 protein

RHT renal homotransplantation

RHTC rural health training center

rH-TNF recombinant human tumor necrosis factor

rh-tPA recombinant human tissue plasminogen activator

rhTPO recombinant human thrombopoietin

RHU registered health underwriter; rheumatology

rHuEPO recombinant human erythropoietin

rHuGCF recombinant human granulocyte colony stimulating factor

rhuMAb recombinant human monoclonal antibody

rHuTNF recombinant human tumor-necrosis factor

RHV right hepatic vein

rHV recombinant hirudin variant

RI radiation intensity; radioactive isotope; radioimmunology; recession index; recombinant inbred [strain]; recurrent inhibition;

refractive index; regenerative index; regional ileitis; regional information system; regular insulin; relative intensity; release inhibition; remission induction; renal index; renal insufficiency; replicative intermediate; resistive index; respiratory illness; respiratory index; response interval; reticulocyte index; retroactive inhibition; retroactive interference; ribosome; rosette index (or inhibition)

R_I intracellular resistivity

R_i internal resistivity

r_i intraclass correlation coefficient

RIA radioimmunoassay; reference information model; reversible ischemic attack

RIA-DA radioimmunoassay double antibody [test]

RIAS Roter Interactional Analysis System

Rib riboflavin; ribose

RIBA recombinant immunoblot assay

ribotyping ribonucleic acid [RNA]-typing

RIBS Rutherford ion backscattering

RIC right internal carotid [artery]; right interventricular coronary [artery]; Royal Institute of Chemistry

RICE replicating and integrating controlled expression [bacterial gene identification]; rest, ice, compression, and elevation

R_{ICF} intracellular fluid resistance

RICM right intercostal margin

RiCoF ristocetin cofactor

RICP recurrent intrahepatic cholestasis of pregnancy

RICU respiratory intensive care unit

RID radial immunodiffusion; reduced interference distribution; remission-inducing drug; ruptured intervertebral disc

RIDDOR Reporting of Injuries, Diseases, and Dangerous Occurrences Regulations [UK]

RIE reactive ion etching

RIF radiation-induced fibrosis; radiological interface; release-inhibiting factor; rifabutin; rifampin; right iliac fossa; rosette-inhibiting factor

RIFA radioiodinated fatty acid

RIFC rat intrinsic factor concentrate

RIFLE risk factor and life expectancy

rIFN recombinant interferon

RIFS remedial investigation/feasibility study

RIG rabies immune globulin; rat insuloma gene

RIGH rabies immune globulin, human

RIGHT [Ce]rivastatin Gemfibrozil Hyperlipidemia Treatment [study]

RIH right inguinal hernia

RIHD radiation-induced heart disease

RIHSA radioactive iodinated human serum albumin

RIKEN Institute of Physical and Clinical Research [database, Japan]

rIL recombinant interleukin

RILT rabbit ileal loop test

RIM radioisotope medicine; recurrent induced malaria; reference information model; relative-intensity measure

RIMA reverse inhibitor of monoamino oxidase A; right internal mammary artery

riMLF rostral interstitial median longitudinal fasciculus

RIMR Rockefeller Institute for Medical Research

RIMS resonance ionization mass spectrometry

RIN radiation-induced neoplasm; radioisotope nephrography; rat insulinoma

R_{in} input resistance

RINB Reitan-Indiana Neuropsychological Battery

RIND reversible ischemic neurologic deficit

RINN recommended international nonproprietary name

RIO right inferior oblique

RIOMV Rio Mamore virus

RIOSV Rio Secundo virus

RIP radioimmunoprecipitation; reflex inhibiting pattern; repeat-induced point [mutation]; respiratory inductance plethysmography

RIPA radioimmunoprecipitation assay

RIPH Royal Institute of Public Health

RIPHH Royal Institute of Public Health and Hygiene

RIPP resistive-intermittent positive pressure

RIPV right inferior pulmonary vein

RIR relative incidence rates; right interior rectus [muscle]

RIRB radioiodinated rose bengal

RIRL retrograde intrarenal lipotripsy

RIRS retrograde intrarenal surgery

RIS radiology information system; rapid immunofluorescence staining; relative intensity score; resonance ionization spectroscopy

R$_{is}$ resistivity of the interstitium

r$_{is}$ interstitial resistance

RISA radioactive iodinated serum albumin; radioimmunosorbent assay

RISC Radiology Information System Consortium; reduced instruction set chip [microprocessor]; reduced instruction set computing; Research Group on Instability in Coronary Artery Disease [study]

RISK Risk Intervention Skills Study

RIS/PACS radiological information system/picture archiving and communication system

RIST radioimmunosorbent test

RIT radioimmune trypsin; radioimmunotherapy; radioiodinated triolein; radioiodine treatment; rosette inhibition titer

RITA Randomised Intervention Treatment of Angina [UK]; right internal thoracic artery

RITC rhodamine isothiocyanate

RITED Italian Registry of Echo-Dobutamine [tests]

RIU radioactive iodine uptake; refractive index unit

RIV retinal image velocity

RIVC right inferior vena cava

RIVD ruptured intervertebral disc

RJA regurgitant jet area

RK rabbit kidney; radial keratotomy; reductase kinase; rhodopsin kinase; right kidney

R$_k$ [heart function] restitution constant

RKG radiocardiogram

RKH Rokitansky-Küster-Hauser [syndrome]

RKM rokitamycin

RKV rabbit kidney vacuolating [virus]

RKY roentgen kymography

RL radial line; radiation laboratory; reduction level; relaxation labeling; renal dysplasia-limb defects [syndrome]; resistive load; reticular lamina; right lateral; right leg; right lung; Ringer's lactate [solution]; run length

R&L right and left

R$_L$ lung resistance

RLA Ranchos de los Amigos [Cognitive Functioning Scale]; right lung apices

RLC residual lung capacity

RLD related living donor; ruptured lumbar disc

RLE right lower extremity

RLF retrolental fibroplasia; right lateral femoral

RLG regional librarians group

RLGS restriction landmark genomic scanning

rliPCR restriction cleavage, self-ligation, inverse polymerase chain reaction

RLIU regional library and information unit

RLL right lobe of liver; right lower limb; right lower lobe; run length limited

RLLS relative laser light scattering

RLM right lower medial

rLM recombinant *Listeria monocytogenes*

RLMA reinforced laryngeal mask airway

RLN recurrent laryngeal nerve; regional lymph node; relaxin

RLNC regional lymph node cell

RLND regional lymph node dissection

RLO residual lymphatic output

RLP radiation leukemia protection; ribosome-like particle

RLPV right lower pulmonary vein

RLQ right lower quadrant

RLR right lateral rectus [muscle]

RLS recursive least square; restless leg syndrome; Ringer lactate solution; Roussy-Levy syndrome; run-length statistics

RLSB right lower scapular border

R-Lsh right-left shunt

RLSL recursive least square lattice

RLT ralitoline

RLU relative light unit

RLV Rauscher leukemia virus

RLWD routine laboratory work done

RLX relaxin

RLXH relaxin H

RLZ right lower zone

RM mutant reverse; radical mastectomy; random migration; radon monitor; range of movement; red marrow; reference material; relative magnitude; relative mobility; rehabilitation medicine; reinforced maneuver; resistive movement; respiratory movement; respiratory muscle; restoration-maximization [algorithm]; Riehl melanosis; risk management; routine management; ruptured membranes

Rm relative mobility; remission

R$_m$ membrane resistance

r$_m$ membrane resistance per unit length

rm remission; room

1RM one-repetition maximum

RMA rapid membrane assay; refuses medical advice; Registered Medical Assistant; relative medullary area; right mentoanterior [fetal position]

RMANOVA repeated measures analysis of variance

RMAT rapid microagglutination test

Rmax maximum resistance

R$_{max}$ maximum response

Rmax,L maximum resistance, lung

Rmax,w maximum resistance, chest wall

RMB right mainstem bronchus

RMBF regional myocardial blood flow

RMC reticular magnocellular [nucleus]; right middle cerebral [artery]; Rozsos microcholecystectomy

RMCA right middle cerebral artery

RMCH rod monochromacy or monochromatism

RMCL recommended maximum contaminant level; right midclavicular line

RMD retromanubrial dullness

RMDP Resource Mothers Development Project

RME rapid maxillary expansion; reasonable maximum exposure; receptor-mediated endocytosis; resting metabolic expenditure; right mediolateral episiotomy

RMEC regional medical education center

RMED rural medical education [program]

RMF recursive median filter; right middle finger

RMI recent myocardial infarction; remote method invocation; reticulocyte maturity index

R-MIM refined message information model

Rmin,L minimum resistance, lung

Rmin,rs minimum resistance, respiratory system

RMK rhesus monkey kidney

RML radiation myeloid leukemia; regional medical library; right mediolateral; right middle lobe

RMLB right middle lobe bronchus

RMLS right middle lobe syndrome

RMLV Rauscher murine leukemia virus

RMM rapid micromedia method

RMN Registered Mental Nurse

RMO Regional Medical Officer; Resident Medical Officer

RMP rapidly miscible pool; Regional Medical Program; regional myocardial infarction; resting membrane potential; ribulose monophosphate pathway; rifampin; right mentoposterior [fetal position]; risk management planning or program

RMPA Royal Medico-Psychological Association

RMR relative maximum respone; repair-misrepair model; resting metabolic rate; right medial rectus [muscle]

RMRS Regenstrief Medical Record System

RMS rectal morphine sulfate [suppository]; red man syndrome; repetitive motion syndrome; residual mean square; resource management system; respiratory muscle strength; rhabdomyosarcoma; rheumatic mitral stenosis; rhodomyosarcoma; rigid man syndrome; root-mean-square

rms root-mean-square

RMSA regulator of mitotic spindle assembly; rhabdomyosarcoma, alveolar

RMSa rhabdomyosarcoma

RMSCR rhabdomyosarcoma chromosomal region

RMSD root-mean-square deviation

RMSE, rmse root-mean-square error

RMSF Rocky Mountain spotted fever

RMSS Ruvalcaba-Myhre-Smith syndrome

RMSSD root mean square of successive differences

RMT Registered Music Therapist; relative medullary thickness; retromolar trigone; right mentotransverse [fetal position]

RMUI relief medication unit index

RMuLV Rauscher murine leukemia virus

RMV respiratory minute volume

RMZ right midzone

RN narrower semantic relationship [UMLS]; radionuclide; red nucleus; Registered Nurse; registry number; residual nitrogen; reticular nucleus

Rn radon

RNA radionuclide angiography; Registered Nurse Anesthetist; ribonucleic acid; rough, noncapsulated, avirulent [bacterial culture]

RNAA radiochemical neutron activation analysis

RNA-BP ribonucleic acid-binding protein

RNAi ribonucleic acid interference

RNAP ribonucleic acid polymerase

RNAse, RNase ribonuclease

RNase P ribonuclease P

RNasin ribonuclease inhibitor

RNC repressing nucleoprotein complexes

RN-C registered nurse-certification

RNCG relative negative charge

RNCM registered nurse case manager

RND radical neck dissection; radionuclide dacryography; reactive neurotic depression; respiratory nursing diagnosis

RNFL retinal nerve fiber layer

RNFP Registered Nurse Fellowship Program

RNGF rhodamine–nerve growth factor [conjugate]

RNI reactive nitrogen intermediate

RNIB Royal National Institute for the Blind

RNICU regional neonatal intensive care unit

RNID Royal National Institute for the Deaf

RNINMEGLA rat integral membrane glycoprotein

RNP ribonucleoprotein

RNP-CS ribonucleoprotein consensus sequence

RNR ribonucleotide reductase

RNS reactive nitrogen species; reference normal serum; repetitive nerve stimulation; replacement normal saline [solution]; ribonuclease

RNSC radionuclide superior cavography

Rnt roentgenology

RNTMI transfer ribonucleic acid initiator methionine

rNTP ribonuclease-5′-triphosphate

RNV radionuclide venography; radionuclide ventriculogram or ventriculography

RNVG radionuclide ventriculography

RO radiation oncology; radiation output; ratio of; relative odds; renal osteodystrophy; reverse osmosis; Ritter-Oleson [technique]; routine order; rule out

ro radius of orifice

R/O, r/o rule out

ROA regurgitant orifice area; right occipitoanterior [fetal position]

ROAD reversible obstructive airways disease

ROAT renal organic anion transporter; repeat open application test

ROATS rabbit ovarian antitumor serum

rob robertsonian translocation

ROBCAD robotic computer-assisted diagnosis

ROBUST Recanalization of Occluded Bypass Graft with Prolonged Urokinase Infusion Site Trial

ROC receiver operating characteristic; receiver operating curve; receptor-operated channels; relative operating characteristic; resident on call; residual organic carbon; right outer canthus

ROCFT Rey-Osterreich complex figure test

ROCK Rho-associated kinase

ROCKET Regionally Organized Cardiac Key European Trial

rOCT rat organic cation transporter

ROCV Rocio virus

ROD record of decision

RODA rapid opioid detoxification under general anesthesia

RODEO rotating delivery of excitation off resonance

rOEF regional oxygen extraction fraction

roent roentgenology

ROESY rotating frame Overhauser effect spectroscopy

ROGAD radiation oncology greater area database

ROH rat ovarian hyperemia [test]

ROI range of interest; reactive oxygen intermediate; region of interest; right occipitolateral [fetal position]

ROIH right oblique inguinal hernia

ROJM range of joint motion

ROLL radioguided occult lesion localization

ROM range of motion; reactive oxygen metabolite; read only memory; reduction of movement; regional office manual; removal of metal [pins or plates in orthopedic surgery]; rupture of membranes

Rom Romberg [sign]

rom reciprocal ohm meter

ROMAS Romanian Multicenter Study

ROM CP range of motion complete and painfree

ROMI rating of medication influence; rule out myocardial infarct

ROMIO Rule Out Myocardial Infarct Observation [study]

ROMS radiation oncology management system

ROOF retro-orbital orbicular fat

ROP removal of pins or plates; removal of plaster [of Paris]; retinopathy of prematurity; right occipitoposterior [fetal position]

RO PACS radiation oncology picture archiving and communication system

ROPE respiratory-ordered phase encoding

ROPS rollover protective structure

ROR reactive oxygen radicals; risk odds ratio

Ror Rorschach [test]

ROS reactive oxygen species; reflectance optical shield; relative outcome score; review of systems; rod outer segment

RoS rostral sulcus

ROSC return of spontaneous circulation

ROSETTA Routine vs Selective Exercise Treadmill Test after Angioplasty [trial]

ROSP rod outer segment protein

ROSS radiotherapy oncology support system; review of subjective symptoms

ROSTER Rotational Atherectomy vs Balloon Angioplasty for In-stent Restenosis [trial]

ROT real oxygen transport; remedial occupational therapy; right occipito-transverse [fetal position]

rot rotating, rotation

ROTA rotablator atherectomy

ROTACS rotational angioplasty catheter system

ROTASTENT Rotational Atherectomy with Adjunctive Stenting [trial]

ROU recurrent oral ulcer

R$_{out}$ outflow resistance

ROW Rendu-Osler-Weber [syndrome]; rest of the world

ROXIS Roxithromycin in Ischemic Syndromes [study]

RP radial pulse; radical prostatectomy; radiographic planimetry; radiopharmaceutical; rapid processing [of film]; rapid prototyping; Raynaud phenomenon; reactive protein; readiness potential; recessive partitioning; recreation and pastime; rectal prolapse; re-entrant pathway; refractory period; regulatory protein; relapsing polychondritis; relative power or potency;

reperfusion; replication protein; resident physician; respiratory rate; responsible party; rest pain; resting position; resting potential; resting pressure; retinitis pigmentosa; retinitis proliferans; retrograde pyelogram; retroperitoneal; reverse phase; rheumatoid polyarthritis; ribonucleoprotein; ribose phosphate; ribosomal protein; Roswell Park [genome database]

R5P ribose-5-phosphate

R/P respiratory pulse [rate]

Rp peripheral resistance

R$_p$ pulmonary resistance

RPA radial photon absorptiometry; replication protein A; resultant physiologic acceleration; retroperitoneal approach; reverse passive anaphylaxis; right pulmonary artery

r-PA reteplase

rPAF receptor for platelet-activating factor

RPAHPET Royal Prince Albert Hospital Positron Emission Tomography [study]

RPase ribonucleic acid polymerase

RPC reactive perforating collagenosis; relapsing polychondritis; relative proliferative capacity; remote procedure call

RPCA reverse passive cutaneous anaphylaxis

RPCF, RPCFT Reiter protein complement fixation [test]

RPCGN rapidly progressive crescenting glomerulonephritis

RPCH rural primary care hospital

RPD removable partial denture

R-PDQ revised prescreening developmental questionnaire

RPE rate of perceived exertion; recurrent pulmonary embolism; retinal pigment epithelium; ribulose 5-phosphate 3-epimerase

RPEP rabies post-exposure prophylaxis

RPET rapid partial exchange transfusion

RPF relaxed pelvic floor; renal plasma flow; retroperitoneal fibrosis

RPG radiation protection guide; Report Program Generator [PC language]; retrograde pyelogram; rheoplethysmography; right paracolic gutter

RPGMEC Regional Postgraduate Medical Education Committee

RPGN rapidly progressive glomerulonephritis

RPGR retinitis pigmentosa guanosine triphosphatase regulator [gene]
RPh Registered Pharmacist
RPHA reversed passive hemagglutination
RPHAMFCA reversed passive hemagglutination by miniature centrifugal fast analysis
RP-HPLC, rpHPLC reverse phase high-performance liquid chromatography
RPI regional perfusion index; relative percentage index; reticulocyte production index, ribose 5-phosphate isomerase
RPIPP reverse phase ion-pair partition
RPK ribosephosphate kinase
RPLAD retroperitoneal lymphadenectomy
RPLC reverse phase liquid chromatography
RPLD repair of potentially lethal damage
RPLND retroperitoneal lymph node dissection
RPM Rapid Pharmaceutical Management; rapid processing mode; revolutions per minute; robust point matching [algorithm]
rpm rapid processing mode; revolutions per minute
RPMD rheumatic pain modulation disorder
RPMI Roswell Park Memorial Institute [medium]
RPMS resource and patient management system
RPO right posterior oblique
RPP heart rate-systolic blood pressure product; rate-pressure produce; retropubic prostatectomy
RPPA reverse-phase protein microarray
RPPI role perception picture inventory
RPPR red cell precursor production rate
RPR rapid plasmin reagin [test]; Reiter protein reagin
RPr retinitis proliferans; rotational panoramic radiography
RPRC regional primate research center
RPRCT rapid plasma reagin cord test
RPRF rapidly progressive renal failure
Rp:Rs pulmonary-to-systemic vascular resistance
RPS renal pressor substance; reverse pivot shift; revolutions per second
rps revolutions per second
RPS-BLAST reverse position-specific iterated basic local alignment search tool

RPSM residency program in social medicine
RPSP reference preparation for serum proteins
RPS4Y ribosomal protein S4, Y-linked
RPT rapid pull-through; refractory period of transmission; Registered Physical Therapist; renal parenchymal thickness; rifapentine
RPTA renal percutaneous transluminal angioplasty
RPTC regional poisoning treatment center
Rptd ruptured
RPTK receptor protein tyrosine kinase
RPTP receptor protein tyrosine phosphatase
RPV raccoon parvovirus; rinderpest virus; right portal vein; right pulmonary vein
RPVC resource provider of virtual center [telemedicine]
RPVP right posterior ventricular pre-excitation
RQ recovery quotient; [Hazardous Substance] Reportable Quantities [List]; reportable quantity; respiratory quotient; risk-adjusted quantity
RQDS Revised Quantified Denver Scale of Communication
RQL rejectable quality level
RR radiation reaction; radiation response; rate ratio; rational recovery [group]; recovery room; recurrence risk; reference reagent; regulatory region; relative resistance; relative response; relative risk; renin release; resistant relapse; respiratory rate; respiratory reserve; response rate; results reporting [system]; retinal reflex; rheumatoid rosette; ribonucleotide reductase; risk ratio; Riva-Rocci [sphygmomanometer]; Ross River [virus]; ruthenium red
Rr respiratory rate
R&R rate and rhythm; rest and recuperation; rotablator and restenosis
RRA radioreceptor assay; registered record administrator
RRAC Research Realignment Advisory Committee
RRBAT relative rigid body accuracy test
RRC residency review committee; risk reduction component; routine respiratory care; Royal Red Cross; rural referral center
RRC-EM residency review committee for emergency medicine

RRDS radiation-resistant deoxyribonucleic acid [DNA] synthesis

RRE radiation-related eosinophilia; Rev response element

RRE, RR&E round, regular, and equal [pupils]

RRF ragged red fiber; residual renal function; ribosome recycling factor; rigid rectus femoris [muscle]

RRFC renal reserve filtration capacity

RR-HPO rapid recompression-high pressure oxygen

RRI recurrent respiratory infection; reflex relaxation index; relative response index

RRIS recurrent respiratory infection syndrome

RRL rabbit reticulocyte lysate; Registered Record Librarian

RRM ribonucleic acid [RNA] recognition motif; ribonucleotide reductase M

RRMS relapsing-remitting multiple sclerosis

RRN returning [for advanced studies] registered nurse

rRNA ribosomal ribonucleic acid

rRNP ribosomal ribonucleoprotein

RRP relative refractory period

RRPCE Reduction of Recurrence and Prevention of Cerebral Emboli [study]

RRpm respiratory rate per minute

RRR regular rhythm and rate; relative risk reduction; renin release rate (or ratio)

RR&R regular rate and rhythm

RRS result reporting [clinical data] repository system; retrorectal space; Richards-Rundle syndrome

R$_{RS}$ respiratory system resistance

RRT random response technique; recommended replacement time [pacemaker]; Registered Respiratory Therapist; relative retention time; renal replacement therapy; retrieved related term

RRU respiratory resistance unit

RRV Ross River virus

RRV-TV tetravalent rhesus-human rotavirus vaccine

RS radioscaphoid; radiosurgery; random sample; rating schedule; Raynaud syndrome; reaction stimulus; recipient's serum; rectal sinus; rectal suppository; rectosigmoid; reducing substance; Reed-Sternberg [cell]; reinforcing stimulus; Reiter syndrome; relative stimulus; remote sensing; remote site; renal specialist; respiratory system; respiratory syncytial [virus]; response to stimulus; resting subject; reticulated siderocyte; retinoschisis; Rett syndrome; review of symptoms; Reye syndrome; right sacrum; Reykjavik Study [coronary diseases in Icelandic males]; ribonucleic acid [RNA] synthetase; right septum; right side; right stellate [ganglion]; Ringer solution; Roberts syndrome; Rous sarcoma

Rs *Rauwolfia serpentina*; systemic resistance

R/s roentgens per second

r$_s$ rank correlation coefficient

RSA rabbit serum albumin; regular spiking activity; relative specific activity; relative standard accuracy; respiratory sinus arrhythmia; right sacroanterior [fetal position]; right subclavian artery; roentgenographic stereogrammetric analysis

Rsa systemic arterial resistance

RSAC regular source of ambulatory care

RSB reticulocyte standard buffer; right sternal border

RSBD REM sleep behavior disorder

RSC rat spleen cell; rested state contraction; reversible sickle-cell; right subclavian

RSCA reference strand mediated conformational analysis

RScA right scapuloanterior [fetal position]

RSCAAL remote sensing chemical agent alarm

RSCN Registered Sick Children's Nurse

RScP right scapuloposterior [fetal position]

RSD rad surface dose; reflex sympathetic dystrophy; relative standard deviation

RSDS reflex sympathetic dystrophy syndrome

RSE rapid spin-echo; reconstruction squared error; refractory status epilepticus; relative standard error

RSEP right somatosensory evoked potential

RSES Rosenberg Self-Esteem Scale

RSF rich [molecular genetics] sequence format

RSG rosiglitazone

RSGP revised scaled gradient projection [radiotherapy]

RSH Royal Society of Health

RSHT regular SNOMED hierarchies table

RSI rapid-sequence induction; rapid sequence intubation; repetition strain injury; repetitive stress injury; Rush Sexual Inventory

RSIC Radiation Shielding Information Center

RSIL respiratory and systemic infection laboratory

R-SIRS Revised Seriousness of Illness Rating Scale

RSIVP rapid-sequence intravenous pyelography

RSK ribosomal S6 kinase

RSL right sacrolateral [fetal position]

RSLD repair of sublethal damage

RSLT test result [UMLS]

RSM risk screening model; Royal Society of Medicine

RSMR relative standard mortality rate

RSN restin; right substantia nigra

RSNA Radiological Society of North America; renal sympathetic nerve activity

RSO radiation safety officer; Resident Surgical Officer; right superior oblique [muscle]

rSO₂ regional oxygen saturation

RSP rapid straight pacing; rat serum protein; recurrent spontaneous pneumothorax; removable silicone plug; respirable suspended particulate; ribose-5-phosphatase; right sacroposterior [fetal position]

RSPAC remote sensing public access center

RSPCA Royal Society for the Prevention of Cruelty to Animals

RS-PCR ribonucleic acid [RNA] specific template polymerase chain reaction

RS₃PE remitting seronegative symmetrical synovitis with pitting edema

RSPH Royal Society for the Promotion of Health

RSPK recurrent spontaneous psychokinesis

RSPV right superior pulmonary vein

RSR rectosphincteric reflex response-stimulus ratio; regular sinus rhythm; relative survival rate; right superior rectus [muscle]

rSr an electrocardiographic complex

RSS rat stomach strip; recombination signal sequence; rectosigmoidoscopy; repetitive stress syndrome; rotary subluxation of the sphenoid; Russell-Silver syndrome; Russian spring-summer [encephalitis]

RSSE Russian spring-summer encephalitis

RSSI received signal strength indication

RSSR relative slow sinus rate

RST radiosensitivity test; rapid surfactant test; reagin screen test; repeated significance test; right sacrotransverse [fetal position]; rubrospinal tract

R$_{st}$ in paper or thin layer chromatography, the distance that a spot of a substance has moved, relative to a reference standard spot

RSTD rectal-skin temperature difference

R-step restoration step

rSTERN recurrent spatiotemporal neuron

RSTI Radiological Service Training Institute

RSTL relaxed skin tension lines

RSTMH Royal Society of Tropical Medicine and Hygiene

RSTS retropharyngeal soft tissue space; Rubinstein-Taybi syndrome

RSTV Rost Island virus

RSU radiological sciences unit

RSV regurgitant stroke volume; respiratory syncytial virus; right subclavian vein; Rous sarcoma virus

RSVC right superior vena cava

RSVP rejuvenation with sparing of vascular perforators; retired senior volunteer program

RSV-Pr-C Rous sarcoma virus (Prague C)

RSV-SR-D Rous sarcoma virus (Schmidt-Ruppin D)

RSV-SR-B Rous sarcoma virus (Schmidt-Ruppin B)

RT rabbit trachea; radiologic technologist; radiotelemetry; radiotherapy; random transfusion; radium therapy; rapid tranquilization; rational therapy; reaction time; reading test; real time; reciprocating tachycardia; recovery time; recreational therapy; rectal temperature; red tetrazolium; red-top; reduction time; reference terminology; Registered Technician; related term [UMLS]; relaxation time; renal transplantation; repetition time; [heart] repolarization time; resistance transfer; respiratory therapist/therapy; response time; rest tremor; retransformation; retrieved term; reverse transcriptase; reverse transcription; right; right thigh; robust take; room temperature; Rubinstein-Taybi [syndrome]

RT3, rT₃ reverse triiodothyronine

RT₉₀ time to 90% relaxation

Rt right; total resistance

rT recurrent tumor [TNM (tumor-node-metastasis) classification]; ribothymidine

rt right; room temperature

RTA ray tracing algorithm; renal tubular acidosis; reverse transcriptase assay; road traffic accident

RTAD renal tubular acidification defect

rTag recombinant small T-antigen

rTAP recombinant tick anticoagulant peptide

RT(ARRT) Radiologic Technologist certified by the American Registry of Radiologic Technologists

RTAS radiology telephone access system

RTC rape treatment center; regional tuberculosis center; renal tubular cell; residential treatment center; return to clinic; reverse thrust catheter

rtc return to clinic

RTCL Radiotherapy Command Language

rTCMS repetitive transcranial magnetic stimulation

RT-CT radiotherapy dedicated computed tomography

RTD real time 3-dimensional [ultrasound]; renal tubular dysplasia or dysgenesis defect; resonant tunneling device; routine test dilution

Rtd retarded

RTE Registry of Toxic Effects

RTEC Regional Technology and Education Consortium

RTECS Registry of Toxic Effects of Chemical Substances [NLM database]

RTF resistance transfer factor; respiratory tract fluid; rich text format

RTG radioactive thermal generator; renal threshold of glucose

RTG-2 rainbow trout gonadal tissue cells

RTH resistance to thyroid hormone

RTI reproductive tract infection; respiratory tract infection; retrograde tracheal intubation; reverse transcriptase inhibition

RTK receptor-tyrosine kinase; rhabdoid tumor of the kidney

rtl rectal

rt lat right lateral

RTM registered trademark

rTMS repetitive transcranial magnetic stimulation

RTN renal tubular necrosis

RTn reverse transcription intermediate

RT(N)(ARRT) Radiologic Technologist (Nuclear Medicine) certified by the American Registry of Radiologic Technologists

RTNet radiotherapy networking system

rTNF recombinant tumor necrosis factor

RTO return to office; right toeoff

RTOG radiation therapy oncology group

RTP radiation treatment planning; radiotherapy treatment planning; renal transplantation patient; reverse transcriptase-producing [agent]

rTPA, rtPA, rt-PA recombinant tissue plasminogen activator

RT-PACS radiotherapy picture archival and communication system

RT-PCR reverse transcriptase polymerase chain reaction [PCR]

RTPV radiation therapy planning and verification; RT parvovirus

RTR Recreational Therapist, Registered; red blood cell turnover rate; retention time ratio

RT(R)(ARRT) Registered Technologist (Radiography) certified by the American Registry of Radiologic Technologists

RT-RH reverse transcriptase–ribonuclease H

RTRR return to recovery room

RTS rapid throughput screening; real time scan; Rett syndrome; Revised Trauma Score; right toestrike; Rothmund-Thomson syndrome; Rubinstein-Taybi syndrome

RTSS rest technetium-99m sestamibi scan

RTT round trip time

RT(T)(ARRT) Radiologic Technologist (Radiation Therapy) certified by the American Registry of Radiologic Technologists

RTTP radiation therapy treatment planning

RTU real-time ultrasonography; relative time unit; renal transplantation unit

RT₃U resin triiodothyronine uptake

RTUI respiratory therapy utilization index

RTV resistance-to-voltage [converter]; rhinotracheitis virus; room temperature vulcanization

RTW return to work

RTX robustotoxin

RU radioulnar; rat unit; reading unit; residual urine; resin uptake; resistance unit; retrograde urogram; right upper; roentgen unit

ru radiation unit

RU-1 human embryonic lung fibroblasts

RU-486 mifepristone

RUA reduced under anesthesia

RUBV rubella virus

RUC rapid update cycle

RUD recurrent ulcer of the duodenal bulb; repeating unit domain

RUE right upper extremity

RUG resource utilization group; retrograde urethrography

RUL right upper eyelid; right upper lateral; right upper limb; right upper lobe

RuMP ribulose monophosphate pathway

RUOQ right upper outer quadrant

RUP right upper pole

Ru1,5P ribulose-1,5-biphosphate

Ru5P ribulose-5-phosphate

rupt ruptured

RUPV right upper pulmonary vein

RUQ right upper quadrant

RUR resin-uptake ratio

RURTI recurrent upper respiratory tract infection

RUS radioulnar synostosis; real-time ultrasonography

RUSB right upper sternal border

RUSP right ventricular systolic pressure

RUT rapid urease test

RUTH Raloxifene Use for the Heart [study]

RUV residual urine volume

RUX right upper extremity

RUZ right upper zone

RV ranavirus; random variable; rat virus; Rauscher virus; rectovaginal; regurgitant [stroke] volume; reinforcement value; renal vein; reovirus; residual volume; respiratory volume; retroventral; retroversion; retrovesical; retrovirus; return visit; rhabdovirus; rheumatoid vasculitis; rhinovirus; right ventricle, right ventricular; rotavirus; rubella vaccine; rubella virus; Russell viper

R/V, R&V record and verify

R$_V$ radius of view

Rv venous resistance

RVA rabies vaccine activated; recombinant virus assay; re-entrant ventricular arrhythmia; right ventricle activation;

right ventricular apex; right vertebral artery

RV-A Rotavirus A

RVAD right ventricular assist device

RVAW right ventricle anterior wall

RVB red venous blood

RV-B Rotavirus B

RVBF reversed vertebral blood flow

RVC reason for visit classification; rectovaginal constriction

RV-C Rotavirus C

RVD regulatory [fluid] volume decrease; relative vertebral density; relative vessel diameter; relative volume decrease; right ventricular dimension; right ventricular dysplasia

RV-D Rotavirus D

RVDC right ventricular diastolic collapse

RVDO right ventricular diastolic overload

RVDV right ventricular diastolic volume

RVE right ventricular enlargement

RV-E Rotavirus E

RVECP right ventricular endocardial potential

RVED right ventricular end-diastolic [pressure]

RVEDD right ventricular end-diastolic diameter

RVEDP right ventricular end-diastolic pressure

RVEDV right ventricular end-diastolic volume

RVEDVI right ventricular end-diastolic volume index

RVEF right ventricular ejection fraction; right ventricular end-flow

RVESV right ventricular end-systolic volume

RVET right ventricular ejection time

RVF renal vascular failure; residual volume fraction; Rift Valley fever; right ventricular failure; right visual field

RV-F Rotavirus F

RVFP right ventricular filling pressure

RVFV Rift Valley fever virus

RVG right ventral gluteus [muscle]; right visceral ganglion; radionuclide ventriculography

RV-G Rotavirus G

RVH renal vascular hypertension, renovascular hypertension; right ventricular hypertrophy

RVHD rheumatic valvular heart disease

RVHR renovascular hypertensive rat

RVI relative value index; right ventricle infarction

RVID right ventricular internal dimension

RVIT right ventricular inflow tract

RV-IVRT right ventricular isovolumic relaxation time

RVL right vastus lateralis

RVLG right ventrolateral gluteal

RVLM rostral ventrolateral medulla

RVM right ventricular mass; right ventricular mean

RVMM rostral ventromedial medulla

RVO Regional Veterinary Officer; relaxed vaginal outlet; right ventricular outflow

RVOT right ventricular outflow tract

RVP red veterinary petrolatum; resting venous pressure; right ventricular pressure

RVPEP right ventricular pre-ejection period

RVPFR right ventricular peak filling rate

RVP/LVP right ventricular pressure/left ventricular pressure [ratio]

RVPRA renal vein plasma renin activity

RVR reduced vascular response; renal vascular resistance; repetitive ventricular response; resistance to venous return

RVRA renal vein renin activity, renal venous renin assay

RVRC renal vein renin concentration

RVS rectovaginal space; relative value scale/study; reported visual sensation; retrovaginal space

RVSO right ventricular stroke output

RVSV right ventricular stroke volume

RVSW right ventricular stroke work

RVSWI right ventricular stroke work index

RVT renal vein thrombosis

RVTE recurring venous thromboembolism

RV/TLC residual volume/total lung capacity

RVU relative value unit

RVV right ventricular volume; rubella vaccine-like virus; Russell viper venom

rVV recombinant vaccinia virus

RVVO right ventricular volume overload

RVVT Russell viper venom time

RVW right ventricular wall

RVWT right ventricle wall thickness

RW radiological warfare; ragweed; respiratory work; Romano-Ward [syndrome]; round window

R-W Rideal-Walker [coefficient]; Romano-Ward [syndrome]

R/W return to work

RWAGE ragweed antigen E

RWC receiving water concentration; regional weaning center

RWIS restraint and water immersion stress

RWJF Robert Wood Johnson Foundation

RWM regional wall motion

RWMA regional wall motion abnormality

RWP ragweed pollen; R-wave progression

RWS radiology work station; ragweed sensitivity

RWT random walk theory [fluorescent imaging]; relative wall thickness

RWV rotating-wall vessel

RX rapid exchange; reaction; residual tumor not assessed [TNM (tumor-node-metastasis) classification]

Rx drug; medication; pharmacy; prescribe, prescription; prescription drug; take [Lat. *recipe*]; therapy; treatment

RXLI recessive X-linked ichthyosis

RXN reaction

RXR retinoid X receptor

RXRA retinoid X receptor alpha

RXRE retinoic X response element

RXRG retinoid X receptor gamma

RXT right exotropia

R-Y Roux-en-Y [anastomosis]

RYD ryanodine

RYR, Ryr ryanodine receptor

S

S apparent power; in electrocardiography, a negative deflection that follows an R wave [wave]; entropy; exposure time; half [Lat. *semis*]; left [Lat. *sinister*]; mean dose per unit cumulated activity; the midpoint of the sella turcica [point]; sacral; saline; *Salmonella*; saturated; scanning [pacemaker]; *Schistosoma*; schizophrenia; scleral [tumor invasion]; second; section; sedimentation coefficient; sella [turcica]; semilente [insulin]; senile, senility; sensation; sensitivity; septum; serine; serum; serum marker; *Shigella*; siderocyte; siemens; sigmoid; signature [prescription]; silicate; slope; single; slow accelerator; small; smooth [colony]; soft [diet]; solid; soluble; solute; sone [unit]; space; spatial; specificity; spherical; *Spirillum*; spleen; spontaneous; standard normal deviation; *Staphylococcus*; stem [cell]; stimulus; *Streptococcus*; streptomycin; subject; subjective findings; substrate; sulfur; sum of an arithmetic series; supravergence; surface; surgery; suture; Svedberg [unit]; swine; Swiss [mouse]; synthesis; systole; without [Lat. *sine*]

S0 scleral invasion not assessed [TNM (tumor-node-metastasis) classification]

S₁ first stimulus

s⁻¹ per second

S1–S5 first to fifth sacral nerves

S₁–S₄ first to fourth heart sounds

S2 supernatant, pure

s² sample variance [statistics]

4S Scandinavian Simvastatin Survival Study Group

S-100 marker protein for peripheral nervous system tumors containing α and β chains

s atomic orbital with angular momentum quantum number 0; distance; left [Lat. *sinister*]; length of path; sample standard deviation; satellite [chromosome]; scruple; second; section; sedimentation coefficient; sensation; series; signed; suckling

s̄ specific heat capacity; without [Lat. *sine*]

s⁻¹ cycles per second

s² sample variance

Σ see *sigma*

σ see *sigma*

SA sacro-anterior; salicylamide; salicylic acid; saline [solution]; salt added; sarcoidosis; sarcoma; scalenus anticus; secondary amenorrhea; secondary anemia; secondary arrest; self-administration; self-agglutination; self-analysis; semen analysis; sensitizing antibody; serratus anterior [muscle]; serum albumin; serum aldolase; sexual abuse; sexual addict; sexual assault; short acting; short axis; sialic acid; sialoadenectomy; signal averaged [ECG]; simian adenovirus; simulated annealing [algorithm]; sinoatrial; sinus arrest; sinus arrhythmia; skeletal age; skin-adipose [unit]; sleep apnea; slightly active; slowly adapting [receptor]; soluble in alkaline medium; Spanish American; specific activity; spectrum analysis; sperm abnormality; spiking activity; spinal abscess; spinal anesthesia; splenic artery; stable angina; standard accuracy; *Staphylococcus aureus*; status asthmaticus; stimulus artifact; Stokes-Adams [syndrome]; streptavidin; subarachnoid; substance abuse; succinylacetone; suicide alert; suicide attempt; surface antigen; surface area; surgery and anesthesia; surgical assistant; suspended animation; suspicious area; sustained action; sympathetic activity; symptom analysis; synthetic aperture; system administrator; systemic aspergillosis

S-A sinoatrial; sinoauricular

S&A sickness and accident [insurance]; sugar and acetone

S/A stent-to-artery [ratio]

Sa the most anterior point of the anterior contour of the sella turcica [point]; saline; *Staphylococcus aureus*

sA statampere

SAA serum amyloid A; serum amyloid-associated [protein]; severe aplastic anemia; starch ampicillin agar

SAAP selective aortic arch perfusion

SAAQ signal averaged acoustic quantification

SAARD slow-acting antirheumatic drug

SAAS Substance Abuse Attitude Survey

SAAST self-administered alcohol screening test

SAB Scientific Advisory Board; serum albumin; signal above baseline; significant asymptomatic bacteriuria; sinoatrial block; Society of American Bacteriologists; spontaneous abortion; subarachnoid block

SAb spontaneous abortion

SABER Stent-assisted Balloon Angioplasty and Its Effects on Restenosis [study]

SABOV Sabo virus

SABV Saboya virus

SABP spontaneous acute bacterial peritonitis; systolic arterial blood pressure

SAC saccharin; sacrum; screening and acute care; seasonal acute conjunctivitis; Self-Assessment of Communication [scale]; serum aminoglycoside concentration; short-arm cast; sideline assessment of concussion; small accessory chromosome; social activity [scale]; splinting for acute closure; stable access cannula; stretch-activated channel [heart contraction]; subarea advisory council; substance abuse counselor; symptomatic anomaly complex

SAC$_{cat}$ stretch-activated channel-cations [heart contraction]

sacch saccharin

SACD subacute combined degeneration

SACE serum angiotensin-converting enzyme

SACH small animal care hospital; solid ankle cushioned heel

SACK suppression of asymmetric cell kinetics

SACNAS Society for the Advancement of Chicanos and Native Americans in Science

SaCO$_2$ alveolar carbon dioxide saturation

SACS secondary anticoagulation system

SACSF subarachnoid cerebrospinal fluid

SACT sinoatrial conduction time

SAD Scale of Anxiety and Depression; seasonal affective disorder; Self-Assessment Depression [scale]; sino-aortic denervation; small airway disease; source-to-axis distance; sugar, acetone, and diacetic acid; suppressor-activating determinant

SADD Short-Alcohol Dependence Data [questionnaire]; standardized assessment of depressive disorders; Students Against Drunk Driving

SADDAN severe achondroplasia with developmental delay and acanthosis nigricans

SADIA small angle double incidence angiography

SADL simulated activities of daily living

SADR suspected adverse drug reaction

SADS Schedule for Affective Disorders and Schizophrenia; self-accelerating decomposition temperature; Sudden Adult Death Survey; sudden arrhythmic death syndrome

SADS-C Schedule for Affective Disorders and Schizophrenia-Change

SADS-L Schedule for Affective Disorders and Schizophrenia-Lifetime

SADT Stetson Auditory Discrimination Test

SAdV simian adenovirus

SAE serious adverse event; sexual assault evaluation; short above-elbow [cast]; specific action exercise; subcortical arteriosclerotic encephalopathy; supported arm exercise

SAEB sinoatrial entrance block

SAECG, SaECG signal averaged electrocardiogram

SAED semiautomatic external defibrillator

SAEFVSS Serious Adverse Events Following Vaccination Surveillance Scheme [Australia]

SAEM Society for Academic Emergency Medicine

SAEP *Salmonella abortus equi* pyrogen

SAF scrapie-associated fibrils; self-articulating femoral; serum accelerator factor; simultaneous auditory feedback; standard analytic file [Medicare]

SAFA soluble antigen fluorescent antibody

SAFE Safety After Fifty Evaluation [study]; surgery, antibiotics, face-washing, environmental change [trachoma]

SAFE-PACE Syncope and Falls in the Elderly-Role of Pacemaker [study]

SAFHS sonic-accelerated fracture-healing system

SAFIRE-D Symptomatic Atrial Fibrillation Investigation and Randomized Evaluation of Dofetilide [study]

SAFTEE-GI systematic assessment for treatment emergent events-general inquiry

SAFTEE-SI systematic assessment for treatment emergent events-systematic inquiry

SAFV Saint-Floris virus

SAG salicyl acyl glucuronide; sodium antimony gluconate; sonoangiography; streptavidin-gold; superantigen; Swiss agammaglobulinemia

sag sagittal

SAGE Serial Analysis of Gene Expression [database]; Systematic Assessment of Geriatric Drug Use via Epidemiology [study]

SAGES signal-averaged electrocardiographic [ECG] study

SAGM sodium chloride, adenine, glucose, mannitol

SAH *S*-adenosyl-L-homocysteine; subarachnoid hemorrhage

SAHA seborrhea-hypertrichosis/hirsutism-alopecia [syndrome]

SAHCS Streptokinase-Aspirin-Heparin Collaborative Study

SAHH *S*-adenosylhomocysteine hydrolase

SAHIGES *Staphylococcus aureus* hyperimmunoglobulinemia E syndrome

SA-HRP streptavidin-conjugated horse radish peroxidase

SAHS San Antonio Heart Study; sleep apnea-hypersomnolence [syndrome]

SAHV St Abb's Head virus

SAI Self-Analysis Inventory; Sexual Arousability Inventory; Social Adequacy Index; suppressor of anchorage independence; systemic active immunotherapy

SAIC Science Applications International Corporation [database]

SAICAR sylaminoimidazole carboxylase

SAID specific adaptation to imposed demand [principle]

SAIDS sexually acquired immunodeficiency syndrome; simian acquired immune deficiency syndrome

SAIMS student applicant information management system

SAKV Sakhalin virus

SAL sensorineural activity level; sterility assurance level; suction-assisted lipectomy

Sal salicylate, salicylic; *Salmonella*

sAl serum aluminum [level]

sal salicylate, salicylic; saline; saliva

SALAD Surgery vs Angioplasty for Proximal Left Anterior Descending Coronary Artery Stenosis [trial]

Salm *Salmonella*

SALP salpingectomy; salpingography; serum alkaline phosphatase

Salpx salpingectomy

SALT skin-associated lymphoid tissue; Swedish Aspirin in Low Dose Trial

SALTS Strategic Alternatives with Ticlopidine in Stenting [study]

SALV Salehebad virus

SAM *S*-adenosyl-L-methionine; scanning acoustic microscope; self-assembled monolayer; senescence accelerated mouse; sex arousal mechanism; short-arc motion; staphylococcal absorption method; subject area model; substrate adhesion molecule; sulfated acid mucopolysaccharide; surface active material; system for assembling markers; systolic anterior motion

SAMA schizoaffective mania mainly affective [type]; Student American Medical Association

SAMD *S*-adenosyl-L-methionine decarboxylase

SAM-DC *S*-adenosyl-L-methionine decarboxylase

SAMe *S*-adenosyl-L-methionine

SAMHSA Substance Abuse and Mental Health Services Administration

SAMI Streptokinase and Angioplasty in Myocardial Infarction [trial]; Streptokinase in Acute Myocardial Infarction [study]; Students for Advancement of Medical Instrumentation

SAMII Survey of Acute Myocardial Ischemia and Infarction [study]

SAMIT Streptokinase and Angioplasty Myocardial Infarction Trial

SAMMEC Smoking-Attributable Mortality, Morbidity, and Economic Costs [study]

SAMO Senior Administrative Medical Officer

SAMPLE Study on Ambulatory Monitoring of Pressure and Lisinopril Evaluation

SAMS Society for Advanced Medical Systems; substrate adhesion molecule

S-AMY serum amylase

SAN sinoatrial node; sinoauricular node; slept all night; solitary autonomous nodule; storage area network

SANA sinoatrial node artery

Sanat sanatorium

SANDR sinoatrial nodal reentry

SANE sexual assault nurse examiner

sang sanguineous

SANGUIS Safe and Good Use of Blood in Surgery [study]

sanit sanitary, sanitation

SANS scale for the assessment of negative symptoms

SANV Sango virus

SANWS sinoatrial node weakness syndrome

SAO small airway obstruction; splanchnic artery occlusion; subvalvular aortic obstruction

S$_{AO_2}$ oxygen saturation in alveolar gas

SaO$_2$ oxygen saturation

S$_{aO_2}$ oxygen saturation in arterial blood

SAP sensory action potential; serum acid phosphatase; serum alkaline phosphatase; serum amyloid P; shrimp alkaline phosphatase; situs ambiguus with polysplenia; sphingolipid activator protein; stable angina pectoris; *Staphylococcus aureus* protease; subjective and physical [findings]; surfactant-associated protein; systemic arterial pressure; systolic arterial pressure

SAPA scan along polygonal approximation; spatial average pulse average

SAPALDIA Swiss Study of Air Pollution and Lung Diseases in Adults

SAPAT Swedish Angina Pectoris Aspirin Trial

SAPD short action potential duration; signal averaged P-wave duration; sphingolipid activator protein deficiency

SAPF simultaneous anterior and posterior [spinal] fusion

saph saphenous

SAPHO synovitis-acne-pustulosis hyperostosis-osteomyelitis [syndrome]

SAPK stress-activated protein kinase

SA-PMP streptavidin-paramagnetic particle

SAPPHIRE Stanford Asian Pacific Program in Hypertension and Insulin Resistance

SAPS simplified acute physiology score; *Staphylococcus aureus* protease sensitivity

SAPV Sapphire virus

SAPX salivary peroxidase

SAQ saquinavir; self-applied questionnaire; short arc quadriceps [muscle]

SAQC statistical analysis of quality control

SAR scaffold attachment region [genomic sequencing]; scatter/air ratio [radiation]; seasonal allergic rhinitis; sexual attitude reassessment; slowly adapting receptor; specific absorption rate; structure-activity relationship; supplied air respirator; supra-aortic ridge; supra-aortic ring; synthetic aperture radar

SARA sexually acquired reactive arthritis; Superfund Amendments and Reauthorization

SARB Statistical Application and Research Branch [FDA]

SARI serotonin-2 antagonist reuptake inhibitor

SARS San Antonio Rotablator study; severe acute respiratory syndrome

SART simultaneous algebraic reconstruction technique

SARV Santa Rosa virus

SAS sarcoma amplified sequence; Scandinavian Angiopeptin Study; sedation-agitation scale; Scottish Ambulance Service; self-rating anxiety scale; short arm splint; Sklar Aphasia Scale; severe aortic stenosis; sleep apnea syndrome; small animal surgery; small aorta syndrome; social adjustment scale; sodium amylosulfate; space-adaptation syndrome; specific activity scale; statistical analysis system; sterile aqueous solution; sterile aqueous suspension; subaortic stenosis; subarachnoid space; sulfasalazine; supravalvular aortic stenosis; surface-active substance; synchronous atrial stimulation

SASA solvent-accessible surface area

SASD State Ambulatory Surgery Databases

SASMAS skin-adipose superficial musculoaponeurotic system

SASP salicylazosulfapyridine

SASPP syndrome of absence of septum pellucidum with preencephaly

SASS Syngen Acute Stroke Study

SAS-SR social adjustment scale, self-report

SASSY Seniors Active Spirits Staying Young [program]

SAST selective arterial secretin injection test; Self-administered Alcoholism Screening Test; serum aspartate aminotransferase

SAT saliva alcohol test; Saruplase Alteplase Study; satellite; satisfactibility; saturated, saturation; serum antitrypsin; shifting attention; single-agent chemotherapy; slide agglutination test; sodium ammonium thiosulfate; spermatogenic activity test; spontaneous activity test; subacute thrombosis; subacute thyroiditis; subcutaneous adipose tissue; sulfate adenyltransferase; symptomless autoimmune thyroiditis; systematic assertive therapy; systematic axis transform; systolic acceleration time

Sat, sat saturation, saturated

SATA spatial average, temporal average

SATB special aptitude test battery

satd saturated

SATE Safety Antiarrhythmic Trial Evaluation

SATL surgical Achilles tendon lengthening

SATP spatial average temporal peak

SATS substance, amount ingested, time ingested, symptoms

SATSA Swedish Adoption-Twin Study of Aging

SATT Scottish Adjuvant Tamoxifen Trial

SATV Sathuperi virus

SAU statistical analysis unit

SAUDIS Sudden and Unexpected Death in Sports [study]

SAV San Angelo virus; sequential atrioventricular [pacing]; Sikhote-Alyn virus

SAVD spontaneous assisted vaginal delivery

SAVE saved-young-life equivalent; sudden A-ventilatory event; Survival and Ventricular Enlargement [trial]

SAVED saphenous vein de novo

SAW surface acoustic wave

SAX short axis; surface antigen, X-linked

SAx short axis

SAX-APEX short-axis plane, apical

SAX-MV short-axis, mitral valve

SAX-PM short-axis plane, papillary muscle

SB Bachelor of Science [L. *Scientiae Baccalaureus*]; Schwartz-Bartter [syndrome]; serum bilirubin; shortness of breath; sick bay; sideroblast; single blind [study]; single breath; sinus bradycardia; small bowel; sodium balance; sodium bisulfite; Southern blotting; soybean; spike burst; spina bifida; spontaneous blastogenesis; spontaneous breathing; standard [hospital] bed;

Stanford-Binet [Intelligence Scale]; stereotyped behavior; sternal border; stillbirth; Sudan black [stain]; surface binding

S-B Sengstaken-Blakemore [tube]; suppression burst

Sb strabismus

sb stilb

SBA serum bactericidal activity; serum bile acid; soybean agglutinin; spina bifida aperta

SBAHC school-based adolescent health care

SBB stimulation-bound behavior

SBBT specialist in blood bank technology

SBC school-based clinic; Schwarz's bayesian criterion; serum bactericidal concentration; strict bed confinement

SBCS Stockholm Breast Cancer Study

SBD selective bowel decontamination; senile brain disease

S-BD seizure-brain damage

SbDH sorbitol dehydrogenase

SBDX scanning beam digital x-ray

SBE breast self-examination; short below-elbow [cast]; shortness of breath on exertion; small bowel enema; small bowel enteroscopy; subacute bacterial endocarditis

SBEH social behavior [UMLS]

SBET Society for Biomedical Engineering Technicians

SBEPI sinusoidal blipped echo-planar imaging

S/β sickle cell beta-thalassemia

SBF serologic-blocking factor; skin blood flow; specific blocking factor; splanchnic blood flow; systemic blood flow

SBFT small bowel follow-through

SBG selenite brilliant green

SBH Sabra hypertensive [rat]; sea-blue histiocyte; small basophilic hemocyte

SBHC school-based health center

SBI shape-based interpolation

SBIAB secondary bacterial infection acute bronchitis

SBIS Stanford-Binet Intelligence Scale

SBL soybean lecithin

sBL sporadic Burkitt lymphoma

SBLA sarcoma, breast and brain tumors, leukemia, laryngeal and lung cancer, and adrenal cortical carcinoma

SB-LM Stanford-Binet Intelligence Test-Form LM

SBM scientific basis of medicine; sexual intercourse between men; Solomon-Bloembergen-Morgan [equation]
SBMA spinal bulbar muscular atrophy
SBN State Board of Nursing
SBN$_2$ single-breath nitrogen [test]
SBNS Society of British Neurological Surgeons
SBNT single-breath nitrogen test
SBNW single-breath nitrogen washout
SBO small bowel obstruction; spina bifida occulta
SBOM soybean oil meal
SBP schizobipolar; serotonin-binding protein; spontaneous bacterial peritonitis; steroid-binding plasma [protein]; sulfobromophthalein; symmetric biphasic; systemic blood pressure; systolic blood pressure
SBQ Smoking Behavior Questionnaire
SBR small bowel resection; small box respirator; spleen-to-body [weight] ratio; strict bed rest; styrene-butadiene rubber
SBRN sensory branch of radial nerve
SBRS senior biomedical research service
SBRT split beam rotation therapy
SBS secondary bilateral synchrony; shaken baby syndrome; short bowel syndrome; sick building syndrome; sinobronchial syndrome; skull base surgery; small bowel series; social breakdown syndrome; straight back syndrome; substrate-binding strand
SBSP simultaneous bilateral spontaneous pneumothorax
SBSS Seligmann's buffered salt solution
SBT sequence-based typing; serum bactericidal titer; single-breath test; sulbactam
SBTI soybean trypsin inhibitor
SBTPE State Boards Test Pool Examination
SBTT small bowel transit time
SBV singular binocular vision; soilborne virus
SB^V pentavalent antimonial
SBW standard body weight
SC conditioned stimulus; sacrococcygeal; Sanitary Corps; sarcomatous component; scalenus [muscle]; scan computer; scapula; Schüller-Christian [disease]; Schwann cell; Schwarz criterion; sciatica; science; sclerosing cholangitis; secondary cleavage; secretory component; self care; semicircular; semilunar valve closure; serum complement; serum creatinine; service-connected; sex chromatin; Sézary cell; short circuit; sick call; sickle cell; sieving coefficient; sigmoid colon; silicone-coated; single chemical; skin conduction; slice collimation; slow component; Snellen chart; sodium citrate; soluble complex; special care; specialty clinic; spinal canal; spinal cord; squamous carcinoma; start conversion; statistical control; stepped care; sternoclavicular; stratum corneum; subcellular; subclavian; subcorneal; subcortical; subcostal; subcutaneous [JCAHO unapproved abbreviation]; subtotal colectomy; succinylcholine; sugar-coated; sulfur-containing; supercoil cruciform [deoxyribonucleic acid, DNA]; supercomputing; superior colliculus; supportive care; supraclavicular; surface colony; surface cooling; switching circuit; systemic candidiasis; systolic click
S/C subcutaneous; sugar-coated [pill]
S-C sickle cell
S&C sclerae and conjunctivae
Sc scandium; scapula; science, scientific; screening
sC statcoulomb
sc subcutaneous
SCA self-care agency; senescent cell antigen; severe congenital anomaly; sickle-cell anemia; single-camera autostereoscopic [imaging]; single-channel analyzer; sperm-coating antigen; spinocerebellar ataxia; starburst calcification; steroidal-cell antibody; subclavian artery; superior cerebellar artery; suppressor cell activity; survivor of cardiac arrest
Sca-1 stem cell antigen 1
SCAA Skin Care Association of America; sporadic cerebral amyloid angiopathy
SCABG single coronary artery bypass
SCAD short chain acyl-coenzyme A dehydrogenase; spontaneous coronary artery dissection
SCAG Sandoz Clinical Assessment-Geriatric [Rating]
SCAI Society for Cardiac Angiography and Interventions
SCAM statistical classification of activities of molecules
SCAMC Symposium on Computer Applications in Medical Care

SCAMIA Symposium on Computer Applications in Medical Care

SCAMIN Self-Concept and Motivation Inventory

SCAMP Stanford Coronary Artery Monitoring Project

SCAN Schedules for Clinical Assessment of Neuropsychiatry; suspected child abuse and neglect; systolic coronary artery narrowing

SCAP scapula

SCAR sequence characterized amplified region; severe cutaneous adverse reactions; Society for Computer Application in Radiology

SCARF skeletal abnormalities, cutis laxa, craniostenosis, psychomotor retardation, facial abnormalities [syndrome]

SCARI Spinal Cord Injury Assessment of Risk Index

SCARMD severe childhood autosomal recessive muscular dystrophy

SCAT sheep cell agglutination test; sickle cell anemia test; Simvastatin and Enalapril Coronary Atherosclerosis Trial; Sports Competition Anxiety Test

SCAV Sunday Canyon virus

SCAVF spinal cord arteriovenous fistula

SCAVM spinal cord arteriovenous malformation

SCB strictly confined to bed

SCBA self-contained breathing apparatus

SCBE single contrast barium enema

SCBF spinal cord blood flow

SCBG symmetric calcification of the basal cerebral ganglia

SCBH systemic cutaneous basophil hypersensitivity

SCBP stratum corneum basic protein

SCC self-care center; sequential combination chemotherapy; services for crippled children; short-course chemotherapy; sickle cell disease; side chain cleavage; small-cell carcinoma; small cleaved cell; spinal cord compression; standardized coding and classification; squamous cell carcinoma; symptom cluster constraint

SC4C subcostal four-chamber [view]

SCCA single-cell cytotoxicity assay; small-cell carcinoma

SCCB small-cell carcinoma of the bronchus

SCCC squamous cell cervical carcinoma

SCCH sternocostoclavicular hyperostosis

SCCHN squamous cell carcinoma of the head and neck

SCCHO sternocostoclavicular hyperostosis

SCCL small cell carcinoma of the lung

SCCM Sertoli cell culture medium; Society of Critical Care Medicine

SCCT severe cerebrocranial trauma

SCD scleroderma; sequential compression device; service-connected disability; sickle-cell disease; spinocerebellar degeneration; subacute combined degeneration; subacute coronary disease; sudden cardiac death; sudden coronary death; support clinical database; systemic carnitine deficiency

ScD Doctor of Science

SCDA situational control of daily activities [scale]

ScDA right scapuloanterior [fetal position, Lat. *scapulodextra anterior*]

SCDF skin condition data form

SCD-HeFT Sudden Cardiac Death in Heart Failure: Trial of Prophylactic Amiodarone vs Implantable Defibrillator Therapy

SCDNT self-care deficit nursing theory

ScDP right scapuloposterior [fetal position, Lat. *scapulodextra posterior*]

SCE secretory carcinoma of the endometrium; serious cardiac event; sister chromatid exchange; split hand-cleft lip/palate ectodermal [dysplasia]; subcutaneous emphysema

SCe somatic cell

SCED single case experimental design

SCEP sandwich counterelectrophoresis; spinal cord evoked potential

SCER sister chromatid exchange rate

SCES subjective computer experience scale

SCETI Stanford Computer-based Educator Training Intervention

SceTy1V *Saccharomyces cerevisiae* Ty1 virus

SceTy2V *Saccharomyces cerevisiae* Ty2 virus

SceTy3V *Saccharomyces cerevisiae* Ty3 virus

SceTy4V *Saccharomyces cerevisiae* Ty4 virus

SceTy5V *Saccharomyces cerevisiae* Ty5 virus

SCF sinusoid containing blood flow; Skin Cancer Foundation; stem cell factor; subcostal frontal [view]

SCFA short-chain fatty acid

SCFE slipped capital femoral epiphysis

SCG scaled conjugate gradient; serum chemistry graft; serum chemogram; sodium cromoglycate; superior cervical ganglion

SCGE single-cell gel electrophoresis

SCH student contact hour; succinylcholine

SCh succinylchloride; succinylcholine

SChE serum cholinesterase

S/CHIP State Children's Health Insurance Program

schiz schizophrenia

SCHL subcapsular hematoma of the liver

SCI Science Citation Index; Scottish Care Information; serial communication interface; spinal cord injury; structured clinical interview

Sci science, scientific

SCID severe combined immunodeficiency [syndrome]; soft copy image display; Structured Clinical Interview for DSM IV [diagnosis]

SCIDS severe combined immunodeficiency syndrome

SCIDX severe combined immunodeficiency disease, X-linked

SCIEH Scottish Centre for Infection and Environmental Health

SCII Strong-Campbell Interest Inventory

SCIM spinal cord injury medicine

SCINT, scint scintigraphy

SCIS spinal cord injury service

SCIU spinal cord injury unit

SCIV subcutaneous intravenous; Subcutaneous vs Intravenous Heparin in Deep Venous Thrombosis [study]

SCIWORA spinal cord injury without radiographic abnormality

SCJ squamocolumnar junction; sternoclavicular joint; sternocostal joint

sCJD sporadic Creutzfeldt-Jakob disease

SCK serum creatine kinase

SCL scleroderma; serum copper level; sinus cycle length; skin conductance level; soft contact lens; stromal cell line; subcostal lateral [view]; symptom checklist; syndrome checklist

SCL-90 symptom checklist 90

scl sclerosis, sclerotic, sclerosed

ScLA left scapuloanterior [fetal position, Lat. *scapulolaeva anterior*]

SCLBCL secondary cutaneous large B-cell lymphoma

SCLC small cell lung carcinoma

SCLD sickle-cell chronic lung disease

SCLE subacute cutaneous lupus erythematosus

scler sclerosis, scleroderma

SCLH subcortical laminar heterotopia

ScLP left scapuloposterior [fetal position, Lat. *scapulolaeva posterior*]

SCL-90-R symptom checklist 90, revised

SCLS systemic capillary leak syndrome

SCM scanning capacitance microscopy; Schwann cell membrane; sensation, circulation, and motion; single chip microcomputer; Society of Computer Medicine; soluble cytotoxic medium; spleen cell-conditioned medium; split cord malformation; spondylitic caudal myelopathy; State Certified Midwife; streptococcal cell membrane; sternocleidomastoid; subclavius muscle; subcutaneous mastectomy; supernumerary marker chromosome; surface-connecting membrane

SCMC spontaneous cell-mediated cytotoxicity

SCMO Senior Clerical Medical Officer

SCN coagulase-negative *Staphylococcus*; severe chronic neutropenia; special care nursing; suprachiasmatic nucleus

SCN1A sodium channel, neuronal alpha-subunit type 1

SCN5A sodium channel gene

SCNS subcutaneous nerve stimulation

SCNT somatic cell nuclear transfer

ScNV-20S *Saccharomyces cerevisiae* narnavirus 20S

ScNV-23S *Saccharomyces cerevisiae* narnavirus 23S

SCO sclerocystic ovary; somatic crossing-over; subcommissural organ

SCOP scopolamine; structural classification of proteins; systematic classification of proteins

SCOPE Scientific Committee on Problems of the Environment; Study of Cognition and Prognosis in the Elderly; Surveillance and Control of Pathogens of Epidemiologic Importance [study]

SCOPEG symmetric, centrally-ordered, phase encoded group [imaging]

SCOPME Standing Committee on Postgraduate Medical and Dental Education [UK]

SCOR Specialized Center for Research [NIH]

SCORES Stent Comparative Restenosis [trial]

SCOT social construction of technology; subcostal [right ventricle] outflow [view]

SCP single-celled protein; smoking cessation program; sodium cellulose phosphate; soluble cytoplasmic protein; specialty care physician; standard care plan; sterol carrier protein; submucous cleft palate; superior cerebral peduncle

scp spherical candle power

SCPE simplified collective protective equipment

SCPK serum creatine phosphokinase

SCPL supracricoid partial laryngectomy

SCPM somatic crossover point mapping

SCPN serum carboxypeptidase N

SCPNT Southern California Postrotary Nystagmus Test

SCPR standard cardiopulmonary resuscitation

S-CPR standard post-compression remodeling

SCPS Skin Cancer Prevention Study

SCPT schizophrenic chronic paranoid type

SCR Schick conversion rate; short consensus repeat; silicon-controlled rectifier; skin conductance response; slow-cycling rhodopsin; spondylitic caudal radiculopathy

SCr, Scr serum creatinine

sCR1 soluble complement receptor type 1

scr scruple

SCRAM speech-controlled respirometer for ambulation measurement

SCRAS Sheehan clinician-rated anxiety scale

SCRF surface coil rotating frame; Systematized Nomenclature in Medicine Cross-Reference Field

SCRIP Stanford Coronary Risk Intervention Project

SCRIPPS Scripps Coronary Radiation to Inhibit Proliferation Post-stenting [trial]

SCRIPT Smoking Cessation-Reduction in Pregnancy Trial

scRNA small cytoplasmic ribonucleic acid

SCRT stereotactic conformation radiotherapy

SCS Saethre-Chotzen syndrome; Seven Country Study; shared computer system; silicon-controlled switch; slow channel syndrome; Society of Clinical Surgery; specialized chromatin structure; spinal canal stenosis; spinal cord stimulation; splatter control shield; splint classification system [American Association of Hand Therapists, ASHT]; synovial chondrosarcoma; systolic click syndrome

SCSA sperm chromatin structure assay; subcostal short axis

SCSB static charge sensitive bed

SCSI small computer system interface

SCSIT Southern California Sensory Integration Test

SCSR standard cervical spine radiography

SCT salmon calcitonin; secretin; Sertoli cell tumor; sex chromatin test; sexual compatibility test; sickle-cell trait; solid cystic tumor; sperm cytotoxicity; spiral computed tomography; spinocervicothalamic; staphylococcal clumping test; star cancellation test; stem cell transplantation; sugar-coated tablet

S-CT spiral computed tomography

S_{CT} serum creatinine

SCTA spiral computed tomography angiography

SCTAT sex cord tumor with annular tubules

SCTN South Carolina Telemedicine Network

SCTR secretin receptor

SCTx spinal cervical traction

SCU self-care unit; special care unit

SCUBA self-contained underwater breathing apparatus

SCUD septicemic cutaneous ulcerative disease

SCUF slow continuous ultrafiltration therapy

SCUP Skin Cancer Utrecht-Philadelphia [Utrecht and Philadelphia study on UVR-caused cancer]

SCU-PA single-chain urokinase plasminogen activator

SCUT schizophrenic chronic undifferentiated type

SCV sensory nerve conduction velocity; smooth, capsulated, virulent; subclavian vein; squamous cell carcinoma of the vulva

ScV *Saccharomyces cerevisiae* virus

ScV-BC *Saccharomyces cerevisiae* virus L-BC

SCV-CPR simultaneous compression ventilation-cardiopulmonary resuscitation

SCVIR Society of Cardiovascular and Interventional Radiology

ScV-L-A *Saccharomyces cerevisiae* virus L-A

SCWM subcortical white matter

SCZ schizophrenia

SD Sandhoff disease; selective decontamination; semi-dry; senile dementia; septal defect; serologically defined; serologically detectable; serologically determined; serum defect; Shine-Dalgarno [sequence]; short dialysis; shoulder disarticulation; Shy-Draper [syndrome]; skin destruction; skin dose; solvent/detergent; somatization disorder; spatial deconvolution; spatial embedding dimension; speech delay; sphincter dilatation; spontaneous delivery; sporadic depression; Sprague-Dawley [rat]; spreading depression; stable disease; standard definition; standard deviation; statistical documentation; Stensen duct; Still disease; stone disintegration; straight drainage; strength duration; streptodornase; structural deterioration; sudden death; superoxide dismutase; synchronous detector; systolic discharge

S-D sickle-cell hemoglobin D; suicide-depression

S/D sharp/dull; Shine-Dalgarno [region]; systolic/diastolic

Sd standard; standard deviation of differences of sample [statistics]; stimulus drive

S^d discriminative stimulus

SDA right sacroanterior [fetal position, Lat. *sacrodextra anterior*]; Sabouraud dextrose agar; serotonin-dopamine antagonist; sialodacryoadenitis; specific dynamic action; strand displacement amplification; structural displacement amplification; succinic dehydrogenase activity

SDAT senile dementia of Alzheimer type; surface digitalization accuracy test

SDAV sialodacryoadenitis virus

SDAVF spinal dural arteriovenous fistula

SDB shared database; sleep-disordered breathing

SDBP seated (or standing, or supine) diastolic blood pressure

SDC serum digoxin concentration; Smith delay compensator; sodium deoxycholate; sodium dichromate; subacute combined degeneration; subclavian hemodialysis catheter; succinyldicholine; syndectan; symptomatic developmental complex

SDCL symptom distress check list

SDCN N-syndectan, neural syndectan

SDD selective decontamination of the digestive tract; Skeletal Dysplasia Diagnostician [database]; sporadic depressive disease; sterile dry dressing

SDDS 2-sulfamoyl-4,4'-diaminodiphenyl-sulfone

SDE simulation development environment; specific dynamic effect; standard-dose epinephrine; structured data entry; subdural empyema

SDEEG sterotactic depth electroencephalography

SDES symptomatic diffuse esophageal spasm

SDF slow death factor; standard data format; stress distribution factor; stromal-derived factor; structured data file

SDFV Syr-Daria Valley virus

SDG sucrose density gradient

SDGF schwannoma-derived growth factor

SDH serine dehydratase; sorbitol dehydrogenase; spinal dorsal horn; subdural hematoma; succinate dehydrogenase

SDHD sudden death heart disease

SDI selective dissemination of information; standard deviation interval; survey diagnostic instrument

SDIF standard generalized markup language document interchange format

SDIHD sudden death ischemic heart disease

SDILINE Selective Dissemination of Information Online [data bank]

SDIS Stockholm Diabetes Intervention Study

SDL serum digoxin level; speech discrimination level

sdl sideline; subline

SDM semantic data model; sensory detection method; sparse distributed memory; standard deviation of the mean; system of decision making; system development method; Systematized Nomenclature in Medicine [SNOMED] Digital Imaging and Communications in Medicine [DICOM] Microglossary

SDMD sulfadimethoxine

SDMS Society of Diagnostic Medical Sonographers

SDN sexually dimorphic nucleus

SDNF sliding discrete Fourier transform narrow band filter

SDNV Serra do Navio virus

SDO standards development organization; sudden dosage onset

SDP right sacroposterior [fetal position, Lat. *sacrodextra posterior*]; shared decision-making program; signal density plot

SDR shared data research; Skeletal Dysplasia Registry; spontaneously diabetic rat; standardized disease ratio; surgical dressing room

SDRI small, deep, recent infarct

SDRS social dysfunction rating scale

SDS same day surgery; school dental services; selective digestive decontamination; self-rating depression scale; sensory deprivation syndrome; sexual differentiation scale; short depression screen; Shy-Drager syndrome; single-dose suppression; sodium dodecylsulfate; specific diagnosis service; squamous [cell carcinoma] dataset; standard deviation score; sudden death syndrome; sulfadiazine silver; sustained depolarizing shift

SDSEM spinocerebellar degeneration-slow eye movements [syndrome]

SD-SK streptodornase-streptokinase

SDSL symmetrical digital single line

SDS/PAGE, SDS-PGE sodium dodecylsulfate–polyacrylamide gel electrophoresis

SDT sensory detection theory; right sacrotransverse [fetal position, Lat. *sacrodextra transversa*]; signal detection theory; single-donor transfusion; speech detection threshold

SD-T spatial deconvolution transformation

SD$_t$ standard deviation of total scores

SDU standard deviation unit; step-down unit

SDUB short double upright brace

SDW spin density-weighted; system development workbench

SDYS Simpson dysmorphia syndrome

SE saline enema; sanitary engineering; self efficacy; serum; Shannon entropy; side effect; sleep efficiency; smoke exposure; socio-economic; solid extract; sphenoethmoidal; spherical equivalent; spin-echo; spongiform encephalopathy; Spurway-Eddowes [syndrome]; standard error; staphylococcal endotoxin; staphylococcal enterotoxin; starch equivalent; Starr-Edwards [prosthesis]; status epilepticus; subclinical encephalopathy; subendothelial; subependymal nodule; sulfoethyl; systematic error

S&E safety and efficiency

S-E socio-economic; spin-echo [imaging]; substantial equivalence

Se secretion; selenium

S$_e$ external skeleton

SE early systolic wave

SEA sheep erythrocyte agglutination; shock-elicited aggression; soluble egg antigen; spatial envelope area; spinal epidural abscess; spontaneous electrical activity; staphylococcal enterotoxin A

SEAC Spongiform Encephalopathy Advisory Committee

SEADS Self-Efficacy and Dyspnea Strategies Scale

SEADS-C Self-Efficacy and Dyspnea Strategies-Confidence [subscale]

SEAL steric and electrostatic alignment

SEAP secreted alkaline phosphatase

SEARCH Study of the Effectiveness of Additional Reductions of Cholesterol and Homocysteine

SEAT sheep erythrocyte agglutination test

SEB seborrhea; staphylococcal enterotoxin B

SE(b) standard error of regression coefficient [statistics]

SEBA staphylococcal enterotoxin B antiserum

SEBI stereotactic external beam irradiation

SEBL self-emptying blind loop

SEBM Society of Experimental Biology and Medicine

SEBOV Sudan Ebola virus

SEC screening end-code; secretin; *S*-ethylcysteine; Singapore epidemic conjunctivitis; size-exclusion chromatography; soft elastic capsule; spontaneous echo contrast [echocardiography]; swollen endothelial cell

Sec Seconal; selenocysteine

sec second; secondary; section

sec-Bu sec-butyl

SeCD service for the care of drug addicts

SECG stress electrocardiography

SECON sequential continuity

SECORDS South-Eastern Consortium on Racial Differences in Stroke

SECRET stiffness of joint, elderly individuals, constitutional symptoms, arthritis, elevated erythrocyte sedimentation rate, temporal arthritis [in polymyalgia rheumatica]

SECSY spin echo correlated spectroscopy

sect section

SECURE Study to Evaluate Carotid Ultrasound Changes with Ramipril and Vitamin E

SED sedimentation rate; skin erythema dose; standard erythema dose; spondyloepiphyseal dysplasia; standard error of deviation; staphylococcal enterotoxin D

sed sedimentation; stool [Lat. *sedes*]

SEDL spondyloepiphyseal dysplasia, late

sed rt sedimentation rate

SEDT spondyloepiphyseal dysplasia tarda

SEDT-PA spondyloepiphyseal dysplasia tarda-progressive arthropathy

SEE standard error of estimate; staphylococcal enterotoxin E

SEEG stereotactic electroencephalography

SEER Surveillance Epidemiology and End Results [program of the National Cancer Institute]

SEF somatosensory evoked magnetic field; spectral edge frequency; staphylococcal enterotoxin F; structured encounter form; suction effusion fluid

SEG segment; soft elastic gelatin; sonoencephalogram

segm segment, segmented

SEGNE secretory granules of neural and endocrine [cells]

Se-GSH-Px selenium cofactor for glutathione peroxidase

SEH spinal epidural hemorrhage; subependymal hemorrhage

SEI Self-Esteem Inventory

S-EIA stick-enzyme immunoassay

SEISMED secure environment for information system in medicine

SE/IVH subependymal/intraventricular hemorrhage

SEL serum ethanol level

SELCA Smooth Excimer Laser Coronary Angioplasty [study]

SELDI surface-enhanced laser desorption ionization [mass spectrometry]

SELDI-TOF surface-enhanced laser desorption-ionization time of flight [mass spectrometry]

SELEX systemic evolution of ligands by experimental enrichment

SELF Self-Evaluation of Life Function [scale]

Sel Pt select patients

SELV Seletar virus

SEM sample evaluation method; scanning electron microphotography; scanning electron microscopy; secondary enrichment medium; standard error of measurement; standard error of the mean; stochastic expectation-maximization [algorithm]; structural equation modeling; systolic ejection murmur

sem half [Lat. *semis*]; semen, seminal

SEMD spondyloepimetaphyseal dysplasia

SEMDIT spondyloepimetaphyseal dysplasia, Irapa type

SEMDJL spondyloepimetaphyseal dysplasia with joint laxity

Semf seminal fluid

SEMG semenogelin; surface electromyography

sEMG surface electromyography

SEMI subendocardial myocardial infarction; subendocardial myocardial injury

SemNet semantic network [UMLS]

SEMSOB Stanford Self-Efficacy for Managing Shortness of Breath

SEN scalp-ear-nipple [syndrome]; State Enrolled Nurse

sen sensitive, sensitivity

SENDCAP St. Mary's Ealing, Northwick Park Diabetes Cardiovascular Prevention [study]

SENIC Study of the Efficacy of Nosocomial Infection Control

SENS sensitivity or sensitization; Stewart evaluation of nursing scale

Sens sensitivity

sens sensation, sensorium, sensory

SENSOR Sentinel Event Notification System for Occupational Risks

SENTAC Society for ENT [ear, nose, throat] Advances in Children

SEOV Seoul virus

SEP self-evaluation process; sensory-evoked potential; separation [of ghosts]; septum; somatosensory evoked potential; sperm entry point; spinal evoked potential; standard error of prediction; surface epithelium; syringe exchange program; systolic ejection period

sEP single evoked potential

separ separately, separation

SE(p1–p2) standard error of the difference of two proportions [statistics]

SEPS subfascial endoscopic perforate ligation; Submaximal Exercise Performance Substudy

SEPT septum

SEPV Sepik virus

SEQ side effects questionnaire

seq sequence; sequel, sequela, sequelae; sequestrum

SEQOL [Bypass Angioplasty Revascularization Investigation] Substudy of Economics and Quality of Life

SER sarcoplasmic/endoplasmic reticulum; sebum excretion rate; sensitizer enhancement ratio; sensory evoked response; service; smooth endoplasmic reticulum; smooth-surface endoplasmic reticulum; somatosensory evoked response; subendocardial resection; supination, external rotation [fracture]; surgical emergency room; systolic ejection rate

S/ER sero/endoplasmic reticulum

Ser serine; serology; serous; service

sER smooth endoplasmic reticulum

ser series, serial; serine

SERC State Emergency Response Commission

SERCA2 sarcoplasmic/endoplasmic reticulum Ca^{2-}

SerCl serum chloride

SERHOLD National Biomedical Serials Holding Database

SER-IV supination external rotation, type 4 fracture

SERLINE Serials Online [NLM database]

SERM selective estrogen receptor modulator

sero, serol serological, serology

SERPIN serpine protease inhibitor

SERS Stimulus Evaluation/Response Selection [test]

SERT sustained ethanol release tube

serv keep, preserve [Lat. *serva*]; service

SERVHEL Service and Health Records

SES Society of Eye Surgeons; socioeconomic status; spatial emotional stimulus; sphenoethmoidal suture; subendothelial space

SESAM Study in Europe of Saruplase and Alteplase in Myocardial Infarction

SESAP Surgical Educational and Self-Assessment Program

SESE somatosensory evoked spike epilepsy

SET secure electronic transaction; single electron transistor; surrogate embryo transfer; systolic ejection time

SET-N software evaluation tool for nursing

SETTS subjective experience of therapeutic touch survey

SEV 1–18, 125, 203 Simian enterovirus 1–18, 125, 203

SeV Sendai virus

sev severe; severed

SEW slice excitation wave

SEWHO shoulder-elbow-wrist-hand orthosis

SE(x) standard error of the mean [statistics]

SF Sabin-Feldman [test]; safety factor; salt-free; scarlet fever; scatter factor; screen film; seminal fluid; serosal fluid; serum factor; serum ferritin; serum fibrinogen; sham feeding; shell fragment; shunt flow; sickle cell-hemoglobin F [disease]; simian foam-virus; skin fibroblast; skinfold; soft feces; spinal fluid; spontaneous fibrillation; stable factor; Steel factor; sterile female; steroidogenic factor; stress formula; sugar-free; superior facet; suppressor factor; suprasternal fossa; surviving fraction; Svedberg flotation [unit]; swine fever; symptom-free; synovial fluid

S1F Steel factor

SF-36 short-form health survey [36 items]

Sf spinal fluid; *Streptococcus faecalis*

Sf Svedberg flotation unit

SFA saturated fatty acid; seminal fluid assay; serum folic acid; skinfold anthropometry; stimulated fibrinolytic activity; superior femoral artery

SFAP single-fiber action potential

SFB Sanfilippo syndrome type B; saphenofemoral bypass; surgical foreign body

SFBL self-filling blind loop

SFC soluble fibrin complex; soluble fibrin-fibrinogen complex; spinal fluid count

SFCP Stanford Five City Project

SFD silo filler's disease; skin-film distance; small for dates; source-film distance; spectral frequency distribution

SFE slipped femoral epiphysis

SFEMG single fiber electromyography

SFFA serum free fatty acid

SFFF sedimentation field flow fractionation

SFFV spleen focus-forming virus

SFG spotted fever group; subglottic foreign body

SFH schizophrenia family history; serum-free hemoglobin; stroma-free hemoglobin

SF/HGF scatter factor/hepatocyte growth factor

SFI Sexual Function Index; Social Function Index

SFIS structural family interaction scale

SFJT saphenofemoral junction thrombophlebitis

SFL scalar fuzzy logic; synovial fluid lymphocyte

SFM scanning force microscopy; Schimmelpenning-Fuerstein-Mims [syndrome]; self-fitting face mask; serum-free medium; solution-focused management; streptozocin, 5-fluorouracil, and mitomycin C

SFMC soluble fibrin monomer complex

SFMS Smith-Fineman-Myers syndrome

SFNM standard finite normal mixture

SFNV Sabin virus; Sandfly fever Naples virus

SFO subfornical organ

SFP screen filtration pressure; simultaneous foveal perception; spinal fluid pressure; stopped flow pressure

SFR screen filtration resistance; stenosis flow reserve; stroke with full recovery

SFS serial foveal seizures; skin and fascia stapler; social functioning schedule; sodium formaldehydesulfoxylate; spatial frequency spectrum; split function study

SFSV Sandfly fever Sicilian virus

SFT Sabin-Feldman test; second field tumor; sensory feedback therapy; skinfold thickness

SFTP secure file transfer protocol [telemedicine]

SFU surgical follow-up

SFV Semliki Forest virus; shipping fever virus; Shope fibroma virus; simian foamy virus; squirrel fibroma virus; swine fever virus

SFV 1, 3 simian foamy virus 1, 3

SFW sexual function of women; shell fragment wound; slow-filling wave

SG Sachs-Georgi [test]; salivary gland; serum globulin; serum glucose; signs; skin graft; soluble gelatin; specific gravity; subgluteal; substantia gelatinosa; succinimidyl glutamate; Surgeon General

sg specific gravity; subgenomic

SGA small for gestational age

sGAG sulfated glycosaminoglycan

SGAP superior gluteal artery perforator [flap]

SG$_{AW}$ specific airway conductance

SGB Simpson-Golabi-Behmel [syndrome]; sparsely granulated basophil

SGBS Simpson-Golabi-Behmel syndrome

SGC soluble guanylate cyclase; spermicide-germicide compound; Swan-Ganz catheter

SGCA subependymal giant cell astrocytoma

SGCRC German Study Group on Colo-Rectal Carcinoma

SGD *Saccharomyces* Genome Database; specific granule deficiency

SGE secondary generalized epilepsy

SGF sarcoma growth factor; skeletal growth factor

SGH subgluteal hematoma

SGL salivary gland lymphocyte; supraglottic laryngectomy

sgl sugarless

SGLD spatial gray level dependence

SGLT sodium-dependent glucose transporter

SGM Society for General Microbiology

SGML standard generalized markup language

SGNE secretory granule neuroendocrine [protein]

SGO Surgeon General's Office; surgery, gynecology, and obstetrics

SGOT serum glutamate oxaloacetate transaminase (aspartate aminotransferase)

SGP scaled gradient projection [radiotherapy]; serine glycerophosphatide; sialoglycoprotein; Society of General Physiologists; soluble glycoprotein; sulfated glycoprotein

SGPA salivary gland pleomorphic adenoma

SGPT serum glutamate pyruvate transaminase (alanine aminotransferase)

SGR Sachs-Georgi reaction; Shwartzman generalized reaction; skin galvanic reflex; submandibular gland renin; substantia gelatinosa Rolandi

sgRNA subgenomic ribonucleic acid [RNA]

SGS Schinzel-Giedion syndrome

SGSG Scandinavian Glioma Study Group

S-Gt Sachs-Georgi test

SGTT standard glucose tolerance test

SGTX surugatoxin; *Scodra griseipes* toxin

SGV salivary gland virus; selective gastric vagotomy; short gastric vessel

SGVHD syngeneic graft-versus-host disease

SH Salter-Harris [fracture]; Schönlein-Henoch [purpura]; self-help; serum hepatitis; sexual harassment; sex hormone; Sherman [rat]; sick in hospital; sinus histiocytosis; social history; somatotropic hormone; spontaneously hypertensive [rat]; standard heparin; state hospital; sulfhydryl; surgical history; symptomatic hypoglycemia; syndrome of hyporeninemic hypoaldosteronism; systemic hyperthermia

S/H sample and hold

S&H speech and hearing

Sh sheep; Sherwood number; *Shigella*; shoulder

sh shoulder

SHA secure hashing algorithm; simple highest avidity; Southern hybridization analysis; staphylococcal hemagglutinating antibody; strategic hospital alliance

sHa suckling hamster

SHAA serum hepatitis associated antigen; Society of Hearing Aid Audiologists

SHAA-Ab serum hepatitis associated antigen antibody

SHAFT sad, hostile, anxious, frustrating, tenacious [patient]

SHAp stoichiometric hydroxyapatite

SHAPE Screening Health Assessment and Preventive Education [program]; Stress, Health and Physical Evaluation [program]; Study of Heparin and Actilyse Processed Electronically

SHARE source of help in airing and resolving experiences; Study of Heart Assessment and Risk in Ethnic Groups

SHARK Stroke, Hypertension and Recurrence in Kyushu [study]

SHARP school health additional referral program; Scottish Heart and Arterial Disease Risk Prevention [program]; Subcutaneous Heparin in Angioplasty Restenosis Prevention [trial]

SHAV Shamonda virus

SHAVE Steerable Housing for Atherovascular Excision

SHB sequential hemibody [irradiation]

S-Hb sulfhemoglobin

SHBD serum hydroxybutyric dehydrogenase

SHBG sex hormone binding globulin

SHC self-help class

SHCC State Health Coordinating Council

SHCO sulfated hydrogenated castor oil

SHD satellite hemodialysis [telemedicine]; sudden heart death

SHE Syrian hamster embryo

SHEA Society for Hospital Epidemiology of America

SHEENT skin, head, eyes, ears, nose, and throat

SHEP Systolic Hypertension in the Elderly Program

SHF simian hemorrhagic fever; subfulminant hepatic failure; superhigh frequency

shf super-high frequency

SHFD split hand/foot deformity

ShFM shear force microscopy

SHFV Simian hemorrhagic fever virus

SHG sonohysterography; synthetic human gastrin

SHH sonic hedgehog [gene]; syndrome of hyporeninemic hypoaldosternonism

Shh sonic hedgehog

SHHD Scottish Home and Health Department

SHHH self-help for hard of hearing

SHHS Scottish Heart Health Study; Sleep Heart Health Study

SHHV Society for Health and Human Values

SHI severe head injury
Shig *Shigella*
SHIN skilled home health nursing
SHINE Strategic Health Informatics Network in Europe
SHIPS Shiga Pravastatin Study
SHIV Shiant Islands virus
SHL sensorineural hearing loss
SHLA soluble human lymphocyte antigen
SHLD shoulder
SHML sinus histiocytosis with massive lymphadenopathy
SHMO Senior Hospital Medical Officer
SHMO, S/HMO social health maintenance organization
SHMT serine-hydroxymethyl transferase
SHN spontaneous hemorrhagic necrosis; subacute hepatic necrosis
SHO secondary hypertrophic osteoarthropathy; Senior House Officer; simple harmonic oscillator
SHOCK Should We Emergently Revascularize Occluded Coronaries for Cardiogenic Shock? [international randomized trial]
SHOP State Hospital Data Project
SHORT, S-H-O-R-T short stature, hyperextensibility of joints or hernia or both, ocular depression, Rieger anomaly, teething delayed
short-FRAME short stature-facial anomalies-Rieger anomaly-midline anomalies-enamel defects [syndrome]
SHOT serious hazards of transfusion; Shunt Occlusion Trial
SHOV Shokwe virus
SHP Schönlein-Henoch purpura; secondary hyperparathyroidism; Skaraborg Hypertension Project; state health plan
SHPDA State Health Planning and Development Agency
sHPT secondary hyperparathyroidism
SHR spontaneously hypertensive rat
SHRED Sedatives and Hemodynamics During Rapid-Sequence Intubation in the Emergency Department [trial]
SHRS scanned handwritten record system
SHRSP stroke-prone spontaneously hypertensive rat
SHS Sayre head sling; sheep hemolysate supernatant; Strong Heart Study; Sutterland-Haan syndrome
SHSF split hand-split foot [malformation]

SHSP spontaneously hypertensive stroke-prone [rat]
SHSS Stanford Hypnotic Susceptibility Scale
SHT simple hypocalcemic tetany; subcutaneous histamine test
SHTTP secure hypertext transport protocol
SHUA System for Hospital Uniform Accounting
SHUR System for Hospital Uniform Reporting
SHUV Shuni virus
SHV simian herpes virus; Southampton virus
SHVRC Shiley Heart Valve Research Center [project]
SI International System of Units [Fr. *Système International d'Unités*]; sacroiliac; saline infusion; saline injection; saturation index; self-inflicted; sensory integration; septic inflammation; serious illness; serum iron; severity index; sex inventory; shock index; signal intensity; Singh Index; single injection; sinus irregularities; small intestine; social interaction; soluble insulin; special intervention; spirochetosis icterohaemorrhagica; stability index; stimulation index; stress incontinence; stroke index; structured interview; sucrase isomaltase; sulfoxidation index; superior-inferior; suppression index; syncytium-inducer
S/I superior/inferior
S&I suction and irrigation
Si the most anterior point on the lower contour of the sella turcica [point]; silicon
SIA serum inhibitory activity; small intestine atresia; stress-induced analgesia; stress-induced anesthesia; stretch-induced arrhythmia; subacute infectious arthritis
SIADH syndrome of inappropriate secretion of antidiuretic hormone
SIAM Streptokinase in Acute Myocardial Infarction [study]
SIB self-inflating bulb; self-injurious behavior; sibling in semantic hierarchy [UMLS]; Swiss Institute for Bioinformatics
sib, sibs sibling, siblings
SIB X, SIB$_X$ extended siblings in semantic hierarchy [UMLS]

SIC serum insulin concentration; Standard Industrial Classification

SICCO Stenting in Chronic Coronary Occlusion [study]

SICD serum isocitrate dehydrogenase

SICU spinal intensive care unit; surgical intensive care unit

SID focal spot to imaging-plane distance; selective intestinal decontamination; single intradermal [test]; Society for Investigative Dermatology; source-image distance; source-isocenter distance; standard imaging display; state inpatient database; stress-induced [heart] depolarization; strong ion difference; sucrase-isomaltase deficiency; sudden inexplicable death; sudden infant death; suggested indication of diagnosis; systemic inflammatory disease

SIDAM Structured Interview for the Diagnosis of Dementia of the Alzheimer Type, Multiinfarct Dementia, and Dementias of Other Etiology

SIDS sudden infant death syndrome; sulfo-iduronate sulfatase

SIE sis-inducible element; stroke in evolution

SIEA superficial inferior epigastric artery

SIEB Systematized Nomenclature of Medicine [SNOMED] International Editorial Board

SIECUS Sex Information and Education Council of the United States

SIESTA Snooze-induced Excitation of Sympathetically Triggered Activity [study]

SIF sacral insufficiency fracture; serum-inhibition factor

SIFT selector ion flow tube

SIG small inducible gene

SIg, sIg surface immunoglobulin

sig sigmoidoscopy; significant

SIgA, S-IgA secretory immunoglobulin A

SIGH-D Structured Interview for the Hamilton Depression Scale

SIgM, S-IgM secretory immunoglobulin M

SigInt signal intelligence

Σ Greek capital letter *sigma*; syphilis; summation of series

σ Greek lowercase letter *sigma*; conductivity; cross section; millisecond; molecular type or bond; population standard deviation; stress; surface tension; wave number

SIGMAV Sigma virus

sigmo sigmoidoscope or sigmoidoscopy

SIGN Scottish Intercollegiate Guideline Network

SIH stimulation-induced hypalgesia; stress-induced hyperthermia; suction-induced hypoxemia

SIHDSPS Stockholm Ischemic Heart Disease Secondary Prevention Study

SIHE spontaneous intramural hematoma of the esophagus

SI-HRDS structured interview Hamilton rating scale for depression

SII self-inflicted injury

SIJ sacroiliac joint

SIL soluble interleukin; speech interference level; squamous intraepithelial lesion

SILD Sequenced Inventory of Language Development

SIM selected ion monitoring; small intestine mesentery; Society of Industrial Microbiology; specialized intestinal metaplasia; subscriber identity module [telemedicine]

SIMA single internal mammary artery; Stenting vs Internal Mammary Artery for Single Left Anterior Descending Arterial Lesion [trial]

SIMD single instruction multiple data

SIMP Schmele instrument to measure the process of nursing care; simulation of initial medical problem

SIMP-C Schmele instrument to measure the process of nursing care

SIMP-H Schmele instrument to measure the process of nursing care in home care

SIMPLE symbolic interactive modeling package and learning environment

SIMS secondary ion mass spectroscopy; situational information management system

simul simultaneously

SIMV Simbu virus; synchronized intermittent mandatory ventilation; synchronized intermittent mechanical ventilation

SIN salpingitis isthmica nodosa; self-inactivating; Sindbis [virus]

SINE short interspersed element [gene coding]

SIN-FM Short Indexed Nomenclature-Family Medicine

SINS Semi-Structured Intelligent Navigation System

SINV Sindbis virus
SIO sacroiliac orthosis
SIOP International Society of Pediatric Oncology
SIP saturation inversion projection; Short Inventory of Problems; Sickness Impact Profile; slow inhibitory potential; stroke in progression; summarized intensity projection [computer-assisted radiography]; surface inductive plethysmography
SIPA shear-induced platelet aggregation
SIPS Strategy for Intracoronary Ultrasound-guided Percutaneous Transluminal Coronary Angioplasty and Stenting [trial]
sIPTH serum immunoreactive parathyroid hormone
SIQ Symptom Interpretation Questionnaire
SIQR semi-interquartile range
SIR short intergenic region; single isomorphous replacement; specific immune release; standardized incidence ratio; stroke index ratio; syndrome of immediate reactivities
SIRA Scientific Instrument Research Association
SIRE short interspersed repetitive element
SIREF specific immune response enhancing factor
SIRF severely impaired renal function; significant intrarenal fragments
SIRIS sputter-initiated resonance ionization spectroscopy
SIRS soluble immune response suppressor; Structured Interview of Reported Symptoms; systemic inflammatory response syndrome
SiRV simian rotavirus
SiRV-SA11 simian rotavirus SA11
SIS semantic indexing system; serotonin irritation syndrome; simian sarcoma; simulator-induced syndrome; small intestinal submucosa; social information system; specialized information system; spontaneous interictal spike; sterile injectable solution; sterile injectable suspension; supplemental information seeking; Surgical Infections Society; surgical information system
SISA Stenting in Small Arteries [trial]
SISAMI Silent Ischemia in Survivors of Acute Myocardial Infarction [study]

SISCOM subtraction ictal single proton emission computed tomography coregistered to magnetic resonance imaging [MRI]
SISH Stage I Systolic Hypertension in the Elderly [study]
SISI short increment sensitivity index
SISO single input single output
SISS Sentinel Injury Surveillance System [for Gunshot and Stab Wounds]; small inducible secreted substances
SISTEMI Southern Italian Study on Thrombolysis Early in Myocardial Infarction
SISV, SiSV simian sarcoma virus
SIT serum inhibiting titer; sit down; Slosson Intelligence Test; specific immunotherapy; sperm immobilization test; strategic intermittent therapy; suggested immobilization test
SITHS Swedish Secure Internet Within Healthcare
SITS supraspinatus, infraspinatus, teres minor, subscapularis [shoulder muscles comprising the rotator cuff]
SIV simian immunodeficiency virus; Sprague-Dawley-Ivanovas [rat]
SIV-agm simian immunodeficiency virus African green monkey
SIV-agm.3 simian immunodeficiency virus African green monkey 3
SIV-agm.155 simian immunodeficiency virus African green monkey 155
SIV-agm.gr simian immunodeficiency virus African green monkey gr-1
SIV-agm.sab simian immunodeficiency virus African green monkey Sab 1
SIV-agm.tan simian immunodeficiency virus African green monkey Tan 1
SIV-agm.TYO simian immunodeficiency virus African green monkey TYO
SIV-cpz simian immunodeficiency virus chimpanzee
SIV-mac simian immunodeficiency virus rhesus *(Maccaca mulatta)*
SIV-mnd simian immunodeficiency virus mandrill
SIV-mne simian immunodeficiency virus pig-tailed macaque
SIV-rcm simian immunodeficiency virus red capped mangabey
SIV-sm simian immunodeficiency virus sooty mangabey

SIV-stm simian immunodeficiency virus stump-tailed macaque

SIV-syk simian immunodeficiency virus Sykes monkey

SIW self-inflicted wound

SIWIP self-induced water intoxication and psychosis

SIWIS self-induced water intoxication and schizophrenic disorders

S$_J$ Jaccard coefficient

SJA Schwartz-Jampel-Aberfeld [syndrome]

SJAV Sandjimba virus

S$_{jb}$O$_2$ jugular bulb venous oxygen saturation

SjO$_2$ jugular vein oxygen saturation

SJR Shinowara-Jones-Reinhart [unit]

SJS Schwartz-Jampel syndrome; Stevens-Johnson syndrome; stiff joint syndrome; Swyer-James syndrome

SjS Sjögren syndrome

SJV San Juan virus

SjVO$_2$ jugular venous oxygen saturation

SK seborrheic keratosis; senile keratosis; Sloan-Kettering [Institute for Cancer Research]; spontaneous killer [cell]; squamous keratin; state of knowledge; streptokinase; swine kidney

Sk skin

SKA supracondylar knee-ankle [orthosis]

SKALP skin-derived antileukoproteinase

SKAT Sex Knowledge and Attitude Test

SKDAMI Streptokinase plus Desmopressin in Acute Myocardial Infarction [study]

skel skeleton, skeletal

SKHYDIP Skara Hypertension and Diabetes Project

SKI Sloan-Kettering Institute

SKL serum killing level

SkM skeletal muscle

SKR semantic knowledge representation

SKSD, SK-SD streptokinase-streptodornase

SKT skin temperature

sk trx skeletal traction

SKY spectral karyotyping

SL sarcolemma; scapholunar, scapholunate; sclerosing leukoencephalopathy; secondary leukemia; segment length; sensation level; sensory latency; septal leaflet; short-leg [brace]; Sibley-Lehninger [unit]; signal level; Sinding-Larsen [syndrome]; Sjögren-Larsson [syndrome]; slit lamp; small lymphocyte; sodium lactate; solidified liquid; sound level; SPECIALIST Lexicon [UMLS]; Stein-Leventhal [syndrome]; streptolysin; sublingual; sway length

S$_L$ systolic wave, latent

S/L sublingual

Sl Steel [mouse]

sl in a broad sense [Lat. *sensu lato*]; stemline; sublingual

SLA left sacroanterior [fetal position, Lat. *sacrolaeva anterior*]; single-cell liquid cytotoxic assay; slide latex agglutination; soluble liver antigen; stereo lithography; superficial linear array; surfactant-like activity

SL$_A$ segment length, anterior

SLAC scapholunate advanced collapse [wrist]

SLAM scanning laser acoustic microscope; systemic lupus erythematosus activity measure

SLAP serum leucine aminopeptidase; superior labrum anterior to posterior

SLAT simultaneous laryngoscopy and abdominal thrusts

SLB short-leg brace

SLBP stem-loop binding protein

SLC short-leg cast

SLCC short-leg cylinder cast

SLCISC Salt Lake City Information Service Center [VA]

SLD scapholunar dissociation; sublethal damage

SLD, SLDH serum lactate dehydrogenase

SLDR sublethal damage repair

SLE slit lamp examination; St. Louis encephalitis; systemic lupus erythematosus

SLEA sheep erythrocyte antibody

SLEDAI systemic lupus erythematosus disease activity index

SLEP short latent evoked potential

sLex sialyl Lewis x

SLEV St. Louis encephalitis virus

SLF steel factor

SL-GXT symptom-limited graded exercise test

SLHR sex-linked hypophosphatemic rickets

SLHT straight line Hough transform

SLI selective lymphoid irradiation; somatostatin-like immunoreactivity; specific language impairment; splenic localization index

SL₁ segment length, inferior

SLIC scanning liquid ionization chamber; Scottish Library and Information Council

SLIDRC Student Loan Interest Deduction Restoration Coalition

SLIP serial line interface protocol; sliding linear investigative platform [for analysis of lower limb stability]

SLIR somatostatin-like immunoreactivity

SLJD Sinding-Larsen-Johanssen disease

SLK superior limbic keratoconjunctivitis

SLKC superior limbic keratoconjunctivitis

SLL small lymphocytic lymphoma

SL_L segment length, lateral

SLM sound level meter

SLMC spontaneous lymphocyte-mediated cytotoxicity

SLN sentinel lymph node; sublentiform nucleus; superior laryngeal nerve; SYBYL line notation

SLNV Saintpaulia leaf necrosis virus

SLNWBC short-leg nonweightbearing cast

SLNWC short-leg nonwalking cast

SLO scanning laser ophthalmoscopy; Smith-Lemli-Opitz syndrome; streptolysin O

SLOS Smith-Lemli-Opitz syndrome

S-LOST sulfur mustard, for Lommel and Steinkopf

SLP left sacroposterior [fetal position, Lat. *sacrolaeva posterior*]; segmental limb systolic pressure; sex-limited protein; single locus probe; short luteal phase; speech language pathologist; subluxation of the patella

slp sex-limited protein

SLPI salivary leukocyte protease inhibitor; secretory leukocyte protease inhibitor

SLPP serum lipophosphoprotein

SLR Shwartzman local reaction; single lens reflex; stent-like result; straight leg raising

SLRROM shoulder lateral rotation range of motion

SLRT straight leg raising test

SLS Seattle Longitudinal Study; segment long-spacing; short-leg splint; single leg separation; single limb support; Sjögren-Larsson syndrome; sodium lauryl phosphate; stagnant loop syndrome; Stein-Leventhal syndrome; synthetic lethal screening

SL_S segment length, septal

SLT left sacrotransverse [fetal position, Lat. *sacrolaeva transversa*]; single lumen tube; single lung transplantation; smokeless tobacco; solid logic technology

SLTEC/VTEC Shigella-like toxin (verotoxin) producing *Escherichia coli*

SLUD salivation, lacrimation, urination, defecation

SLUDGE salivation, lacrimation, urination, defecation, gastrointestinal upset, emesis

SLV semilatent virus; symptomless virus

SLVDS San Luis Valley Diabetes Study

SLWC short-leg walking cast

SM Master of Science [L. *Scientiae Magister*]; sadomasochism; segmental mastectomy; self-monitoring; sensitivity matrix; serum; silicon microphysiometer; simple mastectomy; skim milk; smooth muscle; somatomedin; space medicine; sphingomyelin; splenic macrophage; splenomegaly; sports medicine; storage manager [database module]; streptomycin; Strümpell-Marie [syndrome]; submandibular; submaxillary; submucous; suckling mouse; sucrose medium; suction method; sulfomethyl; superior mesenteric; surgical microscope; surrogate mother; sustained medication; symptoms; synaptic membrane; synovial membrane; systolic motion; systolic murmur

S/M sadomasochism

Sm samarium; *Serratia marcescens*; Smith [antigen]

sM small membrane [protein]; suckling mouse

sm smear

SMA sequential multichannel autoanalyzer; shape memory alloy; simultaneous multichannel autoanalyzer; smooth muscle antibody; Society for Medical Anthropology; somatomedin A; spinal muscular atrophy; spontaneous motor activity; standard method agar; superior mesenteric artery; supplementary motor area; symptomatic morphologic anomaly

SM-A somatomedin A

SMA-6 Sequential Multiple Analysis for six different serum tests

SMABF superior mesenteric artery blood flow

SMAC Sequential Multiple Analyzer Computer

SMAE superior mesenteric artery embolism

SMAF smooth muscle activating factor; specific macrophage arming factor

SMAG Special Medical Advisory Group

SMAL serum methyl alcohol level

sm an small animal

SMAO superior mesenteric artery occlusion

SMAP systemic mean arterial pressure

SMART Self-measurement for Assessment of the Response to Trandolapril [study]; semantic adaptive resonance theory; simultaneous multiple angle reconstruction technique; small volume multiple noncoplanar arc radiotherapy; sperm microaspiration retrieval technique; Study of Medicine vs Angioplasty Reperfusion Trial; Study of Microstent's Ability to Limit Restenosis Trial

SMARTT Serum Markers, Acute Myocardial Infarction, and Rapid Treatment Trial

SMAS submuscular aponeurotic system; superficial musculo-aponeurotic system; superior mesenteric artery syndrome

SMASH Swiss Multicenter Evaluation of Early Angioplasty for Shock [following myocardial infarction]; Sydney Men and Sexual Health [study]

SMAST Short Michigan Alcoholism Screening Test

SMATS Seek Medical Attention in Time Study

SMB selected mucosal biopsy; standard mineral base

sMb suckling mouse brain

SMBFT small bowel follow-through

SMBG self-monitoring of blood glucose

SMC Scientific Manpower Commission; smooth muscle cell; somatomedin C; succinylmonocholine; supernumerary marker chromosome; suture-mediated closure

SM-C, Sm-C somatomedin C

SMCA smooth muscle contracting agent; suckling mouse cataract agent

SMCC succininamidyl-4-(N-maleimidomethyl)cyclohexane-1-carboxylate

SMCD senile macular choroidal degeneration; systemic mast cell disease; systemic meningococcal disease

SM-C/IGF somatomedin C/insulin-like growth factor

SMCR Smith-Magenis chromosome region; 5-sulfoxymethylchrysene

SmCS smart classification

SMD senile macular degeneration; severe mental disorder; spondylometaphyseal dysplasia; submanubrial dullness

SMDA Safe Medical Devices Act [of 1990]; starch methylenedianiline

SMDC sodium-N-methyl dithiocarbamate; standards for medical device communication

SMDM Society for Medical Decision Making

SMDP semi-Markov decision process

SMDS secondary myelodysplastic syndrome; switched multimegabit data service

SME severe myoclonic epilepsy

SMED spondylometaphyseal dysplasia

SMEDI stillbirth-mummification, embryonic death, infertility [syndrome]

SMEI severe myoclonic epilepsy of infancy

SMEM supplemented Eagle minimum essential medium

SMF selected minerals in food; streptozocin, mitomycin C, and 5-fluorouracil; submembrane region containing thrombosthenin filaments; substructural molecular fragment

smf sodium motive force

SMFM shear modulation force microscopy

SMFP state medical facilities plan

SMG specialty medical group; submandibular gland

SmG supramarginal gyrus

SMH state mental hospital; strongyloidiasis with massive hyperinfection

SMHA state mental health agency

SMHC smooth muscle heavy chain myosin

SMI Self-Motivation Inventory; senior medical investigator; severe mental impairment; silent myocardial infarction; stress myocardial image; Style of Mind Inventory; supplementary medical insurance; sustained maximum inspiration

SmIg surface membrane immunoglobulin

SMILE So Much Improvement with a Little Exercise [program]; Survival of Myocardial Infarction: Long-term Evaluation [study]

SMISS Silent Myocardial Ischemia Stress Study

SMK structured meta knowledge

SML smouldering leukemia

SMM scintimammography; smoldering multiple myeloma

SMMD specimen mass measurement device

SMMHC smooth muscle myosin heavy chain

SMMSE Standardized Mini-Mental State Examination

SMN second malignant neoplasm; stathmin; surgical microscope navigator; survival motor neuron

SMN^T telemeric survival motor neuron

SMNB submaximal neuromuscular block

SMO second medical opinion; senior medical officer; surveillance medical officer

SMOH Senior Medical Officer of Health; Society of Medical Officers of Health

SMON subacute myeloopticoneuropathy

SMP slow moving protease; standard medical practice; submitochondrial particle; sulfamethoxypyrazine; symmetric multiprocessor; sympathetically maintained pain

SMPC summary of product characteristics

SMPR small mannose 6-phosphate receptor

SMPV superior mesenteric portal vein

SMR scatter maximum ratio; senior medical resident; sensorimotor rhythm; severe mental retardation; sexual maturity rating; significantly lower mortality rate; skeletal muscle relaxant; somnolent metabolic rate; standardized mortality ratio; stroke with minimum residuum; submucosal resection

SMRR submucosal resection and rhinoplasty

SMRT silencing mediator of retinoid and thyroid receptors

SMRV squirrel monkey retrovirus

SMS scalable modeling system; senior medical student; serial motor seizures; Shared Medical Systems; short messaging system; Simvastatin Multicenter Study; Smith-Magenis syndrome; somatostatin; stiff-man syndrome; supplemental minimum sodium

SMSA standard metropolitan statistical area

SMSV San Miguel sea lion virus

SMT Spanish Multicentre Study; spontaneous mammary tumor; stereotactic mesencephalic tractomy; Stockholm Metoprolol Trial; surface mouth technology

SMTP simple mail transfer protocol

S-MUAP surface-detected motor unit action potential

SMuLV Scripps murine leukemia virus

SMV skeletal muscle ventricle; superior mesenteric vein

SMWHS Seattle Midlife Women's Health Study

SMX, SMZ sulfamethoxazole

SN school nurse; sclerema neonatorum; scrub nurse; Semantic Network [UMLS]; sensorineural; sensory neuron; serum neutralization; sinus node; spontaneous nystagmus; staff nurse; stromal nodule; student nurse; subnormal; substantia nigra; supernatant; suprasternal notch

S/N signal/noise [ratio]; supernatant

Sn subnasale

sn small nucleolar

SNA specimen not available; Student Nurses Association; sympathetic nerve activity

SNa serum sodium concentration

SNagg serum normal agglutinator

SNAP Score for Neonatal Acute Physiology [study]; sensory nerve action potential; *S*-nitroso-*N*-acetylpenicillamine; soluble *N*-ethylmaleimide-sensitive fusion protein attachment protein; Stanford Nutrition Action Program

SNaP Study of Sodium and Blood Pressure

SNAPE Study of Nicorandil in Angina Pectoris in the Elderly

SNARE soluble *N*-ethylmaleimide-sensitive fusion protein attachment protein receptor

SNARL suggested no adverse response level

SNB scalene node biopsy

SNC spontaneous neonatal chylothorax

SNCL sinus node cycle length

SNCS sensory nerve conduction studies

SNCV sensory nerve conduction velocity

SND scatterer number density; sinus node dysfunction; striatonigral degeneration; sympathetic nerve discharge; systematic nodal dissection

SNDA Student National Dental Association

SNDO Standard Nomenclature of Diseases and Operations

SNE sinus node electrogram; subacute necrotizing encephalomyelography

SNES suprascapular nerve entrapment syndrome

SNF sinus node formation; skilled nursing facility

SNGBF single nephron glomerular blood flow

SNGFR single nephron glomerular filtration rate

SNHL sensorineural hearing loss

SNIPA seronegative inflammatory polyarthritis

SNIVT Society of Non-Invasive Vascular Technology

SNJ nevus sebaceous of Jadassohn

SNK Student-Newman-Keuls [procedure]

SNM Society of Nuclear Medicine; sulfanilamide

SNMA Student National Medical Association

SNMP simple network management protocol

SNMT Society of Nuclear Medical Technologists

sno small nucleolar

SNOBOL String-Oriented Symbolic Language

SNODO Standard Nomenclature of Diseases and Operations

SNOMED Systematized Nomenclature of Medicine

SNOMED CMT Systematized Nomenclature of Medicine—Convergent Medical Terminology

SNOMED CT Systematized Nomenclature of Medicine—Clinical Terminology

SNOMED RT Systematized Nomenclature of Medicine—Reference Terminology

SNOMED RT/CMT Systematized Nomenclature of Medicine—Reference Terminology/Convergent Medical Terminology

SNOP Systematized Nomenclature of Pathology

snoRNA small nucleolar ribonucleic acid [RNA]

snoRNP small nucleolar ribonucleoprotein [RNP]

SNP school nurse practitioner; single nucleotide polymorphism; sinonasal papilloma; sinus node potential; sodium nitroprusside

S-NPI start nuclear polymorphism index

SNPV single nucleopolyhedrovirus

SNR selective nerve root [block]; semantic network relationship [UMLS]; signal-to-noise ratio; substantia nigra zona reticulata; supernumerary rib

Snr substantia nigra zona reticulata

SNRB selective nerve root block

snRNA small nuclear ribonucleic acid; small nucleolar ribonucleic acid [RNA]

SNRI selective serotonin-norepinephrine reuptake inhibitor

snRNP small nuclear ribonucleoprotein [RNP]; small nuclear ribonucleoprotein particle

snRP small nuclear ribonucleoprotein polypeptide

SNR$_{Pix}$ signal to noise ratio per pixel

snRPB small nuclear ribonucleoprotein polypeptide B

snRPN small nuclear ribonucleoprotein polypeptide N

SNRT sinus node recovery time

SNRTd sinus node recovery time, direct measuring

SNRTi sinus node recovery time, indirect measuring

SNS Senior Nursing Sister; Society of Neurological Surgeons; supplementary nursing system; sympathetic nervous system

SNSA seronegative spondyloarthropathy

S-NSE serum neuron-specific enolase

SNST sciatic nerve stretch test

SNT sinuses, nose, and throat; spectral noise threshold

SNU skilled nursing unit

SNuPD single nucleotide primer extension

SNV Sin nombre virus; spleen necrosis virus

SNVDO Standard Nomenclature of Veterinary Diseases and Operations

SNW slow negative wave

SO salpingo-oophorectomy; Schlatter-Osgood [test]; second opinion; sex offender; shoulder orthosis; site of origin; slow oxidative; spheno-occipital [synchondrosis]; spinal orthosis; sphincter of Oddi;

S&O salpingo-oophorectomy

SO$_2$ oxygen saturation

SOA serum opsonic activity; shortness of air; spinal opioid anesthesia; stimulus onset asynchrony; swelling of ankles

SoA symptoms of asthma

SOAA signed out against advice

SOAMA signed out against medical advice

SOA-MCA superficial occipital artery to middle cerebral artery

SOAP subjective, objective, assessment, and plan [problem-oriented record]

SOAPIE subjective, objective, assessment, plan, implementation, and evaluation [problem-oriented record]

SOAR Safety of Orbofiban in Acute Coronary Research [study]

SOB see order blank; shortness of breath; stool occult blood

SOBOE shortness of breath on exertion

SOBP spread out Bragg peak [radiotherapy]

SOC self-organized criticality; sequential oral contraceptive; Standard Occupational Classification; standards of care; state of consciousness; store-operated [ion] channel; surgical overhead canopy; synovial osteochondromatosis; syphilitic osteochondritis; system-on-a-chip

SoC state of consciousness

SOCIAIDS Study of Cardiac Involvement in Acquired Immunodeficiency Syndrome [AIDS]

SoCPA stage of change for physical activity

SocSec Social Security

SocServ social services

SOCRATES Study of Coronary Revascularization and Therapeutic Evaluations

SOCS1 suppressor of cytokine signaling 1

S-OCT serum ornithine carbamyl transferase

SOD septo-optic dysplasia; sphincter of Oddi dysfunction; superoxide dismutase

sod sodium

SODAS spheroidal oral drug absorption system

sod bicarb sodium bicarbonate

SODF sperm outer defense fiber

SODH sorbitol dehydrogenase

SOF Study of Osteoporotic Fractures [in association with strokes]; superior orbital fissure

SOFA sequential organ failure assessment

SOFLC self-organizing fuzzy logic control

SOFM self-organization feature map

SOG supraorbital groove

SOH sympathetic orthostatic hypotension

SOHN supraoptic hypothalamic nucleus

SOHND supraomohyoid neck dissection

SOHO self-organizing, holarchic, open; Solar and Heliospheric Observatory [spacecraft data]

SOI severity of illness; signal of interest

SOL solution; space-occupying lesion

sol soluble, solution

SOLD Stenting after Optimal Lesion Debulking [trial]

SOLEC stand on one leg eyes closed

Soln, sol'n solution

SOLVD Studies of Left Ventricular Dysfunction

SOM secretory otitis media; self-organizing map [clustering complex data sets]; sensitivity of method; serous otitis media; somatotropin; state operations manual; superior oblique muscle; suppurative otitis media; supraorbital margin; sustained outward movement [heart]

SOMA Student Osteopathic Medical Association; subjective, objective, management, and analytic [scale]

somat somatic

SOMI sternal occipital mandibular immobilization

SOMIN school of medicine information network

SON superior olivary nucleus; supraoptic nucleus

SONET synchronous optical network transmission

SONH spontaneous osteonecrosis of the hip

SONK spontaneous osteonecrosis of the knee

SOO structured office oral [examination]

SOOF suborbital orbicular fat

SOP service-object pair; standard operating procedure

SoP standard of performance

SOPA Survey of Pain Attitudes; syndrome of primary aldosteronism

SOPCA sporadic olivopontocerebellar ataxia

SOPED Shock Outcome Prediction in the Emergency Department [score]

SOPHE Society for Public Health Education

SOPI service object pair instance

SOPO set of possible occurrences

SOQ Suicide Opinion Questionnaire

SOR stimulus-organism response; successive over-relaxation [algorithm in imaging]; superoxide release

SOr supraorbitale

sOR stratified odds ratio

Sorb, sorb sorbitol

SORD sorbitol dehydrogenase

SOREM sleep onset rapid eye movement

SORF spliceable open-reading frame

SOS self-obtained smear; son of sevenless; Southern Oxidant Study; speed of sound; supplemental oxygen system; surgery on site; Swedish Obesity Study

SoS Stent or Surgery [study]

SOSA Student Osteopathic Surgical Association

SOSF single organ system failure

SOT sensory organization test; systemic oxygen transport

SOWS subjective opiate withdrawal scale

SP sacroposterior; sacrum to pubis; salivary progesterone; schizotypal personality; secretory piece; semi-private [room]; senile plaque; sepiapterin; septal pore; septum pellucidum; sequence processor [radiotherapy]; sequential pulse; serine/proline [rich protein]; seropositive; serum protein; shunt pressure; shunt procedure; silent period; skin potential; sleep deprivation; slow pathway [heart electrical activity]; small protein; smoothed periodogram; soft palate; solid phase; spastic paraplegia; specific protocol; spectrogram; speech pathology; spiramycin; spirometry; spleen; spontaneous proliferation; standards of performance; standard practice; standard procedure; standardized patient; standardized-patient [assessment]; staphylococcal protease; *Staphylococcus pneumoniae*; status post; steady potential; stimulus to P-wave [ECG]; stool preservative; storage phosphor [radiography]; subliminal

perception; substance P; sulfadoxine-pyrimethamine; sulfapyridine; sulfopropyl; summating potential; superimposed pressure; suprapatellar; suprapubic; surface polypeptide; surfactant protein; symphysis pubis; synthase phosphatase; systolic pressure

Sp the most posterior point on the posterior contour of the sella turcica; sleep spindle; species; specific; specimen; sphenoid; spine; *Spirillum*; summation potential

S/P, s/p status, post[operative]

S7P sedoheptulose-7-phosphate

S$_p$ pooled standard deviation [statistics]

sP senile parkinsonism; structural protein

sp space; species; specific; spine, spinal; spirit

SPA salt-poor albumin; scalable [computer] processor architecture; sheep pulmonary adenomatosis; single photon absorptiometry; spastic ataxia; sperm penetration assay; spinal progressive amyotrophy; spondyloarthropathy; spontaneous platelet aggregation; staphylococcal protein A; student progress assessment; suprapubic aspiration; surface polypeptide, anonymous

SP-A surfactant protein A

SPA-Acad Acadian spastic ataxia

SPACE single potential analysis of cavernous electrical activity

SPACELINE Space Life Science Online

sp act specific activity

SPACTO Stent vs Percutaneous Angioplasty in Chronic Total Occlusion [trial]

SPAD stenosing peripheral arterial disease

SPAF spontaneous paroxysmal atrial fibrillation; Stroke Prevention in Atrial Fibrillation [trial]

SPAF TEE Stroke Prevention in Atrial Fibrillation-Transesophageal Echo [study]

SPAG small particle aerosol generator

SPAI steroid protein activity index

SPAM scanning photoacoustic microscopy

SPAMM spatial modulation of magnetization

sp an spinal anesthesia

sPAP systolic pulmonary artery pressure

SPAR sensitivity prediction by acoustic reflex

SPARC cysteine-rich acidic secreted protein; Space Physics and Aeronomy Research Collaboratory; Stroke Prevention Assessment of Risk and Community [trial]

SPARS spatially resolved spectrometry

SPAT slow paroxysmal atrial tachycardia; spatial concept [UMLS]

SPB sinking pre-beta-lipoprotein

SP-B surfactant protein B

SPBI serum protein-bound iodine

SPBMD spinal bone mineral density

SPC salicylamide, phenacetin, and caffeine; scaphopisocapitate; seropositive carrier; single palmar crease; single photoelectron count; soy phosphatidylcholine; spleen cell; standard plate count; statistical process control; summary of [pharmaceutical] product characteristics; synthetizing protein complex

SP-C surfactant protein C

SPCA serum prothrombin conversion accelerator; Society for Prevention of Cruelty to Animals; systemic pulmonary collateral artery

SPCC Spill Prevention, Control, and Countermeasure [plan]

SPCD syndrome of primary ciliary dyskinesia

Sp Cd, sp cd spinal cord

SPCG spectral phonocardiography

SPD schizotypal personality disorder; sociopathic personality disorder; specific paroxysmal discharge; spermidine; standard peak dilution; sterile processing department; storage pool deficiency

SPDC strio-pallido-dentate calcinosis

SPDT single pole double throw

SpDur spike duration

SPE septic pulmonary edema; serum protein electrolytes; serum protein electrophoresis; streptococcal pyrogenic exotoxin; sucrose polyester; sustained physical exercise

SPEA strength Pareto evolutionary approach algorithm

SPEAK spectral peak [strategy]

SPEAR selective parenteral and enteral anti-sepsis regimen

SPE-C streptococcal pyrogenic exotoxin C

Spec specialist, specialty; specificity

spec special; specific; specificity; specimen

spec gr specific gravity

SPECT single photon emission computed tomography

SPEED Strategies for Patency Enhancement in the Emergency Department [study]

sPEEP spontaneous peak end-expiratory pressure

SPEG serum protein electrophoretogram

SPEL syndactyly-polydactyly-earlobe [syndrome]

SPEM smooth pursuit eye movement

SPEP serum protein electrophoresis; Structured Patient Education Programme

SPERM spastic paraplegia-epilepsy-mental retardation [syndrome]

SPET single photon emission tomography; Surgical Procedure Entry Tool

SPF skin protection factor; specific pathogen–free; spectrophotofluorometer; S-phase fraction; split products of fibrin; standard perfusion fluid; Stuart-Prower factor; sun protection factor; systemic pulmonary fistula

Sp Fl, sp fl spinal fluid

SPG serine phosphoglyceride; spastic paraplegia; sphenopalatine ganglion; splenoportography; sucrose, phosphate, and glutamate; symmetrical peripheral gangrene

SpG specific gravity

spg sponge

SPGA Bovarnik solution; sucrose, phosphate, glutamate, and albumin

SPGR spoiled gradient [echo]

SpGr, sp gr specific gravity

SPGX spastic paraplegia, X-linked

SPGY spermatogenesis on Y

SPH secondary pulmonary hemosiderosis; severely and profoundly handicapped; spherocyte; spherocytosis; sphingomyelin

Sph sphenoidale; sphingomyelin

sph spherical; spherical lens; spheroid

SPHS Saskatoon Pregnancy and Health Study

sp ht specific heat

SPI selective protein index; Self-Perception Inventory; serum-precipitable iodine; serum protein index; Shipley Personal Inventory; speech processor interface; standardized-patient instructor; standards for pediatric immunization; structured pain interview; Study of Perioperative Ischemia; subclinical papillomavirus infection

SPI 1, 2 *Salmonella* pathogenicity island 1, 2

SPIA solid-phase immunoabsorption; solid-phase immunoassay

SPICE Simulation Program with Integrated Circuit Emphasis; Study of Patients Intolerant to Converting Enzyme Inhibitors

SPICED TEAS Study of Pacemakers and Implantable Cardioverter Defibrillator Triggering by Electronic Article Surveillance Devices

SPICU surgical pulmonary intensive care unit

SPID summed pain intensity difference

SPIDERS Secondary Prevention of Ischemic Disease by Estrogen Replacement or Statins

SPIE International Society for Optical Engineering

SPIF solid-phase immunoassay fluorescence

SPIH superimposed pregnancy-induced hypertension

SPIHT set partitioning in hierarchical tree

SPIN skeletal plan instantiation; Social Phobia Inventory

spin spine, spinal

SPINAF Stroke Prevention in Nonrheumatic Atrial Fibrillation [study]

SPIO superparamagnetic iron oxide

SPIR Study of Perioperative Ischemia Research

spir spiral; spirit

SPIRIT Salvage from Perindopril in Reperfused Infarction Trial; Stroke Prevention in Reversible Ischemia Trial

SPJ saphenopopliteal junction

SPK serum pyruvate kinase; simultaneous pancreas-kidney [transplantation]; superficial punctate keratitis

SPL skin potential level; sound pressure level; splanchnic; spontaneous lesion; staphylococcal phage lysate; superior parietal lobule; surfactant proteolipid

SPLATT split anterior tibial tendon

sPLM sleep-related periodic leg movements

SPLV serum parvovirus-like virus

SPlw long window spectrogram

SPM scanning probe microscopy; shocks per minute; spatiotemporal population map; spermine; statistical parametric mapping; subhuman primate model; suspended particulate matter; synaptic plasma membrane

SpM spiriformis medialis [nucleus]

spm spermatogonial metaphase

SPMA spinal progressive muscular atrophy

SPMD single program multiple data

SPMMV Sweet potato mild mottle virus

SPMR standard proportionate mortality ratio (or rate)

SPMS secondary progressive multiple sclerosis

SPMSQ Short Portable Mental Status Questionnaire

SPmv medium window spectrogram

S-PMVT sustained polymorphic ventricular fibrillation

SPN senior plan network; sialophorin; solitary pulmonary nodule; supplemental parenteral nutrition; sympathetic preganglionic neuron

SpnCbT spinocerebellar tract

SpO₂ functional oxygen saturation; pulse oximetry

SPOCS Surgical Planning and Organization Computer System

SPOD spouse's perception of disease

spon, spont spontaneous

SPONASTRIME spondylar and nasal alterations with striated metaphyses; spondylar changes-nasal anomaly-associated metaphyses [dysplasia]

SPOOL simultaneous peripheral operation on-line

SPOP sequential paired opposed plaque [technique]

SPORE Specialized Programs of Research Excellence [study]

SPORT Stent Implantation Postrotational Atherectomy Trial

SPOV Spondweni virus

SPP plural of *species*; Sexuality Preference Profile; skin perfusion pressure; small plaque parapsoriasis; suprapubic prostatectomy

spp plural of *species*

SPPF standard portable patient file

SPPK striate palmoplantar keratoderma

Sp Pn, Sp Pnx spontaneous pneumothorax

SPPP, sppp plural of *subspecies*

SPPS single photon planar scintigraphy; solid phase peptide synthesis; stable plasma protein solution

SPPT superprecipitation response

SPPX X-linked spastic paraplegia

SPR scanned projection radiography; selected primer; sepiapterin reductase; serial probe recognition; skin potential response; specific pathogen free; Society for Pediatric Radiology; Society for Pediatric Research; solid phase radioimmunoassay; substance P receptor; superior peroneal retinaculum

Spr scan projection radiography

spr sprain

SPRAS Sheehan patient rated anxiety scale

SPRCA solid phase red cell adherence assay

SPRIA solid phase radioimmunoassay

SPRINT Secondary Prevention of Reinfarction Israeli Nifedipine Trial

SPROM spontaneous premature rupture of membrane

SPRR small proline-rich protein

SPRRA small proline-rich protein A

SPRRB small proline-rich protein B

SPRRC small proline-rich protein C

SPRS Sixty Plus Reinfarction Study

SPRT sequential probability ratio test; Sixty Plus Reinfarction Trial

SPS scapuloperoneal syndrome; shoulder pain and stiffness; simple partial seizures; slow-progressive schizophrenia; Society of Pelvic Surgeons; sodium polyanethol sulfonate; sodium polystyrene; sound production sample; spermidine synthase; stimulated protein synthesis; Stockholm Prospective Study; Suicide Probability Scale; systemic progressive sclerosis

SpS sphenoid sinus

sPSGL, (s)PSGL soluble P-selectin glycoprotein ligand

spSHR stroke-prone spontaneously hypertensive rat

SPSS Statistical Package for the Social Sciences [Australia]

SPST Symonds Picture-Story Test

SPsw short window spectrogram

SPT second primary tumor; secretin-pancreazymin [test]; single patch technique; single patient trial; sleep period time; spectrin; standard psychometric test; station pull-through [technique]

SpT spinal tap

SPTA spatial peak temporal average; spectrin alpha

SPTAN spectrin alpha, nonerythroid

Sp tap spinal tap

SPTI systolic pressure time index

SPTS subjective posttraumatic syndrome

SPTx static pelvic traction

SPU short procedure unit; Society of Pediatric Urology; standardized photometric unit

SPV selective proximal vagotomy; Shope papillomavirus; sulfophosphovanillin; systolic pressure variation

SPW subxiphoid pericardial window

SPWVD smooth pseudo-Winger-Ville distribution [heart rate signal]

SPYWS Stroke Prevention in Young Women Study

SPZ sulfinpyrazone

SQ social quotient; status quo; subcutaneous [JCAHO unapproved abbreviation]; survey question; symptom questionnaire

Sq subcutaneous

sq square; squamous

SQC statistical quality control

sq cell ca squamous cell carcinoma

SQI signal quality index

SQL standard query language; structured query language

SQP sequential quadratic programming

S–QRS stimulus to QRS interval [ECG]

sq rt square root

SQUID superconducting quantum interference device

SR sample response; sarcoplasmic reticulum; saturation recovery; scanning radiometer; screen; secretion rate; sedimentation rate; seizure resistant; selection relaxation [algorithm]; self-recording; senior resident; sensitivity response; sensitization response; service record; sex ratio; shorthair [guinea pig]; short range; side rails; sigma reaction; silicone rubber; sinus rhythm; skin resistance; sleep and rest; slow release; smooth-rough [colony]; sparse representation; spatial resolution [imaging]; specific release; specific [airway] resistance; specific response; splenorenal; spontaneous respiration; steroid resistance; stimulus-response; stomach rumble; stress related; stress relaxation; stretch reflex; sulfonamide-resistant; superior rectus; surface rendering [visualization]; surface roughness; sustained release; suture removal; synchronization ratio; systemic reaction; systemic resistance; systems research; systems review

S-R smooth-rough [bacteria]; stimulus-response

Sr strontium

sr steradian

SRA segmental renal artery; serum renin activity; spleen repopulating activity

SRAM static random access memory

SR$_{AW}$, SR$_{aw}$ specific airway resistance

SRB sulforhodamine B

SRBC sheep red blood cells

SRBD sleep-related breathing disorder

SRBSDS short range biological standoff detection system

SRC sedimented red cells; sheep red cells; signed reaction center; steroid receptor

src Rous sarcoma oncogene

SRCA specific red cell adherence

SRCBC serum reserve cholesterol binding capacity

SR/CP schizophrenic reaction, chronic paranoid

SRD service-related disability; Society for the Relief of Distress; Society for the Right to Die; sodium-restricted diet; specific reading disability; sustained rate duration

SRDS severe respiratory distress syndrome

SRDT single radial diffusion test

SRE Schedule of Recent Experiences; standard regression effect; sterol regulatory element

SREBP sterol regulatory element binding protein

sREM stage rapid eye movement

SRF semirigid fiberglass cast; serum responsive factor; service response force; severe renal failure; skin reactive factor; somatotropin-releasing factor; split renal function; subretinal fluid

SRFA selective restriction fragment amplification

SRF-A slow-reacting factor-anaphylaxis

SRFS split renal function study

SRG specialty review group

SRH single radial hemolysis; somatotropin-releasing hormone; spontaneously responding hyperthyroidism; stigmata of recent hemorrhage

SRI serotonin reuptake inhibitor; severe renal insufficiency; sorcin; Stanford Research Institute; strain rate imaging; structured review instrument

SRID single radial immunodiffusion

SRIF somatotropin-release inhibiting factor

SRLE schedule of recent life events

SRM spontaneous rupture of membranes; Standard Reference Material; superior rectus muscle

SRMD stress-related mucosal damage

SRN State Registered Nurse

sRNA soluble ribonucleic acid

SRNG sustained release nitroglycerin

SRNS steroid-responsive nephrotic syndrome

SRO sex-ratio organism; single room occupancy; smallest region of overlap; Steele-Richardson-Olszewski [syndrome]

SROC summary receiver operating characteristic

SROM spontaneous rupture of membrane

SRP scientific review panel; short rib-polydactyly [syndrome]; signal recognition particle; Society for Radiological Protection; sponsoring residency program; State Registered Physiotherapist; synchronized retroperfusion

SRPG simulated respiratory pattern generator

SRPR signal recognition particle receptor

SRPS short rib-polydactyly syndrome

SRQ Self-Reporting Questionnaire

SRR short R–R interval [ECG]; stabilized relative response; standardized rate ratio; surgery recovery room

SRRS Social Readjustment Rating Scale

SR-RSV Schmidt-Ruppin Rous sarcoma virus

SRS schizophrenic residual state; sequential retrieval system; sex reassignment surgery; silencing regulatory sequences; Silver-Russell syndrome; simple repeat sequence; slow-reacting substance; Snyder-Robinson syndrome; Social and Rehabilitation Service; somatostatin receptor scintigraphy; social relationship scale; spermidine synthase; standard rating scale; stereotactic radiosurgery; suppressor of rad six [locus]; Symptom Rating Scale

SRSA, SRS-A slow-reacting substance of anaphylaxis

SRSCB six random systematic core biopsy

SRSV small round structured virus

SRT sedimentation rate test; simple reaction time; sinus node recovery time; sitting root test; Sorbinil Retinopathy Trial; speech reception test; speech reception threshold; spontaneously resolving thyrotoxicosis; surfactant replacement therapy; sustained-release theophylline; symptom rating test

SRU sample ratio units; side rails up; solitary rectal ulcer; structural repeating unit

SRUS solitary rectal ulcer syndrome

SRV Schmidt-Ruppin virus; sheep retrovirus; simian retrovirus; small round virus; superior radicular vein

SRV 1, 2 simian retrovirus 1, 2

SRVT sustained re-entrant ventricular tachyarrhythmia

SRW short ragweed [test]

SRWS super radiology work station

SRY sex-determining region on Y chromosome

SS disulfide; sacrosciatic; saline soak; saline solution; saliva sample; saliva substitute; *Salmonella-Shigella* [agar]; salt substitute; saturated solution; Schizophrenia Subscale; Seckel syndrome; seizure-sensitive; selective shunt; serum sickness; Sézary syndrome; shear stress; short sleep; short stature; siblings; sickle cell; side-to-side; signs and symptoms; single-stranded; Sjögren syndrome; skull series [radiographs]; soapsuds; Social Security; social services; somatostatin; Spanish-speaking; sparingly soluble; spatial separation; stainless steel; standard score; statistically significant; steady state; steam sterilization; sterile solution; steroid sensitivity; Stickler syndrome; stimulus separation; stromal sarcoma; structural key; subaortic stenosis; subscapular; subspinale; substernal; succinimidyl succinate; suction socket; sum of squares; supersaturated; support and stimulation; Sweet syndrome; synchronous sampling; systemic sclerosis

S/S salt substitute; signs/symptoms

S&S signs and symptoms

Ss *Shigella sonnei*; subjects

ss single-stranded

SSA salicylsalicylic acid; sicca syndrome A; single-stranded annealing; skin-sensitizing antibody; skin sympathetic activity; Sjögren syndrome A; Smith surface antigen; Social Security Administration; Social Security Act; social service agency; sperm-specific antiserum; stochastic simulated annealing [imaging]; sulfosalicylic acid

SSA1 Smallest Space Analysis

SSAA sicca syndrome associated antigen A; Sjögren syndrome-associated antigen A; syringomyelia secondary to arachnoid adhesions

SSAV simian sarcoma-associated virus

SSB short spike burst; sicca syndrome B; single-strand break; single-stranded binding [protein]; stereospecific binding

SS-B Sjögren syndrome B

ssb single-strand break

SSBE short-segment Barrett's esophagus

SSBG sex steroid-binding globulin; social services block grant

SSC salt sodium citrate; single-stripe colitis; single-strand conformational [analysis]; sister strand crossover; skin-to-skin care; somatic stem cell; somatosensory cortex; standard saline citrate; standard sodium citrate; syngeneic spleen cell

SSc systemic scleroderma; systemic sclerosis

SSCA single-strand conformational analysis; spontaneous suppressor cell activity

SSCCS slow spinal cord compression syndrome

ss(c)DNA single-stranded circular deoxyribonucleic acid

SsCEP somatosensory cortical evoked potential

SSCF sleep stage change frequency

SSCI Social Science Citation Index

SSCP single-strand conformation polymorphism, single-stranded conformational polymorphism

SSCPA single-stranded conformational polymorphism analysis

SSCr stainless steel crown

SSCT stereotactic subcaudate tractotomy

SSD shaded surface display; silver sulfadiazine; single saturating dose; solid-state detector; Social Security disability; source-skin distance; source-surface distance; speech-sound discrimination;

squared sum of intensity differences; succinate semialdehyde dehydrogenase; sum of square deviations; syndrome of sudden death

ssD-BP single-stranded D-sequence binding protein

SSDBS symptom schedule for the diagnosis of borderline schizophrenia

SSDD steroid sulfatase deficiency disease

SSDI Social Security Disability Income; striatal or striatocapsular small deep infarction; Supplemental Security Disability Income

ssDNA single-stranded deoxyribonucleic acid [DNA]

SSDS stepping source dosimetry system [radiotherapy]

SSE saline solution enema; skin self-examination; soapsuds enema; steady state exercise; subacute spongiform encephalopathy

SSEA stage-specific embryonic antigen

SSEP somatosensory evoked potential; steady-state evoked potential

SSER somatosensory evoked response

SSES Sexual Self-Efficacy Scale

SSF septic scarlet fever; solid state fermentation; soluble suppressor factor; supplemental sensory feedback

SSFP steady state free precession

SSFSE single shot fast spin-echo [MRI]

SSG sublabial salivary gland

SSH spinal subdural hemorrhage; suppressive subtractive hybridization

SSHM Society for the Social History of Medicine [UK]

SSHL severe sensorineural hearing

SSI segmental sequential irradiation; severity score index; shoulder subluxation inhibition; small-scale integration; Social Security increment; somatic symptom index; Somatic Symptom Inventory; strength-strain index; subshock insulin; supplemental security income; surgical site infection; synchronous serial interface; System Sign Inventory

SSIDS sibling of sudden infant death syndrome [victim]

SSIE Smithsonian Science Information Exchange

SSISS Statewide Sentinel Immunisation Surveillance System

SSKI saturated solution of potassium iodide

SSL secure sockets layer; skin surface lipid; sufficient sleep; suppressor of stem loop

SSLI serum sickness-like illness

SSM skin-sparing mastectomy; solid-state microscopy; subsynaptic membrane; superficial spreading melanoma; system status management

SSMS saturated solution of magnesium iodide

SSN [computer-assisted] surgical segment navigator; severely subnormal; Social Security Number; subacute sensory neuropathy; suprasternal notch

SSNHL sudden sensorineural hearing loss

SSNS steroid-sensitive nephrotic syndrome

SSO sequence-specific oligonucleotide [probe]; Society of Surgical Oncology; special sense organ

SSOP Second Surgical Opinion Program; sequence-specific oligonucleotide probe

SSP Sanarelli-Shwartzman phenomenon; Scottish Society of Physicians; sequence-specific primers; site-specific psoralen; slice sensitivity profile; solute-solvent property; sporozoite surface protein; stereotactic surface projection; subacute sclerosing panencephalitis; subspecies; supersensitivity perception

ssp subspecies

SSPCP service-specific practice cost percentage

SSPE salt sodium phosphate ethylenediamine tetraacetic acid [EDTA]; subacute sclerosing panencephalitis

SSPG steady state plasma glucose

SSPI steady state plasma insulin

SSPL saturation sound pressure level

SSPP subsynaptic plate perforation

SSPS side-to-side portacaval shunt

SS-PSE Schizophrenic Subscale of the Present State Examination

SSQ sequential scalar quantization; Social Support Questionnaire

SSQS security related software quality standard [healthcare]

SSR signal sequence receptor; single sequence repeat; site-specific recombination; solar simulated radiation; somatosensory response; steady state response; sudomotor skin response; surgical supply room; sympathetic skin response

SSr single-strand region

SSrA single-strand region A

SSrB single-strand region B

SSRE shear stress response element

SSRI selective serotonin reuptake inhibitor

ssRNA single-stranded ribonucleic acid

SSS scalded skin syndrome; secondary Sjögren syndrome; sick sinus syndrome; specific soluble substance; Stanford Sleepiness Scale; sterile saline soak; subclavian steal syndrome; subscapular skinfold; superior sagittal sinus; systemic sicca syndrome

SSSA skin sympathetic sudomotor activity

SSSD Spanish Study on Sudden Death

SSSI Siegel Scale of Support for Innovation

SSSIII specific soluble substance III [in *Streptococcus pneumoniae* polysaccharide]

SSSS Scandinavian Simvastatin Survival Study; staphylococcal scalded skin syndrome

SSST superior sagittal sinus thrombosis

SS-STP sum of squares simultaneous test procedure

SSSV superior sagittal sinus velocity

SST skin and soft tissue; sodium sulfite titration; somatostatin

SSTI skin and soft tissue infection

SSTL site-specific target level

SSTR somatostatin receptor

SSU Saybolt Seconds Universal; self-service unit; sterile supply unit

ssu small subunit

SSV Schoolman-Schwartz virus; simian sarcoma virus

SSVEP steady-state visual evoked potential

SSW slow spike wave; spike and sharp waves [EEG]

SSX sulfisoxazole

SSYM sign or symptom [UMLS]

ST [heat]-stable enterotoxin; esotropia; scala tympani; scaphotrapezoid; sclerotherapy; sedimentation time; semantic type [UMLS]; semitendinosus; sensory threshold; septal thickness; serum transferrin; settling time; sharp transients [EEG]; shock therapy; sickle [cell] thalassemia; sincerity test; sinus tachycardia; sinus tympani; skin temperature; skin test; skin thickness; slight trace; slow twitch; soft tissue; solid tumor; spastic torticollis; speech therapist; sphincter tone; split thickness; stable toxin; standard test; starting time; stent thrombosis; sternothyroid; stimulus; store; stress test; stretcher; stria terminalis; striation; string data; sublingual tablet; subtalar; subtotal; sulcus terminalis; sulfotransferase; surface tension; surgical technologist; surgical therapy; surgical tracheostomy; surgical treatment; survival time; syndrome of the trephined; systolic time

S(T) signal-to-symbol translator

S/T spontaneous/timed [device]

S&T science and technology

S-T [*segment*] in electrocardiography, the portion of the segment between the end of the S wave and the beginning of the T wave; sickle-cell thalassemia

St, st let it stand [Lat. *stet*]; let them stand [Lat. *stent*]; stage [of disease]; status; stere; sterile; stimulation; stokes; stone [unit]; straight; stroke; stomach; stomion; subtype

sT tumor surgery [TNM (tumor-node-metastasis) classification: **sT0** surgery not done, **sT1** complete resection, **sT2** resection, 50% to 90%, **sT3** resection 5% to 50%, **sT4** biopsy, and **sT5** shunting]

STA second trimester abortion; serum thrombotic accelerator; superficial temporal artery

Sta staphylion

stab stabilization; stab neutrophil

STACK Sequence Tag Alignment Consensus Knowledge-base

STAG slow-target attaching globulin; split-thickness autogenous graft; striped tag myocardial tagging [system]

STAI State Trait Anxiety Inventory

STA-MCA superficial temporal artery to middle cerebral artery

STAMI Stenting for Acute Myocardial Infarction [study]

STAMP Systemic Thrombolysis in Acute Myocardial Infarction with Prourokinase and Urokinase [trial]

STAND sutures to ambulate and discharge

STANDOUT soft thresholding and depth cueing of unspecified techniques

StanPsych standard psychiatric [nomenclature]

Staph, staph *Staphylococcus*

STAPPA State and Territorial Air Pollution Program Administration

STAR Specialty Training and Advanced Research [NIH]; Staphylokinase Recombinant Trial; Study of Tranexamic Acid after Aneurysm Rupture

StAR steroidogenic acute regulatory [protein]

STARNET South Texas Ambulatory Research Network

STARS Standard Treatment with Activase to Reverse Stroke [study]; Stent Anticoagulation Regimen Study; Stent Anticoagulation Restenosis Study; Stent Antithrombolytic Regimen Study; St. Thomas Atherosclerosis Regression Study

START Saruplase and Taprostene Acute Reocclusion Trial; selective tubal assessment to refine reproductive therapy; simple triage and rapid treatment; Stent vs Angioplasty Restenosis Trial; Stent vs Directional Coronary Atherectomy Randomized Trial; St. Thomas Atherosclerosis Regression Trial; Study of Thrombolytic Therapy with Additional Response Following Taprostene; Study of Titration and Response to Tiazac; systemic arterial system

STAR TAP science, technology, and research transit access point

STARTTS Service for the Treatment and Rehabilitation of Torture and Trauma Survivors [Australia]

STAS sporadic testicular agenesis syndrome

STAT immediately [Lat. *statim*]; signal transducer and activator of transcription; state-trait anxiety inventory; Stent Thrombosis after Ticlopidine [study]; stop teenage addiction to tobacco; Stroke Treatment with Ancrod Trial

Stat statistics, statistical

stat immediately [Lat. *statim*]; radiation emanation unit [German]

STAT-CHF Survival Trial of Antiarrhythmic Therapy in Congestive Heart Failure

STATH statherin

STATRS Stent Antithrombotic Regimen Study

STB super tropical bleach

Stb stillborn

STC sarcomatoid thymic carcinoma; serum theophylline concentration; sexually transmitted condition; soft tissue calcification; specialized treatment center; stanniocalcin; stroke treatment center; subtotal colectomy

STD selective T-cell defect; sexually transmitted disease; short-term disability; skin-to-tumor distance; skin test dose; sodium tetradecyl sulfate; source-tray distance; standardized terminology dialogue; standard test dose; ST segment depression [ECG]

Std Standard

std saturated; standard deviation; standardized

STDH skin test for delayed hypersensitivity

STD-MIS Sexually Transmitted Diseases-Management Information System

STE Scholars for Teaching Excellence

STEAM stimulated echo acquisition mode

STEC Shiga toxin-producing *Escherichia coli*

STEL short-term exposure limit

STEM scanning transmission electron microscope; Society of Teachers of Emergency Medicine

STEN staphylococcal toxic epidermal necrolysis

sten stenosis, stenosed

STENT-BY Stent vs Bypass Surgery for Vessels Undergoing Abrupt Closure [trial]

STENTIM Stenting in Acute Myocardial Infarction [study]

STEP Sequential Test of Educational Progress; simultaneous transmission-emission protocol; Study of Taprostene in Elective Percutaneous Transluminal Coronary Angioplasty

STEPHY Starnberg Trial on Epidemiology of Parkinsonism and Hypertension in the Elderly

STEPS Significance of Transesophageal Electrocardiographic Findings in Prevention of Stroke [study]

STEREO Stents and ReoPro [trial]

stereo stereogram

STESS Subjective (or Subject's) Treatment Emergent Symptom Scale

STET submaximal treadmill exercise test

STEV short-term exposure value

STF serum thymus factor; slow-twitch fiber; special tube feeding; stefin; Stoffel [buffer]; sudden transient freezing

STFeSV Snyder-Theilen feline sarcoma virus

STFM Society of Teachers of Family Medicine

STFT short-time Fourier transform; silicon thin-film transistor

STG short-term goal; split-thickness graft; superior temporal gyrus

STH somatotropic hormone; subtotal hysterectomy

STh sickle cell thalassemia

ST/HR ST segment [ECG] depression with exercise divided by changes in heart rate

STHRF somatotropic hormone releasing factor

STI Scientific and Technical Information; serum trypsin inhibitor; sexually transmitted infection; soybean trypsin inhibitor; structured [cyclic antiretroviral] therapy interruption; systolic time interval

STI-571 imatinib mesylate

STIC Science and Technology Information Center; serum trypsin inhibition capacity; solid-state transducer intracompartment

STILE Surgery vs Thrombolysis for Ischemic Lower Extremity [trial]

stillb stillborn

STIM state transition information model

stim stimulated, stimulation; stimulus

STIMIS Study of Time Intervals in Myocardial Ischaemic Syndromes

STIMS Swedish Ticlodipine Multicenter Study

STIMULATE Speech, Text, Image, and Multimedia Advanced Technology Effort

STIPAS Safety Study of Tirilazad Mesylate in Patients with Acute Ischemic Stroke

STIR short tau inversion recovery

STJ subtalar joint

STK stem cell tyrosine kinase; streptokinase

STL serum theophylline level; standard template library; status thymicolymphaticus; stereolithography; swelling, tenderness, and limited motion

STLI subtotal lymphoid irradiation

STLIS South Thames Library Information Service

ST-LMA stylet-laryngeal mask airway

STLOM swelling, tenderness, and limitation of motion

STLS subacute thyroiditis-like syndrome

STLV simian T-lymphotropic virus

STLV 1, 2, 3 simian T-lymphotropic virus 1, 2, 3

STM *Salmonella typhimurium*; scanning tunneling microscope; short-term memory; signature-tagged mutagenesis; specimen transport medium; streptomycin

STMS short test of mental status

sTMS single-pulse transcranial magnetic stimulation

STMV Santarem virus

STMY stromelysin

STN [computer-assisted] surgical tool navigator; streptozocin; subthalamic nucleus; supratrochlear nucleus

sTNF soluble tumor necrosis factor

sTNFr soluble tumor necrosis factor receptor

sTNM tumor node metastasis [TNM] staging

STNR symmetric tonic neck reflex

STNV satellite tobacco necrosis virus

STO store

STO-3G Slater-type orbital comprising 3 gaussians

stom stomach

STONE Shanghai Trial of Nifedipine in the Elderly

STOP Shunt Thrombotic Occlusion Prevention by Picotamide [study]; Stenting for Total Occlusion and Restenosis Prevention [study]; Stroke Prevention in Sickle Cell Disease [study]; Study of Hypertension in the Elderly [Sweden] or Swedish Trial in Old Patients with Hypertension; surgical termination of pregnancy; Swedish Trial in Older Patients

STOP 2 Swedish Trial in Old Patients with Hypertension 2

STOP-AF Systematic Trial of Pacing to Prevent Atrial Fibrillation

STOP-Hypertension Swedish Trial in Older Patients with Hypertension

STOP IT Sites Testing Osteoporosis Prevention Intervention Treatment

STOPP Selling Teens on Pregnancy Prevention [study]

STOR summary time-oriented record

STORCH syphilis, toxoplasmosis, rubella, cytomegalovirus, and herpesvirus

STP phenol-preferring sulfotransferase; scientifically treated petroleum; short-term potentiation; sodium thiopental; standard temperature and pressure; standard temperature and pulse; stiripentol; strategic technology planning

ST$_p$ settling time per patient

STPB skin transient pulse blood

STPD short time Page distribution

STPS specific thalamic projection system

STQ superior temporal quadrant

STR short tandem repeat; soft tissue relaxation; statherin; stirred tank reactor; string matching

Str, str *Streptococcus*

strab strabismus

STRATIFY St. Thomas' Risk Assessment Tool in Falling Elderly Patients

STRATUS Study to Determine Rotablator and Transluminal Angioplasty Strategy

Strep *Streptococcus*; streptomycin

STRESS Stent Restenosis Study

STRETCH Symptom Tolerability Response to Exercise Trial of Candesartan Cilexetil in Patients with Heart Failure

STRICU shock, trauma, and respiratory intensive care unit

STRIP Special Turku Coronary Risk Factor Intervention Project [for babies]

s-TRSV substrate of tobacco ringspot virus

STRT simultaneous thermoradiotherapy; skin temperature recovery time

struct structure, structural

STRUT stent treatment region assessed by ultrasound tomography

STS self-tensioning suture; sequence-tagged site; sequence target site; serologic test for syphilis; side-to-side [anastomosis]; sodium tetradecyl sulfate; sodium thiosulfate; soft tissue sarcoma; standard test for syphilis; stand up; staphylococcal toxic syndrome; steroid sulfatase; subtrapezial space

STSA Southern Thoracic Surgical Association

STSD Spanish Trial on Sudden Death

STSE split-thickness skin excision

STSG split-thickness skin graft

STSS staphylococcal toxic shock syndrome

STT scaphotrapeziotrapezoid [joint]; serial thrombin time; short term test; skin temperature test; space-time toolkit

STU skin test unit

STUR Student Team Utilizing Research [project]

STV short term variability; spontaneous tidal volume; superior temporal vein

STVA subtotal villose atrophy

STVS short-term visual storage

STX saxitoxin; syntaxin

Stx Shiga toxin

STY semantic type [UMLS]

STZ streptozocin; streptozyme

SU salicyluric acid; secretory unit; sensation unit; solar urticaria; sorbent unit; spectrophotometric unit; status uncertain; subunit; sulfonamide; sulfonylurea; supine; surface

Su sulfonamide; supine

SUA serum uric acid; single umbilical artery; single unit activity

subac subacute

subclav subclavian; subclavicular

subcut subcutaneous

subling sublingual

SubN subthalamic nucleus

subq subcutaneous

SUBS substance [UMLS]

subsp subspecies

substd substandard

suc suction

Succ succinate, succinic

SUD skin unit dose; sudden unexpected death

SUDAAN survey data analysis

SUDEP sudden unexpected death in epilepsy

SUDH succinyldehydrogenase

SUDI sudden unexpected death in infancy

SUDS single use diagnostic system

SUFE slipped upper femoral epiphysis

SuHV suid herpesvirus

SUI stress urinary incontinence; string unique identifier [UMLS]

SUID sudden unexplained infant death

sulf sulfate

sulfa sulfonamide

SULF-PRIM sulfamethoxazole and trimethoprim

SUMA sporadic ulcerating and mutilating acropathy

SUMAA scalable unstructured mesh algorithms and applications

SUMD Scale to Assess Unawareness in Mental Disorder

SUMIT streptokinase-urokinase myocardial infarct test

SUMMIT Stanford University Medical Media and Information Technology

SUMSE stroke unit mental status examination

SUN serum urea nitrogen; standard unit of nomenclature

SUO syncope of unknown origin

SUP schizo-unipolar; supination

sup above [Lat. *supra*]; superficial; superior; supinator; supine

supin supination, supine

supp suppository

suppl supplement, supplementary

SUPPORT Study to Understand Prognoses and Preferences for Outcomes and Risks of Treatment

suppos suppository

SUR sulfonylurea receptor; suramin

SurDx surgical diagnosis

SURE Serial Ultrasound Analysis of Restenosis [study]

SURF surfeit

SURFnet Netherlands Network

SURG, Surg surgery, surgical, surgeon

SurPROC surgical procedure

SURS solitary ulcer of rectum syndrome; Surveillance and Utilization Review System

SURVS-TB Surveillance System for Tuberculosis

SUS Saybolt Universal Seconds; solitary ulcer syndrome; stained urinary sediment; suppressor sensitive

SUSHI Stent Use Is Superior for Hospitalized Infarction Patients [study]

susp suspension, suspended

SUTAMI Saruplase and Urokinase in the Treatment of Acute Myocardial Infarction [trial]

SUTI symptomatic urinary tract infection

SUUD sudden unexpected unexplained death

SUV small unilamellar vessel; standard uptake value

SUVIMAX Supplemental Vitamins, Minerals and Anti-Oxidants [trial]

S-UVT sustained uniform ventricular tachycardia

SUX succinylcholine

SUZI subzonal insemination

SV sample volume; saphenous vein; Sapporo virus; sarcoma virus; satellite virus; scattering volume; selective vagotomy; semilunar valve; seminal vesicle; severe; sigmoid volvulus; simian virus; single ventricle; sinus venosus; snake venom; splenic vein; spontaneous ventilation; starting volume; streak virus; stroke volume; subclavian vein; subventricular; supravital; symptomless virus; synaptic vesicle; syncytial virus; systolic velocity

S/V surface/volume ratio

SV2 synaptic vesicle protein 2

SV-5, -10, -12, -40, -41 simian virus 5, 10, 12, 40, 41

SV$_{40}$ simian vacuolating virus 40

Sv sievert

sv sievert; single vibration

SVA selective vagotomy and antrectomy; selective visceral angiography; sequential ventriculoatrial [pacing]; subtotal villous atrophy

SVAS supravalvular aortic stenosis; supraventricular aortic stenosis

SVAT synaptic vesicle amine transformer

SVB saphenous vein bypass

SVBG saphenous vein bypass grafting

SVC saphenous vein cutdown; segmental venous capacitance; selective venous catheterization; slow vital capacity; spatially varying classification; subclavian vein catheterization; superior vena cava; support vector classification; supraventricular crest; supraventricular extrasystole

SVCCS superior vena cava compression syndrome

SVCG spatial vectorcardiogram

SVCO superior vena-caval obstruction

SVCP Special Virus Cancer Program

SVCR segmental venous capacitance ratio

SVCS superior vena cava syndrome

SVD single vessel disease; singular value decomposition; small vessel disease; spontaneous vaginal delivery; spontaneous vertex delivery; swine vesicular disease

SVE slow volume encephalography; soluble viral extract; spontaneous ventricular event; sterile vaginal examination

SVG saphenous vein graft; scalable vector graphics; scatter and veiling glare; seminal vesiculography

SVGA super video graphics array

SVH saphenous vein harvesting

SV-HUC simian virus-human uro-epithelial cell

SVI seminal vesicle invasion; slow virus infection; small volume infusion; stroke volume index; systolic velocity integral

SVL seminal HIV-1 viral load; superficial vastus lateralis

SVM seminal vesicle microsome; support vector machine; syncytiovascular membrane

SVMP snake venom metalloprotease

SVMT synaptic vesicle monoamine transformer

SVN selectively vulnerable neurons; sinuvertebral nerve; small volume nebulizer

SvO$_2$ venous oxygen saturation

SVOC semivolatile organic compound

SVOM sequential volitional oral movement

SVP selective vagotomy and pyloroplasty; small volume parenteral [infusion]; standing venous pressure; superior vascular plexus

SVPB supraventricular premature beat

SVPC supraventricular premature complex

SVPD snake venom phosphodiesterase

SV40-PML simian vacuolating virus 40 of progressive multifocal leukoencephalopathy

SVR sequential vascular response; stroke volume ratio; support vector regression; sustained viral response; systemic vascular resistance

SVRI systemic vascular resistance index

SVS slit ventricle syndrome; Society for Vascular Surgery

SVT sinoventricular tachycardia; subclavian vein thrombosis; supraventricular tachyarrhythmia; supraventricular tachycardia; sustained ventricular tachycardia

SVTh subvalvular thickening

SVTS Sotalol Ventricular Tachycardia Study

SVV Sal Vieja virus

SW seriously wounded; short waves; sinewave; slow wave; soap and water; social worker; spike wave; spiral wound; stab wound; sterile water; stroke work; Sturge-Weber [syndrome]; Swiss Webster [mouse]

S/W spike wave

Sw swine

SWA seriously wounded in action; slow-wave activity

SWAIDS social workers in acquired immunodeficiency syndrome [AIDS]

SWAP short wavelength automated perimetry

SWAT stationary wavelet transform; Stroke Prevention with Warfarin or Aspirin Trial

SWC submaximal working capacity

S&WC spike and wave complex [EEG]

SWCM social work case manager

SWD short wave diathermy

SWE slow wave encephalography

SWEET Square Wave Endurance Exercise Trial

SWEHSLinC South West England Health Services Library and Information Network

SWG silkworm gut; standard wire gauge; stimulus waveform generator

SWI sterile water for injection; stroke work index; surgical wound infection

SWICE South-West Information for Clinical Effectiveness [UK]

SWIFT Should We Intervene Following Thrombolysis? [study]

SWIM sperm-washing insemination method

SWIORA spinal cord injury without radiologic abnormality

SWISH Swedish Isradipine Study in Hypertension

SWISSI Swiss Interventional Study in Silent Ischemia

SWL shock wave lithotripsy

SWM segmental wall motion

SWMA segmental wall motion analysis

SWMF Semmes-Weinstein monofilament

SWNT single-walled carbon nanotube

SWO superficial white onychomycosis

SWOG South West Oncology Group

SWOOP South Wilshire Out of Hours Project

SWORD Survival with Oral D-Sotalol [study]; surveillance of work-related and occupational respiratory diseases

SWOT Strengths-Weaknesses-Opportunities-Threats [analysis]
SWPV swinepox virus
SWR serum Wassermann reaction; slow wave ratio; surgical wound infection rate
SWRF square wave response function
SWRLIN South and West Regional Library Information Network [UK]
SWS slow-wave sleep; spike-wave stupor; steroid-wasting syndrome; Sturge-Weber syndrome
SWT sine-wave threshold
SWU septic work-up
SwV swine calicivirus
SX scleral invasion cannot be assessed [TNM (tumor-node-metastasis) classification]
Sx suction
Sx, S$_x$ signs; symptoms
s$_x$ standard deviation of sampling distribution [statistics]
SXA single-energy x-ray absorptiometry, single x-ray absorptiometry
SXCT spiral x-ray computed tomography
SXR skull x-ray [examination]; steroid and xenobiotic receptor
Sxr sex reversal
Sxs serological sex-specific [antigen]
SXT sulfamethoxazole-trimethoprim [mixture]
SY spectroscopy; syphilis, syphilitic
SYA subacute yellow atrophy
SYB synaptobrevin
SYDS stomach yin deficiency syndrome
sym symmetrical; symptom

sympath sympathetic
symph symphysis
SYMPHONY Sibrafiban vs Aspirin to Yield Maximum Protection from Ischemic Heart Events Postacute Coronary Syndromes [trial]
sympt symptom
SYN synapse; synovitis
syn synergistic; synonym; synovial
SYNBIAPACE synchronous biatrial pacing therapy
synd syndrome
SYNDIKATE synthesis of distributed knowledge acquired from text
Synf synovial fluid
SynText symbolic text [processor]
SYP synaptophysin
syph syphilis, syphilitic
SYR Syrian [hamster]
syr syrup [Lat. *syrupus*]; syringe
SYREC symmetric recombinant [virus]
SYS stretching-yawning syndrome; systemic
sys system, systemic; systolic
SYS-BP systolic blood pressure
syst system; systole, systolic
SYST-CHINA Systolic Hypertension in Elderly Chinese Trial
SYST-EUR Systolic Hypertension in Europeans Study
SYT synaptotagmin
SZ schizophrenia; streptozocin
Sz seizure; schizophrenia
SZN streptozocin

T

T absolute temperature; an electrocardiographic wave corresponding to the repolarization of the ventricles [wave]; large T [antigen]; life [time]; period [time]; primary tumor [TNM (tumor-node-metastasis) classification: **T0** no evidence of primary tumor, **T1 to T4** tumors in progressing sizes, and **TX** no evidence of primary tumor]; ribosylthymine; tablespoonful; *Taenia*; tamoxifen; telomere or terminal banding; temperature; temporal electrode placement in electroencephalography; temporary; tenderness; tension [intraocular]; tera- [trillion]; tesla; testosterone; tetra; tetracycline; theophylline; therapy; thoracic; thorax; threatened [animal]; threonine; thrombosis; thrombus; thymidine; thymine; thymus [cell]; thymus-derived; thyroid; tidal gas; tidal volume; time; timed [device]; tincture; tissue; tocopherol; topical; torque; total; toxicity; training [group]; transition; transducer; transmittance; transverse; treatment; *Treponema*; triangulation number; *Trichophyton*; triggered [pacemaker]; tritium; tryptamine; *Trypanosoma*; tuberculin; tuberculosis; tumor; turnkey system; type

T- tera- [10^{12}]

T0 no evidence of primary tumor [TNM (tumor-node-metastasis) classification]

T$_{1/2}$ half-life

T1 breast tumor smaller than 2 cm [TNM (tumor-node-metastasis) classification]; longitudinal relaxation time

T-1, T-2, T-3 first, second, and third stages of decreased intraocular tension

T$_1$ spin-lattice or longitudinal relaxation time; time at the beginning of inspiration; tricuspid first sound; tricuspid valve closure sound

T + 1, T + 2, T + 3 first, second, and third stages of increased intraocular tension

T1–4 presence of tumors progressing in size, number, and penetration [TNM (tumor-node-metastasis) classification]

T1–T12 first to twelfth thoracic vertebrae

T2 breast tumor 2.0 to 5.0 cm [TNM (tumor-node-metastasis) classification]; transverse relaxation time

T$_2$ diiodothyronine; spin-spin or transverse relaxation time

T2*, T$_2$* effective transverse relaxation time

2,4,5-T 2,4,5-trichlorophenoxyacetic acid

T3 breast tumor larger than 5.0 cm [TNM (tumor-node-metastasis) classification]

T$_3$ triiodothyronine

T4 breast tumor of any size with extension to chest wall and skin [TNM (tumor-node-metastasis) classification]

T$_4$ thyroxine

T-7 free thyroxine factor

T$_{90}$ time required for 90% mortality in a population of microorganisms exposed to a toxic agent

t duration; small T [antigen]; Student *t* test; teaspoonful; temperature; temporal; terminal; tertiary; test of significance; three times [Lat. *ter*]; time; tissue; tonne; transformer; translocation

t *t* value from *t* distribution [statistics]

t′ time after infusion

t$_{1/2}$ half-life

t$_2$ time at the end of inspiration

τ see *tau*

Θ see *theta*

θ see *theta*

TA alkaline tuberculin; arterial tension; axillary temperature; tactile afferent; Takayasu arteritis; technology assessment; teichoic acid; temporal abstraction; temporal arteritis; terminal antrum; therapeutic abortion; thermophilic *Actinomyces*; thymocytotoxic autoantibody; thyroarytenoid; thyroglobulin autoprecipitation; thyroid antibody; thyroid autoimmunity; tibialis anterior [muscle]; tissue adhesive; titratable acid; total alkaloids; total antibody; toxic adenoma; toxin-antitoxin; traffic accident; transactional analysis; transaldolase; transaminase; transantral; transplantation antigen; transposition of aorta; trapped air; triamcinolone acetonide; tricuspid atresia; trophoblast antigen; true anomaly; truncus arteriosus; tryptamine; tryptose agar; tube agglutination; tumor-associated; typical absences

T-A toxin-antitoxin; transfusion-associated

T&A tonsillectomy and adenoidectomy; tonsils and adenoids

T/A time and amount

TA-4 tumor-associated antigen 4

Ta tantalum; tarsal

T1a breast tumor 0.1 to 0.5 cm [TNM (tumor-node-metastasis) classification]

T4a breast tumor with extension to chest wall [TNM (tumor-node-metastasis) classification]

t_α t value corresponding to specified tail area α [statistics]

TAA thioacetamide; thoracic aortic aneurysm; total ankle arthroplasty; transverse aortic arch; tumor-associated antigen

TAAF thromboplastic activity of the amniotic fluid

TA-AIDS transfusion-associated acquired immunodeficiency syndrome

TAB tape-automated bonding; total autonomic blockage; typhoid, paratyphoid A, and paratyphoid B [vaccine]

TAb therapeutic abortion

tab tablet

TABC total aerobic bacteria count; typhoid, paratyphoid A, paratyphoid B, and paratyphoid C [vaccine]

TABP type A behavior pattern

Tabs tablets

T_{abs} absorption time

TABT typhoid, paratyphoid A, paratyphoid B, and tetanus toxoid [vaccine]

TABTD typhoid, paratyphoid A, paratyphoid B, tetanus toxoid, and diphtheria toxoid [vaccine]

TABV Tamana bat virus

TAC tachykinin; terminal antrum contraction; tetracaine, adrenalin, and cocaine; time-activity curve; total abdominal colectomy; total aganglionosis coli; total allergen content; transient aplastic crisis; triamcinolone cream; truncus arteriosus communis

TAC-1 tachykinin-1

TAC-2 tachykinin-2

TACC thoracic aorta cross-clamping

TACE chlorotrianicene; teichoic acid crude extract; transarterial chemoembolization; tumor-necrosis factor alpha converting enzyme

tachy tachycardia

TACIP Triflusal, Aspirin, Cerebral Infarction Prevention [study]

TACR tachykinin receptor

TACS Thrombolysis and Angioplasty in Cardiogenic Shock [study]

TACSV Triticum aestivum chlorotic spot virus

TACT thermoacoustic computed tomography; Ticlopidine Angioplasty Coronary Trial; Ticlopidine vs Placebo for Prevention of Acute Closure After Angioplasty Trial; tuned aperture computed tomography

TACTICS Thrombolysis and Counterpulsation to Improve Cardiogenic Shock Survival [trial]

TACTICS-TIMI 18 Treat Angina with Aggrastat and Determine Cost of Therapy with an Invasive or Conservative Strategy-Thrombolysis in Myocardial Infarction [trial]

TAD test of auditory discrimination; thoracic asphyxiant dystrophy; tobacco, alcohol, and drugs; Traffic Accident Deformity [scale]; transactivation domain; transient acantholytic dermatosis

TADAC therapeutic abortion, dilatation, aspiration, curettage

TAdV Turkey adenovirus

TADv 1, 2 Turkey adenovirus 1, 2

TAE transcatheter arterial embolism; triacetate ethylenediamine tetraacetic acid [EDTA]

TAF albumose-free tuberculin [Ger. *Tuberculin Albumose frei*]; tissue angiogenesis factor; total abdominal fat; toxin-antitoxin floccules; toxoid-antitoxin floccules; tracheobronchial aspiration fluid; transcriptional activation factor [genetics]; trypsin-aldehyde-fuchsin; tumor angiogenesis factor

TAFU tumor abrasion with focused ultrasound

TAG target attaching globulin; technical advisory group; thymine, adenine, and guanine

TAg large T-antigen

Tag T-antigen

TAGH triiodothyronine, amino acids, glucagon, and heparin

TAGV Taggert virus

TAGVHD transfusion-associated graft-versus-host disease

TAH total abdominal hysterectomy; total artificial heart

TAH BSO total abdominal hysterectomy and bilateral salpingo-oophorectomy

TAHIV transfusion-acquired human immunodeficiency virus [HIV]

TAHSC Toronto Academic Health Science Council

TAHV Tahyna virus

TAI Test Anxiety Inventory

TAIAV Taiassui virus

TAIM Trial of Antihypertensive Intervention and Management

TAIS time assessment interview schedule

TAIST Tinzaparin in Acute Stroke Trial

TAIV Tai virus

TAL T-cell acute leukemia; tendon of Achilles lengthening; thick ascending limb [of Henle's loop]; thymic alymphoplasia; total arm length; tumor-associated lymphocyte

talc talcum

TALH thick ascending limb of Henle's loop

TALL theoretical annual loss of life

TALL, T-ALL T-cell acute lymphoblastic leukemia

TALLA T-cell acute lymphoblastic leukemia antigen

TAM tamoxifen; technological acceptance model; technology acceptance model; technology assessment method; teen-age mother; tele-alarm management; thermoacidurans agar modified; thymidine analog mutation; time-averaged mean; total active motion; Total Atherosclerosis Management [study]; toxin-antitoxoid mixture; transient abnormal myelopoiesis

TAME *N*-alpha-tosyl-1-arginine methyl ester

TAMI Thrombolysis and Angioplasty in Myocardial Infarction [study]; transmural anterior myocardial infarction

TAMIS Telemetric Automated Microbial Identification System

TamMV Tamarillo mosaic virus

TAMRA tetramethylrhodamine

TAMV Tamiami virus; temporal average maximal velocity [Doppler]

TAN total adenine nucleotide; total ammonia nitrogen

tan tandem translocation; tangent

TANet Taiwan Network

TANI total axial [lymph] node irradiation

TANV Tanapox virus; Tanga virus

TAO thromboangiitis obliterans; triacetyloleandomycin

TAP technology architecture project; tick anticoagulant peptide; total access plus [computer-based system]; toxicological agent protection or protective; transesophageal atrial pacing; transluminal angioplasty; transmembrane action potential; transporter in antigen processing; trypsinogen-activating peptide

TAPA target of antiproliferative antibody

TAPE temporary atrial pacemaker electrode

TAPIRSS Triflusal vs Aspirin in Preventing Infarction: Randomized Stroke Study

TAPS The Akita Pathology Study; Teenage Attitude and Practices Study; trial assessment procedure scale

TAPVC total anomalous pulmonary venous connection

TAPVD total anomalous pulmonary venous drainage

TAPVR total anomalous pulmonary venous return

Taq *Thermus aquaticus*

taq DNA *Thermus aquaticus* deoxyribonucleic acid [DNA]

TAQW transient abnormal Q wave

TAR thoracic aortic rupture; thrombocytopenia with absent radii [syndrome]; tissue-air ratio; total abortion rate; transactivation response; transanal resection; transaxillary resection; treatment authorization request

TARA total articular replacement arthroplasty; tumor-associated rejection antigen

TARGET Do Tirofiban and ReoPro Give Similar Efficacy Outcomes Trial

TARP total atrial refractory period

TAR/PD target nursing hours per patient/day

TARS threonyl transfer ribonucleic acid [RNA] synthetase

TAS tetanus antitoxin serum; therapeutic activities specialist; thoracoabdominal syndrome; transcription-based amplification system; traumatic apallic syndrome

TASA tumor-associated surface antigen

TASC tele-archive service center [imaging]; time-accumulating sub-surface contaminant; Trial of Angioplasty and Stents in Canada

Tase tryptophan synthetase

TASH Transcoronary Ablation of Septum Hypertrophy [study]

TASMAN Thrombolysis Anticoagulant Study: Mediterranean, Australia, New Zealand

TASO The Acquired Immunodeficiency Syndrome [AIDS] Support Organisation [Australia]

TASS thyrotoxicosis-Addison disease-Sjögren syndrome-sarcoidosis [syndrome]; Ticlopidine Aspirin Stroke Study

TASTE Ticlopidine Aspirin Stent Evaluation

TAstV Turkey astrovirus

TAT tandem autotransplantation; tetanus antitoxin; thematic apperception test; thematic aptitude test; thrombin-antithrombin complex; thromboplastin activation test; total adipose tissue; total antitryptic activity; toxin-antitoxin; transactivator; transaxial tomography; transplantation-associated thrombocytopenia; tray agglutination test; *Treponema* antibody test; tumor activity test; turnaround time; twin arginine translocation; tyrosine aminotransferase

TATA Pribnow [box]; tumor-associated transplantation antigen

TATD tyrosine aminotransferase deficiency

TATI tumor-associated trypsin inhibitor

TATR tyrosine aminotransferase regulator

TATRC Telemedicine and Advanced Technology Research Center

TATST tetanus antitoxin skin test

TATV Tataguine virus

τ Greek lowercase letter *tau*; life [of radioisotope]; relaxation time; shear stress; spectral transmittance; transmission coefficient

TAUSA Thrombolysis and Angioplasty in Unstable Angina [trial]

TAV transcutaneous aortovelography; trapped air volume

TaV *Thosea asigna* virus

TAVB total atrioventricular block

TAX Taxol

TB Taussig-Bing [syndrome]; terabyte; term birth; terminal bronchiole; terminal bronchus; thromboxane B; thymol blue; tissue bank; toluidine blue; total base; total bilirubin; total body; tracheobronchial; tracheal bronchiolar [region]; tracheobronchitis; trapezoid body; tub bath; triple [gene] block; tubercle bacillus; tuberculin; tuberculosis; tumor bank; tumor-bearing

T$_B$ total buffer

TB$^+$ tuberculosis positive

TB$^-$ tuberculosis negative

Tb Tbilisi [phage]; terabit [trillion bits]; terbium; tubercle bacillus; tuberculosis

T$_b$ biological half-life; body temperature

T1b breast tumor 0.5 to 1.0 cm [TNM (tumor-node-metastasis) classification]

T4b breast tumor with edema (including peau d'orange) or skin ulceration or satellite nodules [TNM (tumor-node-metastasis) classification]

tb tuberculosis

TBA target [hospital] bed occupation; tertiary butylacetate; testosterone-binding affinity; tetrabutylammonium; thiobarbituric acid; to be absorbed; to be added; total bile acids; trypsin-binding activity; tubercle bacillus; tumor-bearing animal

TBAB tryptose blood agar base

TBAF tetrabutylammonium fluoride

TBAN transbronchial aspiration needle

TBARS thiobarbituric acid reactive substance

TBB transbronchial biopsy

TBBA total body bone ash

TBBM total body bone minerals

TBBx transbronchial biopsy

TBC thyroxine-binding coagulin; total body calcium; total body carbon; total body clearance; tuberculosis

Tbc tubercle bacillus; tuberculosis

TBCa total body calcium

TBCl total body chlorine

TBD total body density; Toxicology Data Base

TBE tick-borne encephalitis; triborate ethylenediamine tetraacetic acid [EDTA]; tris-borate ethylenediamine tetraacetic acid [EDTA]; tuberculin bacillin emulsion

TBEV tick-borne encephalitis virus

TBF total body fat

TBFB tracheobronchial foreign body

TBFM total body fat mass

TBFVL tidal breathing flow-volume loops

TBG beta-thromboglobulin; testosterone-binding globulin; thyroglobulin; thyroid-binding globulin; thyroxine-binding globulin; tracheobronchography; tris-buffered Gey solution

TBGI thyroxine-binding globulin index

TBGP total blood granulocyte pool

TBH total body hematocrit

tBHP terbutyl hydroperoxide

TBHQ tertiary butylhydroquinone

TBHT total-body hyperthermia

TBI thyroid-binding index; thyroxine-binding index; tooth-brushing instruction; total-body irradiation; traumatic brain injury

TBII thyroid-stimulating hormone-binding inhibitory immunoglobulin

TBil, T bili total bilirubin

TBIM thoracic bioimpedance monitoring

TBK total body potassium

tbl tablet

TBLB transbronchial lung biopsy

TBLC term birth, living child

TBLI term birth, living infant

TBLTM total body lean tissue mass

TBM thrombomodulin; total body mass; tracheobronchiomegaly; trophoblastic basement membrane; tuberculous meningitis; tubular basement membrane

TBMC total body mineral content

TBMN thin basement membrane nephropathy

TBN bacillus emulsion; temporal belief network; total body nitrogen

Tb.N trabecular number

TBNA total body neutron activation; transbronchial needle aspiration; treated but not admitted

TBNa total body sodium

TBNAA total body neutron activation analysis

TBO total blood out

TBP bithional; testosterone-binding protein; thyroxine-binding protein; total body protein; total bypass; tributyl phosphate; tuberculous peritonitis

TBPA thyroxine-binding prealbumin

TBPr total body protein

Tbps terabits [trillion bits] per second

TBPT total body protein turnover

TBR tumor-bearing rabbit

TB-RD tuberculosis and respiratory disease

TBS total body solids; total body solute; total body surface; total burn size; Townes-Brocks syndrome; tracheobronchial submucosa; tracheobronchoscopy; tribromosalicylanilide; triethanolamine-buffered saline; tris-buffered saline

tbs, tbsp tablespoon

TBSA total body surface area

TBS-G tris-buffered saline with glycerol

Tb.Sp trabecular separation

TBST tris-buffered saline tween

TBSV tomato bushy stunt virus

TBT tolbutamide test; tracheobronchial toilet; tracheobronchial tree; transcervical balloon tuboplasty; tributyltin

TBTC Tuberculosis Trials Consortium

TBTO tributyltin oxide

TBTT tuberculin time test

TBTV Timboteua virus

TBV total blood volume; trabecular bone volume

TBW total body water; total body weight

TBX thromboxane; total body irradiation

TBXA2 thromboxane A2

TBXAS thromboxane A synthase

TBZ tetrabenazine; thiabendazole

TC talocalcaneal; tandem colonoscopy; target cell; taurocholate; temperature compensation; teratocarcinoma; terminal cancer; tertiary cleavage; testicular cancer; tetanic contraction; tetracycline; theca cell; therapeutic community; thermal conductivity; thermocouple; thoracic cage; thoracic compression; thorax circumference; throat culture; thyrocalcitonin; time constant; tissue culture; to contain; total calcium; total capacity; total cholesterol; total colonoscopy; total correction; toxic concentration; transcobalamin; transcriptase complex; transcutaneous; transhepatic cholangiography; transmission control; transplant center; transverse colon; Treacher Collins [syndrome]; true channel; true conjugate; tuberculin contagiosum; tubocurarine; tumor cell; tumor of cerebrum; type and crossmatch

T&C turn and cough; type and crossmatch

T₄(C) serum thyroxine measured by column chromatography

TC₅₀ median toxic concentration; threshold concentration

Tc correlation time; Tanimoto coefficient; technetium; tetracycline; transcobalamin

T^c cytotoxic T cell, cytotoxic T lymphocyte

T_c critical temperature; cytotoxic T cell, cytotoxic T lymphocyte; the generation time of a cell cycle; tricuspid closure

T1c breast tumor 1.0 to 2.0 cm [TNM (tumor-node-metastasis) classification]

t(°C) temperature on the Celsius scale

tc transcutaneous; translational control

TCA T-cell A locus; tentorium cerebelli attachment; terminal cancer; tetracyclic antidepressant; thyrocalcitonin; topological constraint algorithm; total cholic acid; total circulating albumin; total circulatory arrest; total colonic agangliosis; transcondylar axis; tricalcium aluminate; tricarboxylic acid; trichloroacetic acid; tricyclic antidepressant; thyrocalcitonin

TCAB 3,3′,4,4′-tetrachloroazobenzene

TCABG triple coronary artery bypass graft

TCAD tricyclic antidepressant

TCADA Texas Council on Alcohol and Drug Abuse

tCAF tonic cortical activation function

TCAG triple coronary artery graft

TCAId trichloroacetaldehyde

TCAOB 3,3′,4,4′-tetrachloroazoxybenzene

TCAP trimethyl-cetyl-ammonium pentachlorophenate

TCAR T-cell antigen receptor

TCAT transmission computer-assisted tomography

TCB tetrachlorobiphenyl; total cardiopulmonary bypass transcatheter biopsy; transabdominal chorionic biopsy; trusted computing base; tumor cell burden

TcB transcutaneous bilirubin

TCBF total cerebral blood flow

TCBS thiosulfate-citrate-bile salts-sucrose [agar]

TCC terminal complement complex; thromboplastic cell component; transcatheter closure; transitional-cell carcinoma; transmission control computer [imaging]; trauma center coordination or coordinator; trichlorocarbanilide, triclocarban

Tcc triclocarban

TCCA, TCCAV transitional cell cancer-associated [virus]

TCCD transcranial color-coded Doppler

TCCDS transitional cell carcinoma dataset

TCCL T-cell chronic lymphoblastic leukemia

TCCS transcranial color-coded sonography

TCCU&C therapeutic care, understanding and control

TCD tapetochoroidal dystrophy; T-cell depletion; thermal conductivity detector; tissue culture dose; transcranial Doppler [ultrasound or sonography]; transverse cardiac diameter; tumoricidal dose

TCD$_{50}$ median tissue culture dose; tissue culture infectious dose

TCDB turn, cough, deep breathe

TcdB *Clostridium difficile* toxin B

TCDC taurochenodeoxycholate

TCDD 2,3,7,8-tetrachlorodibenzo-*p*-dioxin; threshold contrast detail detectability

TCDF 2,3,7-tetrachlorodibenzofuran

TCE T-cell enriched; tetrachlorodiphenyl ethane; total colon examination; trichloroethane; trichloroethylene

TCED$_{50}$ 50% tissue effective dose

TCES transcutaneous cranial electrical stimulation

TCESOM trichloroethylene-extracted soybean oil meal

TCET transcerebral electrotherapy

TCF T-cell factor; teleconsultation folder; tetanic contraction fatigue; tissue coding factor; total coronary flow; transcription factor; Treacher Collins-Franceschetti [syndrome]

T-CFC T-colony forming cell

TCFU tumor colony-forming unit

TCG therapeutic care-general; time-compensated gain; Thromboprophylaxis Collaborative Group

TCGF T-cell growth factor

TCH tanned-cell hemagglutination; thiophen-2-carboxylic acid hydrazide; total circulating hemoglobin; turn, cough, hyperventilate

TC/HDL total cholesterol/high density lipoproteins [ratio]

TChE total cholinesterase

TCI temporal continuity index; To Come In [open heart surgery program at Cleveland Clinic]; total cerebral ischemia; transient cerebral ischemia; transitory cognitive impairment; transcobalamin I

TCi teracurie

TCID tissue culture infectious dose; tissue culture infective dose; tissue culture inoculated dose

TCID$_{50}$ median tissue culture infective dose; 50% tissue culture infective dose

TCIE transient cerebral ischemic episode

TCII transcobalamin II

TCIII transcobalamin III

TCIMC Trauma Center Information Management Center

TCI_{pr} temporal continuity index for providers

TCI_{pt} temporal continuity index for patients

TCIS T-cell immunodeficiency syndrome; total corrected increment score; transitional carcinoma in situ

TCL tachycardia cycle length; T-cell leukemia; T-cell lymphoma; thermochemiluminescence; tibial collateral ligament; total capacity of the lung; transcallosal latency; transverse carpal ligament; triazine chlorguanide

T-CLL T-cell chronic lymphatic leukemia

TC_{Lo} toxic concentration low

TCLP toxicity characteristic leachate procedure [Environmental Protection Agency, EPA]

TCM tissue culture medium; traditional Chinese medicine; transcutaneous monitor

T&CM type and crossmatch

Tc 99m technetium-99m

TCMA transcortical motor aphasia

TCMI traditional Chinese medicine informatics

Tc 99m MDP technetium-99m methylene diphosphonate

TCMP thematic content modification program

TCMS transcranial magnetic stimulation

TCMV Tacaiuma virus

TCMZ trichloromethiazide

TCN tetracycline; transcobalamin

Tc NM tumor with lymph node metastases

TCNS transcutaneous nerve stimulation/stimulator

TCNV terminal contingent negative variation

TCO transcutaneous oximetry

T_{CO2} total carbon dioxide

TCoV Turkey coronavirus

TCP T-complex protein; therapeutic care-psychosocial; therapeutic class profile; therapeutic continuous penicillin; thienylcyclohexylpiperidine; thrombocytopenia; tibial hole coronal positioning; tissue culture treated plastic; tissue or tumor control probability [radiotherapy]; total cardiopulmonary [connection]; total circulating protein; toxin-coregulated pilus; transcutaneous pacemaker; transcutaneous pacing; transmission control protocol; tranylcypromine; tricalcium phosphate; trichlorophenol; tricresyl phosphate; tropical calcific pancreatitis; tumor control probability

TCPA tetrachlorophthalic anhydride

tcPCO₂, tcpCO₂ transcutaneous partial pressure of carbon dioxide

TCPD₅₀ 50% tissue culture protective dose

TCP/IP transmission control protocol/Internet protocol

TCPL tricalcium-phosphate-lysine

tcPO₂, tcpO₂ transcutaneous partial pressure of oxygen

tcP_{O2}, tcPO₂ transcutaneous oxygen pressure

2,4,5-TCPPA 2-(2,4,5-trichlorophenoxy)-propionic acid

TCPS total cavopulmonary shunt

TCR T-cell reactivity; T-cell receptor; T-cell rosette; thalamocortical relay; total cytoplasmic ribosome; transcriptional control center; transcription-coupled [deoxyribonucleic acid, DNA] repair; trauma center record; true count rate; turn, cough, and rebreathe

TcR T-cell receptor

TCRA T-cell receptor alpha

TCRB T-cell receptor beta

TCRD T-cell receptor delta

TCRG T-cell receptor gamma

tcRNA translational control ribonucleic acid

TCRP total cellular receptor pool

TCRV Tacaribe virus; tissue culture rinderpest vaccine

TCRZ T-cell receptor Z

TCS T-cell supernatant; temporal control structure; tethered cord syndrome; total coronary score; transcranial [magnetic] stimulation; Treacher Collins syndrome

TCSA tetrachlorosalicylanilide

TCSEC trusted computer system evaluation criteria

TCSF T-colony-stimulating factor

TcsL *Clostridium sordelli* lethal toxin

TCSPC time-correlated single photon count

TCT thrombin clotting time; thyrocalcitonin; trachial cytotoxin; transcardial catheter therapy; transmission computed tomography

Tct tincture

tcTOFA time constrained time-of-flight absorbance

TCU timing control unit; trauma care unit; treatment control unit

TCV thoracic cage volume; three concept view

TCW time coincidence window

TD tabes dorsalis; tardive dyskinesia; T-cell dependent [antigen]; temporal embedding dimension; temporary disability; terminal device; tetanus and diphtheria [toxoid]; tetrodotoxin; thanatophoric dwarfism; thanatophoric dysplasia; therapy discontinued; thermal dilution; thoracic duct; three times per day; threshold of detectability; threshold of discomfort; threshold dose; thymus-dependent; time delay; time dictionary; timed disintegration; tocopherol deficiency; to deliver; tone decay; torsion dystonia; total disability; total discrimination; totally disabled; total dose; Tourette disorder; toxic dose; topic-specific document; tracheal diameter; transdermal; transverse diameter; traveler's diarrhea; treatment discontinued; tumor dose; typhoid dysentery

T-D T-cell dependent [antigen]

T/D treatment discontinued

T$_D$ the time required to double the number of cells in a given population; thermal death time

TD$_{01}$ toxic dose, 1% response

T2D type 2 diabetes

T$_4$(D) serum thyroxine measured by displacement analysis

TD$_{50}$ median toxic dose

TD$_{99}$ toxic dose, 99% response

Td doubling time; tetanus-diphtheria toxoid

T1d inflammatory breast carcinoma [TNM (tumor-node-metastasis) classification]

TDA thyroid-stimulating hormone-displacing antibody

TDADF transform domain adaptive filter

TDAF transform domain adaptive filter

TDAP thoracodorsal artery perforator flap

TDB terminologic database; Toxicology Data Bank

T$_{db}$ dry-bulb temperature

TDC taurodeoxycholic acid; thermal dilution catheter; time-density curve [computed tomography]; total dietary calories

T&DC transmural and diagnostic center

Td-CIA T-cell-derived colony-inhibiting activity

TDCO thermodilution cardiac output [measurement]

TDD telecommunication device for the deaf; tetradecadiene; thoracic duct drainage; total digitalizing dose; toxic doses of drugs; transverse digital deficiency

TDE tetrachlorodiphenylethane; total digestible energy; triethylene glycol diglycidyl

TDF tenofovir; testis-determining factor; thoracic duct fistula; thoracic duct flow; thoracodorsal flap; time-dose fractionation; tissue-damaging factor; tumor dose fractionation

TdF thymidine deoxyribose

TDFA testis-determining factor, autosomal

TDFX testis-determining factor X

TDGF teratocarcinoma-derived growth factor

TDH high toxic dose; thermostable direct hemolysin; thoracic disc herniation; threonine dehydrogenase

T/DHT testosterone/dihydrotestosterone ratio

TDI temperature difference integration; three-dimensional interlocking [hip]; time-delay integration; tissue Doppler imaging; tolerable daily intake; toluene 2,4-diisocyanate; total dose infusion; total dose insulin

TDL tegmental dorsolateral [nucleus]; template definition language; thoracic duct lymph; thymus-dependent lymphocyte; toxic dose level

TDLU terminal ductal lobular unit

TDM therapeutic drug monitoring

TD-MCT time-domain microwave computed tomography

TDMS Trex digital mammography system

TDMV Tindholmur virus

TDN Therapeutics Development Network; total digestible nutrients

tDNA transfer deoxyribonucleic acid

TDNN time-delay neural network

TDO tricho-dento-osseous [syndrome]; tryptophan 2,3-dioxygenase

TDP thermal death point; thoracic duct pressure; thymidine diphosphate; total degradation products

TdP torsades de pointes

TDR Tropical Disease Research [WHO]

TDRA theory of dual radiation action

TDS temperature, depth, salinity; thiamine disulfide; total dissolved solids; transduodenal sphincteroplasty

TDSD transient digestive system disorder

TDSNV Trager duck spleen necrosis virus

TDT terminal deoxynucleotidyltransferase; thermal death time; tone decay test; tumor doubling time

TdT terminal deoxynucleotidyl transferase

TdTase terminal deoxynucleotide transferase

T$_{DTH}$ delayed type hypersensitivity T lymphocyte

TDYV Tamdy virus

TDZ thymus-dependent zone

TE echo-time; expiratory time; tennis elbow; test ear; tetanus; tetracycline; threshold energy; thromboembolism; thymus epithelium; thyrotoxic exophthalmos; tick-borne encephalitis; time estimation; tissue engineering; tissue-equivalent; tonsillectomy; tooth extracted; total estrogen; toxic epidermolysis; toxic equivalent; *Toxoplasma* encephalitis; trace element; tracheoesophageal; transepithelial; transesophageal echocardiography; transposable element [DNA]; treadmill exercise; trial error; trichoepithelioma; tris-ethylenediamine tetraacetic acid

T-E echo time

T&E testing and evaluation; trial and error

T$_E$ effector T lymphocyte; exhalation time; expiratory phase time

Te effective half-life; tellurium; tetanic contraction; tetanus

TEA temporal external artery; tetraethylammonium; thermal energy analyzer; thromboendarterectomy; total elbow arthroplasty; triethanolamine

TEAB tetraethylammonium bromide

TEAC tetraethylammonium chloride

TEAE triethylammonioethyl

TEAF trimethylammonium formate

TEAHAT Thrombolysis Early in Acute Heart Attack Trial

TEAM techniques for effective alcohol management; Thrombolytic Trial of Eminase in Acute Myocardial Infarction; Total Evaluation and Acceptance Methodology; Training in Expanded Auxiliary Management; total exposure assessment method; transfemoral endovascular aneurysm management

TEAS telemetric electrode array system

teasp teaspoon

TEB thoracic electrical bioimpedance

TEBG, TeBG testosterone-estradiol-binding globulin

TEBV tissue-engineered blood vessel

TEC tissue engineered construct; total electron count; total eosinophil count; total exchange capacity; transient erythroblastopenia of childhood; transluminal extraction catheter; trauma and emergency center

TECBEST Transluminal Extraction Catheter Before Stent [study]

tecMAAP template endonuclear cleavage multiple arbitrary amplicon profiling

TECP tetrachloropropane

TECSAC tele-collaboration for signal analysis in cardiology

TECSS The European Coronary Surgery Study

TECU thermoelectric cooling unit

TECV traumatic epiphyseal coxa vara

TED Tasks of Emotional Development; threshold erythema dose; thromboembolic disease

TEDS anti-embolism stockings

TEE thermic effect of exercise; total energy expenditure; transesophageal echocardiography; tyrosine ethyl ester

TEEP tetraethyl pyrophosphate

TEER transepithelial electrical resistance

TEF thermic effect of food; thoraco-epigastric flap; thyrotroph embryonic factor; toxic equivalency factor; tracheoesophageal fistula; transcriptional enhancer factor; trunk extension-flexion [unit]

T$_{eff}$ effective half-life

TEFRA Tax Equity and Fiscal Responsibility Act

TEFS transmural electrical field stimulation

TEG thromboelastogram

TEGDMA tetraethylene glycol dimethacrylate

TEHIP Toxicology and Environmental Health Program

TEIB triethyleneiminobenzoquinone

TEK total exchangeable potassium

TEL tetraethyl lead

TELV Turkey entero-like virus

TEM transmission electron microscope/microscopy; triethylenemelamine

TEMED tetramethylethylenediamine

TEMP temporal concept [UMLS]

temp temperature; temple, temporal

TEMS tactical emergency medical services; Trimetazidine European Multicentre Study

TEN titanium elastic nail; total enteral nutrition; total excretory nitrogen; toxic epidermal necrolysis; transepidermal neurostimulation; Trans-European Network

TENa total exchangeable sodium

TENS toxic epidermal necrolysis syndrome; transcutaneous electrical nerve stimulation

TeNT tetanus neurotoxin

TENV Tensaw virus

TEOAE transient evoked oto-acoustic emissions

TEP tetraethylpyrophosphate; tracheoesophageal puncture; transepithelial potential; transesophageal pacing; triethylphosphate

TEPA triethylenephosphamide

TEPH total end-prosthetic hip implantation

TEPP tetraethyl pyrophosphate; triethylene pyrophosphate

TEPR toward an electronic patient record

t₁/₂eq equilibration half-life

TER teratogen; terminology; total endoplasmic reticulum; transcapillary escape rate; transepithelial resistance

ter rub [Lat. *tere*]; terminal [end of chromosome]; terminal or end; terminus; ternary; tertiary; three times; threefold

term terminal

TERT total end range time

tert tertiary

TERV Termeil virus

TES thymic epithelial supernatant; toxic epidemic syndrome; *Toxocara canis* excretory/secretory [antigen]; transcutaneous electrical stimulation; transmural electrical stimulation; tutorial evaluation system

TeS terminology server

TESA testicular sperm aspiration

TESE testicular sperm extraction

TESPA thiotepa

TESS Toxic Exposure Surveillance System; Treatment Emergent Symptom Scale; Tirilazad Efficacy Stroke Study

TEST Timolol, Encainide, Sotalol Trial

TET tetracycline; total ejection time; total exchange thyroxine; treadmill exercise test

Tet tetralogy of Fallot

tet tetanus; tetracycline

TETA triethylenetetramine

TETD tetraethylthiuram disulfide

TETEV Tete virus

tetʳ tetracycline resistance

tet tox tetanus toxoid

TEV tadpole edema virus; talipes equinovarus; tissue-engineered vessel

TeV temperate virus

TEVC two electrode voltage

TEVG tissue engineered vascular graft

TEWL transepidermal water loss

TEWM tissue engineered blood vessel wall model

TexCAPS Texas Coronary Atherosclerosis Prevention Study

TEZ transthoracic electric impedance respirogram

TF free thyroxine; tactile fremitus; tail flick [reflex]; temperature factor; term formula [infant feeding]; term frequency; testicular feminization; tetralogy of Fallot; thymol flocculation; thymus factor; time frequency; tissue-damaging factor; tissue factor; to follow; total flow; transcription factor; transfer factor; transferrin; transformation frequency; transfrontal; tube feeding; tuberculin filtrate; tubular fluid; tuning fork; typhoid fever

T/F time/frequency

t(°F) temperature on the Fahrenheit scale

Tf transferrin

T_f freezing temperature

t-f time-frequency [distribution]

TFA thigh-foot angle; tibio-femoral angle; total fatty acids; transfatty acid; transverse fascicular area; trifluoroacetic acid

TFIIIA transcription factor IIIA

TFAV Thiafora virus

TFB transformation buffer

TFC common form of transferrin; threadable fusion cage; triangular fibrocartilage

TFCC triangular fibrocartilage complex

TFD target-film distance; time-frequency distribution; time-frequency domain; Transcriptional Factor Database

TFd dialyzable transfer factor

TFE polytetrafluoroethylene; transcription factor for immunoglobulin heavy chain enhancer

TFF tube-fed food

TFI thoracic fluid index; transient forebrain ischemia

TFIID transcription factor IID

TFJ tibiofemoral joint

TFJA tibiofemoral joint abduction

t-FLAS turbo-fast low angle shot [MRI]

TFM testicular feminization male; testicular feminization mutation; total fluid movement; transmission electron microscopy

TFMoV Taro feathery mottle virus

TFMPP 1-(trifluoromethylphenyl)-piperazine

TFN total fecal nitrogen; transferrin

TFO triplex-forming oligonucleotide

TFP tubular fluid plasma

TFPI tissue factor pathway inhibitor

TFPZ trifluoperazine

TFR time-frequency representation; time to full repolarization; total fertility rate; total flow resistance; traditional functional retraining; transferrin receptor

TFS testicular feminization syndrome; thyroid function study; tube-fed saline

T1FS T1-weighted fat-suppressed [image]

TFT thin-film transistor; thrombus formation time; thyroid function test; tight filum terminale; trifluorothymidine

TFTP trivial file transfer protocol [software]

TFUN tissue function [UMLS]

TFV Telok Forest virus; tick fever virus

TFX toxic effects

TG temperature gradient; tendon graft; testosterone glucuronide; tetraglycine; thioglucose; thioglycolate; thioguanine; thromboglobulin; thyroglobulin; tocogram; total gastrectomy; toxic goiter; transglutaminase; transmissible gastroenteritis; treated group; triacylglycerol; trigeminal ganglion; triglyceride; tumor growth

6-TG thioguanine

Tg generation time; thyroglobulin; *Toxoplasma gondii*; transglycosylation

T$_g$ glass transition temperature; globe temperature

tG$_1$ the time required to complete the G$_1$ phase of the cell cycle

tG$_2$ the time required to complete the G$_2$ phase of the cell cycle

TGA taurocholate gelatin agar; thyroglobulin activity; total glycoalkaloids; total gonadotropin activity; transient global amnesia; transposition of great arteries; tumor glycoprotein assay

TgAb thyroglobulin antibody

TGAI technical grade active ingredient

TGAR total graft area rejected

TGase transglutaminase

TGB thromboglobulin beta; tiagabine

tGB triangular Gregory-Bézier [patches]

TGBG dimethylglyoxal bis-guanylhydrazone

TGC time gain compensation

TGD thermal-green dye

TG-DPC temperature gradient deoxyribonucleic acid [DNA] probe chromatography

TGE theoretical growth evaluation; transmissible gastroenteritis; tryptone glucose extract

TGEV transmissible gastroenteritis virus

TGF T-cell growth factor; therapeutic gain factor; transforming growth factor; tuboglomerular feedback; tumor growth factor

TG-F transforming growth factor

TGFA transforming growth factor alpha; triglyceride fatty acid

TGFb transforming growth factor beta

TGG turkey gamma globulin

TGI tracheal gas insufflation

TGL triglyceride; triglyceride lipase

TGMV Tomato golden mosaic virus

TGN thioguanine nucleotide; trans-Golgi network

TGP tobacco glycoprotein

TGPV total glucose in venous plasma

TgPVR transgenic mice that express human cellular receptor for poliovirus

TGR transgenic rat

6-TGR 6-thioguanine riboside

TGS tincture of green soap

TGs triglycerides

TGT thromboplastin generation test/time; tolbutamide-glucagon test

TGV thoracic gas volume; thoracic great vessel; transposition of great vessels

TGY tryptone glucose yeast [agar]

TGYA tryptone glucose yeast agar

TH tension headache; tetrahydrocortisol; T helper [cell]; theophylline; thiohydantoin; thorax; thrill; thyrohyoid; thyroid hormone; topical hypothermia; total hysterectomy; triquetrohamate; tyrosine hydrolase; tyrosine hydroxylase

T_H T-helper [lymphocyte]

Th T-helper [lymphocyte]; thenar; therapist; therapy; thoracic, thorax; thorium; throat

T_h hypothermic temperature; T-helper [lymphocyte]

th thenar; thermic; thoracic; thyroid; transhepatic

THA tacrine; tetrahydroaminoacridine; thiacetazone; total hip arthroplasty; total hydroxyapatite; *Treponema* hemagglutination

ThA thoracic aorta

THAIV Thailand virus

THAL thalassemia

THAM tris(hydroxymethyl)aminomethane

THAMES Tenormin in Hypertension and Myocardial Ischemia Epidemiological Study

THAT Thrombolysis in Myocardial Infarction Trial

THB tetrahydrobiopterin; thrombocyte B; Todd-Hewitt broth; total heart beats

THb total hemoglobin

THBD thrombomodulin

THBI thyroid hormone binding inhibitor

THBP 7,8,9,10-tetrahydrobenzo[a]-pyrene; thyroid hormone binding protein

THBS thrombospondin

THC teen health clinic; tentative human consensus; terpin hydrate and codeine; tetrahydrocannabinol; tetrahydrocortisol; thiocarbanidin; thrombocytopenia; transhepatic cholangiogram; transplantable hepatocellular carcinoma

THCA alpha-trihydroxy-5-beta-cholestannic acid

THD Thomsen disease; transverse heart diameter

Thd ribothymidine

THDOC tetrahydrodeoxycorticosterone

THE tetrahydrocortisone E; tonic hind limb extension; transhepatic embolization; transhiatal esophagectomy; tropical hypereosinophilia

T-HELPER, T-Helper [computer-assisted] therapy helper; therapy helper

theor theory, theoretical

THER therapeutic procedure [UMLS]

ther therapy, therapeutic; thermometer

therap therapy, therapeutic

THERAPIS telecommunication-helped radiotherapy planning and information system

ther ex therapeutic exercise

therm thermal; thermometer

Θ Greek capital letter *theta*; thermodynamic temperature

θ Greek lowercase letter *theta*; an angular coordinate variable; customary temperature; temperature interval

ThETT thallium stress test

THEV Tehran virus

THF tetrahydrocortisone F; tetrahydrofolate; tetrahydrofolic [acid]; tetrahydrofuran; thymic humoral factor

THFA tetrahydrofolic acid; tetrahydrofurfuryl alcohol

Thg thyroglobulin

THH telangiectasia hereditaria haemorrhagica; trichohyalin

THI transient hypogammaglobulinemia of infancy

Thi thiamine

Thio-TEPA thiotriethylenephosphamide

THIP tetrahydroisoxazolopyridinol

THIS Tissue Plasminogen Activator Heparin Interaction Study; total hospital information system

THIV Thimiri virus

THL trichohyalin

THM total heme mass

TH_2O titrated water

Thor thoracic

thor thoracic, thorax

THORP titanium hollow reconstruction plate

thou thousandth

THOV Thogoto virus

THP Tamm-Horsfall protein; tetrahydropapaveroline; tetrakis(hydroxymethyl)-phosphonium; tissue hydrostatic pressure; total hip replacement; total hydroxyproline; transthoracic portography; trihexyphenidyl

Thp T-cell helper precursor

THPA tetrahydropteric acid

THPC tetrakis(hydroxymethyl)phosphonium chloride

THPP thiamine pyrophosphate; trihydroxy propriophenone

ThPP thiamine pyrophosphate

tHPT tertiary hyperparathyroidism

THPV transhepatic portal vein

THQ tetraquinone

THR targeted heart rate; threonine; thyroid hormone receptor; total hip replacement; transhepatic resistance

Thr thrill; threonine

thr threonine; thyroid, thyroidectomy

THRA thyroid hormone receptor alpha

THRF thyrotropic hormone-releasing factor

THRIFT Thromboembolism Risk Factors Study

THRM thrombomodulin

ThrO thrombotic occlusion

throm, thromb thrombosis, thrombus

THRV Thormódseyjarlettur virus

THS Teebe hypertelorism syndrome; tetrahydro-compound S; thrombohemorrhagic syndrome; Tolosa-Hunt syndrome; Tromsø Study; Turkish Heart Study

THSC totipotent hematopoietic stem cell; totipotential stem cell

THTH thyrotropic hormone

THU tetrahydrouridine

THUG thyroid uptake gradient

THV Turkey hepatitis virus

ThV thebesian valve; Theilovirus

THVO terminal hepatic vein obliteration; terminal hepatic vein obstruction

Thx thromboxane

THY thymosin

Thy thymine

thy thymectomy, thymus

THYB thymosin beta

THz terahertz

TI inversion time; T-cell independent [antigen]; temporal integration; term importance; terminal ileum; thalassemia intermedia; therapeutic index; thoracic index; thymus-independent; thymus irradiation; time interval; tonic immobility; topical irritation; total iron; transcallosally mediated inhibition; transient inward [current]; transischial; translational inhibition; transverse inlet; tricuspid incompetence; tricuspid insufficiency; tumor induction

T$_I$ inspiration time

T-I T-cell independent [antigen]

Ti titanium; translation imitation

TIA topical irritation arthritis; tracheoinnominate artery; transient ischemic attack; tumor-induced angiogenesis; turbidimetric immunoassay

TIA + CE transient ischemic attack plus carotid endarterectomy

TIAFO toe-inhibiting ankle-foot arthrosis

TIAH total implantation of artificial heart

TIB tibia; time in bed; tumor immunology bank

TIBA 2,3,5-triiodobenzoic acid

TIBBS Total Ischaemic Burden Bisoprolol Study

TIBC total iron-binding capacity

TIBET Total Ischemic Burden European Trial

TIBS Trends in Biochemical Sciences

T-IBS T-cell immunoblastic sarcoma

TIBV Tibrogargan virus

TIC total ion current; Toxicology Information Center; trypsin inhibitory capability; tubulointerstitial cell; tumor-inducing complex

TICA traumatic intracranial aneurysm; trichloroacetic acid

TICC time from cessation of contraception to conception

TICO Thrombolysis in Coronary Occlusion [study]

TICU trauma intensive care unit

TID time interval difference [imaging]; titrated initial dose; trusted image discrimination

TIDA tuberoinfundibular dopaminergic system

TIDAL Team Interactive Decision Analysis [software]

TIDE Technology Initiative for Disabled and Elderly People [Europe]

TIDES Transdermal Intermittent Dosing Evaluation Study

TIE transient ischemic episode

TIF tumor-inducing factor; tumor-infiltrating [lymphocyte]; tumor-inhibiting factor

TIG Thrombosis Interest Group [study]

TIG, Tig tetanus immunoglobulin

TIGER/Line Topologically Integrated Geographic Encoding and Referencing System

TIGR The Institute for Genome Research

TIH time interval histogram

TIIAP technical information infrastructure assistance program

TIL tumor-infiltrating leukocyte; tumor-infiltrating lymphocyte

TILLV Tillamook virus

TILV Tilligerry virus

TIM transthoracic intracardiac monitoring; Triflusal in Myocardial Infarction [study]; triose phosphate isomerase

TIMAD Ticlodipine in Micro-angiopathy of Diabetes [study]

TIMC tumor-induced marrow cytotoxicity

TIME Teaching Immunization for Medical Education [study]; Treatment of Infarcting Myocardium Early [trials]

TIMED Trials to Investigate Morning vs Evening Dosing [nisoldipine in hypertension]

TIMI thrombolysis in myocardial infarction; transmural inferior myocardial infarction

TIMIIIIA Thrombolysis in Myocardial Ischemia [trial]

TIMIIIIB Thrombolysis in Myocardial Infarction [trial]

TIMI-7 Thrombin Inhibition in Myocardial Ischemia [trial]

TIMI-9 Thrombolysis and Thrombin Inhibition in Myocardial Infarction [trial]

TIMIKO Thrombolysis in Myocardial Infarction in Korea [study]

TIMP tissue inhibitor of metalloproteinases

TIMS Tertatolol International Multicentre Study; Tuberculosis Information Management System

TIMV Timbo virus

TIN tubulointerstitial nephropathy

tinc, tinct tincture

T$_{inf}$ infusion time

TINU tubulo-interstitial nephritis-uveitis [syndrome]

TINV Tinarov virus

TIOD total iodine organification defect

TIP telemedicine instrumentation pack; terminal interface processor; thermal inactivation point; Toxicology Information Program; translation-inhibiting protein; tumor-inhibiting principle

TIPE Thrombolysis in Pulmonary Embolism [study]; Thrombolysis in Peripheral Embolism [study]

TIPI time-insensitive predictive instrument

TIPJ terminal interphalangeal joint

TIPPS tetraiodophenylphthalein sodium

TIPS Transjugular Intrahepatic Portacaval Shunt [study]; transjugular intrahepatic portosystemic shunt

TIPSS transjugular intrahepatic portosystemic stent shunt

TIQ tetrahydroisoquinoline

TIR terminal innervation ratio; terminal inverted repeat [DNA]; totally immunoreactive

TIRES transient infrared emission spectroscopy

TIS telemedicine information service; tetracycline-induced steatosis; titanium interbody spacer; transdermal infusion system; triage illness scale; trypsin-insoluble segment; tumor in situ

Tis tumor in situ

TISP total immunoreactive serum pepsinogen

TISS Therapeutic Intervention Scoring System; Ticlodipine Indobufen Stroke Study

TIT *Treponema* immobilization test

TIT, TITh triiodothyronine

TIU trypsin-inhibiting unit

TIUP term intrauterine pregnancy

TIUV total intrauterine volume

TIV tomographic image visualization; total intracranial volume

TIVA total intravenous anesthesia

TIVC thoracic inferior vena cava

TIVT Thrombolysis in Deep Vein Thrombosis [study]

TIW three times a week [JCAHO unapproved abbreviation]

TJ tetrajoule; thigh junction; triceps jerk

TJA total joint arthroplasty

TJR total joint replacement

TK thermokeratoplasty; through knee; thymidine kinase; transketolase; triose-kinase; tyrosine kinase

T(°K) absolute temperature on the Kelvin scale

tk thymidine kinase

TKA total knee arthroplasty; transketolase activity; trochanter, knee, ankle

TKase thymidine kinase

TKB tutor knowledge base

TKC torticollis-keloids-cryptorchidism [syndrome]

TKCR torticollis-keloids-cryptorchidism-renal dysplasia [syndrome]

TKD thymidine kinase deficiency; tokodynamometer

TKG tokodynagraph

TKLI tachykinin-like immunoreactivity

TKO to keep open

TKPV Turkeypox virus

TKR total knee replacement

TKT transketolase

TL temporal lobe; terminal latency; terminal lumen; thermolabile; thermoluminescence; thoracolumbar; threat to life; thymus-leukemia [antigen]; thymus lymphocyte; thymus lymphoma; time lapse; time-limited; tolerance limit; total laryngectomy; total lipids; total lung [capacity]; true lumen; tubal ligation

T-L thoracolumbar; thymus-dependent lymphocyte

TL$_{50}$ median tolerance limit

Tl thallium

TLA thymus leukemia antigen; tissue lactase activity; tongue-to-lip adhesion; translaryngeal aspiration; translumbar aortogram; transluminal angioplasty

t$_{lag}$ lag-time

TLAA T-lymphocyte-associated antigen

TLam thoracic laminectomy

TLAV Tlacotalpan virus

TLC telephone-linked care; tender loving care; thin-layer chromatography; threshold limit concentration; total L-chain concentration; total library computerization; total lung capacity; total lung compliance; total lymphocyte count; transverse loop colostomy

Tl$_{CO}$ transfer factor for lung carbon monoxide

TLD thermoluminescent dosimeter; thermoluminescent dosimetry; thoracic lymphatic duct; tumor lethal dose

T/LD$_{100}$ minimum dose causing 100% deaths or malformations

TLE temporal lobe epilepsy; thin-layer electrophoresis; total lipid extract

TLF total linear filtration; truncated Lévy flight

TLI thymidine labeling index; total lymphatic irradiation; transmitted light intensity; trypsin-like immune activity; Tucker-Lewis index

TLL T-cell leukemia or lymphoma; tissue lesion load

TLm median tolerance limit

TLMV TTV-like minivirus

TLPD thoracolaryngopelvic dysplasia

TLQ total living quotient

TLR tapetal-like reflex; target lesion revascularization; toll-like receptor; tonic labyrinthine reflex

TLS thoracolumbosacral; total least squares; Tourette-like syndrome; translaminar screw; tumor lysis syndrome

TLSER theoretical linear solvation energy relationship

TLSO thoracolumbosacral orthosis

TLSQL time-line standard query language

TLSSO thoracolumbosacral spinal orthosis

TLT tryptophan load test

TLTP Teaching and Learning Technology Programme [UK]

TLV threshold limit value; tidal liquid ventilation; T-lymphotropic virus; total lung volume

TLV-BLV threshold limit value-biological

TLV-C threshold limit value-ceiling

TLV-STEL threshold limit value-short term exposure limit

TLV-TWA threshold limit value-weighted value

TLW total lung water

TLX trophoblast-lymphocyte cross-reactivity

TM technology management; tectorial membrane; temperature by mouth; temporalis muscle; temporomandibular; tender midline; tendomyopathy; teres major; thalassemia major; Thayer-Martin [medium]; thrombomodulin; time and materials; time-motion; tobramycin; torus mandibularis; total mortality; trabecular network; trademark; traditional medicine; transatrial membranotomy; transitional mucosa; transmediastinal; transmembrane; transmetatarsal; transport mechanism; transport medium; transverse myelitis; tropical medicine; tropomyosin; tuberculous meningitis; twitch movement; tympanic membrane

T-M Thayer-Martin [medium]

T&M type and crossmatch

Tm temperature; thulium; tubular maximum excretory capacity of kidneys

T_m melting temperature; membrane immunoglobulin heavy chain polypeptide; temperature midpoint; tubular maximum excretory capacity of kidneys

tM the time required to complete the M phase of the cell cycle

tm transport medium; true mean

TMA tetramethylammonium; thrombotic microangiopathy; thyroid microsomal antibody; transcortical mixed aphasia; transcription-mediated amplification; transmetatarsal amputation; trimellitic anhydride; trimethoxyamphetamine; trimethoxyphenyl aminopropane; trimethylamine; true metatarsus adductus

TMACl tetramethylammonium chloride

TMAH trimethylphenylammonium (anilinium) hydroxide

TMAI trimethylphenylammonium (anilinium) iodide

TMAO trimethylamine *N*-oxide

TMAP transmembrane action potential

TMAS Taylor Manifest Anxiety Scale

T_{max} maximum threshold; time to maximum [concentration]

TMB transient monocular blindness

TMB4 *N,N′*-trimethylenebis(pyridine-4-aldoxime bromide)

TMBA trimethoxybenzaldehyde

TMBF transmural blood flow

TMBJ thermoplastic Minerva body jacket

TMC transmyocardial mechanical channeling; triamcinolone and terramycin capsules

TMD temporomandibular disorder; transient myeloproliferative disease; transmembrane domain; trimethadione

t-MDS therapy-related myelodysplastic syndrome

TME total metabolizable energy; transmissible mink encephalopathy; transmural enteritis; trapezium-metacarpal eburnation

TMEP telangiectasia macularis eruptiva perstans

TMET treadmill exercise test

TMEV Tembe virus; Theiler murine encephalomyelitis virus

TMF transformed mink fibroblast; transmitral flow

TM_g maximum tubular reabsorption rate for glucose

TMH tetramethylammonium hydroxide

TM-HSA trimellityl-human serum albumin

TMI testing motor impairment; total medical record; threatened myocardial infarction; transmural myocardial infarction

TMIC Toxic Materials Information Center

T1mic breast tumor microinvasion of less than 0.1 cm [TNM (tumor-node-metastasis) classification]

TMIF tumor-cell migratory inhibition factor

TMIS Technicon Medical Information System

TMJ temporomandibular joint; trapeziometacarpal joint

TMJS temporomandibular joint syndrome

TMK thymidylate kinase

TML terminal midline; terminal motor latency; tetramethyl lead

TMLR transmyocardial laser revascularization

TMM tissue mimicking material

TMN thin membrane nephropathy; tumor-node-metastasis

TMNST tethered median nerve stress test

TMP 2,2,4,4-tetramethylpentane; thiamine monophosphate; thymidine monophosphate; thymidine-5′-monophosphate; thymolphthalein monophosphate; transmembrane potential; transmembrane pressure; trimethaphan; trimethoprim; trimethylpsoralen

TM_{PAH} maximum tubular excretory capacity for para-aminohippuric acid

TMPD tetramethyl-*p*-phenylinediamine

TMPDS temporomandibular pain and dysfunction syndrome; thiamine monophosphate disulfide

TMP-SMX trimethoprim-sulfamethoxazole

TMR the medical record; tissue maximum ratio; topical magnetic resonance; trainable mentally retarded; transmyocardial revascularization

TMRM tetramethylrhodamine

TMS telematic monitoring service [telemedicine]; thallium myocardial scintigraphy; The Muscatine Study; thread mate system; thymidylate synthase; total morbidity score; transcranial magnetic stimulation; trapezoidocephaly-multiple synostosis [syndrome]; trimethylsilane

TMSE Thai Mental State Examination

TMST treadmill stem test

TMT tarsometatarsal; thiol methyltransferase; Trail-Making Test; treadmill test; trimethyllin

TMTD tetramethylthiuram disulfide

TMTJ tarsometatarsal joint

TMTX trimetrexate

TMU tetramethyl urea

TMUV Tembusu virus

TMV tobacco mosaic virus

TMX tamoxifen

TMZ transformation zone

TN talonavicular; tarsonavicular; team nursing; temperature normal; tenascin; test negative; trigeminal nucleus; total negatives; toxin neutralization; trigeminal neuralgia; trochlear nucleus; true negative

T/N tar and nicotine

T₄N normal serum thyroxine

Tn normal intraocular tension; transposon; troponin

TnI troponin I

TNA total nutrient admixture; trinitrotoluene

TNB transnasal butorphanol

TNBP tri-*n*-butyl phosphate

TnC troponin C

TND term normal delivery

t-NE total norepinephrine

TNEE titrated norepinephrine excretion

TNF true negative fraction; tumor necrosis factor

TNFA tumor necrosis factor alpha

TNFAIP tumor necrosis factor, alpha-induced protein

TNFAR tumor necrosis factor alpha receptor

TNFB tumor necrosis factor beta

TNFBR tumor necrosis factor beta receptor

TNFR1 tumor necrosis factor type 1 receptor

TNFr tumor necrosis factor receptor

TNG trinitroglycerin

tng tongue

tNGF truncated nerve growth factor

TnGV *Trichoplusia ni* granulovirus

TNH teaching nursing home; transient neonatal hyperammonemia

T-NHL T-cell-derived non-Hodgkin leukemia

TNHP teaching nursing home program

TNI total nodal irradiation

TNM primary tumor, regional nodes, metastases [tumor staging and coding]; thyroid node metastases; tumor node metastasis

TNMR tritium nuclear magnetic resonance

TNP total net positive; trinitrophenyl

TNPACK truncated Newton program package

TNP-KLH trinitrophenyl keyhole limpet hemocyanin

TNP-LPS trinitrophenyl-lipopolysaccharide

TNR tonic neck reflex; true negative rate

TNS total nuclear score; transcutaneous nerve stimulation; tumor necrosis serum

TNT tetranitroblue tetrazolium; Transderm-Nitro Trial; Treatment to New Target [study of effectiveness of atorvastatin in coronary heart disease]; 2,4,6-trinitrotoluene

TnT troponin T

TNTC too numerous to count

TNV tobacco necrosis virus

TO old tuberculin; oral temperature; original tuberculin; target organ; telephone order; thoracic orthosis; thromboangiitis obliterans; thrombotic occlusion; tincture of opium; total obstruction; tracheoesophageal; treatment object; tubo-ovarian; turnover

T(O) oral temperature

TO₂ oxygen transport

Tₒ tricuspid opening

to tincture of opium

TOA total quality assessment; tubo-ovarian abscess

TOAP thioguanine, Oncovin, cytosine arabinoside, and prednisone

TOAST Treatment of Acute Stroke Trial; Trial of Org 10172 in Acute Stroke Trial

TOAT The Open Artery Trial

TOB tobramycin

TOBEC total body electrical conductivity [test]

TobRV tobacco ringspot virus

TOC total Organic carbon

TOCC Total Occlusion of Coronary Arteries, Chronic [study]

TOCP tri-*o*-cresyl phosphate

TOCSY total correlation spectroscopy

TOD right eye tension [Lat. *oculus dexter*]; target organ damage; target organ disease; Time-Oriented Data [Bank]; titanium optimized design [plate]

TOD/CCD target organ disease/clinical cardiovascular disease

TODS toxic organic dust syndrome

TOE tender on examination; tracheoesophageal; transesophageal echography; transferred nuclear Overhauser effect

TOEFL Test of English as a Foreign Language [for foreign medical graduates]

TOES toxic oil epidemic syndrome

TOF tetralogy of Fallot; time-of-flight; train of four [monitor]; tracheo[o]esophageal fistula

ToF time-of-flight

TOFA time-of-flight absorbance; time-of-flight and abstinence [imaging]

T of F tetralogy of Fallot

TOFHLA test of functional health literacy in adults

TOFMS, TOF-MS time-of-flight mass spectrometry

TOFS total organ failure score

TOH transient osteoporosis of hip; tower of Hanoi [neurophysiological test]

TOHP Trial of Hypertension Prevention

TOL trial of labor

tol tolerance, tolerated

TOLB, tolb tolbutamine

TOLC Treatment of Low-density Lipoprotein-bound Cholesterol [study]

TOLD top-level driver

TOM toxic oxygen metabolite

TOMA tri-octylmethylammonium chloride

TOMAS torsional ocular movement analysis system

TOMHS Treatment of Mild Hypertension Study

TOMI turkey ovomucoid inhibitor

TOMIIS Total Occlusion Postmyocardial Infarction Intervention Study

Tomo tomogram, tomography

tomos tomograms

TOMS The Oklahoma Marker Study

TON traumatic optic neuropathy

TONE tilted optimized nonsaturating excitation; Trial of Nonpharmacologic Interventions in the Elderly

tonoc tonight

TOP termination of pregnancy; Thrombolysis in Old Patients [study]; topoisomerase

top topical

TOPAS Thrombolysis or Peripheral Arterial Surgery [study]

TOPCAD topical prevention or conception and disease

TOPLIT Transluminal Extraction Catheter or Percutaneous Transluminal Coronary Angioplasty in Thrombus [study]

TOPS Take Off Pounds Sensibly [program]; Thrombolysis in Old Patients Study; Treatment of Post-thrombolytic Stenosis [study]

TOPV Topografov virus; trivalent oral poliovaccine

TORCH toxoplasmosis, other [congenital syphilis and viruses], rubella, cytomegalovirus, and herpes simplex virus

ToRCHeS toxoplasmosis, rubella, cytomegalovirus, herpes, syphilis

TORCHS toxoplasmosis, other diseases, rubella, cytomegalovirus infections, herpes simplex, syphilis

TORP total ossicular replacement prosthesis

torr mm Hg pressure

TOS thoracic outlet syndrome; toxic oil syndrome

TOSCA Total Occlusion Study in Canada

TOSV Toscana virus

TOT The Oslo Trial; total operating time; tubal ovum transfer

TOTAL Total Occlusion Trial with Angioplasty by Using Laser Guidewire

TOTP tri-*o*-tolyl phosphate

TOV trial of voiding

TOVA test of variables of attention; trigger of ventricular arrhythmia

TOWARD Toyama Warfarin Rational Dosage [study]

Tox, tox toxicity, toxic

TOXICON Toxicology Conversational Online Network [NLM database]

TOXLINE Toxicology Information On-Line [NLM database]

TOXLIT Toxicology Literature [NLM database]

TOXNET Toxicology Data Network [NLM database]

TP temperature and pressure; temperature probe; template; temporal peak; temporoparietal; tender point; tension pneumothorax; terminal phalanx; terminal protein; testosterone propionate; thick padding; thin-plate; threshold potential; thrombocytopenic purpura; thrombophlebitis; thromboxane prostaglandin; thymic polypeptide; thymidine phosphorylase; thymopentin; thymopoietin; thymus polypeptide; thymus protein; tissue pressure; Todd palsy; toe pressure; torsades de pointes; torus palatinus; total population; total positives; total protein; transaction processing; transforming principle; transition point; transpyloric; transverse polarization; transverse process; transverse propagation; treating physician; treatment period; treatment progress; treatment protocol; *Treponema pallidum*; triazolophthalazine; trigger point; triphosphate; true positive; tryptophan; tryptophan pyrrolase; tube precipitin; tuberculin precipitate; tumor protein

6-TP 6-thiopurine

T&P temperature and pressure; temperature and pulse

T+P temperature and pulse

Tp primary transmission; time of preparation; *Treponema pallidum*; tryptophan

T$_p$ physical half-life

TPA tannic acid, polyphosphomolybdic acid, and amino acid; 12-*O*-tetradecanoylphorbol-13-acetate; third-party administrator; thrombotic pulmonary artery; tissue plasminogen activator; tissue polypeptide antigen; total parenteral alimentation; *Treponema pallidum* agglutination; tumor polypeptide antigen

t-PA tissue plasminogen activator

TPAC torso phased array coil

TPAI tissue plasminogen activator inhibitor

TPase thymidine phosphorylase

TPASK Tissue Plasminogen Activator vs Streptokinase [trial]

TPAT Tissue Plasminogen Activator, Toronto Trial

TPB tetraphenyl borate; tryptone phosphate broth

TPBF total pulmonary blood flow

TPBG trophoblast glycoprotein

TPBS three-phase bone scintigraphy; three-phase radionuclide bone scanning

TPC thromboplastic plasma component; thyroid papillary carcinoma; time to peak contrast; total patient care; total plasma catecholamines; total plasma cholesterol;

total plate count; *Treponema pallidum* complement

TPCF *Treponema pallidum* complement fixation

TPCV total packed cell volume

TPD temporary partial disability; thiamine propyl disulfide; tripotassium phenolphthalein disulfate; tumor-producing dose

TP-DNA template deoxyribonucleic acid [DNA]

TPDS tropical pancreatic diabetes syndrome

TPE therapeutic plasma exchange; totally protected environment; tris-phosphate ethylenediamine tetraacetic acid [EDTA]; typhoid-parathyroid enteritis

T^{Pe} expiratory pause time

T$_{peak}$ time-to-peak

TPEV 1, 2 Turkey pseudoenteritis virus 1, 2

TPEY tellurite polymyxin egg yolk [agar]

TPF thymus permeability factor; thymus to peak flow; true positive fraction

TPFR time to peak filling rate

TPG transmembrane potential gradient; transplacental gradient; transpulmonary gradient; tryptophan peptone glucose [broth]

TPGS E-alpha-tocopheryl polyethylene glycol succinate; Talairach Proportional Grid System

TPGYT trypticase-peptone-glucose-yeast extract-trypsin [medium]

TPH transplacental hemorrhage; tryptophan hydroxylase

TpH tryptophane hydroxylase

TPHA *Treponema pallidum* hemagglutination

TPHU Tropical Public Health Unit [Australia]

TPI Thrombolytic Predictive Instrument [project]; time period integrator; treponemal immobilization test; *Treponema pallidum* immobilization; triose phosphate isomerase

T^{Pi} inspiratory pause time

TPIA *Treponema pallidum* immune adherence

TPIIA time of postexpiratory inspiratory activity

TPK tyrosine protein kinase

TPL third party liability; titanium proximal loading; tumor progression locus; tyrosine phenol-lyase

tpl transplantation, transplanted

TPLL T-cell prolymphocytic leukemia

TPLSM two-photon laser scanning microscopy

TPLV transient pulmonary vascular lability

TPM temporary pacemaker; thrombophlebitis migrans; topiramate; total particulate matter; total passive motion; triphenylmethane; tropomyosin; turning-point morphology

TPMT thiopurine methyltransferase

TPMV Thottapalayam virus

TPN thalamic projection neuron; total parenteral nutrition; transition protein; triphosphopyridine nucleotide

TPNH reduced triphosphopyridine nucleotide

TPO thrombopoietin; thyroid peroxidase; tryptophan peroxidase

Tpo thrombopoietin

TPP tetraphenylporphyrin; thiamine pyrophosphate; transpulmonary pressure; treadmill performance test; tripeptidyl peptidase; triphenyl phosphite

TPPase thiamine pyrophosphatase

TPPD thoracic-pelvic-phalangeal dystrophy

TPPI time proportional phase incrementation

TPPN total peripheral parenteral nutrition

TPQ Threshold Planning Quantity

TPR temperature, pulse, and respiration; testosterone production rate; tetraricopeptide repeat; third party reimbursement; tissue phantom ratio; total peripheral resistance; total pulmonary resistance; true positive rate; tumor potentiating region; true positive rate

TPRI total peripheral resistance index

TPS thin-plate-spline; time to peak shortening; topical skin protectant; treatment planning system; trypsin; tryptase; tumor polysaccharide substance

TPSE 2-(p-triphenyl)sulfonylethanol

TPST true positive stress test; tyrosyl protein sulfotransferase

TPT tetraphenyl tetrazolium; Thrombosis Prevention Trial; time to peak tension; topotecan; total protein tuberculin; triphalangeal thumb; typhoid-paratyphoid [vaccine]

TPTE 2-(p-triphenyl)thioethanol

TPTX thyro-parathyroidectomized

TPTZ tripyridyltriazine

TPV tetanus-pertussis vaccine; tipranavir

TPVR total peripheral vascular resistance; total pulmonary vascular resistance

TPVS transhepatic portal venous sampling

TPX testis-specific protein

TPZ thioproperazine

TQ tocopherolquinone; tourniquet

TQD target quit date [smoking cessation]

TQFCOSY triple-quantum filtered correlated spectroscopy

TQI total quality improvement

TQM total quality management

TQS Terminology Query Service

TR recovery time; rectal temperature; repetition time; residual tuberculin; terminal repeat; tetrazolium reduction; therapeutic radiology; therapeutic ratio; therapeutic recreation; thrombin receptor; thyroid [hormone] receptor; time release; time to relengthening; total resistance; total response; trachea; transfusion reaction; transmission rate; transrectal; tricuspid regurgitation; Trinder reagent; tuberculin R [new tuberculin]; tuberculin residue; turbidity-reducing; turnover ratio

T:R thickness to radius [ratio]

T&R treated and released

T/R transmission/[frequency] response

TR₉₀ time to 90 percent relengthening

T(°R) absolute temperature on the Rankine scale

Tr trace; tragion; transferrin; trypsin

Tᵣ radiologic half-life; retention time

tr tincture; trace; traction; transaldolase; trauma, traumatic; tremor; triradial

TRA total renin activity; tumor-resistant antigen

tra transfer

TRAb thyrotoxin receptor antibody

TRABS thiobarbituric reactive substance

TRAC tool for referral assessment of continuity [of health]

trac traction

TRACE Trandolapril Cardiac Evaluation [trial]

trach trachea, tracheal, tracheostomy

TRAJ time repetitive ankle jerk

TRALI transfusion-related acute lung injury

TRALT transfusion-related acute lung injury

TRAM transport remote acquisition monitor; transverse rectus abdominis muscle; Treatment Rating Assessment Matrix; Treatment Response Assessment Method; trisaminomethane

TRAMAH trauma resources allocation model for ambulances and hospitals

TRAMPE tricho-rhino-auriculophalangeal multiple exostoses

TRANDA Trandolapril Andalusian Study

trans transfer; transference; transverse

TRANSAX translation of axes [cause of death data]

trans D transverse diameter

TRANSFAIR Transfatty Acids in Food in Europe [study]

transm transmission, transmitted

transpl transplantation, transplanted

TRAP carpal tunnel syndrome, Raynaud phenomenon, aching muscles, proximal muscle weakness [rheumatic disorders associated with hypothyroidism]; tartrate-resistant acid phosphatase; telomeric repeat amplification protocol; transport and rapid accessioning for additional procedures; triiodothyronine receptor auxiliary protein; Twin Reversed Arterial Perfusion [study]

TrAP transcriptional activator protein

trap trapezius

TRAPIST Trapidil vs Placebo to Prevent In-Stent Intimal Hyperplasia [study]

TRAS transplanted renal artery stenosis

TraSH transposition-site hybridization; transposon site hybridization

TRASHES tuberculosis, radiotherapy, ankylosing spondylitis, histoplasmosis, extrinsic allergic alveolitis, silicosis [chest x-ray findings]

traum trauma, traumatic

TRB terbutalone; tropanyl benzylate

TRBF total renal blood flow

TRBV Tribec virus

TRC tanned red cell; therapeutic residential center; T lymphocyte antigen receptor; total renin concentration; total respiratory conductance; total ridge count

TRCA tanned red cell agglutination

TRCF transcription repair coupling factor

TRCH tanned red cell hemagglutination

TRCHI tanned red cell hemagglutination inhibition

TRCV total red cell volume

TRD tongue-retaining device; traumatic rupture of diaphragm

TRDN transient respiratory distress of the newborn

TRE target registration error; thymic reticuloendothelial; thyroid hormone response; triplet rapid expansion; true radiation emission

TREA triethanolamine

TREAT Tranilast Restenosis Following Angioplasty Trial

treat treatment

TRECs T-cell receptor rearrangement excision circles

TREND Trial on Reversing Endothelial Dysfunction

Trend Trendelenburg [position]

TRENT Trial of Early Nifedipine Treatment of Acute Myocardial Infarction

Trep *Treponema*

TRF targeted ribonucleic acid [RNA] fingerprinting; T-cell replacing factor; thymus replacing factor; thyrotropin-releasing factor; transferrin; tubular rejection fraction

TRFC total rosette-forming cell

TRG T-cell rearranging gene; transfer ribonucleic acid glycine

TRH tension-reducing hypothesis; thyrotropin-releasing hormone

TRHR thyrotropin-releasing hormone receptor

TRH-ST thyrotropin-releasing hormone stimulation test

TRI tetrazolium reduction inhibition; Thyroid Research Institute; total response index; Toxic Chemical Release Inventory [NLM database]; tubuloreticular inclusion

tri tricentric

T₃RIA, T₃(RIA) triiodothyronine radioimmunoassay

T₄RIA, T₄(RIA) thyroxine radioimmunoassay

TRIAC 3,5,3′-triiodothyroacetic acid

TRIADS time resolved imaging by automatic data segmentation

TRIC Thrombolysis with Recombinant Tissue Plasminogen Activator During

Instability in Coronary Artery Disease [trial]; trachoma inclusion conjunctivitis [organism]

TRICB trichlorobiphenyl

TRICC Transfusion Requirements in Critical Care [trial]

Trich *Trichomonas*

TRIFACTS Toxic Chemical Release Inventory Facts

trig trigger; triglycerides; trigonum

TRIM Thrombin Inhibition in Myocardial Ischemia [study]

TRIMIS Tri-Service Medical Information Systems [Department of Defense]

TRIMM Triggers and Mechanisms of Myocardial Infarction [study]

TRINS totally reversible ischemic neurological symptoms

TRIPS Trade-Related Aspects of Intellectual Property

TRIS tris-(hydroxymethyl)-aminomethane

TRISS trauma and injury severity score

TRIT triiodothyronine

trit triturate

TRITC tetrarhodamine isothiocyanate

TRK transketolase; tyrosine kinase

TRL transfer ribonucleic acid leucine

TRLP triglyceride-rich lipoprotein

TRM traditional medicines; transplant-related mortality

TRMA thiamine-responsive megaloblastic anemia

TR-MALLS time-resolved multi-angle laser light scattering

TRMC trimethylrhodamino-isothiocyanate

TRMI transfer ribonucleic acid initiator methionine

TRML, Trml terminal

TRM-SMX trimethoprim-sulfamethoxazole

TRMV Trombetas virus

TRN tegmental reticular nucleus

tRNA transfer ribonucleic acid

tRNA GLU transfer ribonucleic acid glutamic acid

tRNA-i(met) transfer ribonucleic acid initiator methionine

tRNA-SER transfer ribonucleic acid serine

TRNG tetracycline-resistant *Neisseria gonorrhoeae*

TRNOE transfer nuclear Overhauser effect

TRNS transfer ribonucleic acid serine

TRO tissue reflectance oximetry

Troch trochanter

TROM torque range of motion

Trop tropical

TROPCAB total revascularization off pump by coronary artery bypass

TROPHY Treatment Effects of Lisinopril vs Hydrochlorothiazide in Obese Patients with Hypertension [trial]; Treatment of Obese Patients with Hypertension [trial]; Trial of Preventing Hypertension

TRP peak through response phase; total refractory period; transfer ribonucleic acid proline; transient receptor potential; trichorhinophalangeal [syndrome]; tubular reabsorption of phosphate; tyrosine-related protein

TrP tricuspid valve

Trp, trp tryptophan

TRPA tryptophan-rich prealbumin

TrPl treatment plan

TRPM testosterone-repressed prostate message

TRPO tryptophan oxygenase

TRPS trichorhinophalangeal syndrome

TRPT theoretical renal phosphorus threshold

TRR temporal representation and reasoning; total respiratory resistance

TRS task routing system; testicular regression syndrome; total reducing sugars; tubuloreticular structure

TrS trauma surgery

TRST triage risk screening tool

TRSV tobacco ringspot virus

TRT thoracic radiotherapy; transfer ribonucleic acid threonine

TR/TE repetition time/echo time

T-RTS triage-revised trauma score

TRTV Turkey rhinotracheitis virus

TRU task-related unit; turbidity-reducing unit

T$_3$RU triiodothyronine resin uptake

TRUS transrectal ultrasonography

TRUSP transrectal ultrasonography of prostate

TRUST Trial in United Kingdom for Stroke Treatment

TRUV Trubanaman virus

TRV Tanjong Rabok virus; tobacco rattle virus

TrV Triatoma virus

TRVV total right ventricular volume

TRX thioredoxin

trx traction

Tryp tryptophan

TS Takayasu syndrome; Tay-Sachs [disease]; telemedicine system; temperature sensitivity; temperature sensor; temperature, skin; temporal stem; tensile strength; test solution; thermal stability; thoracic surgery; thymidylate synthase; time scale; tissue space; total solids [in urine]; Tourette syndrome; toxic substance; toxic syndrome; tracheal sound; trachomatous scarring; transferrin saturation; transition; transitional sleep; transsexual; transverse section; transverse sinus; trauma score; treadmill score; triceps surae; tricuspid stenosis; triple strength; tropical sprue; Troyer syndrome; trypticase soy [plate]; T suppressor [cell]; tuberous sclerosis; tumor-specific; Turner syndrome; type-specific

T/S transverse section

T+S type and screen

Ts skin temperature; tosylate

T$_s$ secreted immunoglobulin heavy chain polypeptide; stimulus timing; T-cell suppressor; T suppressor [cell]

T$_s$1, T$_s$3 suppressor T lymphocyte subpopulations 1 and 3

tS time required to complete the S phase of the cell cycle

ts temperature sensitivity

ts, tsp teaspoon

TSA technical surgical assistance; time series analysis; toluene sulfonic acid; total shoulder arthroplasty; total solute absorption; toxic shock antigen; transcortical sensory aphasia; trypticase-soy agar; tumor-specific antigen; tumor surface antigen; type-specific antibody

T$_4$SA thyroxine-specific activity

TSAb thyroid-stimulating antibody

TSAP toxic-shock-associated protein; transport services access point

TSAS total severity assessment score

TSAT tube slide agglutination test

TSB total serum bilirubin; trypticase soy broth; tryptone soy broth

TSBA total serum bile acids

TSBB transtracheal selective bronchial brushing

TSC technetium sulfur colloid; thiazide-sensitive sodium-chloride cotransporter; thiosemicarbazide; total static compliance; total symptom complex; transient sponta-

neous circulation; transverse spinal sclerosis; tuberous sclerosis complex

TSCA Toxic Substances Control Act

TSCOHS Tri-Service Comprehensive Oral Health Survey

TSCS Tennessee Self-Concept Scale

TSD target site duplication [DNA]; target-skin distance; Tay-Sachs disease; theory of signal detectability; thermionic selective detector; traditional stripchart display

TSE testicular self-examination; time since exposure; tissue-specific extinguisher; total skin electron; total skin examination; transcutaneous spinal electroanesthesia; transmissible spongiform encephalopathy; trisodium edetate; turbo-spin echo

TSEB total skin electron beam

T sect transverse section

TSEM transmission scanning electron microscopy

TSES Target Symptom Evaluation Scale

T-set tracheotomy set

TSF T cell suppressor factor; testicular feminization syndrome; thrombopoiesis-stimulating factor; total systemic flow; triceps skinfold

T$_s$F T cell suppressor factor

TSG tumor suppressor gene

TSG, TSGP tumor-specific glycoprotein

TSGE temperature sweep gel electrophoresis

TSH thyroid-stimulating hormone; transient synovitis of the hip

TSHA thyroid-stimulating hormone, alpha chain

TSHB thyroid-stimulating hormone, beta chain

TSHR thyroid-stimulating hormone receptor

TSH-RF thyroid-stimulating hormone-releasing factor

TSH-RH thyroid-stimulating hormone-releasing hormone

TSHW Thyroid Study in Healthy Women

TSI thyroid stimulating immunoglobulin; triple sugar iron [agar]

TSIA total small intestine allotransplantation; triple sugar iron agar

tSIDS totally unexplained sudden infant death syndrome

TSJ Telemedicine Society of Japan

TSL task specification language; terminal sensory latency; transport layer security [telemedicine]

TSLP thymic stroma-derived lymphopoietin

TSM type-specific M protein

TSMDB Tuberous Sclerosis Mutation Database

TSO transient spastic occlusion; *trans*-stilbene oxide

TSOP time from symptom onset to presentation

TSP tailspin protein; testis-specific protein; thrombin-sensitive protein; thrombospondin; tibial hole sagittal positioning; total serum protein; total sleep period; total suspended particulate [matter]; trisodium phosphate; tropical spastic paraparesis

tsp teaspoon

TSP I thrombospondin type I

TSPA thiotepa

TSPAP total serum prostatic acid phosphatase

TSPL transplant

TSPP tetrasodium pyrophosphate

TSR theophylline sustained release; thyroid to serum ratio; tissue scatter ratio [radiotherapy]; tissue standard ratio [radiotherapy]; total systemic resistance

TSS toxic shock syndrome; tropical splenomegaly syndrome

TSSA tumor-specific cell surface antigen

TSSE toxic shock syndrome exotoxin

TSST toxic shock syndrome toxin

TST thermoregulatory sweat test; thiosulfate sulfur-transferase; thromboplastin screening test; total sleep time; transforming sequence, thyroid; treadmill stress test; triceps skinfold thickness; tricipital skinfold thickness; tuberculin skin test; tumor skin test

TSTA toxoplasmin skin test antigen; tumor-specific tissue antigen; tumor-specific transplantation antigen

TsTX tityustoxin

TSU triple sugar urea [agar]

TSUV Tsuruse virus

TSV total stomach volume; total stroke volume

TSVR total systemic vascular resistance

TSWT tree-structured wavelet transform

TSY trypticase soy yeast

TSYEA trypticase soy yeast enriched agar

TT tablet triturate; talar tilt; tactile tension; tendon of Todaro; tendon transfer; terminal transferase; test tube; testicular torsion; tetanus toxin; tetanus toxoid; tetrathionate; tetrazol; therapeutic touch; thrombin time; thrombolytic therapy; thromboplastin time; thymol turbidity; tibial tubercle; tibial tuberosity; tick typhus; tiger-top; tilt table; tiny T [antigen]; tissue tolerance; tolerance test; tonometry; total thyroidectomy; total thyroxine; total time; total transfer; trabecular thickness; transient tachypnea; transferred to; transit time; transthoracic; transtracheal; treadmill test; trend template; triple therapy; tritiated thymidine; tuberculin test; tuberculoid [in Ridley-Jopling Hansen disease classification]; tube thoracostomy; tumor thrombus; turnover time; tyrosine transaminase

T&T time and temperature; touch and tone

TT$_2$ total diiodothyronine

TT$_3$ total triiodothyronine

TT$_4$ total thyroxine

T$_t$ transition temperature

TTA tetanus toxoid antibody; timed therapeutic absence; tissue texture abnormality; total toe arthroplasty; transtracheal aspiration

tTA tetracycline-controlled transactivator

TTAP threaded titanium acetabular prosthesis

TTATTS Thrombolytic Therapy in Acute Thrombotic/Thromboembolic Stroke [study]

TTB third trimester bleeding

TTC triphenyltetrazolium chloride; T-tube cholangiogram

TTD temporary total disability; tetraethylthiuram disulfide; tissue tolerance dose; transfusion-transmitted disease; transient tic disorder; transverse thoracic diameter; trichothiodystrophy

TTDF time to distant failure

TTE transthoracic echocardiography

TTF thyroid transcription factor; time to failure

TTFD tetrahydrofurfuryldisulfide

TTG T-cell translocation gene; telethermography; tellurite, taurocholate, and gelatin

TTGA tellurite, taurocholate, and gelatin agar

TTH thyrotropic hormone; tritiated thymidine

TTI tension-time index; time-temperature indicator; time-tension index; time-to-intubation; torque-time interval; transtracheal insufflation

TTIdi tension time index diaphragm

TTIM T-cell tumor invasion and metastasis

T-TIME tourniquet time

TTJV transtracheal jet ventilation

TTL total thymus lymphocytes; training test lung; transistor-transistor logic

TTLC true total lung capacity

TTLD terminal transverse limb defect

TTLF time to local failure; transtelephonic monitoring [telemedicine]

TTN titin; transient tachypnea of the newborn

TT$_n$ normal trend template

TTNA transthoracic needle aspiration

TTNAB transthoracic needle aspiration biopsy

TTNB transthoracic needle biopsy

TTO time trade-off [method]

TTO$_2$ transtracheal oxygen

TTOPP Thrombolytic Therapy in Older Patient Population [study]

TTP thiamine triphosphate; thrombotic thrombocytopenic purpura; thymidine triphosphate; time to peak; time to progression; tocopherol transfer protein; transtrabecular plane; tristetraprolin; tritolyl phosphate; trusted third party

TTPA triethylene thiophosphoramide

TTR time in target range; transthoracic resistance; transthyretin; triceps tendon reflex

TTS tarsal tunnel syndrome; temporary threshold shift; The Tromø Study; through the scope; through the skin; tilt table standing; transdermal therapeutic system; twin transfusion syndrome

TTSS type three secretion system

T$_3$/T$_4$ syndrome low triiodothyronine/low thyroxine syndrome

TTT thymol turbidity test; tolbutamide tolerance test; total twitch time; tuberculin tine test

TTTS twin-to-twin transfusion syndrome

TTTT test tube turbidity test; Tokyo Trop-T Trial

TTV tracheal transport velocity; transfusion-transmitted virus

TTVS Transfusion Transmitted Viruses Study

TTWB toe touch weightbearing

TTX tetrodotoxin

TU texture unit [artificial neural network]; thiouracil; thyroid uptake; Todd unit; toxic unit; toxin unit; transmission unit; transurethral; tuberculin unit; turbidity unit

T$_3$U triiodothyronine uptake

TUAV Turuna virus

TUB tubulin

TUBA tubulin alpha

TUBAL tubulin alpha-like

TUBB tubulin beta

tuberc tuberculosis

TUBG tubulin gamma

TUBS traumatic unidirectional Bankart surgical

TUCC Tissue Plasminogen Activator/Urokinase Comparison in China [study]

TUCV Tucunduba virus

TUD total urethral discharge

TUG total urinary gonadotropin

TUGMI Tsukuba University Group for Myocardial Infarction

TUGSE traumatic ulcerative granuloma with stromal eosinophilia

TuHV Tupaiid herpesvirus

TUI transurethral incision; type unique identifier [UMLS]

TUIP trans-urethral incision of prostate

TUL tumescent ultrasound liposculpture

TULIP transurethral ultrasound-guided laser-induced prostatectomy

TULV Tula virus

TUN total urinary nitrogen

TUNEL deoxyuride-5'-triphosphate biotin nick end labeling

TUNV Tunis virus

TUP temporal utility program; transumbilical plane

TUPV Tupaia virus

TUR transurethral resection

TURB, TURBT transurethral resection of bladder [tumor]

turb turbid, turbidity

turboFLASH turbo fast low-angle shot

TURP transurethral resection of the prostate

TURS transurethral resection syndrome

TURV transurethral resection of valves; Turlock virus

TUS trauma ultrasound

TUTase terminal uridylate transferase

TV box turtle virus; talipes varus; target volume [radiotherapy]; television; teschovirus; tetrazolium violet; thoracic vertebra; tickborne virus; tidal volume; tigré virus; *Torovirus*; total volume; toxic vertigo; transumbilical plane; transvaginal; transvenous; transverse; transversion; trial visit; *Trichomonas vaginalis*; tricuspid valve; trivalent; true vertebra; truncal vagotomy; tuberculin volutin; tubovesicular typhoid vaccine; tumor virus

Tv *Trichomonas vaginalis*

TVA truncal vagotomy and antrectomy

TVC timed vital capacity; total viable cells; total volume capacity; transvaginal cone; triple voiding cystogram; true vocal cords

TVCV transvenous cardioversion

TVD transmissible virus dementia; triple vessel disease

TVF tactile vocal fremitus

TVFD time-varying frequency dependence

TVG time-varied gain

TVH total vaginal hysterectomy; turkey virus hepatitis

TVHS transvaginal hysterosonography

TVI time-velocity integral

TVL tenth value layer; tunica vasculosa lentis

TVMF time varying magnetic field

TVOC total volatile organic compound

TVP tensor veli palatini [muscle]; textured vegetable protein; transvenous pacemaker; tricuspid valve prolapse; truncal vagotomy and pyloroplasty

TVR target vessel revascularization; tonic vibratory reflex; total vascular resistance; tricuspid valve replacement; triple valve replacement

TVRE transvaginal resection or endometrium

TVS transvaginal sonography; transvesical sonography

TVSS transient voltage surge suppressor

TVT tension-free vaginal tape; transmissible venereal tumor; tunica vaginalis testis

TVTV Trivittatus virus

TVU total volume of the urine

TVV *Trichomonas vaginalis* virus

TVX tumor virus X

TW tap water; terminal web; test weight; thyroid weight; total body water; traveling wave

Tw twist

TWA time weighted average; total wrist arthroplasty; T wave alternans [ECG]

TWAR Taiwan acute respiratory [*Chlamydia pneumoniae* strain]

T$_{wb}$ wet-bulb temperature

TWBC total white blood cells; total white blood count

TWD total white and differential [cell count]; traveling-wave dielectrophoresis

TWE tap water enema; tepid water enema

TWIST time without symptoms of disease and subjective toxic effects of treatment

TWISTER Trial of Within Stent Treatment of Endoluminal Restenosis

TWL transepidermal water loss

TWS tranquilizer withdrawal syndrome

TWs triphasic waves

TWT The Wellcome Trust; total waiting time

TWWD tap water wet dressing

TX a derivative of contagious tuberculin; no evidence of primary tumor [TNM (tumor-node-metastasis) classification]; tamoxifen; thromboxane; thyroidectomized; transplantation; treatment

T&X type and crossmatch

6TX 6-thioxanthine

Tx transplant or transplantation

Tx, T$_x$ treatment; therapy; traction

tx traction

TXA, TxA thromboxane A

TXA2, TXA$_2$ thromboxane A2 (A$_2$)

TXB2, TXB$_2$ thromboxane B2 (B$_2$)

TXDD transmitted data decoder [telemedicine]

TxDD/T transmitted data decoder/timer [telemedicine]

TXDS qualifying toxic dose

TxDE transmitted data encoder [telemedicine]

TXN thioredoxin

Ty type; typhoid; tyrosine

TYH tyrosine hydrolase

Tymp tympanic, tympanum

TYMS thymidylate synthase

TYMV turnip yellow mosaic virus

Ty-neg tyrosinase negative
Ty-pos tyrosinase positive
Tyr, tyr tyrosine
TyRIA thyroid radioisotope assay
TYRL tyrosinase-like
TYRP tyrosine-related protein

TYUV Tyuleniy virus
TZ zymoplastic tuberculin [the dried residue which is soluble in alcohol, Ger. *Tuberculin zymoplastische*]
$t_{1/2z}$ terminal half-life
TZD thiazolidinedione

U

U congenital limb absence; in electrocardiography, an undulating deflection that follows the T wave; internal energy; International Unit of enzyme activity; Mann-Whitney rank sum statistic; potential difference (in volts); ulcer; ulna; ultralente [insulin]; umbilicus; uncertain; unerupted; unit [JCAHO unapproved abbreviation]; universal application [residency]; unknown; unsharpness; upper; uracil; uranium; urea; urethra; uridine; uridylic acid; urinary concentration; urine; urology; uterus; uvula; volume velocity

U/2 upper half

U/3 upper third

u unified atomic mass unit; velocity

ϒ see *upsilon*

υ see *upsilon*

UA absorption unsharpness; ultra-audible; ultrasonic arteriography; umbilical artery; unauthorized absence; unicystic ameloblastoma; unit of analysis; unstable angina; upper airways; upper arm; uric acid; uridylic acid; urinalysis; urinary aldosterone; uronic acid; uterine activity; uterine aspiration

U/A uric acid; urinalysis

ua urinalysis

UAC umbilical artery catheter; unusual-appearing child

UA/C uric acid/creatinine [ratio]

UAE unilateral absence of excretion; urine albumin excretion

UAEM University Association for Emergency Medicine

UAGA Uniform Anatomical Gift Act

UAI uterine activity interval

UAI-C unprotected anal intercourse with casual partners

UAL ultrasound-assisted liposuction

U-AMY urinary amylase

UAN uric acid nitrogen

UAO upper airway obstruction

UAP unlicensed assistive personnel; unstable angina pectoris; urinary acid phosphatase; urinary alkaline phosphatase

UAPA unilateral absence of pulmonary artery

UAR upper airway resistance; uric acid riboside

UAS upper abdomen surgery; upstream activating sequence; upstream activation site

UAU uterine activity unit

UB ultimobranchial body; Unna boot; upper back; urinary bladder

UB 82 universal billing document [1982]

UBA undenatured bacterial antigen; ureidoisobutyric acid

UBB ubiquitin B

UBBC unsaturated vitamin B_{12} binding capacity

UBC ubiquitin C; University of British Columbia [brace]

UBE ubiquitin-activating enzyme

UBF uterine blood flow

UBG, Ubg urobilinogen

UBI ultraviolet blood irradiation

UBL undifferentiated B-cell lymphoma

UBM ultrasound backscatter microscopy; ultrasound biomicroscopy

UBN urobilin

UBO unidentified bright object

UBP ureteral back pressure

UBPS ultrasound bone profile score

UBS unidentified bright signal

UBT urea breath test

UBW usual body weight

UC ulcerative colitis; ultracentrifugal; umbilical cord; unchanged; unclassifiable; unconscious; undifferentiated carcinoma; undifferentiated cells; unit clerk; unsatisfactory condition; untreated cells; urea clearance; urethral catheterization; urinary catheter; urinary catheterization; urine concentrate; urine culture; usual care; uterine contractions

U&C urethral and cervical; usual and customary

UCA ultrasound contrast agent

UCAID University Corporation for Advanced Internet Development

UCARE, U-CARE Unexplained Cardiac Arrest Registry of Europe

UCB unconjugated bilirubin

UCBC umbilical cord blood culture

UCC Uniform Code Council

UCD urine collection device; user-centered design [information system]; usual childhood diseases
UCDS uniform clinical data set
UCE urea cycle enzymopathy
UCG ultrasonic cardiography; urinary chorionic gonadotropin
UCHD usual childhood diseases
UCI unusual childhood illness; urethral catheter in; urinary catheter in
UCL ulnar collateral ligament; upper collateral ligament; upper confidence limit; upper control limit; urea clearance
UCLP unilateral cleft of lip and palate
UCO ultrasonic cardiac output; urethral catheter out; urinary catheter out
UCOD underlying cause of death
UCP uncoupling protein; urinary coproporphyrin; urinary C-peptide
UCPT urinary coproporphyrin test
UCR unconditioned response; usual, customary, and reasonable [fees]
U_cr urinary creatinine
UCS unconditioned stimulus; ultimate compressive strength; unconscious; uterine compression syndrome
ucs unconscious
UCT ultrasound computed tomography; urological care table
UCTD, uCTD undifferentiated (unclassifiable) connective tissue disease
UCV uncontrolled variable; unconventional viral [disease]
UCVA uncorrected visual acuity
UD ulcerative dermatosis; ulnar deviation; undetermined; underdeveloped; unit dose; urethral dilatation; urethral discharge; uridine diphosphate; uroporphyrinogen decarboxylase; uterine delivery
UD-AHF UD-CG 115 BS in Acute Heart Failure [study]
UDB universal database
UDC usual diseases of childhood
UDCA ursodeoxycholic acid
UDE user defined edge [aortic tomography]
UDF user data file
UDIR underdose isodose range [radiation]
UDKase uridine diphosphate kinase
UDN ulcerative dermal necrosis
UDO undetermined origin
UDP uridine diphosphate; user datagram protocol

UDPG uridine diphosphate glucose; urine diphosphoglucose
UDPGA uridine diphosphate-glucuronic acid
UDPGT uridine diphosphate glucuronosyl transferase
UDP/IP user datagram protocol/Internet protocol
UDR user defined region
UDR-BMD ultradistal radius bone mineral density
UDRP urine diribose phosphate
UDRV ulcerative disease rhabdovirus
UDS ultrasound Doppler sonography; uniform data system; unscheduled deoxyribonucleic acid [DNA] synthesis
UE uncertain etiology; under elbow; uninvolved epidermis; upper esophagus; upper extremity
UEA *Ulex europaeus* agglutinin
UEFFDE upper extremity fitness for duty evaluation
UEG ultrasonic encephalography; unifocal eosinophilic granuloma
UEHB uniform effective health benefits
UEL upper explosive limit
UEM universal electron microscope
UEMC unidentified endosteal marrow cell
UES upper esophageal sphincter
uE_s unconjugated estriol
u/ext upper extremity
UF film unsharpness; ultrafiltrate; ultrafiltration; ultrafine; ultrasonic frequency; unaffected female; uncertainty factor; universal feeder; unknown factor; urinary formaldehyde
Uf ultrafiltration
UFA unesterified fatty acid
UFB urinary fat bodies
UFC ultrafast ceramics; urinary free cortisol
UFCT ultrafast computed tomography
UFD ultrasonic flow detector; unilateral facet dislocation
UFFI urea formaldehyde foam insulation
UFH unfractionated heparin
UFL upper flammable limit; upper frequency limit
UFN unreamed femoral nail
UFOV useful field of view
UFP ultrafiltration pressure
UFR ultrafiltration rate; urine filtration rate; uroflowmetry

uFSH urinary follicle-stimulating hormone

UG geometric unsharpness; urogastrone; urogenital

Ug uracyl glycol

UGCR ultrasound-guided compression repair

UGD urogenital diaphragm

UGDP University Group Diabetes Project

UGDV Uasin Gishu disease virus

UGF unidentified growth factor

UGH uveitis-glaucoma-hyphema [syndrome]

UGH+ uveitis-glaucoma-hyphema plus vitreous hemorrhage [syndrome]

UGI upper gastrointestinal [tract]

UGIH upper gastrointestinal hemorrhage

UGIS upper gastrointestinal series

UGME undergraduate medical education

UGP uridyl diphosphate glucose pyrophosphorylase

UGPA undergraduate grade-point average

UGPP uridyl diphosphate glucose pyrophosphorylase

UGS urogenital sinus

UGSV Uganda S virus

UGT uridine diphosphate-glucuronosyltransferase; urogenital tract; urogenital tuberculosis

UH umbilical hernia; unaffected hemisphere; uncontrolled hemorrhage; unfavorable histology; upper half

UHC university hospital consortium

UHD universal heteroduplex generator; unstable hemoglobin disease

UHDDS uniform hospital discharge data set

UHDRS unified Huntington disease rating scale

UHDS uniform hospital dataset

UHF ultrahigh frequency

UHID universal healthcare identifier

UHIS universal healthcare information system; university hospital information system

UHL universal hypertrichosis lanuginosa

UHMM ultrahigh magnification mammography

UHMW ultrahigh molecular weight

UHMWPE ultrahigh molecular weight polyethylene

UHN unreamed humeral nail

UHR underlying heart rhythm

UHS uncontrolled hemorrhagic shock; university health services

UHSC university health services clinic

UHT ultrahigh temperature

UI urinary incontinence; uroporphyrin isomerase; user interface

U/I unidentified

UIBC unsaturated iron-binding capacity

UICAO unilateral internal carotid artery occlusion

UICC Union Internationale Contre le Cancer [International Union Against Cancer]

UID unique identifier; unique image identifier

UIF undegraded insulin factor

UIL user interface language

UIMS user interface management system

UIP unintended pregnancy; usual interstitial pneumonia

UIQ upper inner quadrant

UIR unsolicited information retrieval

UIS Utilization Information Service

UJT unijunction transistor

UK unknown; uridine kinase; urinary kallikrein; urokinase

UKA unicompartmental knee arthroplasty

UKα urinary kallikrein

UKAEA United Kingdom Atomic Energy Authority

UKase uridine kinase

UKCCSG United Kingdom Children's Cancer Study Group

UK-COMA United Kingdom Committee on Medical Aspects [food and nutrition]

UKCSG United Kingdom Collaborative Study Group [timolol trial]

UKEGNS United Kingdom Epidemiology Group for the Nutrition Society

UKHAS United Kingdom Heart Attack Study

UKHEART United Kingdom Heart Failure Evaluation and Assessment of Risk Trial

UK in USA Urokinase in Unstable Angina [study]

UKM urea kinetic modeling

ukn unknown

UKNCSPAIVS United Kingdom National Collaborative Study of Pulmonary Atresia with Intact Ventricular Septum

UKPACE United Kingdom Pacing and Cardiovascular Events [study]; United Kingdom Pacing and Clinical Events [study]

UKPDS United Kingdom Prospective Diabetes Study

UKSAT United Kingdom Small Aneurysm Trial

UK-TIA United Kingdom Transient Ischemic Attack [aspirin trial]

UKTSSA United Kingdom Transplant Support Service Authority

UL ultrasonic; Underwriters Laboratories; undifferentiated lymphoma; upper limb; upper limit; upper lobe

U&L upper and lower

U/l units per liter

ULAM United Network for Organ Sharing Liver Allocation Model

ULBW ultralow birth weight

ULD Unverricht-Lundborg disease

ULDH urinary lactate dehydrogenase

ULDR ultra-low dose rate

ULF ultralow frequency

ULL ultra-lipo-lift

ULLE upper lid of left eye

ULN upper limits of normal

uln ulna, ulnar

ULP ultra low profile; User Liaison Program [Agency for Healthcare Research and Quality]

ULPA ultra low penetration air filter

ULPE upper lobe pulmonary edema

ULQ upper left quadrant

ULR universal leukoreduction

ULRE upper lid of right eye

ULT ultrahigh temperature

ult ultimate

ULTC urban level trauma center

ULTIMA Unprotected Left Main Trunk Intervention Multicenter Assessment

ULTRA utilizing GFX 2.5 stent in small diameter arteries

UltraSTAR ultrasound structured attribute reporting

ULV ultralow volume

ULvWF unusually large von Willebrand factor

UM movement unsharpness; ultra-rapid metabolizer; unaffected male; upper motor [neuron]; uracil mustard; utilization management

uM, μM micromole, micromolar

UMA ulcerative mutilating acropathy; upright membrane assay; urinary muramidase activity

UMAV Umatilla virus

Umax maximum urinary osmolality

umb umbilicus, umbilical

UMBV Umbre virus

UMC unidimensional chromatography; university medical center

UM-CIDI University of Michigan Composite International Diagnostic Interview

UMCV-TO ulnar motor conduction velocity across thoracic outlet

UMD unmodified domain

UMDNS Universal Medical Device Nomenclature System

UME undergraduate medical education

UMHDS uniform minimum health data set

UMI urinary meconium index

UMIN university medical information network

UMKase uridine monophosphate kinase

UML unified modeling language

UMLS Unified Medical Language System

UMN upper motor neuron

UMNL upper motor neuron lesion

UMNS upper motor neuron syndrome

UMP uridine monophosphate

UMPH uridine 5′-monophosphate phosphohydrolase

UMPK uridine monophosphate kinase

UMPS uridine monophosphate synthase

UMS urethral manipulation syndrome

UMT units of medical time

UN ulnar nerve; undernourished; unilateral neglect; updraft nebulizer; urea nitrogen; urinary nitrogen

UNa, U_{Na} urinary sodium

UNAI Uniform Needs Assessment Instrument for posthospital care

UNAIDS United Nations Acquired Immunodeficiency Syndrome [program]

UNASEM Unstable Angina Study Using Eminase

UNAV Una virus

uncomp uncompensated

uncond unconditioned

UNCV ulnar nerve conduction velocity

undet undetermined

UNDP United Nations Development Program

UNDRO United Nations Disaster Relief Organization

UNE urinary norepinephrine

UNEP United Nations Environmental Programme

UNFPA United Nations Population Fund

UNG uracil deoxyribonucleic acid glycosylase

UNHCR United Nations High Commission on Refugees

UniGene Unique Human Gene Sequence Collection

unilat unilateral

UNIS Urological Nursing Information System

univ universal

unk, unkn unknown

UNL upper normal limit

UNLS Unified Nursing Language System

UNOS United Network for Organ Sharing

UNRPCA Use of Nicardipine to Retard the Progression of Coronary Atherosclerosis [trial]

UNSA Unstable Angina Study

unsat unsatisfactory; unsaturated

UNSCEAR United Nations Scientific Committee on Effects of Atomic Radiation

UNT untreated

UNTS unilateral nevoid telangiectasia syndrome

UNX uninephrectomy

UO under observation; undetermined origin; urethral orifice; urinary output

U/O urinary output

u/o under observation

UOP urinary output

UOQ upper outer quadrant

UOsm urinary osmolality

UOV units of variance

UOX urate oxidase

UP parallax unsharpness; ulcerative proctitis; ultrahigh purity; unipolar; upright posture; ureteropelvic; uridine phosphorylase; uroporphyrin

U/P urine to plasma [ratio]

uPA, u-PA urokinase plasminogen activator

uPAR urokinase type plasminogen activator receptor

UPase uridine phosphorylase

UPC usual provider continuity

UPD ulcerative periodontal disease; uniparental disomy; urinary production

UPDIC Uppsala Prospective Diabetes Control [study]

UPDRS Unified Parkinson Disease Rating Scale

UPEC uropathogenic *Escherichia coli* signature-tagged mutagenesis A

UPEP urinary protein electrophoresis; urine protein electrophoresis

UPET Urokinase Pulmonary Embolism Trial

UPF universal proximal femur [prosthesis]

UPG uroporphyrinogen

UPGMA unweighted pair group method with averages

UPI unique patient identifier; uteroplacental insufficiency; uteroplacental ischemia

UPID uniparental isodisomy

UPIF uniform provider [electronic] interchange format

UPIN universal physician identifier number [Health Care Financing Administration, HCFA]

UPJ ureteropelvic junction

UPJO ureteropelvic junction obstruction

UPL unusual position of limbs

UPOV Upolu virus

UPP urethral pressure profile

UPPP uvulopalatopharyngoplasty

UPPRA upright peripheral plasma renin activity

UPS ultraviolet photoelectron spectroscopy; uninterruptible power supply; uroporphyrinogen synthetase; uterine progesterone system

UPSC uterine papillary serous carcinoma

ϒ Greek capital letter *upsilon*

υ Greek lowercase letter *upsilon*

UPSIT University of Pennsylvania Smell Identification Test

UPSIZE Ultrasound-controlled Percutaneous Transluminal Coronary Angioplasty with Optional Balloon Size [study]

UpU uridyl (3′-5′)uridine

UQ ubiquinone; upper quadrant

UQAC unit quality assurance committee

UQCRC ubiquinol-cytochrome *c* reductase core

UQL unacceptable quality level

UQS upper quadrant syndrome

UR unconditioned reflex; upper respiratory; uridine; urinal; urology; utilization review

Ur urea; urine, urinary

URA unilateral renal agenesis

URA, Ura uracil

URAC Utilization Review Accreditation Commission

URALMI Urokinase and Alteplase in Myocardial Infarction [study]

URC upper rib cage; utilization review committee

URD unrelated donor; unspecified respiratory disease; upper respiratory disease

Urd uridine

ureth urethra

URF unidentified reading frame; uterine relaxing factor

URG urogastrone

URI uniform resource identifier; upper respiratory illness; upper respiratory infection

URISA Urban and Regional Information Systems Association

URK urokinase

URL uniform resource locator; upper rate limit [pacemaker]

URN uniform resource name

U-RNA uridylic acid ribonucleic acid

URO urology; uroporphyrin; uroporphyrinogen; utilization review organization

UROD uroporphyrinogen decarboxylase

URO-GEN urogenital

Urol urology, urologist

UROS uroporphyrinogen synthase

URQ upper right quadrant

URR upstream regulatory region

URS ultrasonic renal scanning; upstream repressing sequence

UR2SV UR2 sarcoma virus

URT upper respiratory tract

URTI upper respiratory tract infection

URUV Urucuri virus

URVD unilateral renovascular disease

US screen unsharpness; ultrasonic, ultrasound, ultrasonography; unconditioned stimulus; unique sequence; unit separator; upper segment; upper strength; urinary sugar; Usher syndrome

US1 Usher syndrome type I

US2 Usher syndrome type II

US3 Usher syndrome type III

US4 Usher syndrome type IV

u/s ultrasonic or ultrasound

US1A Usher syndrome type IA

US2A Usher syndrome type IIA

USAFH United States Air Force Hospital

USAFRHL United States Air Force Radiological Health Laboratory

USAH United States Army Hospital

USAHC United States Army Health Clinic

USAID United States Agency for International Development

USAIDR United States Army Institute of Dental Research

USAM Unified Services Action Model

USAMEDS United States Army Medical Service

USAMRICD United States Army Research Institute of Chemical Defense

USAMRID United States Army Medical Research Institute of Infectious Diseases

USAMRIID United States Army Medical Research Institute for Infectious Diseases

USAMRMC United States Army Medical Research and Materiel Command

USAN United States Adopted Names

USAR urban search and rescue

USASI United States of America Standards Institute

USAT ultrasmall aperture terminal

USB upper sternal border

US1B Usher syndrome type IB

US2B Usher syndrome type IIB

USBS United States Bureau of Standards

USBWC United States Biological Warfare Committee

US1C Usher syndrome type IC

USCA ultrasound contrast agent

USCG ultrasonic cardiography

USCR universal self-care requisites

USCT ultrasound computed tomography

USD United States Dispensary

USDA United States Department of Agriculture

USDHEW United States Department of Health, Education, and Welfare

USDHHS United States Department of Health and Human Services

USE ultrasonic echography

USEIR United States Eye Injury Registry

USF upstream stimulatory factor

USFA United States Fire Administration

USFMG United States foreign medical graduate

USFMS United States foreign medical student

USG ultrasonography; user semantic group

USH Usher syndrome

USH1 Usher syndrome type I

USH1A Usher syndrome type IA

USH1B Usher syndrome type IB

USH1C Usher syndrome type IC

USH2 Usher syndrome type II

USH2A Usher syndrome type IIA

USH2B Usher syndrome type IIB

USH3 Usher syndrome type III

USH4 Usher syndrome type IV

US + HC ultrasound-driven hydrocortisone

USHL United States Hygienic Laboratory

USHMAC United States Health Manpower Advisory Council

USI universal serial interface; urinary stress incontinence

USIA United States Information Agency

USIMG United States citizen international medical school graduate

USL ultrasound lithotripsy

US/LS upper strength/lower strength [ratio]

USMG United States or Canada medical school graduate

USMH United States Marine Hospital

USMLE United States Medical Licensing Examination

USMRID United States Army Medical Research Institute of Infectious Diseases

USN ultrasonic nebulizer; unilateral spatial neglect

USNCHS United States National Center for Health Statistics

USNH United States Naval Hospital

USNRP United States National Reference Preparation

USO unilateral salpingo-oophorectomy

USP United States Pharmacopeia

US + P ultrasound and placebo

USPC United States Pharmacopeia Convention

USPDI United States Pharmacopeia Drug Information

USPET Urokinase Streptokinase Pulmonary Embolism Trial

USPHS United States Public Health Service; United States Physicians' Health Study

USPIO ultrasmall particle superparamagnetic iron oxide

USPSTF United States Preventive Services Task Force

USPTA United States Physical Therapy Association

USR unheated serum reagin

USRDS United States Renal Data System

USS ultrasound scanning; universal spine system; user support system

USUHS Uniformed Services University of the Health Services

USUV Usutu virus

USVH United States Veterans Hospital

USVMD urine specimen volume measuring device

USW ultrashort waves

UT total unsharpness; Ullrich-Turner [syndrome]; Unna-Thost [syndrome]; untested; untreated; urinary tract; urticaria

uT unbound testosterone

UTBG unbound thyroxine-binding globulin

UTC ultrasonic tissue characterization; upper thoracic compression

UTD up to date

UT-ETT ultrathin endotracheal tube

UTI urinary tract infection; urinary trypsin inhibitor

util rev utilization review

UTIV Utinga virus

UTO upper tibial osteotomy; urinary tract obstruction

UTOPIA Utilization of Platelet Inhibition in Angina [trial]

UTP unilateral tension pneumothorax; unshielded twisted pair; uridine triphosphate

UTR untranslated region

UTS Ullrich-Turner syndrome; ulnar tunnel syndrome; ultimate tensile strength

UTTS-ETT two-stage ultrathin-walled endotracheal tube

UTZ ultrasound

UU urinary urea; urine urobilinogen

UUID universal unique identifier

UUKV Uukuniemi virus

UUN urinary urea nitrogen

UUO unilateral urethral obstruction

UUP urinary uroporphyrin

UV ultraviolet; umbilical vein; Uppsala virus; ureterovesical; urinary volume

UVA ultraviolet A; ultraviolet germicidal irradiation; ureterovesical angle
UV-A ultraviolet A
UVAL-MED universal visual associative language for medicine
UVB, UV-B ultraviolet B
UVC Ullucus virus C; ultraviolet C; umbilical venous catheter
UV-C ultraviolet C
UVEB unifocal ventricular ectopic beat
UVER ultraviolet-enhanced reactivation
UVGI ultraviolet germicidal irradiation
UVI ultraviolet irradiation
UVJ ureterovesical junction

UVL ultraviolet light
UVO uvomorulin
UVP ultraviolet photometry
UVR ultraviolet radiation
UVV Utive virus
UW unilateral weakness
UWB unit of whole blood
UWD Urbach-Wiethe disease
UWSC unstimulated whole saliva collection
UWW underwater weight
UX uranium X, proactinium
UYP upper yield point

V

V in cardiography, unipolar chest lead; coefficient of variation; electrical potential [in volts]; in electroencephalography, vertex sharp transient; five; a logical binary relation that is true if any argument is true, and false otherwise; luminous efficiency; potential; potential energy [joules]; vaccinated, vaccine; vagina; valine; valve; vanadium; variable; variation; varnish; vector; vegetarian; vein [Lat. *vena*]; velocity; venom, venomous; venous; venous tumor invasion; ventilation; ventricle; ventricular [fibrillation]; verbal comprehension [factor]; vertebra; vertex; vestibular; *Vibrio*; vincristine; violet; viral [antigen]; virion; virulence; virus; vision; visual acuity; voice; volt; voltage; volume; vomiting

V0 no evidence of venous invasion [TNM (tumor-node-metastasis) classification]

V$_{0.5}$ midpoint voltage

V1 primary visual area; venous [tumor] invasion assessed [TNM (tumor-node-metastasis) classification]

V$_1$ mean flow velocity

V1 to V6 ventral 1 to ventral 6 [chest leads in ECG]

v or [Lat. *vel*]; rate of reaction catalyzed by an enzyme; see [Lat. *vide*]; specific volume; valve; vein [Lat. *vena*]; velocity; venous; ventricular; versus; very; virus; vision; volt; volume

VA alveolar ventilation; vacuum aspiration; valproic acid; vasodilator agent; ventricular aneurysm; ventricular arrhythmia; ventriculoatrial; ventroanterior; Veterans Administration; Veterans Affairs; vincristine, Adriamycin; viral antigen; visual acuity; visual aid; visual axis; volt-ampere; volume-average

V$_A$ alveolar ventilation

V/A volt/ampere

V-A veno-arterial

Va activated factor V

V$_a$ alveolar ventilation

va volt-ampere

VAAE vaccine-associated adverse events

VAB vincristine, actinomycin D, and bleomycin; violent antisocial behavior

VAB-6 vincristine, actinomycin, bleomycin, cisplatin, Cytoxan

VABP venoarterial bypass pumping

VABS Vineland Adaptive Behavior Scales

VAC ventriculoatrial conduction; vincristine, doxorubicin, and cyclophosphamide; virus capsid antigen

vac vacuum

VACA Valvuloplasty and Angioplasty in Congenital Anomalies [registry]

VAcc visual acuity with correction

vacc vaccination

VACO Veterans Affairs Central Office

VACS Veterans Administration Cooperative Study

VACSDM Veterans Affairs Cooperative Study on Glycemic Control and Complications in Non-Insulin Dependent Diabetes Mellitus

VACT Veterans Administration Cooperative Trial

VACTERL vertebral abnormalities, anal atresia, cardiac abnormalities, tracheoesophageal fistula and/or esophageal atresia, renal agenesis and dysplasia, and limb defects [association]

VACV vaccinia virus

VAD venous access device; ventricular assist device; vinblastine and dexamethasone; virus-adjusting diluent; vitamin A deficiency

VaD vascular dementia

VADD vitamin A deficiency disorder

VAE venous air emboli; vertical attachment energy

VA-ECMO venoarterial extracorporeal membrane oxygenation

VAEG visual and auditory environment generator

VAERS Vaccine Adverse Events Reporting System

VAEV Vearoy virus

VAF viral-free antigen

VAG vibroarthrography

vag vagina, vaginal, vaginitis

VAG HYST vaginal hysterectomy

VAH vertebral ankylosing hyperostosis; Veterans Affairs Hospital; virilizing adrenal hyperplasia

VA-HIT Veterans Affairs High-density Lipoprotein Intervention Trial

VAHS virus-associated hemophagocytic syndrome
VAIN vaginal intraepithelial neoplasm
V$_{ak}$ atrial volume constant
VAL valproate
Val valine
val valine; valve
VALE visual acuity, left eye
Val-HeFT Valsartan-Heart Failure Trial
VALIANT Valsartan in Acute Myocardial Infarction [study]
VALID Velocity Assessment for Lesions of Intermediate Severity [trial]
VALID II Velocity Assessment for Lesions of Indeterminate Severity [trial]
ValRS valyl ribonucleic acid [RNA] synthetase
VALUE Valsartan Antihypertensive Long-term Use Evaluation
VAM ventricular arrhythmia monitor; virtual archive manager [database element]
VAMC Veterans Affairs Medical Center
VAMP venous arterial blood management protection system; vincristine, amethopterine, 6-mercaptopurine, and prednisone
VAN value-added network; vein, artery, nerve
VANQWISH Veterans Affairs Non-Q-wave Infarction Strategies In-Hospital [study]
VAP vaginal acid phosphatase; variant angina pectoris; venous access port; ventilator-associated pneumonia; virulence-attenuated pool
vap vapor
VAPP vaccine-associated paralytic poliomyelitis
VAPS visual analog pain score
VAPSE variation affecting protein structure or expression
VAPSHCS Veterans Affairs Puget Sound Health Care System
V$_a$/Q alveolar ventilation/perfusion
VA/Q$_c$ ventilation-perfusion [ratio]
VAR vector autoregressive [model algorithm]; veno-arteriolar reflex; visual-auditory range
Var variable; variant, variation, variety; varicella
var variable; variant, variation, variety; varicose
VARE visual acuity, right eye

VARETA variable-resolution electromagnetic tomography
VA RNA virus-associated ribonucleic acid [RNA]
VARPRO variable projection
VARS valyl-transfer ribonucleic acid synthetase
VARV variola virus
VAS vagal afferents; vascular; vascular access service; ventricular assist system; ventriculo-atrial shunt; Verapamil Angioplasty Study; vesicle attachment site; vestibular aqueduct syndrome; Veterans Adjustment Scale; vibro-acoustic stimulation; viral arthritis syndrome; Visual Analogue Scale
VASC vascular; Verbal Auditory Screen for Children; visual-auditory screening
VAsc visual acuity without correction
vasc vascular
VASD Vascular Access Service Database
VASP vasodilator-stimulated phosphoprotein
VASPNAF Veterans Administration Stroke Prevention in Nonrheumatic Atrial Fibrillation [study]
VAS RAD vascular radiology
VAST visual analysis systems technology
VAST/STT visual analysis systems technology/space-time toolkit
VAT variable antigen type; vaso-occlusive angiotherapy; ventricular accommodation test; ventricular activation time; vesicular amine transformer; video-assisted thoracoscopy; visceral adipose tissue; visual action therapy; visual action time; visual apperception test; vocational apperception test
VATER vertebral defects, imperforate anus, tracheoesophageal fistula, and radial and renal dysplasia
v-ATPase vascular adenosine triphosphatase
VATS Veterans Administration medical center transference syndrome; video-assisted thoracic surgery
VATs surface variable antigen
VATT vascular anatomy teaching tool
VAV variable air volume
VB vaginal bulb; valence bond; venous blood; ventrobasal; Veronal buffer; vertebrobasilar; viable birth; vinblastine; virus buffer; voided bladder
Vb vinblastine

VBAC vaginal birth after cesarean section
VBAIN vertebrobasilar artery insufficiency nystagmus
VBC vincristine, bleomycin, and cisplatin; visualization in biomedical computing; volumetric based capnometry
VBD vanishing bile duct; Veronal-buffered diluent
VBE visualized bronchus endoscope
VBF variable bandwidth filter [ECG]
VBG vagotomy and Billroth gastroenterostomy; venous blood gases; venous bypass graft; vertical-banded gastroplasty
VBI ventral blood island; vertebrobasilar insufficiency; vertebrobasilar ischemia
VBL vinblastine
VbMF vinblastine, methotrexate, 5-fluorouracil
VBNC viable but nonculturable [microorganisms]
vBNS very high bandwidth network service; very high-performance backbone network services
VBOS Veronal-buffered oxalated saline
VBP vagal body paraganglia; venous blood pressure; ventricular premature beat
VBR ventricular brain ratio; vertebral body repositioning
VBS Veronal-buffered saline; vertebrobasilar system
VBS:FBS Veronal-buffered saline-fetal bovine serum
VBWG Vascular Biology Working Group
VBX visual basic controls
VC color vision; variance cardiography; variation coefficient; vascular changes; vasoconstriction; vena cava; venereal case; venous capacitance; ventilatory capacity; ventral column; ventricular contraction; vertebral canal; Veterinary Corps; videocassette; video conference; vincristine; vinyl chloride; virtual coloscopy; virus C; visual capacity; visual cortex; vital capacity; vocal cord
V/C ventilation/circulation [ratio]
Vc vital capacity
V$_c$ volume of [central] compartment
VCA vancomycin, colistin, and anisomycin; viral capsid antigen
VCAM vascular cell adhesion molecule
VCAP vincristine, cyclophosphamide, Adriamycin, and prednisone
VCB ventricular capture beat

vCBF venous cerebral blood flow
VCC vasoconstrictor center; ventral cell column
VC-CFMV volume-controlled constant flow mechanical ventilation
VCD Van Capelle-Durrer [model of cardiac cell depolarization-repolarization]; vibrational circular dichroism
VCE vagina, ectocervix, and endocervix
VCF velocardiofacial [syndrome]; velocity of circumferential fiber [lengthening]; ventricular contractility function
VCFG volume-cycled flow generator
VCF$_{min}$ minimum velocity of circumferential fiber [lengthening]
VCFS velo-cardio-facial syndrome
VCG vectorcardiogram, vectorcardiography; voiding cystourethrography; volumetric cardiogram
VCHS Virginia Center for Health Statistics
VCL vinculin; visual concept library; Voxtool Command Language
VCM vinyl chloride monomer
V$_{cM}$ volume of [central] compartment for metabolite
VCMP vincristine, cyclophosphamide, melphalan, and prednisone
VCN vancomycin, colistomethane, and nystatin; *Vibrio cholerae* neuraminidase
VCO endogenous production of carbon monoxide; voltage-controlled oscillator
V$_{CO}$ endogenous production of carbon monoxide
VCO$_2$ carbon dioxide output; carbon dioxide elimination rate
V$_{CO_2}$ carbon dioxide output
VCP vincristine, cyclophosphamide, and prednisone
VCR vasoconstriction rate; vincristine; volume clearance rate
VCRS virtual center for renal support [telemedicine]; voluntary cardiorespiratory synchronization
VCS vasoconstrictor substance; vesicocervical space; virtual chart system
VCSA viral cell surface antigen
VCSF ventricular cerebrospinal fluid
VCT venous clotting time; voluntary counseling and testing
VCU video conference unit; videocystourethrography; voiding cystourethrogram, voiding cystourethrography

VCUG vesicoureterogram; voiding cysto-urethrogram

VCV vein chlorosis virus; vein clearing virus

VD vapor density; vascular disease; vasodilation, vasodilator; venereal disease; venous dilatation; ventricular dilator; ventrodorsal; verbal dysphasia; vertical deviation; vertical divergence; video-disk; viral diarrhea; voided; volume of dead space; volume of distribution

V&D vomiting and diarrhea

V$_D$ dead space; volume of distribution

Vd value of [drug] distribution; viroid; voided, voiding; volume dead space; volume of distribution

V$_d$ apparent volume of distribution

V$_D$ dead space

VDA virtual DNA analysis; visual discriminatory acuity

VDAC voltage-dependent anion channel

VDB virtual database

VdB van der Bergh [test]

VDBR volume of distribution of bilirubin

VDC vasodilator center

VDCC voltage dependent calcium channel

VDD atrial synchronous ventricular inhibited [pacemaker]; vitamin D-dependent

VDDR vitamin D-dependent rickets

VDE vertical detachment energy

VDEL Venereal Disease Experimental Laboratory

VDEM vasodepressor material

VDF ventricular diastolic fragmentation

VDG, VD-G venereal disease-gonorrhea

vdg voiding

VDH valvular disease of the heart

VDI venous distensibility index; virus defective interfering [particle]

V$_{dia}$ diastolic potential

VDL vasodepressor lipid; visual detection level

VDM vasodepressor material

vDOC virtual distributed online clinic

VDP ventricular premature depolarization

VDR venous diameter ratio; vitamin D receptor

VDRG vitamin D receptor gene

VDRL Venereal Disease Research Laboratory [test for syphilis]

VDRR vitamin D-resistant rickets

VDRS Verdun Depression Rating Scale

VDRT venereal disease reference test

VDS vasodilator substance; vindesine

VDS, VD-S venereal disease-syphilis

VDT vector distance transform; vibration disappearance threshold; visual display terminal; visual distortion test

VDU video display unit

VDV ventricular end-diastolic volume

V$_D$/V$_T$ dead space to tidal volume [ratio]

Vd/Vt dead space ventilation/total ventilation [ratio]

VDWS van der Woude syndrome

VE vaginal examination; valve-equivalent [mechanical]; vascular endothelial; Venezuelan encephalitis; venous emptying; venous extension; ventilation; ventilatory equivalent; ventricular elasticity; ventricular extrasystole; vertex; vesicular exanthema; viral encephalitis; virtual endoscopy; virtual environment; visual efficiency; vitamin E; volume ejection; voluntary effort

V&E Vinethine and ether

V$_E$ environmental variance; respiratory minute volume

V$_E$ minute ventilation

Ve ventilation

V$_e$ volume of effect compartment

VEA ventricular ectopic activity; ventricular ectopic arrhythmia; viral envelope antigen

VEB ventricular ectopic beat

VEC velocity encoding cine [MRI]; virtual environment control [system]

VEcad vascular endothelial cadherin

VECG vector electrocardiogram

VEC-MR velocity encoded cine-magnetic resonance

VECP visually evoked cortical potential

VED vacuum erection device; ventricular ectopic depolarization; virtual environment display [system]; vital exhaustion and depression

VEE vagina, ectocervix, and endocervix; Venezuelan equine encephalomyelitis

VEEV Venezuelan equine encephalitis virus

VEF ventricular ejection fraction; visually evoked field

VEG vegetation; von Egner gland [protein]

VEGAS Vein Graft Angiojet Study; ventricular enlargement with gait apraxia syndrome

VEGF vascular endothelial growth factor

VEGF-A vascular endothelial growth factor type A

VEGP von Ebner gland protein

vehic vehicle

VEI volume [lung] at the end of inspiration

VEINES Venous Insufficiency Epidemiologic and Economic Study

vel, veloc velocity

VELV Vellore virus

VEM vasoexcitor material

VEMR virtual electronic medical record

VENC velocity encoding

vent ventilation; ventral; ventricle, ventricular

vent fib ventricular fibrillation

ventric ventricle

VENUS Very Early Nimodipine Use in Stroke [trial]

VEP visual evoked potential

VEPID video-based electronic portal imaging device

VEPT volume of electrically participating thoracic tissue

VER ventricular evoked response; visual evoked response

Verc vervet (African green monkey) kidney cells

VERDI Verapamil vs Diuretics [trial]

VERDICT Verapamil Digoxin Cardioversion Trial; Veterans Evidence-Based Research, Dissemination, and Implementation Center

VERP visual event related potential

vert vertebra, vertebral

VES virtual endoscope system; viscoelastic substance

ves bladder [Lat. *vesica*]; vesicular; vessel

VESA virtual endoscopy software application

vesic a blister [Lat. *vesicula*]

VEST Vesnarinone Trial

vest vestibular

ves ur urinary bladder [Lat. *vesica urinaria*]

VET ventricular ejection time; vestigial testis

Vet veteran; veterinarian, veterinary

VETF vaccinia early transcription factor

VetMB Bachelor of Veterinary Medicine

Vet Med veterinary medicine

VETS Veterinary Expert Technology System

Vet Sci veterinary science

VEUD virtual emergency and urgency department

VF left leg [electrode]; ventricular fibrillation; ventricular fluid; ventricular flutter; ventricular function; videofluorography; visual field; vitreous fluorophotometry; vocal fremitus

Vf visual frequency

V$_f$ final voltage; variant frequency

vf visual field

VFA volatile fatty acid

VFC vaccine for children; ventricular function curve

VFD vacuum fluorescent display; visual feedback display; visual field defect

VFDP variant familial developmental pattern

VFI venous filling index; visual field intact

V fib ventricular fibrillation

VFID virtual focus-isocenter-distance

VFL ventricular flutter

VFOS vector fast orthogonal search

VFP ventricular filling pressure; ventricular fluid pressure; vocal fold pathology

VFR voiding flow rate

VFS vascular fragility syndrome; very fast sedimentation; visual file system

VFT venous filling time; ventricular fibrillation threshold

VF/VT ventricular fibrillation/ventricular tachycardia

VG van Gieson [stain]; ventricular gallop; volume of gas

V$_G$ genetic variance

VGA video graphics array

VGAS visual grading analysis score

VGAT vesicular gamma aminobutyric acid transporter

VGB vigabatrin

VGCC voltage-gated calcium channels

VGH very good health

vGI ventral giant interneuron

VGM venous graft myringoplasty

VGP viral glycoprotein

VGPO volume-guaranteed pressure options [ventilation]

VGS video game-induced seizures

VH vaginal hysterectomy; venous hematocrit; ventral hippocampus; ventricular hypertrophy; veterans hospital; viral hepatitis; virtual hospital; Visible Human [project]

V_H variable domain of heavy chain; variable heavy chain
Vh volt-hours
VHA Veterans Health Administration; Voluntary Hospital Association
V/Hallu visual hallucinations
VHAS Verapamil in Hypertension Atherosclerosis Study
VHCD virtual health care databank
VHD valvular heart disease; viral hematodepressive disease; Visible Human Dataset
VHDL very high density lipoprotein
V-HeFT Vasodilator Heart Failure Trial; Veterans Administration Heart Failure Trial
VHEV Vilyuisk human encephalomyelitis virus
VHF very high frequency; viral hemorrhagic fever; visual half-field
VHL Virtual Health Library; von Hippel-Lindau [syndrome]
VHN Vickers hardness number
VHP vaporized hydrogen peroxide; Visible Human Project
VHR ventricular heart rate
VHS veterans health study
VHS&RA Veterans Health Service and Research Administration
VHSV viral hemorrhagic septicemia virus
VI Roman numeral six; vaginal irrigation; variable interval; vastus intermedius; ventilation index; virgo intacta; virtual document; virulence, virulent; viscosity index; visual impairment; visual inspection; vitality index; volume index
V_I initial voltage
Vi virulence, virulent
VIA virus inactivating agent; virus infection-associated antigen
VIB viral inclusion body
vib vibration
vib & perc vibration and percussion
VIC valvular interstitial cell; variable impedance characterization; vasoinhibitory center; virtual information center; visual communication therapy; voice intensity control
VICP Vaccine Injury Compensation Program
VI-CTS vibration-induced carpal tunnel syndrome
VID visible iris diameter

VIDA viability identification with dipyridamole-dobutamine administration
VIDE Virus Identification Data Exchange
VIDERO virtual delivery room
VIDRL Victorian Infectious Diseases Reference Laboratory [Australia]
VIF variance inflation factor; virus-induced interferon
VIG, VIg vaccinia immune globulin; vaccinia immunoglobulin
VIGIM intravascular vaccinia immunoglobulin
VIGIV intravenous vaccinia immunoglobulin
VIGOUR Virtual Coordinating Center for Global Collaborative Cardiovascular Research
VIGRE velocity imaging with gradient-recalled echos
VIIag factor VII antigen
VIIIc factor VIII clotting activity
VIII_{vwf} von Willebrand factor
VIL villin
VILI ventilator-induced lung injury
VIM video-intensification microscopy; vimentin
VIN vulvar intraepithelial neoplasm
vin vinyl
VINDICATE vascular, inflammatory/infectious, neoplastic/neurologic/psychiatric, degenerative/dietary, intoxication/idiopathic/iatrogenic, congenital, allergic/autoimmune, trauma, endocrine/metabolic [differential diagnosis mnemonic]
VINV Vinces virus
VIP vaccine information pamphlet; vasoactive intestinal peptide; vasoinhibitory peptide; venous impedance plethysmography; ventricular inotropic parameter; Viability Impact on Prognosis [study]; video interface processor; voluntary interruption of pregnancy
vip vegetative insecticidal enterotoxin
VIPERS Virtual Intelligent Patient Electronic Record System
VIPoma vasoactive intestinal polypeptide-secreting tumor
VIPOR Vermont Integrated Problem-Oriented Record
VIQ Verbal Intelligence Quotient
vIQ virtual inhibitory quotient
VIR virology
Vir virus, viral

vir virulent

VIRTUOS virtual radiotherapy simulation and verification

VIS vaccine information statement; vaginal irrigation smear; value-intensity-strength; venous insufficiency syndrome; vertebral irritation syndrome; visible; visual information storage

vis vision, visual

VISA vancomycin-intermediate *Staphylococcus aureus*

VISC vitreous infusion suction cutter

visc viscera, visceral; viscosity

VISI volar intercalated segment instability

VISIR Verification and Information System in Radiology

VISN veterans integrated service network

VISNA Visna/maedi virus

VISP Vitamin Intervention for Stroke Prevention [trial]

Vit vitamin

vit vital

VITA Vicenza Thrombophilia and Atherosclerosis Project

VITALS vital indicators of teaching and learning success

vit cap vital capacity

VIVAS Vaccination Information Vaccination Administration System

VIVIAN virtual intracranial visualization and navigation

VJ ventriculojugular

VJC ventriculojugularcardiac

VK vervet (African green monkey) kidney cells

VKC vernal keratoconjunctivitis

VKG videokymography

VKH, VKHS Vogt-Koyanagi-Harada [syndrome]

VL left arm [electrode]; vastus lateralis [muscle]; ventralis lateralis [nucleus]; ventrolateral; viral load; visceral leishmaniasis; vision, left [eye]

V$_L$ lung volume; variable domain of the light chain; variable light chain

VLA very late activation [antigen or protein]; virus-like agent

VLAB, VLA-BETA very late activation protein beta

V LACT venous lactate

VLAN virtual online area network

VLAS vector least squares

VLB vinblastine; vincaleukoblastine

VLBR very low birth rate

VLBW very low birth weight

VLC variable length coding

VLCAD very long chain acyl-coenzyme A dehydrogenase

VLCD very low calorie diet

VLCFA very long chain fatty acid

VLD very low density; volume limiter disk

VLDL, VLDLP very low density lipoprotein

VLDLR very low density lipoprotein receptor

VLDL-TG very-low-density lipoprotein-triglyceride complex

V$_{LES}$ volume of lesion

VLF very low frequency

VLG ventral nucleus of the lateral geniculate body

VLH ventrolateral nucleus of the hypothalamus

VLIA virus-like infectious agent

VLIS Virtual Laboratory Information System

VLM ventrolateral medulla; visceral larva migrans

VLO vastus lateralis obliquus

VLP vincristine, L-asparaginase, and prednisone; virus-like particle

VLp virus-like particle

VLPA ventrolateral pressure area

VLR vinleurosine

VLS vascular leak syndrome

VLSI very large scale integration

VLTF vaccinia late transcription factor

VM Valsalva maneuver; vasomotor; ventilator management; ventralis medialis; ventricular mass; ventriculomegaly; ventriculometry; ventromedial; vestibular membrane; video microscopy; viomycin; viral myocarditis; voltmeter

V/m volts per meter

V$_m$ membrane potential; muscle volume; maximum velocity

VMA vanillylmandelic acid; vastus medialis advancement; ventilator management advisor

VMAP, Vmap velocity mapping

VMAT vesicular monoamine transformer

Vmax maximum velocity

V$_{max}$ maximum volume

VMC vasomotor center

VMCG vector magnetocardiogram

VMCHN Victorian Maternal and Child Health Nurses

VMD Doctor of Veterinary Medicine; virtual medical device; vitelliform macular dystrophy

VMDS virtual medical device system

vMDV virulent Marek disease virus

VME Volunteers for Medical Engineering

VMF vasomotor flushing

VMGT Visual Motor Gestalt Test

VMH ventromedial hypothalamus

VMI, VMIT visual-motor integration [test]

VML vector markup language; ventriculo-megaly

VMLS virtual medical library system

VMN ventromedial nucleus

VMO vastus medialis obliquus [muscle]; visiting medical officer

VMP virtual machine platform

VMR vasomotor rhinitis

VMRS Vermont Medical Record System

VMS virtual medical school; virtual memory system; visual memory span

VMST visual motor sequencing test

VMT vasomotor tonus; ventilatory muscle training; ventromedial tegmentum

V$_m$(t) time-averaged membrane potential

V$_m$(x,t) absolute transmembrane potential

VN vesical neck; vestibular nucleus; virus neutralization; visceral nucleus; visiting nurse; vitronectin; vocational nurse; vomeronasal

VNA Visiting Nurse Association

VNDPT visual numerical discrimination pre-test

VNO vomeronasal organ

VNQ variable N-Quoit filter [imaging]

VNR vitronectin receptor

VNRA vitronectin receptor alpha

VNS vagal nerve stimulation; virtual notebook system; visiting nursing service

VNTR variable number of tandem repeats; variable copy number tandem repeats

VO verbal order; volume overload; voluntary opening

V$_o$ rest volume

VO$_2$, V$_{O_2}$ volume of oxygen utilization

Vo standard volume; vascular volume

VOC vaso-occlusive crisis; volatile organic compound

VOCC voltage-operated calcium channel

VOD veno-occlusive disease; video on demand

VOI [Bayesian] value of information; volume of interest

VO$_2$I volume of oxygen utilization index

VoIP voice over Internet protocol

vol volar; volatile; volume; voluntary, volunteer

VOM volt-ohm-milliammeter

VO$_2$ Max, VO$_2$max maximum volume of oxygen utilization

VON Victorian Order of Nurses

V-ONC viral oncogene

v-one viral oncogene

VOO ventricular asynchronous (competitive, fixed-rate) [pacemaker]

vOOMM visual object-oriented matrix model

VOP vaso-occlusive pain; venous occlusion plethysmography

VOPS vector optimal parameter search [algorithm]

VOR vestibulo-ocular reflex; volume of regret

VORd vestibulo-ocular reflex in darkness

VORe vestibulo-ocular reflex enhancement

VORs vestibulo-ocular reflex suppression

VOS videothoracoscopic operator staging; vision, left eye [Lat. *visio, oculus sinister*]

VOT voice onset time

VOTE Value of Transesophageal Echocardiography [study]

VP physiological volume; vapor pressure; Varadi-Papp [orofaciodigital syndrome]; variegate porphyria; vascular permeability; vasopressin; velopharyngeal; venipuncture; venous pressure; ventricular pacing; ventricular pericardium; ventricular premature [beat]; ventroposterior; Ve-Pepsid; verbal paraphrasia; vertex potential; vincristine and prednisone; virion protein; visual presentation; Voges-Proskauer [medium or test]; voiding pressure; volume-pressure; vulnerable period

V/P ventilation/perfusion [ratio]

V&P vagotomy and pyloroplasty

Vp paced ventricular output; peak velocity; peak voltage; phenotype variance; plasma volume; ventricular premature [beat]

vp vapor pressure

VPA valproic acid

VPAP variable positive airway pressure

VPB ventricular premature beat

VPC vapor-phase chromatography; ventricular premature complex; ventricular premature contraction; volume-packed cells; volume percent

VPCT ventricular premature contraction threshold

VPD vaccine-preventable disease; ventricular premature depolarization

VPF vascular permeability factor

VPFRU vapor-protective, flame-resistant undergarment

VPG velopharyngeal gap

VPg genome-linked protein

VPGSS venous pressure gradient support stockings

VPI vapor phase inhibitor; velopharyngeal insufficiency

VPL ventroposterolateral; vertical partial laryngectomy

VPM ventilator pressure manometer; ventroposteromedial

vpm vibrations per minute

VPN ventral pontine nucleus; virtual private network [telemedicine]

VPO velopharyngeal opening; vertical pendular oscillation

VPP Vaccine Provision Project; vacuolar proton pump; viral porcine pneumonia

VPR vascular permeability reaction; ventricular paced rhythm; virtual patient record; Voges-Proskauer reaction; volume/pressure ratio

VPRBC volume of packed red blood cells

VPRC volume of packed red cells

VPRS variable precision rough set [model]

VPS Vasovagal Pacemaker Study; ventriculoperitoneal shunt; verbal pain scale; virtual point source; visual pleural space; volume performance standard

vps vibrations per second

VPT vibratory perception threshold

VQ vector quantization

V/Q ventilation/perfusion [ratio]; voice quality

VQE visa qualifying examination [for foreign medical graduates]

VQI ventilation perfusion index

V-QRS QRS ventricular potential [ECG]

VR right arm [electrode]; Valsalva ratio; valve replacement; valvular regurgitation; vanilloid receptor; variable rate; variable ratio; variable region; vascular resistance;

vasopressin receptor; venous flow reversal; venous reflux; venous resistance; venous return; ventilation rate; ventilation ratio; ventral root; ventricular rale; ventricular response; ventricular rhythm; vesicular rosette; virtual reality; vision, right [eye]; vital records; vocal resonance; vocational rehabilitation; volume ratio; volume regulation; volume rendering [imaging]

2VR double valve replacement

Vr relaxation volume

V2R vasopressin 2 receptor [gene]

VRA visual reinforcement audiometry

VRBC red blood cell volume

VRC Vaccine Research Center; venous renin concentration

VRCP vitreoretinochoroidopathy

VRD ventricular radial dysplasia; viral reference division

VRE vancomycin-resistant enterococcus

VR&E vocational rehabilitation and education

VREF vancomycin-resistant *Enterococcus faecium*

V$_{rest}$ resting potential

VRI viral respiratory infection; virtual reality imaging

VRL lumbar ventral root; vanilloid receptor-like [protein]; Virus Reference Laboratory

VRML Virtual Reality Modeling Language

VRNA viral ribonucleic acid

VRNI neovascular inflammatory vitreoretinopathy

VROM voluntary range of motion

VRP ventral root potential; ventricular refractory period

VRR ventral root reflex

VRS verbal rating scale; Virchow-Robin space

VRSA vancomycin-resistant *Staphylococcus aureus*

VRT vehicle rescue technician; virtual reality therapy; volume ray tracing; volume-rendering technique

VRV ventricular residual volume; viper retrovirus; Virgin River virus

VRX variable resolution x-ray

VS vaccination scar; vaccine serotype; vagal stimulation; vascular surgeon; vasospasm; venesection; ventricular septum; verapamil shock; verification/recording system; vesicular stomatitis; veterinary surgeon; vibration syndrome; virtual simulator; visual storage; vital sign; Vogt-Spielmeyer [syndrome]; volatile solid; volume support; volumetric solution; voluntary sterilization

Vs stressed volume; venesection

Vs vibration second; volt-second

V$_s$ system tissue volume

V x s volts by seconds

vs see above [Lat. *vide supra*]; single vibration; versus; vibration seconds; vital signs

VSA variant-specific surface antigen

VSAT very small aperture terminal

VSAV vesicular stomatitis Alagoas virus

VSBE very short below-elbow [cast]

VSC visual sequence comparison; voluntary surgical contraception

VSCC volume-sensitive chloride channel

VSCT ventral spinocerebellar cell

VSD ventricular septal defect; vesicular stomatitis virus; virtually safe dose

VSFP venous stop flow pressure

VSG variant surface glycoprotein; Vesnarinone Study Group

VSHD ventricular septal heart defect

VSIE volume surface integral equation [method]

VSINC Virus Subcommittee of the International Nomenclature Committee

VSIV vesicular stomatitis Indiana virus

VSM vascular smooth muscle

VSMC vascular smooth muscle cell

VSMS Vineland Social Maturity Scale

vsn vision

VSNJV vesicular stomatitis New Jersey virus

VSO vertical supranuclear ophthalmoplegia

VSOK vital signs normal

VSP variable spine plating; very short patch [deoxyribonucleic acid, DNA, repair]

VSR venous stasis retinopathy; visceral/subcutaneous adipose tissue ratio

VSRA variable speech rate audiometry

VSS vital signs stable

V$_{ss}$ volume at steady state

VST ventral spinothalamic tract; videosee-through; volume-selective excitation

VSTA Virus-Serum-Toxin Act

v-STM vaginal specimen transport medium

VSV vesicular stomatitis virus

VSV-G G protein of Gibbon ape leukemia virus

VSW ventricular stroke work

VT tetrazolium violet; tidal volume; total ventilation; vacuum tube; vacuum tuberculin; vasotonin; velocity of tension; venous thrombosis; ventricular tachyarrhythmia; ventricular tachycardia; verocytotoxin; verotoxin; vibration threshold; vitronectin

V$_T$ tidal volume; T lymphocyte antigen receptor variable region; total ventilation

+VT maximum velocity of tension

−VT decline in velocity of tension

V&T volume and tension

V$_T$ tidal volume

Vt total vascular volume; volume of tissue [compartment]

VTA ventral tegmental area

VTach, Vtach, V tach ventricular tachycardia

VTB virtual tracheobronchoscopy

VTE venous thromboembolism; ventricular tachycardia event

VTEC verotoxin-producing *Escherichia coli*

VTEU Vaccine and Treatment Evaluation Unit

VTG volume thoracic gas

VTI velocity-time integral; volume thickness index

VTK visualization tool kit

VTL ventricular tracking limit

VTM mechanical tidal volume; virus transport medium

VT-MASS Metoprolol and Sotalol for Sustained Ventricular Tachycardia [study]

VTN Vaccine Trials Network; vitronectin

VTOP vaginal termination of pregnancy

VTR variable tandem repeats; vesicular transport system; videotape recording; vitronectin receptor

VTSRS Verdun Target Symptom Rating Scale

VT/VF ventricular tachycardia/ventricular fibrillation

VTVM vacuum tube voltmeter

VTX verocytotoxin; vertex

vtx vertex

VU varicose ulcer; volume unit

vu volume unit

VUC voided urinary cytology

VUD voluntary unrelated donor

VUJ vesico-ureteral junction

VUO vesico-ureteral orifice

VUR vesico-ureteral reflux

V-US volumetric ultrasonography

VUSE variable angle uniform signal excitation

VUV vacuum ultraviolet

VV vaccinia virus; variable volume; varicose veins; venous volume; veno-venous; vertical vein; viper venom; vulva and vagina

2VV double valve replacement

V&V verification and validation

V-V veno-venous [bypass]

vv varicose veins; veins

v/v percent volume in volume

VVAS vertical visual analog scale

VVC vulvovaginal candidiasis

VVD vaginal vertex delivery

VVDL venovenous double-lumen [catheter]

VVFR vesicovaginal fistula repair

VVGF vaccinia virus growth factor

VVI ventricular inhibited [pacemaker]; vocal velocity index

v$_{vk}$ ventricular volume constant

VVLBW very very low birth weight

vvMDV very virulent Marek disease virus

VVol venous volume

VVS vesicovaginal space; vestibulo-vegetative syndrome

VVT ventricular triggered [pacemaker]

VW van der Woude [syndrome]; vascular wall; vessel wall; Volterra-Wiener [approach]; von Willebrand [disease]

v/w volume per weight

vWAg von Willebrand antigen

VWD ventral wall defect

vWD von Willebrand disease

VWDFAg, vWDFAg von Willebrand factor antigen

VWF velocity waveform; vibration-induced white finger; von Willebrand factor; von Willebrand Factor Database

vWF, vWf von Willebrand factor

VWM ventricular wall motion; verbal working memory

vWS van der Woude syndrome; viewing work station; von Willebrand syndrome

VX no evidence of venous invasion [TNM (tumor-node-metastasis) classification]; virus X

Vx vertex

VYS visceral yolk sac

VZ varicella-zoster

V$_z$ volume of distribution in the terminal phase

VZIG, VZIg varicella zoster immunoglobulin

VZV varicella-zoster virus

W

W dominant spotting [mouse]; energy; section modulus; a series of small triangular incisions in plastic surgery [plasty]; tryptophan; tungsten [Ger. *Wolfram*]; wakefulness; ward; water; watt; Weber [test]; week; wehnelt; weight; white; widowed; width; wife; Wilcoxon rank sum statistic; Wistar [rat]; with; word fluency; work; wound

W3 World Wide Web

w velocity (m/s); water; watt; while; with

W+ weakly positive

WA when awake; white adult; Wiskott-Aldrich [syndrome]

W/A watt/ampere

W&A weakness and atrophy

WAAT Warfarin Plus Aspirin vs Aspirin Trial

WAB Western Aphasia Battery

WACS Women's Atherosclerosis Cardiovascular Study

WAF weakness, atrophy, and fasciculation; white adult female

WAFUS Warfarin Anticoagulation Follow-up Study

WAGR Wilms tumor, aniridia, genitourinary abnormalities, and mental retardation

WAI Web Accessibility Initiative

WAIS Wechsler Adult Intelligence Scale; Western Angiographic and Interventional Society; wide area information server; Workplace Advocacy Information System

WAIS-R revised Wechsler Adult Intelligence Scale

WAK wearable artificial kidney

WALK Walking with Angina-Learning Is the Key [program]

WALV Wallal virus

WAM white adult male; work area model; worksheet for ambulatory medicine

WAMMI Website Analysis and Measurement Inventory [Ireland]

WAN wide area network

WANTO WEB-Aided Nursing the Old Information System

WANV Wanowrie virus

WAP wandering atrial pacemaker; whey acid protein; wireless application protocol [telemedicine]

WAR Wasserman antigen reaction; without additional reagents

WARCRY Wegener and Related Diseases Compassionate Regimen Yield [study]

WARDS Welfare of Animals Used for Research in Drugs and Therapy

WARF warfarin [Wisconsin Alumni Research Foundation]

WARIS Warfarin Reinfarction Study

WARIS II Warfarin-Aspirin Reinfarction Study-Norwegian

WARSS Warfarin-Aspirin Recurrent Stroke Study

WARV Warrego virus

WAS weekly activities summary; Wiskott-Aldrich syndrome

WASH Warfarin-Aspirin Study of Heart Failure

WASID Warfarin-Aspirin Symptomatic Intracranial Disease [study]

WASP Weber Advanced Spatial Perception [test]; Wiskott-Aldrich syndrome protein

Wass Wasserman [reaction]

WAT word association test

WATCH Warfarin Antiplatelet Trial in Chronic Heart Failure; Worcester-area Trial for Counseling in Hyperlipidemia

WATSMART Waterloo Spatial Motion Analysis and Recording Technique

WAVE Women's Angiographic Vitamin and Estrogen [trial]

WB waist belt; washable base; washed bladder; water bottle; Wechsler-Bellevue [Scale]; weight-bearing; well baby; Western blot [assay]; wet bulb; whole blood; whole body; Willowbrook [virus]; Wilson-Blair [agar]

Wb weber; well-being

WBA wax bean agglutinin; Western blot assay; whole body activity

Wb/A webers/ampere

WBAPTT whole blood activated partial thromboplastin time

WBC well baby care/clinic; white blood cell; white blood cell count; whole blood cell count

WBCT whole-blood clotting time

WBDC whole-body digital scanner

WBE whole-body extract

WBF whole-blood folate

WBGT wet bulb global temperature

WBH whole-blood hematocrit; whole-body hyperthermia

WBI Web-based instruction [telemedicine]; whole bowel irrigation

WBLT Watson-Barker Listening Test

Wb/m² weber per square meter

WBMP wireless bitmap [telemedicine]

WBN whole-blood nitrogen

WBPTT whole-blood partial thromboplastin time

WBR whole-body radiation

WBRT whole-blood recalcification time; whole breast radiation therapy

WBS Wechsler-Bellevue Scale; whole-blood serum; whole-body scan; Wiedemann-Beckwith syndrome; Williams-Beuren syndrome; withdrawal body shakes

WBT wet bulb temperature

WBV waterborne virus; whole blood volume; whole brain volume

WC waist circumference; ward clerk; warty carcinoma; water closet; Weber-Christian [syndrome]; wheel chair; white cell; white cell casts; white cell count; white child; whooping cough; wild caught [animal]; work capacity; workers' compensation; writer's cramp

WC′ whole complement

W/C watch carefully; wheel chair

W3C World Wide Web Consortium

wc wheel chair

WCB working cell bank

WCC Walker carcinosarcoma cells; white cell count; windowed cross correlation

WCD Weber-Christian disease

W-CDMA wideband-code division multiple access [telemedicine]

WCE whole cell extract; work capacity evaluation

WCGS Western Collaborative Group Study

WCL Wenckebach cycle length; whole cell lysate

w/cm² watts per square centimeter

WCP well characterized product

WCPs whole chromosome paints

WCS white clot syndrome; Wisconsin Card Sort [test]; worst case scenario

WCST Wisconsin Card Sorting Test

WCT wide [QRS] complex tachycardia; word categorization test

WCTU Women's Christian Temperance Union

WCUS Wiktor Stent and Cutting Balloon Angioplasty Study

WD wallerian degeneration; well developed; well differentiated; wet dressing; Whitney Damon [dextrose]; Wilson disease; Winger distribution; with disease; withdraw or withdrawn; without dyskinesia; Wolman disease; wrist disarticulation

W/D warm and dry

Wd ward

wd well developed; wound, wounded

WDCC well-developed collateral circulation

WDG water-dispersible granule

WDHA watery diarrhea, hypokalemia, achlorhydria [syndrome]

WDHH watery diarrhea, hypokalemia, and hypochlorhydria

WDI warfarin dose index; World Drug Index

WDL well-differentiated lymphocytic

WDLL well-differentiated lymphatic lymphoma

WDMF wall-defective microbial forms

WDR wide dynamic range

WDS watery diarrhea syndrome; wet dog shakes [syndrome]

WDSCC well-differentiated squamous cell carcinoma

WDTC well-differentiated thyroid cancer

WDWN, wdwn well developed and well nourished

WE wax ester; Wernicke encephalopathy; western encephalitis; western encephalomyelitis; wound of entry

We weber

WEB Women's Experience with Battering [scale]

WECN Wisconsin Ethics Committee Network

WEDI Workshop for Electronic Data Interchange

WEE western equine encephalitis/encephalomyelitis

WEEV Western equine encephalitis virus

WEL wave equivalent length

WELL-HART Women's Estrogen/Progestin and Lipid-lowering Hormone Atherosclerosis Regression Trial

WELLSTENT-CABG Wellstent European Study on Stenting for Coronary Artery Bypass Grafts

WELV Weldona virus

W3-EMRS World Wide Web Electronic Medical Records System

WENR Workgroup of European Nurse Researchers

WEP wired equivalent privacy [telemedicine]

WER wheal erythema reaction

WES wall echo shadow; wall echo sign; work environment scale; wound evaluation scale

WESDR Wisconsin Epidemiologic Study of Diabetic Retinopathy

WESH West European Study of Health

WESSV Wesselsbron virus

WEST Western European Stent Trial; Women's Estrogen for Stroke Trial

WEXV Wexford virus

WF Weil-Felix reaction; white female; Wistar-Furth [rat]; workflow

W/F, wf white female

WFC workflow cycle

WFD word-finding difficulty

WFDB Waveform Database

WFE Williams flexion exercise

WFI water for injection

WFL within function limits

WFLC weighted frequency Fourier linear combiner [algorithm]

WfMS workflow management system

WFOT World Federation of Occupational Therapists

WFPHA World Federation of Public Health Associations

WFR Weil-Felix reaction; wheal-and-flare reaction

WFRT wide field radiation therapy

WFS Waterhouse-Friderichsen syndrome; World Fertility Survey

WFSL workflow specification language

WFT windowed Fourier transform

WG water gauge; Wegener granulomatosis; Wright-Giemsa [stain]

WGA wheat germ agglutinin

WGE wheat germ extract

WG-RH whole genome radiation hybrid task

WGRV Wongorr virus

WGS whole genome shotgun

wgt weight

WH well hydrated; Werdnig-Hoffmann [syndrome]; whole homogenate; wound healing

Wh watt/hours; white

wh white

w·h watt-hour

WHA warm and humid air; World Health Assembly

WHAP Women's Health Australian Project

WHAS Women's Health and Aging Study; Women's Heart Attack Study

WHAT Worcester Heart Attack Trial

WHAV Whataroa virus

wh ch wheel chair; white child

WHCOA White House Conference on Aging

WHCR Wolf-Hirschhorn chromosome region

WHD Werdnig-Hoffmann disease

WHEASE What Happens Eventually to Asthmatics Sociologically and Epidemiologically? [study]

WHHHIMP Wernicke encephalopathy/withdrawal, hypertensive encephalopathy, hypoglycemia, hypoxemia, intracranial bleeding/infection, meningitis/encephalitis, poison/medication

WHHL Watanaby heritable hyperlipidemia; Watanaby heritable hyperlipidemic [rabbit]

WHI Women's Health Initiative

WHIMS Women's Health Initiative Memory Study

WHIN Wisconsin Health Information Network

WHML Wellcome Historical Medical Library

WHO World Health Organization; wrist-hand orthosis

WHO/ISH World Health Organization/International Society of Hypertension [survey]

whp whirlpool

WHR waist:hips girth ratio

whr watt-hour

WHRC World Health Research Centre

WHS Werdnig-Hoffmann syndrome; Wolf-Hirschhorn syndrome; Women's Health Study

WHT Walsh-Hadamard transform; Warm Heart Trial

WHTVS Women's Health Trial Vanguard Study
WHV woodchuck hepatic virus
WHVP wedged hepatic venous pressure
WHYMPI West Haven-Yale Multidimensional Pain Inventory
WI human embryonic lung cell line; walk-in [patient]; water ingestion; weaning index; Wistar [rat]; World Wide Web [WWW] intervention
WIA wounded in action
WIBC Wiggins Interpersonal Behavior Circle
WIC walk-in clinic; women, infants, and children
WICHEN Western Interstate Commission for Higher Education in Nursing
WIHS Women's Interagency Human Immunodeficiency Virus [HIV] Study
WIL workflow intermediate language
WILLOW Washington Information Looker-upper Layered Over Windows
WIMP windows, icons, menus, pointing
WIN Wallstent in Native Vessel [study]; Weight Control Information Network; Western Institute of Nursing
WINS Wallstent in Saphenous Vein Grafts [study]
WIPI Word Intelligibility Picture Identification
WIR Workgroup on Immunization Registries
WIS Wechsler Intelligence Scale
WISC Wechsler Intelligence Scale for Children
WISCR Wisconsin clinical record
WISC-R Wechsler Intelligence Scale for Children-Revised
WISE Women's Ischemic Syndrome Evaluation
WISH wearable information system for human healthcare
WIST Whitaker Index of Schizophrenic Thinking
WITS Women and Infants Transmission Study
WITT Wittenborn [Psychiatric Rating Scale]
WITV Witwatersrand virus
W-J Woodcock-Johnson [Psychoeducational Battery]
WJG Wilders-Jongsma-van Ginneken [pacemaker model]

WK week; Wernicke-Korsakoff [syndrome]; Wilson-Kimmelstiel [syndrome]; Windkessel [model]
wk weak; week; work
WKD Wilson-Kimmelstiel disease
W/kg watts per kilogram
WKS Wernicke-Korsakoff syndrome
WKY Wistar-Kyoto [rat]
WL waiting list; warning letter; waterload; wavelength; weighted least squares; weight loss; window level [imaging]; withdrawal; Wood's lamp; working level [exposure to radon decay products]; workload
wl wavelength
WLAN wireless local area network
WLE white light endoscopy; wide local excision
WLF whole lymphocytic fraction
WLI weight-length index
WLM white light microscopy; working level month [cumulative exposure to radon]
WLS weighted least square; wet lung syndrome
WLT whole lung tomography
WM Waldenström macroglobulinemia; wall motion; ward manager; warm and moist; Wernicke-Mann [hemiplegia]; wet mount; white male; white matter; whole milk; Wilson-Mikity [syndrome]; working memory
W-M Weill-Marchesani [syndrome]
W/M white male
wm white male; whole milk; whole mount
w/m² watts per square meter
WMA wall motion abnormality; wall motion analysis; World Medical Association
WMBT weighted moving beam therapy
WMC weight-matched control
WMD weapon of mass destruction
WME Williams' medium E
WMF wavelet multiresolution filter; Windows MetaFile
WMH white matter hyperintensities
WMHP Women's Medical Health Page
WML white matter lesion; wireless markup language [telemedicine]
WMO ward medical officer
WMP weight management program
WMR work metabolic rate; World Medical Relief

WMS Wechsler Memory Scale; Weill-Marchesani syndrome; Williams syndrome; workflow management system
WMS-R Wechsler memory scale-revised
WMV Wad Medani virus
WMX whirlpool, massage, exercise
WN, wn well nourished
WNE West Nile encephalitis
WNF well-nourished female
WNL within normal limits
WNM well-nourished male
WNN wavelet neural network
WNPW wide, notched P wave
WNSA weighted negative surface area
WNV West Nile virus
WO wash out; will order; written order
W/O water in oil [emulsion]
w/o without
wo weeks old
WOB work of breathing
WOB$_I$ imposed work of breathing
WOB$_P$ physiologic work of breathing
WOB$_T$ total work of breathing [WOB$_P$ plus WOB$_I$]
WOB$_V$ work of breathing performed by ventilator
WOE wound of entry
WOLF Work, Lipids, Fibrinogen [study]
WONCA World Organization of Family Doctors
WONV Wongal virus
WOOFS Warfarin Optimized Outpatient Follow-up Study
WooV Woot virus
WOP without pain
WORM write once read many times
WOSCOPS West of Scotland Coronary Prevention Study
WOU women's outpatient unit
WOWS weak opiate withdrawal scale
WOX wound of exit
WP wavelet packet; weakly positive; weak-plate; wedge pressure; wet pack; wettable powder; whirlpool; white phosphorus; white pulp; word processor; working point
W/P water/powder ratio
wp wettable powder
WPAI work productivity and activity impairment [questionnaire]
WP-ANAT weak-plate with anatomic information
WPB whirlpool bath

WPCU weighted patient care unit
WPDL workflow process definition language
Wpf wave at a pilot frequency
WPFM Wright peak flow meter
WPk Ward's pack; wet pack
WPPSI Wechsler Preschool and Primary Scale of Intelligence
WPR written progress report
WPRS Wittenborn Psychiatric Rating Scale
WPS wasting pig syndrome
WPW Wolff-Parkinson-White [syndrome]
WQAC ward quality assurance committee
W-QLI Wisconsin quality of life index
WR Wassermann reaction; water retention; weakly reactive; weak response; whole response; Wiedemann-Rautenstrauch [syndrome]; wiping reaction; work rate
W$_R$ radiation weighting factor
Wr wrist; writhe
WRAC wide-ranging aerosol classifier
WRAIN Walter Reed Army Medical Center Institute of Nursing
WRAIR Walter Reed Army Institute for Research
WRAMC Walter Reed Army Medical Center
WRAML Wide Range Assessment of Memory and Learning
WRAT Wide Range Achievement Test
WRBC washed red blood cells
WRC washed red cells; water retention coefficient
WRE wahole ragweed extract
WR HA-NP Western Reserve hemagglutinin and nucleoprotein [replication-competent vaccinia virus]
WRISS Weapons Related Injury Surveillance System
WRIST Washington Radiation for Instent Restenosis Trial
WRK Woodward reagent K
WRLIN Wessex Regional Library and Information Network [UK]
WRMD work-related musculoskeletal disorder
WRMT Woodcock Reading Mastery Test
WRN Werner [syndrome]
WRS Ward-Romano syndrome; war research service; Wiedemann-Rautenstrauch syndrome

WRSI Work-related Strain Inventory
WRSS weighted residual sum of squares
WRVP wedged renal vein pressure
WS Waardenburg syndrome; Wallenberg syndrome; ward secretary; Warkany syndrome; warning stimulus; Warthin-Starry [stain]; water soluble; water swallow; watt-second; Wellens syndrome; Werner syndrome; West syndrome; Wiener spectrum [x-ray]; Wilder silver [stain]; Williams syndrome; Wolfram syndrome; word sense; work station
WSI Waardenburg syndrome type I
W&S wound and skin
W·s watt-second
ws water-soluble
WSA water-soluble antibiotic
WSB wheat-soy blend
WSC water-soluble contrast [medium]
WSDRN Western Satellite Data Relay System
w-sec watt-second
WSL Wesselsbron [virus]
WSM women who have sex with men
WSP withdrawal seizure prone
WSPHU Western Sector Public Health Unit [Australia]
WSQ wavelet scalar quantization
WSR Westergren sedimentation rate; withdrawal seizure resistant
W/sr watts per steradian
WSS Weaver-Smith syndrome; wrinkly skin syndrome
WSW women who have sex with women
WT wall thickness; water temperature; wavelet transform; wild type [strain]; Wilms tumor; wisdom teeth; work therapy
wt weight; white; wild type
WT-1 Wilms tumor gene-1
wtAAV wild type adeno-associated virus
wtAd wild type adenovirus
WTCC wavelet transform cross correlation
WTE whole time equivalent
WTF weight transferral frequency
WTH Women Take Heart [project]
WTO World Trade Organization
WTP willingness to pay
wtPSGL wild type P selectin glycoprotein ligand

WTR waist/thigh circumference ratio
WTS Wilson-Turner syndrome
WTV wound tumor virus
W/U workup
WV walking ventilation; weighting vector; Wrath virus
W/V, w/v percent weight in volume, weight/volume
W^v variable dominant spotting [mouse]
WVD wavelet-vaguelette decomposition; Winger-Ville distribution
WW Weight Watchers; wet weight; whisker weaving; window width [imaging]
W/W, w/w weight; percent weight
WWAV Whitewater Arroyo virus
WWBV Weddel waterborne virus
WWICT Western Washington Intracoronary Streptokinase Trial
WWISK Western Washington Intracoronary Streptokinase Trial
WWIST Western Washington Intravenous Streptokinase Trial
WWIV Western Washington Intravascular Streptokinase Trial
WWIVSK Western Washington Intravenous Streptokinase Trial
WWM world wide microscope
W/wo with or without
WWS Walker-Warburg syndrome; Wieacker-Wolff syndrome; Working Well Study
WWSIMIT Western Washington Streptokinase in Myocardial Infarction Trials
WWU weighted working unit
WWW World Wide Web
WWW-PACS World Wide Web-picture archiving and communication system
WWW VL World Wide Web Virtual Library
WX wound of exit
WxB wax bite
WxP wax pattern
WY women years
WYOV Wyeomyia virus
WYSIWYG what you see is what you get
WZa wide zone alpha
WZS Weissenbacher-Zweymuller syndrome

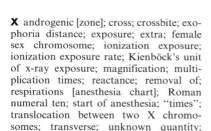

X androgenic [zone]; cross; crossbite; exophoria distance; exposure; extra; female sex chromosome; ionization exposure; ionization exposure rate; Kienböck's unit of x-ray exposure; magnification; multiplication times; reactance; removal of; respirations [anesthesia chart]; Roman numeral ten; start of anesthesia; "times"; translocation between two X chromosomes; transverse; unknown quantity; xanthosine; X unit; xylene

X sample mean

X^2, χ^2 chi-square

X3 orientation as to time, place, and person

x except; extremity; horizontal axis of a rectangular coordinate system; mole fraction; multiplication times; position; roentgen [rays]; sample mean; "times"; unknown factor; xanthine

Ξ see *xi*

ξ see *xi*

XA xanthurenic acid; x-ray analysis

X-A xylene and alcohol

Xa activated factor X; chiasma

Xaa unknown amino acid

XAD External Atrial Defibrillation [trial]

Xam examination

Xan xanthine

Xanth xanthomatosis

Xao xanthosine

XBP xanthophyll-binding protein; X-box binding protein

XBSN X-linked bulbospinal neuropathy

XC, Xc excretory cystogram

X-CAR cross-relational computer-based retention

XCCL exaggerated craniocaudal lateral [view]

XCE X-chromosome controlling element

X-CGD X-linked chronic granulomatous disease

XCMD external [computer] command

Xcv *Xanthomonas campestris vesicatoria*

XD x-ray diffraction

XDH xanthine dehydrogenase

XDP xanthine diphosphate; xeroderma pigmentosum

XDR transducer

Xe electric susceptibility; xenon

XECT, XeCT xenon-enhanced computed tomography

XEF excess ejection fraction

XES x-ray energy spectrometry

Xfb cross-linked Gibrin

XFD x-ray flat detector

XGP xanthogranulomatous pyelonephritis

XGPT xylosylprotein-4-beta-galactosyltransferase

XGRAIL Gene Recognition and Analysis Internet Link X window [client server system]

Xi inactive X chromosome

Ξ Greek capital letter *xi*

ξ Greek lowercase letter *xi*

XIBV Xiburema virus

XIC X chromosome inactivation center; X-inactivation center

X-IEP crossed immunoelectrophoresis

XIMS extensible markup language [XML] information management system

XINV Xingu virus

XIP exchanger inhibitory peptide; x-ray-induced polypeptide; x-ray in plaster

XISHF Xamoterol in Severe Heart Failure [study]

XIST inactive X chromosome specific transcript; X-inactivation specific transcript

XL excess lactate; X-linked [inheritance]; xylose-lysine [agar base]

XLA, X-LA X-linked agammaglobulinemia

XLAS X-linked aqueductal stenosis

XLCM X-linked dilated cardiomyopathy

XLD X-linked dominant; xylose-lysine-deoxycholate [agar]

XLH X-linked hydrocephalus; X-linked hypophosphatemia

XLHED X-linked hypohidrotic ectodermal dysplasia

XLI X-linked ichthyosis

XLMR X-linked mental retardation

XLMTM, XLMTm X-linked myotubular myopathy

XLOS X-linked Opitz syndrome

XLP X-linked lymphoproliferative [syndrome]

XLPD X-linked lymphoproliferative disease
XLR X-linked recessive
XLRP X-linked retinitis pigmentosa
XLS X-linked recessive lymphoproliferative syndrome
XLSP X-linked spastic paraplegia
XM crossmatch
Xm, X^m maternal chromosome X
xma chiasma
X-mas Christmas [factor]
x-mat crossmatch [blood]
X-match crossmatch
XME xenobiotic-metabolizing enzyme
XMI extensible markup language [XML] metadata-interchange [format]
XML extensible markup language
XML-DOM extensible markup language-document object model
XML-DTD extensible markup language-document type definition
XMP xanthine monophosphate
XMMR *Xenopus* molecular marker resource
XMR X-linked mental retardation
XN night blindness
XO presence of only one sex chromosome; xanthine oxidase
XOAD X-linked ocular albinism with deafness
XOAN X-linked ocular albinism of Nettleship-Falls
XOM extraocular movements
XOP x-ray out of plaster
XOR exclusive operating room
XP xanthogranulomatous pyelonephritis; xeroderma pigmentosum
Xp paternal chromosome X; short arm of chromosome X
XPA xeroderma pigmentosum group A
XPC xeroderma pigmentosum group C
XPN xanthogranulomatous pyelonephritis
XPS x-ray photoelectron spectroscopy; x-ray photoemission spectroscopy
XPTB extrapulmonary tuberculosis
Xq long arm of chromosome X
XR extended release; xeroradiography; X-linked recessive [inheritance]; x-ray
x-rays roentgen rays

XRD x-ray diffraction
XRE xenobiotic response element
XRF x-ray fluorescence
XRFDC x-ray film digitization console
XRII x-ray image intensifier
XRMR X-linked recessive mental retardation
XRN X-linked recessive nephrolithiasis
XRS x-ray sensitivity
XRT x-ray therapy
XS cross-section; excessive; xiphisternum
X/S cross-section
xs excess
XSA cross-section area
XSCID X-linked severe combined immunodeficiency [syndrome]
XSCLH X-linked subcortical laminar heterotopia
X-sect cross-section
XSL extensible stylesheet language
XSP xanthoma striatum palmare
XT exotropia
Xt extra toe
Xta chiasmata
Xtab cross-tabulating
XTE xeroderma, talipes, and enamel defect [syndrome]
XTM xanthoma tuberosum multiplex
XTP xanthosine triphosphate
X-TUL external tumescent ultrasound liposculpture
XU excretory urogram; X unit
Xu X-unit
X_u cumulative amount of urine
XUC extended use case [format]
XuMP xylulose monophosphate
Xu5P, Xu5p xylulose-5-phosphate
XX chromosome X disomy; double strength; female chromosome type
46, XX 46 chromosomes, 2 X chromosomes (normal female)
XXL xylocaine
XXX chromosome X trisomy
XXXX chromosome X tetrasomy
XXXXX chromosome X pentasomy
XX/XY sex karyotypes
XY male chromosome type
46, XY 46 chromosomes, 1 X and 1 Y chromosome (normal male)
Xyl xylose

Y

Y a coordinate axis in a plane; electrical admittance; male sex chromosome; tyrosine; year; yellow; *Yersinia*; yield; yttrium
Y̅ mean of y values
Y- yotta- [10^{24}]
y the vertical axis of a rectangular coordinate system
y- yocto- [10^{-24}]
Y see *upsilon*
υ see *upsilon*
YA *Yersinia* arthritis
Y/A years of age
YAC yeast artificial chromosome
YACP young adult chronic patient
YACV Yacaaba virus
YADH yeast alcohol dehydrogenase
YAG yttrium aluminum garnet [laser]
Yahoo Yet Another Hierarchically Officious Oracle [hierarchical subject index to Web sites]
YAOV Yaounde virus
YATAV Yata virus
Yb ytterbium
YBOCS Yale-Brown Obsessive Compulsive Scale
YBV Yug Bogdanovac virus
YCB yeast carbon base
YCMI Yale Center for Medical Informatics
YCT YMCA Cardiac Therapy [program]
YCVDS Yugoslavia Cardiovascular Disease Study
yd yard
YDV yeast-derived hepatitis B vaccine
YDYES yin deficiency yang excess syndrome
YE yeast extract; yellow enzyme
YEH₂ reduced yellow enzyme
YEI *Yersinia enterocolitica* infection
Yel yellow
YF yellow fever
YFI yellow fever immunization

YFMD yellow fever membrane disease
YFV yellow fever virus
YHAP Yale Health and Aging Project
YHV Yaquina Head virus
Y2K year 2000
YKV yokapoxvirus
YLC youngest living child
YLD year lived with disability
YLF yttrium lithium fluoride
YLL years of life lost
YLS years of life saved
YM yeast and mannitol; yeast and mold; Young's modulus
Y$_{max}$ maximum yield
YMB yeast malt broth
YMS Young Men's Survey
YMTV Yaba monkey tumor virus
YNB yeast nitrogen base
YNS yellow nail syndrome
y/o years old
YOB year of birth
Y$_{obs}$ observed value
YOGV Yogue virus
YOKV Yokose virus
Yops *Yersinia* outer membrane proteins
YOS Yale Observation Scale
YP yeast phase; yield pressure
YPA yeast, peptone, and adenine sulfate
YpkA *Yersinia* protein kinase A
YPLL years of potential life lost
yr year
YRBS Youth Risk Behavior Survey
YRD Yangtze River disease
YRRM Y ribonucleic acid [RNA] recognition motif
YS yellow spot; yield strength; yolk sac
ys yellow spot; yolk sac
YSHR younger spontaneously hypertensive rat
YST yolk sac tumor
Y73SV Y73 sarcoma virus
YT, yt yttrium
Y1V Yaba-1 virus
Y7V Yaba-7 virus
yWACC younger woman with aggressive cervical cancer
YWKY younger Wistar-Kyoto rat

Z

Z acoustic impedance; atomic number; complex impedance; contraction [Ger. *Zuckung*]; the disk that separates sarcomeres [Ger. *Zwischenscheibe*]; glutamine; impedance; ionic charge number; no effect; point formed by a line perpendicular to the nasion-menton line through the anterior nasal spine; proton number; section modulus; standardized deviate; standard normal score [statistics]; standard score; zero; zone; a Z-shaped incision in plastic surgery

Z- zetta- [10^{21}]

Z′ , Z″ increasing degrees of contraction

z algebraic unknown or space coordinate; axis of a three-dimensional rectangular coordinate system; catalytic amount; standard normal deviate; zero

z- zepto- [10^{-21}]

ζ see *zeta*

ZAG, ZA2G zinc-alpha-2-glycoprotein

ZAM Zhao-Atlas-Marks [distribution]

ZAP zeta-associated protein; zymosanactivated plasma [rabbit]

ZAPF zinc adequate pair-fed

ZAPS zonal air pollution system

ZAS zymosan-activated autologous serum

ZB zebra body

ZBG zinc-binding group

ZCA zone or cortical abnormality

ZCAP zinc-calcium-phosphorous; oxide [ceramic]

ZCP zinc chloride poisoning

ZD zero defects; zero discharge; zinc deficiency

Z-D Zamorano-Duchovny [digitizer]

ZDDP zinc dialkyldithiophosphate

Z-DNA zig-zag (left-handed helical) deoxyribonucleic acid

ZDO zero differential overlap

ZDS zinc depletion syndrome

ZDV zidovudine

ZE Zollinger-Ellison [syndrome]

ZEBOV Zaire Ebola virus

ZEBRA zero balanced reimbursement account

ZEC Zinsser-Engman-Cole [syndrome]

ZEEP zero end-expiratory pressure

ZEGV Zegla virus

ZEPI zonal echo planar imaging

Z-ERS zeta erythrocyte sedimentation rate

ZES Zollinger-Ellison syndrome; Zutphen Elderly Study

ZEST Zocor Early Start Trial

ζ Greek lowercase letter *zeta*

ZF zero frequency; zinc finger [protein]; zona fasciculata

ZFF zinc fume fever

ZFP zinc finger protein

ZFX X-linked zinc finger protein

Zfy zinc-finger [protein]

ZG zona glomerulosa

ZGM zinc glycinate marker

ZIFT zygote intrafallopian tube transfer

ZIG, ZIg zoster immunoglobulin

ZIKV Zika virus

ZIP zoster immune plasma

ZIRV Zirqa virus

zJ zeptojoule

ZK Zuelzer-Kaplan [syndrome]

ZLS Zimmerman-Laband syndrome

Zm zygomaxillare

ZMA zinc meta-arsenite

ZMC zygomaticomaxillary complex

ZN Ziehl-Neelsen [staining]

ZNF zinc finger [protein]

ZnOE zinc oxide and eugenol

ZNS zonisamide

ZO Zichen-Oppenheim [syndrome]; *Zonula occludens*; Zuelzer-Ogden [syndrome]

Zo impedance; thoracic fluid

ZOA zinc orthoarsenate

ZOE zinc oxide-eugenol

ZOL zoladex

Zool zoology

ZOT *Zonula occludens* toxin

ZP zona pellucida

ZPA zone of polarizing activity

ZPC zero point of change

ZPG zero population growth

ZPO zinc peroxide

ZPP zinc protoporphyrin

ZPT zinc pyridinethione

ZR zona reticularis

Zr zirconium

ZS Zellweger syndrome; Zutphen Study

ZSC zone of slow conduction

ZSR zeta sedimentation ratio

ZSV signature-tagged mutagenesis; zonate spot virus
ZT Zwolle Trial
ZTS zymosan-treated serum
Z-TSP zephiran-trisodium phosphate
ZTT zinc turbidity test
ZTV Zaliv Terpeniya virus
ZVD zidovudine
ZVT Zehlenverbindungstest
ZW Zellweger [syndrome]

ZWCHRS Zellweger cerebrohepatorenal syndrome
ZWOLLE Primary Coronary Angioplasty Compared with Intravenous Streptokinase [trial from Zwolle, The Netherlands]
ZWS Zellweger syndrome
ZXF zero crossing frequency
Zy zygion
ZyC zymosan complement
zyg zygotene
Zz ginger [Lat. *zingibar*]